How to access the supplemental web study guide

We are pleased to provide access to a web study guide that supplements your textbook, *Medical Conditions in the Athlete, Third Edition.* The web study guide contains 18 case studies with questions that allow you to apply strategies taught in the text to the case study scenarios.

Accessing the web study guide is easy!
Follow these steps if you purchased a new book:

1. Visit **www.HumanKinetics.com/MedicalConditionsInTheAthlete**.

2. Click the third edition link next to the corresponding third edition book cover.

3. Click the Sign In link on the left or top of the page. If you do not have an account with Human Kinetics, you will be prompted to create one.

4. If the online product you purchased does not appear in the Ancillary Items box on the left of the page, click the Enter Key Code option in that box. Enter the key code that is printed at the right, including all hyphens. Click the Submit button to unlock your online product.

5. After you have entered your key code the first time, you will never have to enter it again to access this product. Once unlocked, a link to your product will permanently appear in the menu on the left. For future visits, all you need to do is sign in to the textbook's website and follow the link that appears in the left menu!

→ Click the Need Help? button on the textbook's website if you need assistance along the way.

How to access the web study guide if you purchased a used book:

You may purchase access to the web study guide by visiting the text's website, **www.HumanKinetics.com/MedicalConditionsInTheAthlete**, or by calling the following:

800-747-4457 . . . . U.S. customers
800-465-7301 . . . . .Canadian customers
+44 (0) 113 255 5665 . . . . European customers
217-351-5076 . . . . .International customers

For technical support, send an e-mail to:
support@hkusa.com . . . . U.S. and international customers
info@hkcanada.com . . . . Canadian customers
academic@hkeurope.com . . . . European customers

HUMAN KINETICS
The Information Leader in Physical Activity & Health

03-2017

Product: Medical Conditions in the Athlete, Third Edition, web study guide

Key code: WALSH-6VEDPZ-OSG

This unique code allows you access to the web study guide.

Access is provided if you have purchased a new book. Once submitted, the code may not be entered for any other user.

Medical Conditions in the Athlete

THIRD EDITION

Medical Conditions in the Athlete

THIRD EDITION

Katie Walsh Flanagan, EdD, LAT, ATC
East Carolina University

Micki Cuppett, EdD, LAT, ATC

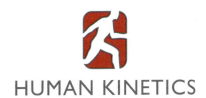

HUMAN KINETICS

Library of Congress Cataloging-in-Publication Data

Names: Cuppett, Micki, author. | Flanagan, Katie Walsh, author.
Title: Medical conditions in the athlete / Katie Walsh Flanagan, Micki
  Cuppett.
Other titles: General medical conditions in the athlete
Description: Third edition. | Champaign, IL : Human Kinetics, [2017] |
  Preceded by General medical conditions in the athlete / Micki Cuppett,
  Katie M. Walsh. 2nd ed. c2012. | Author's names reversed on previous
  editions. | Includes bibliographical references and index.
Identifiers: LCCN 2016029847| ISBN 9781492533504 (print) | ISBN 9781492539094
  (e-book)
Subjects: | MESH: Athletic Injuries | Sports Medicine--methods | Primary
  Health Care
Classification: LCC RC1210 | NLM QT 261 | DDC 617.1/027--dc23 LC record available at https://lccn.loc.gov/2016029847

ISBN: 978-1-4925-3350-4 (print)

This book is a revised edition of *General Medical Conditions in the Athlete, Second Edition,* published in 2012 by Mosby, Inc., an affiliate of Elsevier, Inc.

The web addresses cited in this text were current as of December 2016, unless otherwise noted.

Acquisitions Editor: Joshua J. Stone; **Developmental and Managing Editor:** Amanda S. Ewing; **Copyeditor:** Kevin Campbell; **Proofreader:** Anna Lan Seaman; **Indexer:** Dan Connolly; **Permissions Manager:** Dalene Reeder; **Senior Graphic Designer:** Nancy Rasmus; **Cover Designer:** Keith Blomberg; **Photographs (cover):** © Human Kinetics, blood pressure photo © PhotoDisc; **Photographer (interior):** Neil Bernstein, unless otherwise noted; photographs © Human Kinetics, unless otherwise noted; **Photo Asset Manager:** Laura Fitch; **Visual Production Assistant:** Joyce Brumfield; **Photo Production Manager:** Jason Allen; **Senior Art Manager:** Kelly Hendren; **Printer:** Walsworth

We thank East Carolina University in Greenville, North Carolina, for assistance in providing the location for the photo shoot for this book.

Printed in the United States of America   10 9 8 7 6 5 4 3 2 1

The paper in this book was manufactured using responsible forestry methods.

Human Kinetics
Website: www.HumanKinetics.com

United States: Human Kinetics
P.O. Box 5076
Champaign, IL 61825-5076
800-747-4457
e-mail: info@hkusa.com

Canada: Human Kinetics
475 Devonshire Road Unit 100
Windsor, ON N8Y 2L5
800-465-7301 (in Canada only)
e-mail: info@hkcanada.com

Europe: Human Kinetics
107 Bradford Road
Stanningley
Leeds LS28 6AT, United Kingdom
+44 (0) 113 255 5665
e-mail: hk@hkeurope.com

E6834

This book is dedicated to my mother, Phyllis Fletcher Walsh Kelly, and bonus father, Gerald Kelly, who in their mid-80s have more energy, curiosity, and drive to keep learning than most half their age.

In memory of my mother-in-law, M. Jean Bryce Flanagan, a lifelong nurse who taught me more about patient interaction and humor than any research could have.

And to my husband, Sean Bryce Flanagan, who has made me a better person by being in my life.

–Katie Walsh Flanagan

In memory of my dad, Jim Cuppett, who taught me more than I will ever realize.

To my mom, Annabelle Cuppett, thank you for being a wonderful role model.

To my sons, Derek and Kyle, who literally grew up in the athletic training room and have been an inspiration for me to contribute to the growth of the athletic training profession, if only in this small way.

To Michael Szemeredy, who is always there for me and whose infectious enthusiasm keeps me motivated.

–Micki Cuppett

CONTENTS

CONDITION FINDER

PREFACE

This textbook is designed for the health care provider who works with a physically active population. Providers are referred to variously throughout the text as *athletic trainers, health care providers,* and *clinicians.* We use these multiple titles to help readers to better understand the role they play in identifying and treating the conditions described in this text.

In the past, athletic training programs have tended to concentrate on building the knowledge and skills needed for orthopedic assessment and have provided a systematic overview of athletic injuries. The emphasis has been on teaching students to follow the history, inspection and observation, palpation, special tests (HIPS/HOPS) plan in taking a history, and then to determine how to make decisions about return to play. In these largely orthopedic situations, an injury is usually obvious because it has been witnessed by the athletic trainer, and a thorough history may shed light on the type of damage sustained.

Unlike the typical athletic injury, medical conditions are not always immediately apparent in an assessment. This book is a comprehensive resource for health care students and providers that covers medical conditions by body system, their mechanism of acquisition, signs, symptoms, differential diagnoses, referral, treatment, and return-to-participation criteria. The purpose of this text is not only to provide information but also to help readers to develop a framework for decision making. We assume that readers are versed in basic human anatomy and physiology and can build on that knowledge. The text also includes associated chapters on diagnostic imaging and tests, pharmacology, psychological and substance abuse disorders, and special populations.

The role of a health care provider in caring for physically active people continues to expand to more diverse populations. Today, athletic trainers (ATs) provide orthopedic and medical care to children, teens, young and mature adults, and special needs athletes. In all of these groups, underlying or preexisting medical conditions may be a concern. The AT is often the first person to learn about a medical problem in athletes and thus is in a position to determine if it is a minor illness or a potentially serious medical condition. Therefore it is imperative that those working with active populations be able to recognize and appreciate potentially serious medical conditions and be able to determine when to seek additional medical consultation and care.

The third edition of *Medical Conditions in the Athlete* is a full-color textbook that contains new and updated content and references, as well as updated graphic elements. Our goal in writing the third edition was to expand and update the content from the second edition and to provide current, research-driven assessment and treatment information for medical conditions that affect the physically active population. We wanted to offer a comprehensive reference book on medical conditions in the athlete that can be used by all health care providers.

Organization

This textbook is separated into three parts: "Introduction to Medical Conditions," "Pharmacology and Interventions," and "Medical Conditions by System." Part I begins with an overview of the basic information presented in subsequent chapters, including a discussion of the role of the AT as an initial and primary health care provider for the athlete and the importance of the preparticipation examination (PPE). These introductory chapters also explain communication tools, policies, rules, legal concerns, and regulations associated with medical care, and they stress prevention of disease transmission. Chapter 3 describes the common diagnostic tests and procedures that are mentioned later in the textbook.

Part II contains three chapters relating to pharmacology, therapeutic drug categories, and common invasive procedures seen in the athletic training clinic. With the requirement of a graduate-level degree for athletic trainers on the horizon, it will be important for ATs to know about maintaining a sterile field and the procedures for wound closure, injections, and intravenous administrations. Readers are reminded that some states' practice acts do not allow ATs to perform some of the procedures included in chapter 6.

Part III follows a systematic approach as the chapters address common conditions and diseases by body system. Most chapters follow a simple template, beginning with an overview of the relevant anatomy and physiology as they relate to the body system; then identifying specific conditions; explaining signs and symptoms, including potential differential diagnoses; referral and diagnostic tests; discussing treatment and return to participation; and finally, discussing prognoses and prevention, if applicable. If a condition has related age- or gender-specific considerations, those issues are also discussed. Implications for pediatric and mature athletes are also included when relevant.

Textbook Features

When applicable, we include current National Athletic Trainers' Association (NATA), National Collegiate Athletic Association (NCAA), and National Federation of State High School Associations (NFHS) position statements and references. Content is expanded and reinforced by clinical tips, red flags, and condition highlight elements.

- **Clinical Tips** present key-point-type information to help reinforce student understanding.
- **Red Flags** present warnings to readers.
- **Condition Highlight** spotlights a condition specific to the chapter that is either common or warrants additional emphasis.

More than 300 photos and illustrations enhance the reader's comprehension of anatomy, physiology, and pathophysiology. Pharmacological tables provide easy access to a full range of drug categories with generic and trade names, therapeutic uses, adult dosage information, and possible adverse effects. Important terminology is highlighted throughout the chapters, and a glossary appears at the end of the text.

eBook available at your campus bookstore or HumanKinetics.com

Web Study Guide

Perhaps the most unique feature of this text is the web study guide, which contains 18 case studies. Each case study starts with the history or chief complaint of the person featured in the case study. Most cases are followed by evaluation and treatment notes. Questions then follow that allow students to apply strategies taught in the text to the scenario presented in the case study. The web study guide is available at www.HumanKinetics.com/MedicalConditionsInTheAthlete.

Instructor Resources

Instructors have access to a full array of ancillary materials.

- **Presentation package.** The presentation package includes more than 800 slides that provide detailed lecture notes and select art, photos, and tables from the text. Instructors can modify these slides as needed to best fit their classes and lecture format.
- **Image bank.** The image bank contains most of the art, photos, and tables from the text, which can be used to create custom presentations, student handouts, and other materials.
- **Chapter quizzes.** These ready-made quizzes allow instructors to test students' understanding of the most important chapter concepts.

These ancillaries are available at www.HumanKinetics.com/MedicalConditionsInTheAthlete.

Final Thoughts

We are athletic training educators and practitioners who have pooled our experience and worked with our colleagues in athletic training and medicine to design this textbook and the ancillary resources. We present it to you as an informative and easy-to-use instructional tool for beginning and advanced students, as well as an indispensable reference guide for practitioners in the field. We look forward to your feedback and suggestions for future editions.

ACKNOWLEDGMENTS

We wish to thank the many people who made this project possible. First of all, we thank the current and past chapter contributors for providing their knowledge of the subject matter and expertise in their fields. They took time away from their busy practices and lives to ensure the text's accuracy and currency. We appreciate their spectacular responses to a tight timeline and their ongoing support of the project.

We are forever grateful to the Human Kinetics team that has made publication of this third edition an enjoyable process. Josh Stone, our acquisitions editor, listened to our vision of this latest edition and made our project better. His enthusiasm and vision made this edition a truly different and better textbook. We had the great fortune to work with Amanda Ewing, our "handler," who wore many hats to keep this project on task and looking polished. She is the developmental editor, managing editor, ancillary queen, and Grand Poobah who reviewed our work with fresh eyes and provided excellent suggestions and edits. Her continuous communications, dedication, and patience kept us on task and focused. A thank you will never truly convey our appreciation for her work. We are also thankful to Susi Huls, our instructional designer, who was instrumental in developing and managing the web study guide.

We also thank the athletic training faculty and clinical staff at East Carolina University and the University of South Florida for their patience, advice, and clinical tips while we sought to bring the research to clinical practice. In addition, the faculty at USF Morsani Center for Advanced Health Care and USF College of Medicine were also gracious enough to allow us access to equipment for many of the pictures in this edition.

We also want to recognize the efforts of the past and present undergraduate and graduate athletic training students at East Carolina University and the University of South Florida for their input and assistance. Their comments, suggestions, and energy helped to make this edition stronger. We are grateful for their dedication to athletic training.

This edition would not have been possible without the encouragement and support of our professional colleagues. They provided advice, suggestions, critical appraisal, and challenges. They transformed this text into a user-friendly resource.

Finally, we recognize and appreciate the tenacity of our friendship, which began long ago at a professional meeting and evolved into "Hey, let's do this project!" It has remained strong throughout the pursuit of our vision of improving the educational experience in the field of medicine for the athletic trainer. We have learned that with vision, drive, and determination, anything is possible if good friends keep pulling and pushing each other in the same direction with a common goal.

PART I

Introduction to Medical Conditions

This textbook begins with an overview of the basic information presented in subsequent chapters, including a discussion of the role of the athletic trainer as an initial health care provider. Chapter 1 covers three general categories: communication; prevention of disease transmission; and legal considerations, medical care, and disposition. The communication section recommends open-ended questions and the use of nonverbal techniques to gather the best responses from patients. Proper medical terminology and communication with other health care providers are discussed, as well as the protection of patients' confidentiality. The second part of chapter 1, "Prevention of Disease Transmission," touches on federal regulations, bloodborne pathogens, barriers to disease transmission (such as correct glove use), and disinfection of equipment and facilities. The last section of chapter 1, "Legal Considerations, Medical Care, and Disposition," touches on legal aspects of medical care (or lack thereof), patient-reported outcomes (PROs), and evidence-based medicine as they relate to the ultimate quality of health care. The subject of classifying and tracking (coding) diseases is covered briefly. Finally, the importance of the preparticipation examination (PPE) is reviewed as are the resources to determine whether an athlete qualifies for sport participation.

Chapter 2, "Medical Examination," is the most critical chapter in the text. It discusses the basic evaluation tools that will assist the reader throughout the remainder of the book. Health history, observation and inspection, palpation, and diagnostic tests are thoroughly explained. Photographs and carefully detailed procedures instruct the reader on the use of special equipment and techniques for the medical examination. Topics covered include assessing blood pressure, pulse, respiration, and temperature; using evaluation tools such as stethoscopes, ophthalmoscopes, and otoscopes; and various diagnostic tests such as neurological testing (dermatomes, deep tendon reflex arc, cranial nerve assessment), palpation, percussion, and auscultation.

Chapter 3, "Diagnostic Imaging and Testing," describes various diagnostic imaging procedures (X-rays, radionuclide bone scan, fluoroscopy, CT scan, PET scan, MRI) and their associated risks or side effects as well as many diagnostic testing procedures such as electrocardiography, the Holter monitor, stress tests, and laparoscopy. Many laboratory tests, such as urinalysis, CBC, and lumbar punctures, are described so that readers can tell their patients what to expect.

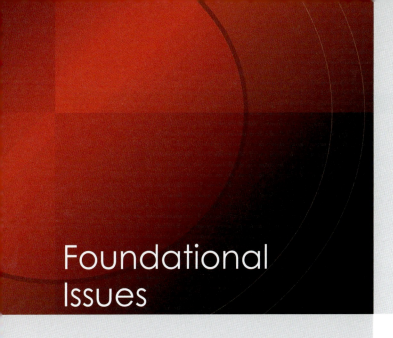

Foundational Issues

1

At the completion of this chapter the reader should be able to do the following:

- Discuss the basic differences between orthopedic and medical assessment.

- Appreciate the athletic trainer as a health care provider in the recognition, referral, and disposition of medical conditions.

- Practice effective communication in the medical assessment of the physically active person.

- Apply principles of disease transmission prevention.

- Implement the regulations and laws that govern the care and privacy of patients.

- Compare CPT and ICD codes to medical conditions.

- Recognize the importance of patient-reported outcomes (PROs) and evidence-based practice (EBP) in the comprehensive evaluation and treatment of a patient's medical condition.

- Explain the purpose of the preparticipation examination (PPE) for athletes, and identify the medical organizations that provide guidelines.

- Differentiate the office visit from the station-based PPE.

This introductory chapter provides an overview of the foundational premises for subsequent chapters in the following broad categories: communication, prevention of disease transmission and legal considerations, medical care, and disposition. It touches on many topics briefly such as medical coding, evidence-based practice, and patient-reported outcomes. Although not covered in depth here, these topics can apply to every chapter, so a quick review of their relevance is important. Chapter 1 also reviews the role of the athletic trainer in the diagnosis and treatment of medical conditions, the importance of effective communication, the prevention of disease transmission, legal concerns, and the administrative aspects of the preparticipation examination (PPE).

Role of the Athletic Trainer in Evaluation of Medical Conditions

Although this text is not exclusively for certified athletic trainers (ATs), they are often the first to detect an athlete's potential medical issue. A brief description of the education and training of ATs is useful here so that readers can understand their role. Athletes who are feeling ill commonly turn to the athletic trainer because the AT is the most accessible health care provider. Athletic trainers establish a rapport with their athletes and are familiar with their medical histories and their normal performance, as well as the demands the sport places on their bodies. This may enable the AT to detect a condition that otherwise might go unnoticed. The AT working with college or professional teams is also responsible for the health care of the entire team while traveling with the team to games and events. Although many athletic issues are orthopedic in nature, the conditions an athletic trainer encounters can also include infections, colds, and other maladies

Certified Athletic Trainers

An athletic trainer is a health care professional who provides services under the direction of or in collaboration with a physician. To enter the profession, candidates must graduate with a degree in athletic training from a Commission on Accreditation of Athletic Training Education (CAATE) accredited athletic training education program. The fall of 2022 will be the last time an undergraduate can enroll in a CAATE-accredited AT program to seek a bachelor's degree in AT and sit for the national Board of Certification (BOC) exam to practice athletic training. After this time, all professional AT programs will be delivered at the master's degree level only. ATs work with physicians in a number of settings, most traditionally in high school, college, professional, and Olympic sports. They can also be found in clinics, hospitals, and industry.

All athletic training students must have a minimum of two years of clinical experience within college credit courses that must be completed with different populations and various levels of risk, including nonorthopedic or medical conditions. The proposed 2019 CAATE standards include additional skills in both emergent and nonemergent medical situations.

- ATs must pass a national certification examination (from the Board of Certification) after college graduation.

- Most states also require state licensure or registration to practice athletic training in that state.

Commission on Accreditation of Athletic Training Education 2015.

---

that need to be identified quickly and treated properly in order for the athlete to perform at optimal levels.

It has been nearly 20 yr since the National Athletic Trainers' Association (NATA) first identified a new series of educational competencies and clinical proficiencies in several areas that were not previously part of an athletic trainer's preparation: pathology of injury and illness, pharmacology, and general medical conditions and disabilities (Commission on Accreditation of Athletic Training Education 2015). These competencies and proficiencies have since then been included in athletic training curricula throughout the United States and have been expanded in subsequent professional requirements.

The athletic trainer continues to assume a greater role in health care of patients, and this places more emphasis on the clinical diagnosis and the coordinated plan of care for patients' medical problems. In part, this is a result of advances in medical science that now enable athletes with medical conditions to compete at the highest levels. It also is the result of expanding employment opportunities for ATs. Athletic trainers are employed in industries, inpatient hospitals, outpatient clinics, and other nontraditional workplaces as well as in the traditional realms of interscholastic, intercollegiate, and professional sport. Athletic trainers work carefully with physicians and see a more diverse population, including pediatric athletes, physically active mature and older adults, and those with physical impairments. Because ATs are health care providers who work with diverse populations, they must be effective communicators. They must be able explain to the pediatric patient her medical condition in terms she would understand and also be able to relay lab and diagnostic reports to other professionals in the medical community.

Athletic trainers can defend their decision to the coach to deny participation to an asthmatic athlete, and they can provide explicit take-home care instructions to the parent of a concussed athlete. All of these transferals of medical knowledge require an ability to accurately relay facts and to respect the intended audience.

Communication in the Medical Field

Effective communication is one of the most critical aspects of evaluating a patient. Communication takes many forms, from the initial encounter with the patient to determining the chief complaint, acquiring critical information, and sharing the findings with the patient and with other health care providers if warranted.

Communication With Patients

Because the medical examination is centered on symptoms, the nature of the initial meeting and the questions asked when acquiring a health or illness history are as critical as the information gained from them. The patient must be comfortable enough to openly discuss his or her symptoms. Effective communication depends on the practitioner's familiarity with the patient, respect for cultural, gender, language, or other potential barriers, and an ability to maintain a pleasant and interested demeanor. One way to promote dialogue between the practitioner and the athlete is to ask open-ended questions, such as "Why have you come to see me today?"

Being empathetic—for example, "That sounds difficult."—and allowing pauses that give the athlete time

Effective Communication With Patients

- Ask open-ended questions.
- Maintain eye contact, if culturally respectful.
- Display an open, relaxed posture.
- Repeat key words spoken by the patient.
- Use simple phrases for encouragement, such as "go on" or "mm-hmmm."

for additional comments can reassure the patient that the clinician is listening carefully. Asking how the patient feels about the symptoms is also appropriate in medical assessment. A good practitioner can summarize and interpret the athlete's comments by saying, "I hear you say…" rather than by empathetically injecting words or opinions into the conversation during the subjective review of symptoms.

Along with verbal communication skills, the health care provider must be sensitive to cultural, ethnic, and gender issues. In certain cultures, touching is impermissible because it violates a personal space. In others, direct eye contact is disrespectful. Knowing the patients or asking them if they are comfortable is a good beginning. A person will more freely give a medical history if the health care provider uses a quiet and private place to communicate.

The health care provider must always be aware of the surroundings when communicating with an athlete about a medical issue. When a practitioner assesses a patient of a different gender, a person of the athlete's gender should be present in the room as well. Using proper draping and maintaining privacy during physical examinations or discussion of private topics are critical.

Communication With Health Professionals

Federal regulations allow health care providers to exchange information about a patient's medical care. This exchange can occur after the patient grants permission under the Health Insurance Portability and Accountability Act (HIPAA). Athletic trainers should be familiar with medical terminology so that they can discuss medical conditions with other health care providers.

Because some communications among health care providers take the form of written notes or electronic records (Electronic Medical Record—EMR), athletic trainers must understand typical medical terminology and standard medical abbreviations. The "Common Medical Terminology" sidebar lists common medical conditions and situations that are used throughout this text.

Medical Referral

People working with injured or ill patients know that a delay in receiving medical attention may result in lasting damage or possible death. Because many team physicians specialize in orthopedic or family practice, ATs should have access to other medical doctors (MDs) or doctors

Common Medical Terminology

adventitious—Coming from an external source; occurring spontaneously

afebrile—Without a fever; also *apyretic*

biopsy—Removal and examination of tissue

comorbid—Two or more possibly unrelated medical conditions existing at the same time

constitutional—Relating to the body as a whole

erythema—Redness of the skin brought about by capillary dilation

febrile—Having a fever

malaise—A general feeling of discomfort or uneasiness; often the first symptom of an illness or infection

morbidity—Consequences of a given illness

mortality—Death from a particular illness or disease

palliative or supportive—Reducing the severity of an illness or treatment of disease without curing it

prodromal—Preillness symptoms

purulent—Pus filled

sequela, sequelae—A condition occurring as a consequence of a given illness or disease

suppurative—Pus forming

CLINICAL TIPS

Knowing the Difference Between a Sign and a Symptom

Although generally mentioned together during the assessment of a medical condition, signs and symptoms are not synonymous.

- *Sign* refers to something that the athletic trainer sees or feels, such as a temperature, respiration, heartbeat, or blood pressure. A sign can be objectively measured or assessed.

- *Symptom* (Sx) refers to something the athlete feels or tells the AT, such as a headache, nausea, dizziness, or pain.

of osteopathy (DOs) for the referral of specific medical conditions in their athlete-patients. ATs should know the differences among the various medical specialties (see table 1.1) in order to direct athletes to the right providers.

Sending an athlete with a concussion to an orthopedic surgeon may not be the most effective (or affordable) referral if the physician does not have training in concussion management. Before making a referral, determine what the physician can contribute to the athlete's well-being and safe return to activity.

Federal Regulations Pertaining to Communication Among Medical Professionals

The right of the athlete to have personal medical information protected against dissemination to outside parties is of the utmost importance. These outside agents may include the media, coaches, or even parents if the athlete is over age 18 and can function as an adult. Although it is common to cite an orthopedic reason for an athlete's inability to participate, many athletes do not explicitly give permission to reveal medical conditions that prevent their full activity. Even when they sign a form that allows medical information to be shared with parties such as coaches, insurance secretaries, professional scouts, and the media, this form typically applies only to injuries

TABLE 1.1 Health Care Providers

Degree	Title	BS/BA	MS/MA	PhD/doctorate	Postgraduate education	Prescribing authority
AT	Athletic trainer	X	X	X		
DC	Doctor of chiropractic	X			+4 yr	
DO	Doctor of osteopathy	X			+7 yr	X
DPM	Doctor of podiatry	X			+4 yr	X
EMT	Emergency medical technician (initial 6 wk course)					
EMT-P	Paramedic (various levels, including intubation or IV administration)					
LPN	Licensed practical nurse (1 yr technical degree)					
MD	Medical doctor	X			+7 yr	X
NP	Nurse practitioner	X	X			X
OT	Occupational therapist	X	X	X		
PA	Physician's assistant (intensive 26 mo program)	X	X	X		X
PhD	Psychologist	X	X	X		
PT	Physical therapist	X	X	X		
PTA	Physical therapy assistant (associate's degree)					
RD	Registered dietitian	X	X			
RN	Registered nurse	X	X	X		

IV = intravenous.

that are orthopedic in nature; it does not cover medical issues such as sexually transmitted infections (STIs) or other diseases. Students in the health care fields must be aware of the regulations for their field. The NATA Code of Ethics and the Board of Certification that oversees the Standards of Professional Practice for certified ATs, for example, both include principles for the preservation of privileged information and requirements for adherence to federal laws (National Athletic Trainers' Association 2013; Board of Certification 2016).

Case law has routinely protected the athlete from violations of patient privacy, citing discrimination and Americans with Disabilities Act protections in cases of athletes with HIV or AIDS (Wong and Apostolopoulou 1999). Disclosure of medical information without a patient's express permission is illegal and falls under two federal acts that govern personal health information (PHI), depending on the age of the athlete: HIPAA and the Family Educational Rights and Privacy Act (FERPA).

HIPAA

HIPAA, also known as *Public Law 104-191*, was implemented in 2003. It is the first federally mandated act to protect patient privacy, oversee medical records, and give patients more control over how and to whom their personal health information is disclosed (United States Department of Health & Human Services 2016). Specifically, the law allows patients to see their medical records and request corrections if factual errors are discovered. It places limits on the use and sharing of PHI outside of health care agencies—for example, with a life insurance company. The act dictates how PHI may be disseminated in given situations, verbally or electronically. The U.S. Department of Health and Human Services Office for Civil Rights provides oversight and enforcement of HIPAA (United States Department of Health & Human Services 2016).

FERPA

FERPA, also known as the *Buckley Amendment*, was created in 1974 to protect the privacy of student education records, and it applies to any school receiving funds from the U.S. Department of Education (United States Department of Education 2016). It functions similarly to HIPAA in that it gives people access to and limits disclosure of their educational records. Parents have a right to inspect a child's educational records until the student is 18 years old. After the student becomes a legal adult and attends a school beyond high school, the rights transfer from the parent to the student. After this, parents have no right to their adult children's educational or medical records unless the children sign a waiver (United States Department of Education 2016).

The act allows only certain parties access to educational records without prior permission in given situations. An example is "appropriate officials in cases of health and safety emergencies" (United States Department of Education 2016). An educational record may contain biographical information, grade point averages, records of student conduct, and test scores. Disclosing without prior consent that a particular athlete weighs a certain amount, is an orphan, took remedial reading classes, or plagiarized is a violation of this act. The consequences of disclosure range from loss of certain federal funds to prosecution of a criminal offense.

Medical Records

Adequate records on the health care of athletes must be kept, and everyone who has access to these records must appreciate and abide by confidentiality and the athletes' right to privacy as well as preserving HIPAA and FERPA confidentiality (National Collegiate Athletic Association 2014). These records must be maintained and stored in areas with limited access in accordance with institutional and state regulatory acts, and they must be safeguarded against improper disclosure at all times. Limited access applies to the monitoring of daily injury reports, the athletes' status, the results of diagnostic tests, and the accessibility of medical files. Even daily treatment logs, e-mails with identifiable information, and fax transmissions must be considered privileged information. Unsecured files, open storage areas, or unprotected computers without password encryption are examples of inappropriate medical record storage.

Abbreviations used among health care workers are considered appropriate and legal methods of keeping notations on medical records. The athletic trainer and other health care providers must be familiar with these abbreviations because they save time and space when writing notes into charts.

Electronic Medical Records

Many companies provide electronic services to update and maintain medical records. Typically, an institution subscribes with a vendor for services to update, repair, and maintain the software and server. The only restrictions are the amount of money the institution has for this type of service and the size of the server it wishes to maintain. Many electronic medical records (EMRs) permit electronic exchange between providers and insurance carriers on secure sites. This allows medical providers at different venues to gain access to provider notes, X-ray and lab results, diagnostic tests, and other information. Some EMRs also provide for communication with patients about appointments, lab and diagnostic results, and any follow-up needs. Often the institution can have the software tailored to meet its specific needs.

Prevention of Disease Transmission

Everyone who works in health care appreciates the need to prevent disease transmission. Protection from infection and maintaining a sanitary environment are two critical elements in caring for patients with illnesses. Another prevention technique is immunization from specific diseases by vaccine. Chapter 15 discusses vaccination as well as established standards for preventing the spread of disease and illnesses.

There are federal mandates that address the prevention and spread of disease. States and institutions may also impose restrictions for safety on their subjects, and health care providers must know the policies and regulations for their own workplaces. Intercollegiate sports medicine guidelines require that all necessary materials, such as barriers, bleach, waste receptacles, and wound coverings, comply with universal precautions and be available to all health care providers (Parsons 2014).

The Occupational Safety and Health Administration (OSHA) sets standards to protect health care workers and their patients. OSHA standards apply only to established relationships between employers and employees and do not extend federal protections to students (United States Department of Labor 2016b). However, students such as those in the health care, who could be exposed to hazardous waste in facilities where they practice or observe, should follow the safety standards set forth by OSHA, receive training, and have ready access to precautionary materials, such as barriers and proper disposal containers.

OSHA can inspect any facility under its auspices without prior notification, and it has the power to suspend or shut down a facility as well as to impose hefty fines for noncompliance with standards (United States Department of Labor 2016b, d). The most familiar OSHA requirement affecting athletic medical care concerns the bloodborne pathogens (BBP) standard. Athletic trainers must be intimately familiar with this standard because athletes often receive open wounds in the course of their activities, with the consequent risk of infection.

Bloodborne Pathogens

The OSHA bloodborne pathogens (BBP) standard is intended to safeguard health care workers against hazards resulting from exposure to infectious body fluids, and it covers anyone who could reasonably anticipate having occupational exposure to infectious waste (e.g., blood). Included in this standard is a description of how to formulate an individualized institutional or setting exposure control plan. A written document outlines steps to take and specific people to call in the event of an exposure to infectious waste. An exposure may range from a needle stick to blood spilled onto intact skin. All health care workers must have an operating knowledge of their employer's plan, access to personal protective equipment, BBP training, and knowledge about whom to contact should an exposure occur (United States Department of Labor 2016d). Typically, these instructions are visibly posted throughout the facility.

The BBP standard uses the phrase *universal precautions* to emphasize that all human waste should be treated as if it were infectious and that health care workers and patients must be protected in every situation in which they might be exposed to body fluid, including contact with mucous membranes in the eyes, mouth, or nose; genital secretions; or blood. Any sharp object that may be contaminated with infectious waste, such as needles, scalpels, or broken glass, is also considered potentially hazardous material (United States Department of Labor 2016d).

CLINICAL TIPS

Handling Infectious Waste

- All infectious waste must be placed in a closeable, leakproof-approved container for storage, transporting, or shipping.
- An OSHA-approved plan for proper disposal of infectious waste bags and sharps units must be on hand and followed.
- Gloves must be worn when personnel handle infectious laundry.
- Laundry contaminated with infectious waste must be separated from other materials to be cleaned.
- Personal protective equipment (gowns, masks, gloves) shall be properly disposed of before leaving the treatment room or on contamination.
- While wearing gloves, personnel may clean bloodstains on material (uniforms, towels) with hydrogen peroxide in cold water and immediately rinse.
- Only red hazardous waste bags should be used to dispose of infectious materials.
- In the absence of antibacterial soap and running water, personnel should use antibacterial wipes or gels to sanitize hands often.
- Personnel should avoid putting ungloved hands to face (eyes, nose, mouth) when around ill patients or when working with infectious waste.

Data from Parsons 2014; United States Department of Labor 2016a-d.

The National Collegiate Athletic Association (NCAA) and National Federation of State High School Associations (NFHS) have explicit regulations that address infection control and bleeding athletes or those with blood on their uniforms (Parsons 2014; Beaschler 2015; National Federation of State High School Associations 2015). These regulations require that a bleeding athlete be removed from activity until the bleeding has been stopped and the wound covered with a dressing sturdy enough to withstand the demands of activity. Soiled uniforms must be cleaned or changed before resumption of activity (Parsons 2014). Again, the requirements of storing and disposing of infectious waste are intended to protect both the athlete and the health care provider and prevent them from transmitting diseases.

Barriers to Disease Transmission

Barriers are devices worn to protect both the health care worker and the patient against the spread of disease. The traditionally accepted barrier is latex gloves, but OSHA also requires access to face and eye protection, gowns, and mouthpieces for resuscitation (Parsons 2014; United States Department of Labor 2016d). Health care workers with allergies to latex must be provided with an alternative material suitable as a barrier against the transmission of BBPs.

CLINICAL TIPS

Correct Glove Use

1. Thoroughly wash all aspects of both hands and fingers, with liberal use of an antibacterial soap and plenty of water.
2. Dry hands with a disposable single-use hand towel.
3. Apply gloves without touching the external surfaces of the gloves.

When the procedure requiring gloves is complete:

1. Use the gloved index finger and thumb of one hand; gently pinch the glove at the wrist and pull toward fingertips.
2. Invert the glove, and remove all but index finger and thumb.
3. Repeat the procedure with the second hand, inverting the glove as it is removed.
4. Fold gloves inside out and dispose of them in a red (OSHA-approved) bag.
5. Thoroughly wash and dry hands as described previously.

All health care workers must have ready access to barriers that fit properly in order to retard infection from hazardous materials. Washing with soap and water is the best way to clean hands before and after glove use. If soap and water are not readily available, commercial disinfectant gels or single-use wipes can sanitize hands.

Workers should remove and properly dispose of soiled barriers before leaving the treatment area. Brightly labeled red infectious waste bags are the most common means of storing such waste until it can be disposed of per OSHA protocol. These bags must be contained in a sturdy, leakproof container with a lid and located in an easily accessible area for all to use.

Sharps Containers

Sharps containers are specifically built, self-contained units that have one-way valves (figure 1.1) and are used to accommodate sharp instruments such as needles and scalpels that may have infectious materials on them. Some sharps containers are locked to a wall so that only an OSHA-approved provider can remove them for proper disposal. These containers should never be opened or overstuffed. Typically, institutions that have sharps containers have a service that maintains them, including scheduled emptying and inspection for safety.

Disinfection

Another component of prevention in the spread of infections is disinfection of surfaces used for examination, and treatment and disinfection of soiled materials, including uniforms and clothing. Disinfection is a critical aspect of every athletic training facility because of its potential to stop the spread of disease. The simple acts of sterilizing

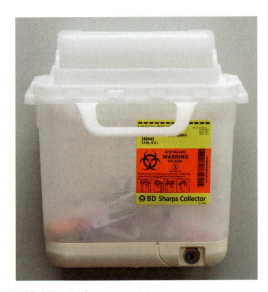

FIGURE 1.1 A sharps container.

treatment tables after use and washing hands often can diminish disease transmission considerably. Many infections, such as hepatitis B, are quite hardy and can live outside the body if not obliterated properly (see chapter 15).

The Environmental Protection Agency (EPA) registers all disinfectants in the United States. The EPA has prior approval on all test methods companies use to determine whether their product is effective against a particular organism (United States Environmental Protection Agency 2016). Disinfectants approved by the EPA have a registration number on the label of the product as well as a list of organisms targeted. To be labeled as "hospital strength" a disinfectant must eradicate 100% of all organisms listed on the label. Household chlorine bleach contains 5.25% active sodium hypochlorite and 94.75% water. Although it is extremely effective against *Staphylococcus* and *Streptococcus* bacteria, *Salmonella, Escherichia coli,* certain fungi, and influenza A and B, it is not a cleaner. The EPA and U.S. Department of Agriculture have deemed chlorine bleach safe for use in food preparation and as a disinfectant. It is registered with the EPA for appropriate use as a hospital disinfectant, and the Centers for Disease Control and Prevention have written guidelines for its use in health care facilities (United States Environmental Protection Agency 2016).

The difference between a disinfectant and a disinfectant-cleaner is that a disinfectant merely kills microorganisms, whereas a combination cleaner removes soils and disinfects in one step. Regulations governing how these cleaners and disinfectants are dispersed include the following: If the material is removed from its original container, it must have all the product information transferred to the second receptacle, including a notation that the cleaner was moved, for example, from a gallon container to a spray bottle (United States Department of Labor 2016a). When sanitizing surfaces soiled with possible BBPs, OSHA recommends properly using barriers, cleaning all blood from the surface and properly disposing of the waste, and then disinfecting the area (United States Department of Labor 2016c).

CLINICAL TIPS

OSHA Mandates on Disinfectant Agents

- Contaminated surfaces must be sprayed to saturation with the disinfectant.
- HIV-1 disinfection requires 30 s of saturation.
- Hepatitis B virus disinfection requires 10 min of saturation.

From United States Department of Labor 2016c.

The *2014–2015 NCAA Sports Medicine Handbook* suggests using a 1:100 ratio of freshly prepared bleach-to-water solution for disinfecting surfaces (Parsons 2014). Calling for a more proactive approach to disinfecting surfaces, the NFHS recommends cleaning equipment and pads weekly with this bleach solution (National Federation of State High School Associations 2015).

Legal Considerations, Medical Care, and Disposition

This section offers a brief overview of several topics relating to medical care. It begins with a short discussion on the legal aspects of providing quality medical care and continues with patient disposition. Patient-reported outcomes (PROs) and evidence-based practice (EBP) are two important components of delivering appropriate care to patients. Entire textbooks have been written on both of these areas, so we only touch upon them here. Next, the classification systems that assist with coding diagnoses and prescribing treatment are discussed. The purpose of this short section is to help you to see the importance of the coding and how it assists with tracking trends and insurance payments. Finally, we discuss the importance and administration of the preparticipation exam for athletes.

Legal Considerations

As with everything else, legal ramifications must be considered when caring for athletes. Health care providers hired to evaluate athletes and prevent illnesses and injuries have a duty to their employers, and subsequently their patients, to render appropriate medical care. The word *duty* here is a legal term, one of the four components considered in proving negligence. Breaching a duty, and therefore causing harm, is negligence. Athletic trainers also have other duties to their athlete-patients. Among them are maintaining skills and knowledge, providing a reasonable standard of care, giving medical referrals if necessary, and upholding patients' right to privacy.

Negligence is conduct that falls below an established and expected standard of care validated by law for the protection of others, which results in physical or mental harm or damage to another. Typically, case law helps us to interpret what the standard of care should be in a given situation. In the case of *Kleinknecht v. Gettysburg College,* the court held that the college had a duty to protect against medical crisis, specifically to adopt a policy that might avoid life-threatening emergencies (1992). In another case, the presence of a qualified medical person at certain practices but not others was not deemed in itself to be a violation of the standard of care owed an athlete

(Kennedy v. Syracuse University 1995). In this situation, the athletic trainer was always present at higher risk sports events. A serious wrist injury occurred at a different venue but was not caused or worsened by the failure of the athletic trainer to habitually attend football practice but not gymnastics. Other recent lawsuits claim death occurred because of failure to recognize athletes suffering from a sickle cell crisis (Price 2005; Fainaru-Wada 2008), permanent disability from returning to play with a concussion (Hetzner 2009), and death resulting from clearing an athlete to play with a concussion (Letchworth 2009).

The privilege of being a certified and state-licensed or registered AT does carry with it certain obligations. Athletic trainers are held to a higher standard than are physical education teachers or personal trainers because of their training, experience, and national certification. Among the critical obligations is establishing and practicing a venue-specific emergency action plan (EAP) to address catastrophic events that may occur within the realm of athletic participation. Components within the EAP include access to early cardiac defibrillation, the presence of or access to a physician, communication between on-site personnel and a medical facility, and transportation to a medical facility (Parsons 2014). The *NCAA Sports Medicine Handbook* is updated annually and specifically discusses the role of the health care provider in many medical aspects of sport, including issues related to bloodborne pathogens, concussions, sickle cell trait, pregnancy, and other conditions. The BOC Standards of Professional Practice has several references to the expected level of care its members should give to patients (Board of Certification 2016). Athletic trainers would be wise to review their job descriptions to clearly delineate their roles and responsibilities and to understand the expected standard of care.

Because most ATs do not see as many medical conditions as they do orthopedic problems, they must also work within established guidelines, such as under the direction of a team physician, especially when working with medical disorders. It is critical to know when a medical condition is beyond the athletic trainer's scope of practice and should be referred.

Patient-Reported Outcomes

Patient-reported outcomes (PROs) are generally used in the clinical setting when data are collected directly from patients. Their purpose is to engage patients as active partners in their own progress and to determine if a given treatment is working. PROs are often presented as scales (Likert 1–5) or numerical sets (1–10) that correlate with how the patient is feeling. Typical sections of a PRO include symptoms, disability (how well the patient is or is not functioning daily), health status, quality of life (QoL), and general health concerns or perceptions.

Each type of health issue can have its own questionnaire. For example, a PRO for a patient with heart valve replacement will be different from one who has chronic psoriasis. Clinical trials use PROs to determine if a given treatment or therapy was effective from the patient's point of view, and often a clinic will tailor a PRO to meet the needs of the patient or condition. There is a lot of research on validating PROs for given conditions. One of the more common valid PROs is the Short-Form 36 (SF-36) that offers 36 short questions pertaining to the patient's health. PROs are critical to the application of evidence-based practice.

Evidence-Based Practice

Evidence-based practice (EBP) entails blending the best research evidence and clinical expertise to make health care decisions. EBP involves the patients' values and preferences to create a complete research–practice–patient circle. This type of practice begins with a patient-centered problem or concern, followed by the creation of a very specific question or desired outcome. The health care provider must then seek appropriate, validated research or resources to assist with research. The health care provider must have a strong grasp of how robust the research is, how valid the instrument or assessment is, and how sensitive or specific the treatment is in working toward the desired outcome. EBP is engaging and promotes curiosity. It involves using best practices for a given condition. Clinicians should encourage patients not only to participate, but also to engage in their own treatment.

Classification and Surveillance Systems

There are two national medical classification systems: one that categorize diseases and conditions (International Classification of Diseases) and another that tracks treatments, procedures, and therapies (Current Procedural Terminology). It is important to be familiar with these classification systems because they are widely used both to track disease trends and types and to follow developments in treatments and therapies. People working in medical offices, hospitals, and clinics will also use the systems to code insurance billing as well as determine trends in treatments.

International Classification of Diseases

In 1983, the United States government mandated a medical classification system that linked diagnosis-related groups for the purpose of cataloging and medical record-keeping. Since then, people responsible for billing and reimbursement have used the International Classification of Diseases (ICD) manual, which is currently in its 10th revision (ICD-10).

The World Health Organization (WHO, Geneva, Switzerland) established the ICD to provide statistical data on the morbidity and mortality of medical conditions. Since 1988, physicians seeking reimbursement for services rendered have been required to submit diagnosis codes for any Medicare patient.

The seven-digit codes are organized in the following manner: There are 22 chapters of codes (chapters I–XXII) that assign specific alphabetic codes and numbers (A00–B99 is in chapter 1; Z00–Z99 is in chapter XXII) to certain tissues, injuries, or causes of death (table 1.2). Chapter I is *Certain Infectious and Parasitic Diseases*, whereas chapters IX and XV are *Diseases of the Circulatory System*, and *Pregnancy, Childbirth, and Puerperium*, respectively. Following the alphabetic letter are the two-digit main codes. Typically, a dot provides separation between the main code and any qualifier. A qualifier can be three to seven digits, alphabetic, numeric, or a combination of both. The qualifier can indicate many things, including etiology, anatomical site, and severity. The ICD is primarily used to diagnose and track conditions, but it helps insurance companies to determine when to cover a given procedure for a given ICD code. For example, a patient with a third sinus infection in a relatively short period may be allowed a CT of the sinuses to determine if there is another underlying condition (Centers for Medicare and Medicaid Services 2015).

Current Procedural Terminology

Unlike the ICD, Current Procedural Terminology (CPT) provides a set of billing codes, descriptions, and guidelines associated with procedures and services used by health care professionals. This manual is published annually in January by the American Medical Association (AMA), and it contains five-digit codes that identify the procedure or service rendered. The CPT is divided into six sections and each has subsections. Like the ICD, there are often numbers following the code with a decimal point to further identify a given service. The use of the plus (+) symbol indicates that procedures were performed in combination (e.g., 97005 is "athletic training evaluation" and could be combined with 97033 "iontophoresis" and 97140 "manual therapy techniques").

Preparticipation Examination

The purpose of a preparticipation examination (PPE) is not only to determine readiness for a specific sport but to identify any potential or correctable conditions that may impair the athlete's ability to fully perform. In general, the PPE is the first interaction a health care provider has with an athlete. This examination is not a true physical but a screening procedure that sheds light on potential problems associated with activity. The American Academy of Family Physicians (AAFP) recommends that all athletes have a PPE for the primary purpose of identifying any medical problems or conditions that could affect participation in sports (American Academy of Family Physicians et al. 2010). Without this examination, an athlete with systemic illnesses or a family history of cardiovascular disease may not be discovered or treated appropriately. The AAFP, along with other medical

TABLE 1.2 **Sample of the Alphanumeric Coding for ICD-10**

Chapter	Code numbers	Description
I	A00–B99	Certain infectious and parasitic diseases
II	C00–D49	Neoplasms
IV	E00–E89	Endocrine, nutritional, and metabolic diseases
V	F01–F99	Mental, behavioral, and neurodevelopmental disorders
VI	G00–G99	Diseases of the nervous system
VII	H00–H59	Diseases of the eye and adnexa
VIII	H60–H95	Diseases of the ear and mastoid process
IX	I00–I99	Diseases of the circulatory system
X	J00–J99	Diseases of the respiratory system
XI	K00–K95	Diseases of the digestive system
XII	L00–L99	Diseases of the skin and subcutaneous tissue
XIV	N00–N99	Diseases of the genitourinary system
XV	O00–O0A	Pregnancy, childbirth, and puerperium
XIX	S00–T88	Injury, poisoning, and certain other consequences of external causes
XX	V00–Y99	External causes of morbidity and mortality

societies, requires the PPE to be signed by either an MD or a DO, although some states or school districts allow a health care provider other than a DO or an MD to administer a PPE.

Student-athletes are required to have a comprehensive PPE on entry into middle or high school or upon transfer to a new school. The AAFP recommends these comprehensive evaluations at 2 to 3 yr intervals for older students, with annual updates on a comprehensive health history, problem-focused areas, and vital signs (American Academy of Family Physicians et al. 2010). Although some in the medical community still contend that PPEs are not thorough enough, especially in the realm of conditions related to sudden death, these evaluations have come a long way from the mass gymnasium physicals of 20 yr ago.

According to the NCAA, a PPE is also required for a student's entrance into the intercollegiate athletics program, and an updated annual health history should follow (Parsons 2014). Although many institutions use this examination largely as a medical history that focuses on orthopedic issues, it is also a venue to address medical problems (American Academy of Family Physicians et al. 2010). According to the NCAA, the college athlete's PPE should answer questions relating to current immunizations, allergies, and illnesses, in addition to containing cardiovascular, neurological, and musculoskeletal system assessments. Together with the American Academy of Pediatrics, the American College of Sports Medicine, the American Medical Society for Sports Medicine, the American Orthopedic Society for Sports Medicine, and the American Osteopathic Academy for Sports Medicine, the AAFP has created a preparticipation physical evaluation that screens for most areas that could affect full participation. This group created the medical history questions, physical examination form, and clearance form for sports PPE found in figure 1.2. (Note the types of history questions asked in figure 1.2, which relate to the various body systems and include mental health.)

Proper administration of the PPE requires good communication skills, which are also critical to the assessment of medical conditions. The health care provider must be aware of tone, body positioning, and language when having a dialogue with athletes.

The NCAA and NFHS are constantly reviewing and updating the PPE process and regulations. The failure of personnel to recognize a sickle-cell trait medical emergency contributed to the recent NCAA ruling that all athletes who are not certain of their status must be tested for sickle-cell as part of the medical examination with the university (Parsons 2014). Changes such as this are intended to provide better care to the student-athlete and to provide health care providers with a medical history that can contribute to safer participation. The current

version of the medical groups' (listed previously) PPE collaboration is displayed in figure 1.2.

While the actual PPE is discussed in detail in chapter 2, here is an overview of the process of establishing and conducting PPEs. It is best that the PPE be conducted at least 6 wk before the onset of the sport season, so physicians have time to order and analyze additional screening tests if necessary. There are two basic types of preparticipation examinations: office visit and station-based. Both have advantages and disadvantages. The office visit is more private and is typically performed by a physician who has a working relationship with the athlete; it is also potentially expensive and rarely covered by insurance, and the examining physician may not be as familiar with the requirements of the sport as would the team physician. In station-based PPEs, athletes move from station to station (medical history, orthopedic evaluation, visual screening, lung and cardiac auscultation). The station-based PPEs often occur as a courtesy or community service from a group of physicians. Although they are cost-effective (nominal fee or free) and feature physicians with different specialties, they are not as private as office visits, and they can be loud or confusing to patients (American Academy of Family Physicians et al. 2010). The traditional station-based PPE ends with a thorough review of the medical history and a final checkout by the team physician. In this scenario, athletes are all seen by the team physician, who has a better appreciation for the rigors of a particular sport than might the athlete's personal physician.

Determining Sport Qualification

There are certain medical conditions (e.g., loss of one paired organ) that may disqualify an athlete from certain sports or from competitive activity altogether. Chapter 8 has extensive information about the *36th Bethesda Conference: Eligibility Recommendations for Competitive Athletes with Cardiovascular Abnormalities*. These recommendations identify safe competitive areas for athletes with specific cardiovascular ailments. Pulmonary insufficiency, certain dermatological conditions, and organ mutations are all conditions that must be addressed on an individual basis with the athlete, parent (if the athlete is younger than 18), medical specialist, and team physician. Ultimately, it is the responsibility of the team physician to determine the level of risk inherent in a given sport for an athlete with a medical condition. If an athlete is not cleared to participate, the physician should provide recommendations to correct any medical condition that can be modified with medication, treatment, or rehabilitation. If the medical situation preventing activity is acute and temporary, a follow-up appointment should be made.

HISTORY FORM

(Note: This form is to be filled out by the patient and parent prior to seeing the physician. The physician should keep this form in the chart.)

Date of Exam _____

Name _____ Date of birth _____

Sex _____ Age _____ Grade _____ School _____ Sport(s) _____

Medicines and Allergies: Please list all of the prescription and over-the-counter medicines and supplements (herbal and nutritional) that you are currently taking

Do you have any allergies? ☐ Yes ☐ No If yes, please identify specific allergy below.
☐ Medicines   ☐ Pollens   ☐ Food   ☐ Stinging Insects

Explain "Yes" answers below. Circle questions you don't know the answers to.

GENERAL QUESTIONS	Yes	No
1. Has a doctor ever denied or restricted your participation in sports for any reason?		
2. Do you have any ongoing medical conditions? If so, please identify below:☐ Asthma ☐ Anemia ☐ Diabetes ☐ Infections Other: _____		
3. Have you ever spent the night in the hospital?		
4. Have you ever had surgery?		
HEART HEALTH QUESTIONS ABOUT YOU	**Yes**	**No**
5. Have you ever passed out or nearly passed out DURING or AFTER exercise?		
6. Have you ever had discomfort, pain, tightness, or pressure in your chest during exercise?		
7. Does your heart ever race or skip beats (irregular beats) during exercise?		
8. Has a doctor ever told you that you have any heart problems? If so, check all that apply:☐ High blood pressure ☐ A heart murmur ☐ High cholesterol ☐ A heart infection ☐ Kawasaki disease Other: _____		
9. Has a doctor ever ordered a test for your heart? (For example, ECG/EKG, echocardiogram)		
10. Do you get lightheaded or feel more short of breath than expected during exercise?		
11. Have you ever had an unexplained seizure?		
12. Do you get more tired or short of breath more quickly than your friends during exercise?		
HEART HEALTH QUESTIONS ABOUT YOUR FAMILY	**Yes**	**No**
13. Has any family member or relative died of heart problems or had an unexpected or unexplained sudden death before age 50 (including drowning, unexplained car accident, or sudden infant death syndrome)?		
14. Does anyone in your family have hypertrophic cardiomyopathy, Marfan syndrome, arrhythmogenic right ventricular cardiomyopathy, long QT syndrome, short QT syndrome, Brugada syndrome, or catecholaminergic polymorphic ventricular tachycardia?		
15. Does anyone in your family have a heart problem, pacemaker, or implanted defibrillator?		
16. Has anyone in your family had unexplained fainting, unexplained seizures, or near drowning?		
BONE AND JOINT QUESTIONS	**Yes**	**No**
17. Have you ever had an injury to a bone, muscle, ligament, or tendon that caused you to miss a practice or a game?		
18. Have you ever had any broken or fractured bones or dislocated joints?		
19. Have you ever had an injury that required x-rays, MRI, CT scan, injections, therapy, a brace, a cast, or crutches?		
20. Have you ever had a stress fracture?		
21. Have you ever been told that you have or have you had an x-ray for neck instability or atlantoaxial instability? (Down syndrome or dwarfism)		
22. Do you regularly use a brace, orthotics, or other assistive device?		
23. Do you have a bone, muscle, or joint injury that bothers you?		
24. Do any of your joints become painful, swollen, feel warm, or look red?		
25. Do you have any history of juvenile arthritis or connective tissue disease?		

MEDICAL QUESTIONS	Yes	No
26. Do you cough, wheeze, or have difficulty breathing during or after exercise?		
27. Have you ever used an inhaler or taken asthma medicine?		
28. Is there anyone in your family who has asthma?		
29. Were you born without or are you missing a kidney, an eye, a testicle (males), your spleen, or any other organ?		
30. Do you have groin pain or a painful bulge or hernia in the groin area?		
31. Have you had infectious mononucleosis (mono) within the last month?		
32. Do you have any rashes, pressure sores, or other skin problems?		
33. Have you had a herpes or MRSA skin infection?		
34. Have you ever had a head injury or concussion?		
35. Have you ever had a hit or blow to the head that caused confusion, prolonged headache, or memory problems?		
36. Do you have a history of seizure disorder?		
37. Do you have headaches with exercise?		
38. Have you ever had numbness, tingling, or weakness in your arms or legs after being hit or falling?		
39. Have you ever been unable to move your arms or legs after being hit or falling?		
40. Have you ever become ill while exercising in the heat?		
41. Do you get frequent muscle cramps when exercising?		
42. Do you or someone in your family have sickle cell trait or disease?		
43. Have you had any problems with your eyes or vision?		
44. Have you had any eye injuries?		
45. Do you wear glasses or contact lenses?		
46. Do you wear protective eyewear, such as goggles or a face shield?		
47. Do you worry about your weight?		
48. Are you trying to or has anyone recommended that you gain or lose weight?		
49. Are you on a special diet or do you avoid certain types of foods?		
50. Have you ever had an eating disorder?		
51. Do you have any concerns that you would like to discuss with a doctor?		
FEMALES ONLY		
52. Have you ever had a menstrual period?		
53. How old were you when you had your first menstrual period?		
54. How many periods have you had in the last 12 months?		

Explain "yes" answers here

_____
_____
_____
_____
_____
_____
_____

I hereby state that, to the best of my knowledge, my answers to the above questions are complete and correct.

Signature of athlete _____ Signature of parent/guardian _____ Date _____

> *continued*

FIGURE 1.2 Preparticipation physical examination (PPE).

From American Academy of Family Physicians, Preparticipation physical examination form, Elk Grove Village, IL: American Academy of Pediatrics: 2010, Copyright © 2010, American Academy of Pediatrics, Reproduced with permission.

THE ATHLETE WITH SPECIAL NEEDS: SUPPLEMENTAL HISTORY FORM

Date of Exam _____

Name _____ Date of birth _____

Sex _____ Age _____ Grade _____ School _____ Sport(s) _____

	Yes	No
1. Type of disability		
2. Date of disability		
3. Classification (if available)		
4. Cause of disability (birth, disease, accident/trauma, other)		
5. List the sports you are interested in playing		
6. Do you regularly use a brace, assistive device, or prosthetic?		
7. Do you use any special brace or assistive device for sports?		
8. Do you have any rashes, pressure sores, or any other skin problems?		
9. Do you have a hearing loss? Do you use a hearing aid?		
10. Do you have a visual impairment?		
11. Do you use any special devices for bowel or bladder function?		
12. Do you have burning or discomfort when urinating?		
13. Have you had autonomic dysreflexia?		
14. Have you ever been diagnosed with a heat-related (hyperthermia) or cold-related (hypothermia) illness?		
15. Do you have muscle spasticity?		
16. Do you have frequent seizures that cannot be controlled by medication?		

Explain "yes" answers here

_____
_____
_____
_____
_____
_____

Please indicate if you have ever had any of the following.

	Yes	No
Atlantoaxial instability		
X-ray evaluation for atlantoaxial instability		
Dislocated joints (more than one)		
Easy bleeding		
Enlarged spleen		
Hepatitis		
Osteopenia or osteoporosis		
Difficulty controlling bowel		
Difficulty controlling bladder		
Numbness or tingling in arms or hands		
Numbness or tingling in legs or feet		
Weakness in arms or hands		
Weakness in legs or feet		
Recent change in coordination		
Recent change in ability to walk		
Spina bifida		
Latex allergy		

Explain "yes" answers here

_____
_____
_____
_____
_____

I hereby state that, to the best of my knowledge, my answers to the above questions are complete and correct.

Signature of athlete _____ Signature of parent/guardian _____ Date _____

FIGURE 1.2 *> continued*

PHYSICAL EXAMINATION FORM

Name _____ Date of birth _____

PHYSICIAN REMINDERS

1. Consider additional questions on more sensitive issues
   - Do you feel stressed out or under a lot of pressure?
   - Do you ever feel sad, hopeless, depressed, or anxious?
   - Do you feel safe at your home or residence?
   - Have you ever tried cigarettes, chewing tobacco, snuff, or dip?
   - During the past 30 days, did you use chewing tobacco, snuff, or dip?
   - Do you drink alcohol or use any other drugs?
   - Have you ever taken anabolic steroids or used any other performance supplement?
   - Have you ever taken any supplements to help you gain or lose weight or improve your performance?
   - Do you wear a seat belt, use a helmet, and use condoms?
2. Consider reviewing questions on cardiovascular symptoms (questions 5–14).

EXAMINATION				
Height		Weight	☐ Male ☐ Female	
BP / (/) Pulse		Vision R 20/	L 20/	Corrected ☐ Y ☐ N

MEDICAL	NORMAL	ABNORMAL FINDINGS
Appearance • Marfan stigmata (kyphoscoliosis, high-arched palate, pectus excavatum, arachnodactyly, arm span > height, hyperlaxity, myopia, MVP, aortic insufficiency)		
Eyes/ears/nose/throat • Pupils equal • Hearing		
Lymph nodes		
Heart ª • Murmurs (auscultation standing, supine, +/- Valsalva) • Location of point of maximal impulse (PMI)		
Pulses • Simultaneous femoral and radial pulses		
Lungs		
Abdomen		
Genitourinary (males only)ᵇ		
Skin • HSV, lesions suggestive of MRSA, tinea corporis		
Neurologic ᶜ		
MUSCULOSKELETAL		
Neck		
Back		
Shoulder/arm		
Elbow/forearm		
Wrist/hand/fingers		
Hip/thigh		
Knee		
Leg/ankle		
Foot/toes		
Functional • Duck-walk, single leg hop		

ªConsider ECG, echocardiogram, and referral to cardiology for abnormal cardiac history or exam.
ᵇConsider GU exam if in private setting. Having third party present is recommended.
ᶜConsider cognitive evaluation or baseline neuropsychiatric testing if a history of significant concussion.

☐ Cleared for all sports without restriction

☐ Cleared for all sports without restriction with recommendations for further evaluation or treatment for _____
_____

☐ Not cleared

      ☐ Pending further evaluation

      ☐ For any sports

      ☐ For certain sports _____

      Reason _____

Recommendations _____
_____

I have examined the above-named student and completed the preparticipation physical evaluation. The athlete does not present apparent clinical contraindications to practice and participate in the sport(s) as outlined above. A copy of the physical exam is on record in my office and can be made available to the school at the request of the parents. If conditions arise after the athlete has been cleared for participation, the physician may rescind the clearance until the problem is resolved and the potential consequences are completely explained to the athlete (and parents/guardians).

Name of physician (print/type) _____ Date _____

Address _____ Phone _____

Signature of physician _____ , MD or DO

FIGURE 1.2 > continued

■ Preparticipation Physical Evaluation
CLEARANCE FORM

Name ______________________ Sex ☐ M ☐ F Age __________ Date of birth __________

☐ Cleared for all sports without restriction

☐ Cleared for all sports without restriction with recommendations for further evaluation or treatment for ______________________

____

☐ Not cleared

☐ Pending further evaluation

☐ For any sports

☐ For certain sports ______________________

Reason ______________________

Recommendations ______________________

____

____

____

____

____

I have examined the above-named student and completed the preparticipation physical evaluation. The athlete does not present apparent clinical contraindications to practice and participate in the sport(s) as outlined above. A copy of the physical exam is on record in my office and can be made available to the school at the request of the parents. If conditions arise after the athlete has been cleared for participation, the physician may rescind the clearance until the problem is resolved and the potential consequences are completely explained to the athlete (and parents/guardians).

Name of physician (print/type) ______________________ Date __________

Address ______________________ Phone __________

Signature of physician ______________________, MD or DO

EMERGENCY INFORMATION

Allergies ______________________

____

____

____

____

____

Other information ______________________

____

____

____

____

____

____

____

____

____

FIGURE 1.2 > *continued*

Summary

The athletic trainer is in a unique position to detect medical conditions in the athlete and to determine the appropriate course of action. Health care providers must be familiar with the techniques for evaluating these conditions and the signs and symptoms that may indicate them. Assessment of medical conditions in athletes requires a slightly different approach from orthopedic assessment. The chief complaint may be largely symptomatic; the athletic trainer must exhibit good communication skills to elicit full disclosure of pertinent information. The PPE may represent the first disclosure of a medical problem, and therefore the form should be carefully crafted and reviewed to ensure that it covers a broad medical spectrum.

Because ill athletes may be a source of infection for others in the program and community, it is important for the athletic trainer to follow OSHA protocols. A knowledge of the recognized standards to prevent disease transmission and correct application of those standards are critical both in caring for the ill athlete and in maintaining a sanitary workplace.

Athletes may be cared for in a school or university setting, but the mandates for a medical facility still need to be followed, including the maintenance of accurate and private records. Federal law requires that records be safely secured and that the contents remain undisclosed to protect the best interests of the athlete. The last part of this chapter discussed the administration of the PPE. It is up to the athletic trainer to determine, in conjunction with the team physician, the best method for conducting a PPE for the school or institution. The results of the PPE will be used to determine readiness for athletic participation.

 Apply It! The case study for this chapter tests how well you know your medical terminology and abbreviations. Read the scenario and answer the questions at www.HumanKinetics.com/MedicalConditionsInTheAthlete.

2

Medical Examination

At the completion of this chapter the reader should be able to do the following:

- Describe a basic general medical examination, including a comprehensive history and physical examination.

- Differentiate between a focal orthopedic examination and a medical examination of conditions that may affect many organ systems.

- Describe and demonstrate the proper use of evaluation tools and techniques for the assessment of general health.

- Apply the basics of palpation, percussion, and auscultation in a general medical examination.

This chapter focuses on the evaluation techniques and equipment used in a medical examination. It introduces the use of the otoscope, ophthalmoscope, and stethoscope; presents basic techniques in palpation, percussion, and auscultation; and discusses general information about normal vital signs. The chapters that follow present a more detailed explanation of both normal and abnormal examination results for each body system. Later chapters also assume that you have reviewed and understood this chapter and are familiar with the equipment and techniques used in a general medical examination.

Examination of the Patient With a Medical Condition

The examination of the patient with a nonorthopedic condition may present the health care provider with a challenge. Often there is no identifiable onset, and there may be few signs that anything is wrong. Each evaluation begins with a thorough history followed by an overall systemic review and, finally, an examination specific to the condition. The examiner must rely heavily on the patient's history to guide the examination. Evaluating a medical condition requires a systematic approach similar to the history, inspection and observation, palpation, and special tests (HIPS/HOPS) of the typical orthopedic evaluation.

Comprehensive Medical History

A medical health history taken to ascertain the extent of a medical condition or illness is vastly different from an orthopedic history. In an athletic injury, the condition is typically contained within one joint, muscle, or bone, and it usually involves only the musculoskeletal system. On the other hand, a medical condition may involve many body systems, may be difficult to describe, and may not be at all obvious. The clinician needs to understand the potential **comorbid** conditions that may exist with a medical condition. The clinician also must understand how the questions asked when taking a health history for a medical condition differ from those for an orthopedic injury. Typical orthopedic questions include the mechanism of injury; sounds associated with the onset (e.g., snap, crunch, pop); and immediate disability associated with the injury, such as swelling, inability to bear weight, deformity, and radiculopathy. Questions in a medical health history review the entire body and include respiratory, gastrointestinal, and neurological symptoms. Questions about symptoms are critical because symptoms cannot be measured objectively, yet they may offer clues about the patient's condition (Longo et al. 2013). The following are several questions to consider asking when taking a history for a medical condition.

- Describe your symptoms.
- How long have you had these symptoms?
- Do your symptoms interfere with activities of daily living?
- Are you currently taking any medications, vitamins, or supplements?
- Do your symptoms tend to occur at a specific time (e.g., after eating, when exercising, after exposure to an allergen, at night)?
- Do your symptoms come and go, or are they constant?
- Are you sleeping well, according to your normal habits?
- Do you feel more fatigued than usual?
- Have you recently changed your diet, medication, activity level, or personal habits?
- Are you under more stress than usual?
- Are you having normal bowel and bladder function? (This may help to determine whether the condition is gastrointestinal.)
- Is there anything else going on that you would like to discuss?

Other aspects of a medical history include duration of signs and symptoms, onset (e.g., rapid, insidious, gradual), and disability from symptoms. Some medical situations may be life-threatening and may require complex information to make a correct but timely decision. The end result for the examiner is a decision about how to treat the patient and when or to whom to refer. A basic upper respiratory infection or cold may be treated with over-the-counter medications, whereas a long-term infection of the respiratory tract or asthma requires physician intervention and medication.

Usually we begin taking a comprehensive medical history by identifying and recording a patient's age and gender. If ethnicity, marital status, occupation, and religion are important to the diagnosis or treatment, they may be documented as well (Longo et al. 2013). Next, the patient's chief complaint is identified, including the present illness, onset, and setting when symptoms were first apparent. Descriptions of the chief complaint that help the examiner include the locations of discomfort; the quality or quantity of symptoms; their frequency, onset, and duration; and any associated factors that aggravate or alleviate symptoms. Patients should be asked whether they are currently using medications, supplements, vitamins, home remedies, or poultices. Also, the examiner needs to know whether the patient has shared or borrowed teammates' or roommates' prescription medications.

The next sections of a comprehensive history for a patient with a medical condition include past medical history, current health status, and family history. Past history incorporates childhood and adult illnesses as well as accidents and injuries. Keep in mind that adult illnesses also may include psychiatric, obstetrical, or gynecological conditions and surgery. Typically, the patient's current health status covers alcohol, drug, and tobacco use; exercise; diet; and immunizations. The examiner asks questions about any history of allergies and specific reactions to the antigens and ensures that the patient is up-to-date with routine screening tests, such as Pap smears and breast and testicular self-examinations. It may also be appropriate to explore the environmental safety of the home and workplace.

A look into the patient's family history may be quite useful in identifying a susceptibility for a given illness or disease and may prove helpful in the examination and care of the patient. Diabetes, heart disease, hypertension, kidney disease, cardiovascular disorders (e.g., deep vein thrombosis [DVT], stroke), allergies, asthma, mental illness, and addictions are all examples of diseases with a

---

CLINICAL TIPS

Chief Complaints

Descriptions important to evaluation are the following:

- Locations of discomfort
- Quality or quantity of symptoms
- Frequency
- Onset
- Duration
- Any associated factors that aggravate or alleviate the symptoms

CLINICAL TIPS

Family Health History

Conditions and diseases that have a genetic tendency include the following:

- Diabetes
- Heart disease
- Hypertension
- Kidney disease
- Cardiovascular disorders (deep vein thrombosis [DVT], myocardial infarction, stroke)
- Allergies
- Asthma
- Mental illness
- Addictions

genetic tendency. The age, current health, cause of death, and age at death of immediate family members are also important in a family health history. Some physicians add another category, personal and social history, to help them understand their patients better. This category covers a patient's education, occupation, significant others, home life, daily activities, hobbies, and important beliefs. Although this information is not critical to diagnosing specific conditions, some physicians believe it profoundly affects their patients' overall health and attitudes toward wellness (Ball et al. 2014).

Review of Body Systems

The review of body systems is the health care provider's primary focus in the evaluation of medical conditions. Indeed, most health care professionals use the comprehensive medical history and review of body systems to assess medical issues. Traditionally, all systems are reviewed, unlike an orthopedic assessment, which focuses on the anatomical area or system believed to be affected. A medical review differs from an orthopedic evaluation in that the examiner may stop after determining there is crepitus rather than continuing to look for ligamentous injury. For example, in an orthopedic injury, if the patient has a clearly displaced fractured femur, the examiner does not continue the initial evaluation to determine whether the anterior cruciate ligament (ACL) is intact.

The goal of the review of body systems during an examination for a general medical condition is to enable the clinician to gather enough information to make an intelligent decision about patient referral and, if necessary, referral to a specific type of practitioner.

The review of systems always begins with a general assessment of the patient's condition: weight and associated changes, fatigue, fever, and any reported sleep disturbances. Then the review continues system by system, starting with the skin and descending from head to toe. When assessing the skin, the examiner looks for obvious rashes, sores, dryness, color change, lumps, or swelling and asks the patient about itching or skin dryness.

A good mnemonic to help you remember the order of the first part of the review of systems is HEENT, which stands for head, eyes, ears, nose, and throat. Beginning with signs and symptoms associated with the head, the examiner asks about the following: headaches, seizures, syncope, tremors, paralysis, or history of a head injury. Essential questions to ask about the eyes concern visual acuity, the need to wear corrective lenses, a surgical history that may include procedures that correct vision, date and results of last eye examination, and any history of redness, tearing, diplopia, floaters, pain, dryness, or disease of the eye.

Questions linked to the ears relate to symptoms of tinnitus, vertigo, earaches, and signs of ear dysfunction, such as discharge. Patients with nasal problems or conditions of the accompanying sinuses can present with discharge, sinus pain, itching, sneezing, or stuffiness, whereas mouth and throat problems are manifested by hoarseness, sores, caries, halitosis, or bleeding gums. Pain or stiffness in the neck can indicate an infectious disease, and enlarged glands are palpable signs of a response to changes in the body. Questions about breast discomfort, lumps, or nipple discharge may be relevant if the examiner is given information that points to pathology of the breast tissue. These questions may be pertinent to both genders.

The review of systems continues with the respiratory, cardiovascular, and gastrointestinal systems and follows the same **cephalocaudal** order. Signs associated with respiratory problems include the presence of excessive sputum, altered respiratory sounds, and hemoptysis. The cardiovascular system encompasses the heart and blood vessels, including blood pressure. Symptoms of cardiovascular anomalies include murmurs, dyspnea, chest pain, vasovagal responses, hypertension, and syncope. Gastrointestinal problems may manifest with symptoms such as heartburn, nausea, constipation, and food intolerance. Signs include vomiting; change in frequency, consistency, and/or color of stools; rectal bleeding; diarrhea; gas; and jaundice (Longo et al. 2013).

Next in this descending order of specific systems come the urinary and gynecological systems. Incontinence, pain, discolored urine, or any change in frequency of urination may indicate genitourinary system pathology. A male patient who complains of penile sores, discharge, or hesitancy in voiding should be referred to a physician.

Gynecological disorders include delayed onset of menses, **oligomenorrhea**, **dysmenorrhea**, **polymenorrhea**, severe cramping, late menstrual period, abnormal pain, discharge, and vaginal sores. The examiner questions the patient about these symptoms if gynecological issues are raised when discussing her current health history.

After the cephalocaudal systems review, the evaluation goes on to other prevalent body systems: peripheral vascular, musculoskeletal, neurological, hematological, endocrine, and psychiatric. Important areas to explore include complaints of loss of sensation in the extremities, pitting edema, soreness and swelling in multiple joints, and abnormal fatigue (Ball et al. 2014). Specific questions about these systems are discussed later in the appropriate chapters. After the review of all systems, the examiner begins a physical examination of the patient.

Physical Examination

Again, the examiner follows the universally accepted cephalocaudal sequence for the physical examination (see the sidebar "Sequence of Symptom Review and Physical Examination"). The general survey includes observation of the patient's apparent state of health, level of consciousness, signs of distress, height and weight, skin color, obvious lesions, and hygiene (Jarvis 2012). These are noted as the patient enters the examination area. The practitioner continues the physical assessment in the same order as the previously described review of systems, beginning with the vital signs and skin and advancing from the head down the body. The proper evaluation tools should be ready to expedite the examination.

Vital Signs

Assessment of all vital signs includes height and weight, blood pressure, heart and respiratory rate and rhythm, and body temperature.

Height and Weight

Recording a patient's height and weight is essential because it provides a baseline for future reference. Height is often critical to athletes but is typically of only mild interest to the health care practitioner. Weight is more critical because a drastic change in weight, whether gain or loss, can indicate a health problem and needs to be followed up in a timely fashion.

Height is typically measured with a stadiometer or, particularly with extremely tall patients, a tape measure fastened to the wall. The patient removes shoes and stands with the back to the stadiometer or wall, placing all weight on the heels. When using a stadiometer, the clinician stands to the side of the patient and raises the stadiometer to the patient's height. The horizontal arm rests at the crown of the patient's head. The height measurement is read on the instrument's vertical scale (figure 2.1). If not using a stadiometer, the athletic trainer

must accurately mark increments on the wall or fasten a tape measure to the wall. The athletic trainer stands to the side of the patient (on a stool if necessary) and uses a flat surface on a sagittal plane along the crown of the patient's head to evenly mark the height measurement on the wall. Height may be recorded as either centimeters or inches and should be indicated as such in the medical record (1 in. equals 2.54 cm).

Normal body weight is measured without shoes or excessive clothing. Weight is a confidential measurement, so the health care practitioner needs to ensure privacy for the patient during weighing when possible. Weight is typically recorded in medical records in kilograms but may also be recorded in pounds (1 kg equals 2.2 lb). During preseason or excessively warm days, take weight measurements several times each day (preexercise and postexercise) to monitor proper hydration levels and to prevent heat-related illnesses (Binkley et al. 2002). Standardization of measurements can be improved by following the same procedures each time height and weight are measured—for example, measuring both height and weight in the morning and having patients wear a standard attire of gym shorts and T-shirt. More accurate

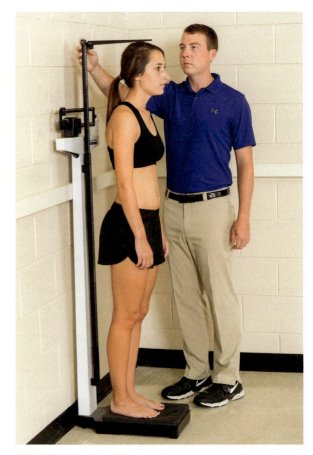

FIGURE 2.1 An athletic trainer measures the patient's height with a stadiometer.

Sequence of Symptom Review and Physical Examination

General
- Fatigue and energy
- Desired weight
- Fever

Diet
- Appetite
- Supplements
- Restrictions

Skin, Hair, Nails
- Appearance
- Color

Head and Neck
- Supple neck
- Headache
- LOC
- Dizziness

Eyes
- Visual acuity
- Corrective lenses
- Visual disturbances

Ears
- Vertigo
- Tinnitus
- Hearing acuity
- Discharge

Nose
- Functional
- Congestions
- History of bleeding

Throat and Mouth
- Hoarseness
- Sore throat
- Dental issues
- Chewing tobacco

Gastrointestinal
- Heartburn
- Vomiting
- Diarrhea
- Constipation

Lymphatic System
- Swelling
- Pitting edema
- Tenderness

Endocrine
- Heat or cold intolerance
- Weight or energy change

Female
- FMP/LMP
- Regularity
- Symptoms

Male
- Testicular pain or swelling

Breasts
- Swelling
- Lumps
- Pain

Chest and Lungs
- SOB
- Dyspnea
- Night sweats
- Cough
- Sputum

Cardiovascular
- Chest pain
- Exercise history
- Exertional SOB

Hematology
- Bruising history

Genitourinary
- Urine frequency, volume, color
- Dysuria

Musculoskeletal
- Joint or muscle pain or swelling
- Neurological symptoms

Mental Status
- Eating, sleeping, social habits
- Mood
- Concentration

FMP = first menstrual period; LMP = last menstrual period; LOC = level of consciousness; SOB = shortness of breath.

---

assessments of body composition exclusive of height and weight charts include hydrostatic weighing, skinfold calipers, bioimpedance, and body mass index (BMI).

Blood Pressure

A stethoscope and sphygmomanometer of the correct size will measure blood pressure properly. This is especially important for the athletic trainer, who often must evaluate extremely muscular or large athletes for whom a regular-size blood pressure cuff is too small. Using a cuff that is too small results in a reading that is incorrect,

indicating abnormally high blood pressure. Normal resting blood pressure is measured after the patient has been resting quietly for a period of time; it is never measured immediately after any exertion, such as practice or hurrying to an appointment (Ball et al. 2014; Bickley 2012).

The patient is positioned in a quiet area with the selected arm free of clothing and positioned so that the brachial artery is roughly at heart level, which can be done by having the patient rest the arm on a table next to the chair. The sphygmomanometer is placed around the upper arm with the lower edge of the cuff about 2.5

Use of Blood Pressure Cuff

- Blood pressure cuffs come in various sizes.
- A cuff that is too small gives an abnormally high blood pressure reading.

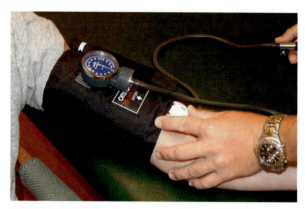

FIGURE 2.2   The sphygmomanometer is used to assess blood pressure.
© Micki Cuppett

cm above the antecubital crease (figure 2.2). The cuff is snugly secured around the arm with the Velcro fasteners, and the aneroid dial is positioned with its face toward the examiner. The diaphragm of the stethoscope is placed lightly over the brachial artery, touching the skin.

The cuff is inflated first to greater than 200 mmHg and then gradually deflated at a rate of 2 to 3 mmHg/s. While deflating the cuff, the examiner listens for two consecutive beats, which will indicate the systolic pressure, and notes the numerical value on the aneroid dial when this occurs. The examiner continues to deflate the blood pressure cuff slowly until the sound becomes muffled and finally disappears. The level at which the sound disappears is the diastolic pressure; this is often referred to as the fifth **Korotkoff sound** (the last of a series of sounds produced by distention of an artery by the cuff). Systolic pressure is related to contraction of the ventricles of the heart, whereas diastolic pressure represents the relaxation of the ventricles. The effect of the cuff on arterial blood flow is related to the auscultatory findings. Table 2.1 lists the phase and quality of each sound. Chapter 8 gives more details on cardiac output and blood pressure, and table 2.2 shows normal and abnormal blood pressure readings for adults.

TABLE 2.1   Understanding Korotkoff Sounds When Assessing Blood Pressure

Phase	Quality	Description	Rationale
Cuff inflated to occlude brachial artery	No sound		Brachial artery is compressed by exceeding the heart's systolic pressure with the cuff inflation, and therefore no blood is flowing under the stethoscope.
I	Tapping	Tapping sound, starting soft and increasing in intensity	As the pressure lessens, an audible sound is created as the blood flows into the brachial artery at a high velocity.
Auscultatory gap (abnormal sound)	No sound	Silence for up to 30–40 mmHg	In a person with hypertension, the sounds may temporarily disappear toward the end of phase I and then reappear in phase II. If undetected, results in falsely low systolic reading or falsely high diastolic reading.
II	Swooshing	Softer murmur follows tapping	Because the artery is still partially occluded, the turbulent blood flow is audible as a swooshing sound.
III	Knocking	Crisp, high-pitched sounds	Sound is created with the less turbulent flow of blood through the artery. Artery closes momentarily during the latter part of diastole.
IV	Abrupt muffling	Sound mutes to a low-pitched, cushioned murmur; blowing quality	Once the artery is no longer occluded, the blood flow changes to a low-pitched murmur.
V	Silence		The disappearance of the last audible sound is called the fifth Korotkoff sound and defines diastolic blood pressure. Silence occurs when blood flow returns to normal velocity.

TABLE 2.2 **Understanding Blood Pressure Readings**

Blood pressure	Systolic (mmHg)	Diastolic (mmHg)
Normal	<120	<80
Prehypertension	120–139	80–89
High blood pressure (hypertension)		
Stage 1 (hypertension)	140–159	90–99
Stage 2 (hypertension)	≥160	≥100
Hypertensive crisis	>180	>110

A physician should evaluate low or high readings.

Modified from American Heart Association, 2016, *What is the AHA recommendation for health blood pressure?* Available: www.heart.org/HEARTORG/Conditions/HighBloodPressure/AboutHighBloodPressure/Understanding-Blood-Pressure-Readings_UCM_301764_Article.jsp#.Vz3cZWPHG9U.

Pulse Rate and Rhythm

The examiner determines the heart rate by feeling the radial pulse with the pads of the index and middle fingers (figure 2.3). Once the pulse is found, the number of beats in 15 s is counted and then multiplied by 4 to estimate the heart rate (a normal, resting heart rate is 60 to 72 beats/min). The pulse is described by its rate, rhythm, and force.

Rate
  Bradycardia: <60 beats/min
  Tachycardia: >100 beats/min

Rhythm
  Sinus arrhythmia: Heart rate speeds up at peak of inspiration and slows to normal with expiration

Force
  4+   Bounding
  3+   Increased
  2+   Normal
  1+   Weak, thready
  Absent

The examiner notes any irregular rhythms and further evaluates by auscultating with the stethoscope at the cardiac apex (Rakel and Rakel 2011), keeping in mind that it is normal for athletes to have bradycardia, that is, a pulse rate of 60 beats/min or less. The pulse is also easily palpable at the carotid artery, the posterior tibial artery, and other pulse points (figure 2.4). Pulse characteristics at the distal extremities give the examiner information about the status of blood flow to those extremities.

Respiratory Rate and Rhythm

Evaluation of respiration includes the rate, effort, and depth of inspiration as well as the ratio of the depth of inspiration to expiration. The rate is quantified by counting the number of respirations in 1 min. The normal respiration rate for an adult is 12 to 20 breaths/min (Rakel and Rakel 2011). When assessing the rate, the examiner evaluates the patient's effort by watching for symmetry and the use of accessory muscles (sternocleidomastoid, trapezius, intercostals) to assist in breathing.

Temperature

Assessment of temperature can be omitted if there is no reason to suspect fever or heat-related illness. It may be

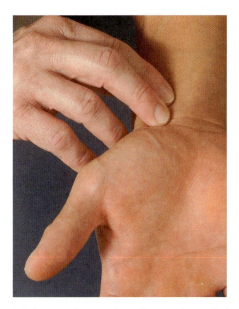

FIGURE 2.3 A pulse can be taken at the radial artery in the wrist.

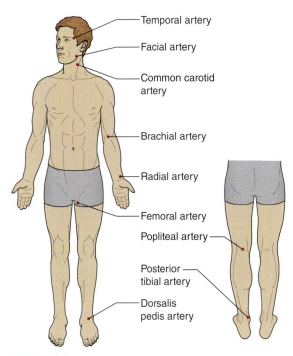

FIGURE 2.4 Common pulse points on the body surface where arterial pulses can be assessed.

wise, however, to record the temperature of any patient presenting with a nonorthopedic complaint because temperature sometimes provides a defining clue to the severity of the condition. Normal temperature fluctuates considerably from the commonly reported oral temperature of 37 °C (98.6 °F) (Ferri 2016); it may be as low as 35.8 °C (96.4 °F) in the early morning hours and as high as 37.3 °C (99.1 °F) in the evening. Rectal temperatures are higher than oral temperatures by 0.4 °C to 0.5 °C, but this difference is also quite variable. In addition, athletes who have just finished a workout, recently experienced a heat modality (e.g., warm whirlpool or Hydrocollator), or drunk a hot beverage can present with a slightly elevated temperature.

It is important to maintain thermometer sanitation. Glass thermometers, although now used less often because of environmental concerns about mercury (Rakel and Rakel 2011), must be sanitized with either alcohol swabs or another approved cleaning medium. Electronic thermometers must be covered by single-use plastic covers to ensure sanitation, and tympanic thermometers likewise must have single-use protective covers.

Oral temperature can be measured with either liquid-filled (mercury or alcohol) glass or electronic thermometers. Care must be taken with the glass thermometer to shake down the mercury to at least 35 °C (96 °F) before inserting it under the tongue; it needs to be left in place for 3 to 5 min for accurate measurement. For those who wish to keep using liquid-filled thermometers, the alcohol-filled type is the standard replacement for the toxic mercury-filled type.

There are several types of electronic thermometers that can be used for rectal, oral, or axillary temperature measurement (figure 2.5), and different technologies

are used in each. Digital heat sensors use electronic heat sensors to detect body temperature, and they may be used in the mouth, armpit, or rectum. A plastic probe cover is always used on electronic heat sensor thermometers. The examiner turns the unit on and places it under the patient's tongue; it generally takes only 10 s to beep, indicating that an accurate reading is available.

The examiner measures rectal temperature, if the patient is unconscious or suspected of having a heat-related illness, to provide a better indicator of core temperature. The patient is placed on the side with the hip flexed. A probe cover is used with an electronic rectal thermometer. The examiner lubricates the tip of the thermometer with petroleum jelly or K-Y jelly before inserting it into the anal canal.

Infrared wave sensors are most commonly used in tympanic thermometers. Tympanic thermometers are increasingly common, are safe, and measure temperature very quickly. However, their reliability has been questioned, especially in the athletic setting or in the assessment of heat-related illness. In suspected heat-related conditions, rectal temperature determination is the

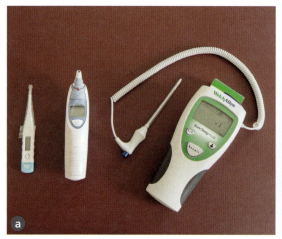 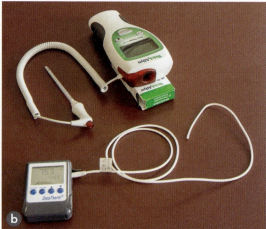

FIGURE 2.5   *(a)* Oral, tympanic, and digital thermometers. Note the blue coloring on the digital oral thermometer. *(b)* Both of these digital thermometers measure rectal (core) temperature. The WelchAllyn unit is interchangeable with the blue oral thermometer. The DataTherm unit is designed to have the sensor remain in the anus while cooling measures are administered to the body.

only method currently shown to reliably measure core temperature. A rectal probe with a remote display will allow the monitoring of core body temperature even while the patient is being cooled in an ice bath (Armstrong et al. 2007; Binkley et al. 2002; Casa 2011; Casa, Guskiewicz, and Anderson 2012; Spring 2015).

To use a tympanic thermometer, the examiner places the covered probe of the thermometer so that the beam has a direct route to the tympanic membrane (figure 2.6). The auditory canal needs to be free of excessive cerumen. Within 2 to 3 s the tympanic temperature will register on the thermometer. Temperatures taken with the tympanic thermometer are generally 0.8 °C (1.4 °F) higher than normal oral temperatures (Ball et al. 2014; Rakel and Rakel 2011). A newer thermometer uses infrared waves to measure the temperature of the temporal artery in the forehead. Its efficacy is still being determined.

Another method sometimes used to measure temperature is the axillary method, in which a thermometer is placed in the axilla for 10 min. This method is most often used with infants, but with tympanic thermometers readily available, it is not used as often as in the past. This method is not as accurate as either oral or rectal temperatures and is often as much as 0.5 °C (32.9 °F) lower than an oral temperature taken simultaneously (Longo et al. 2013).

Evaluation Tools

In addition to the examiner's hands that might be used for palpation, there are several tools that the examiner may use during an examination. In this section we will describe each tool and its proper use. Some of the tools require more practice than others.

Stethoscope

A good-quality acoustic stethoscope is sufficient for most examinations by athletic trainers. More sophisticated stethoscopes (magnetic, electronic, stereophonic, or Doppler) are used to auscultate less obvious sounds. An acoustic stethoscope contains a diaphragm and bell that are heavy enough to lay firmly on the body surface and thick, heavy tubing to conduct the sound (Ball et al. 2014). Earpieces fit snugly and comfortably (figure 2.7).

To correctly use the stethoscope, the examiner holds the end piece between the fingers, pressing the diaphragm (used for high-pitched sounds) firmly against the bare skin. When using the bell (for low-pitched sounds), the examiner holds it lightly on the skin to ensure that the entire bell is in contact with the skin. The tubing should not rub against itself or any other surface because extraneous noises will occur. Similarly, the environment must be quiet and free of noises. The examiner listens not only for the presence or absence of sound but also for intensity, pitch, duration, and quality (Ball et al. 2014).

Ophthalmoscope

The ophthalmoscope is used to view the internal structures of the eye (figure 2.8). The head of the instrument contains a light source, which allows the examiner to

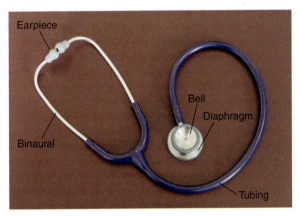

FIGURE 2.7 The parts of an acoustic stethoscope.

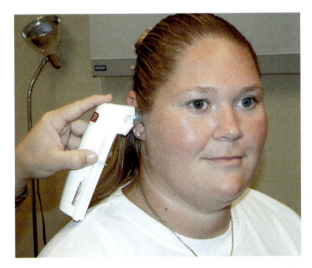

FIGURE 2.6 Tympanic thermometers are increasingly common, are safe, and measure temperature very quickly, but they may not be as reliable as electronic models for assessing heat-related illnesses.
© Micki Cuppett

CLINICAL TIPS
Using a Stethoscope
- The bell is used to hear low-pitched sounds.
- The diaphragm is used to hear high-pitched sounds.

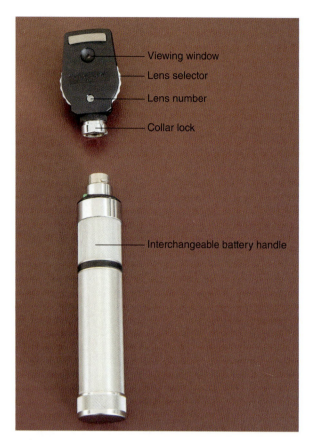

FIGURE 2.8 The parts of an ophthalmoscope.

visualize the inner eye through a series of lenses and apertures to allow for near or far focusing. The most commonly used aperture projects a large, round beam.

Other apertures include the small aperture; the slit-lamp aperture to examine the anterior eye; the red-free filter aperture, which shines a green beam to check the optic disk; and the grid aperture used to estimate the size of fundal lesions (Ball et al. 2014).

The diopter (magnification power of the lens) of the ophthalmoscope may be changed by turning the lens selector or disk to the corresponding magnification (Ball et al. 2014). The black numbers indicate positive magnification power, and the red numbers show the negative. Turning the wheel clockwise selects positive lenses, and rotating it counterclockwise selects negative lenses. Lens numbers range from ±20 to ±140 magnification power. The range of plus and minus lenses can compensate for **myopia** or **hyperopia** in both the examiner and the patient (Ball et al. 2014).

The heads of both the ophthalmoscope and the otoscope (used to view the ears and nose) typically share a common handle containing a rechargeable battery. The heads are interchangeable and can easily be converted from one instrument to the other. To change from an otoscope head to an ophthalmoscope head, the examiner

pushes down on the head that is currently on the handle while turning it to unlock the attachment, inserts the other head, and fastens it to the handle in the same manner.

Both instruments are turned in the same way, namely, by pushing the on/off switch while turning the black rheostat clockwise to the desired intensity of light.

Otoscope

The examiner visualizes the external auditory canal and tympanic membrane with an otoscope (figure 2.9). As described previously, the otoscope usually shares its base and handle with the ophthalmoscope. The otoscope consists of a lamp to direct the light for illumination and disposable speculums, which protect it from contamination. The disposable speculums come in various sizes, and each is attached to the otoscope by placing it and then twisting clockwise approximately one-half turn to secure it on the instrument. The instrument also has a viewing window that magnifies the area being visualized. Some otoscopes also contain a pneumatic attachment used to test the integrity of the tympanic membrane. In addition, the instrument can be used as a nasal speculum.

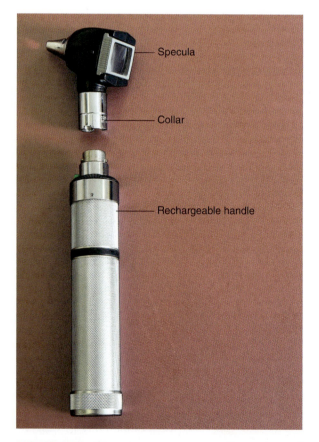

FIGURE 2.9 The otoscope uses various sizes of specula and may have a pneumatic attachment. The chargeable base often enables the otoscope to be interchangeable with the ophthalmoscope.

Tuning Fork

A tuning fork (figure 2.10) is used as a diagnostic tool for many different conditions. The most common uses are to check vibratory sensation or auditory sensitivity. A tuning fork with a frequency of 500 to 1000 Hz mimics the range of normal speech and is used for auditory evaluation (Jarvis 2012). The examiner squeezes the fork or taps the prongs against the opposite hand to activate it while holding the tuning fork at its base.

Snellen Chart

The Snellen chart is a quick and easy-to-use screening tool for distance vision and is used most often during preparticipation examinations to screen a patient's vision. The chart contains graduated sizes of letters with standardized acuity numbers at the end of each line (figure 2.11).

The patient is asked to read the lines of the chart while standing 20 ft away and covering one eye. The number corresponding to the row of the smallest letters the patient can read measures visual acuity. Although the patient is allowed to err in calling out a particular number or letter, two wrong answers on a line indicate inability to correctly read at that distance. Visual acuity is recorded as a fraction, with the numerator of 20 indicating the distance away from the chart and the denominator being the distance at which a person with normal vision should be able to read the lettering (Potter and Perry 2011; Zimmerman, Lust, and Bullimore 2011). A measurement of 20/20 is considered normal vision, with denominators greater than 20 indicating poorer vision. A person with a measurement of 20/200 is considered legally blind. One must remember that this is a screening tool for far visual acuity only and does not measure near vision or dynamic visual acuity. Referral to an optometrist or ophthalmologist for a complete visual assessment may be warranted. A patient who normally wears corrective lenses is screened without those corrective lenses, and the results of the examination are noted as being without corrective lenses.

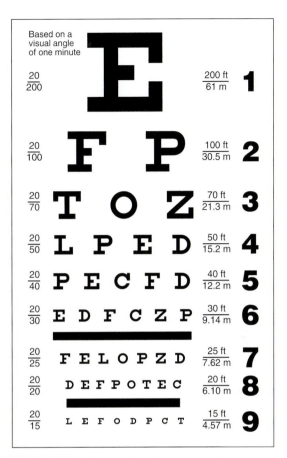

FIGURE 2.11 The Snellen chart is used to measure visual acuity.

Near vision is assessed with the Rosenbaum or Jaeger chart or with a newspaper (Bickley 2012).

Diagnostic Tests

Many common diagnostic tests are used to confirm specific conditions. The health care provider needs to be familiar with these tests, what they are used for, and what the results indicate. Common imaging and diagnostic testing is discussed in detail in chapter 3.

Neurological Testing

Neurological tests provide information about sensory, motor, and deep tendon reflexes, which may indicate pathology associated with the central nervous system or peripheral nerve trauma. The examiner performs neurological testing whenever a patient complains of paresthesia, heightened sensations, or muscular weakness.

A dermatome is a specific area of skin innervated by a dorsal or sensory nerve root. These areas tend to make a circular pattern over the body and are associated with very specific nerve roots (figure 2.12). Myotomes are single muscles or groups of muscles innervated by a

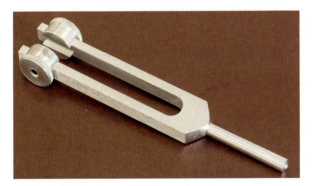

FIGURE 2.10 Tuning forks are used to assess vibratory sensations and to screen for auditory perception.

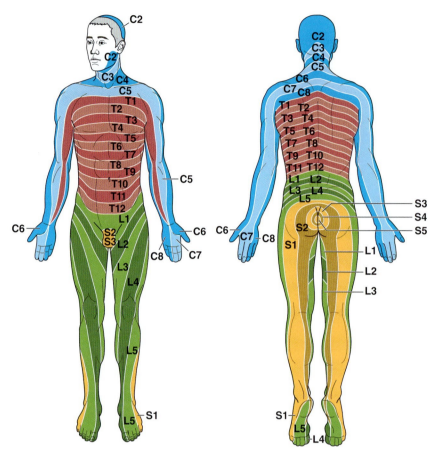

FIGURE 2.12 Dermatomes are areas of the skin supplied by a single nerve or nerve root. Shown here is the distribution of dermatomes throughout the body.

single ventral or motor nerve (Rakel and Rakel 2011). A detailed description of dermatome and myotome evaluation is found in chapter 11.

A deep tendon reflex (DTR) is an involuntary motor reaction to a stimulus. This reflex depends on several conditions, beginning with the hammer stimulus. The dorsal fibers of sensory nerves transmit impulses from the hammer tap on the stretched tendon to sensory receptors in the muscle and along to the spinal cord. In the gray matter of the spinal cord, a flex reaction can occur if the dorsal fibers synapse with the ventral or motor fibers, which in turn travel back to stimulate the muscle to contract (figure 2.13).

This reflex will not occur if the patient's synapses are not functioning correctly or if there is damage to or disease involving either dorsal or ventral nerve fibers. The instruments used to test these pathological conditions are called reflex and neurological hammers. When doing a neurological assessment, test bilaterally to note any differences between sides.

Reflex and Neurological Hammers

The reflex hammer is commonly used to test DTRs. The examiner holds it loosely between the thumb and index finger (figure 2.14a). The wrist is snapped rapidly downward when striking the tendon to elicit the best reflex response. Common locations for DTRs are the insertion of the biceps brachii, distal triceps tendon, distal brachioradialis tendon, patellar tendon, and Achilles tendon. The ulnar aspect of the hand or the fingertips can provide the same effect and may be used in place of the hammer when necessary. DTRs have a common rating scale for responses (table 2.3). When using the reflex hammer, the examiner places the patient in a relaxed position (sitting is best) and provides slight tension on the tendon to be tested. The tendon should be palpated first to make certain you strike it correctly rather than striking the muscle.

A neurological hammer is a reflex hammer that also includes a brush and a sharp implement to use when eliciting the sensations a patient can feel, thereby assessing the integrity of dermatomes (figure 2.14b). Patients close their eyes during the test. This ensures a nondiscriminatory assessment because the patients cannot witness the application of the tool. The pointed end of the tool is used to lightly depress the skin over a given dermatome, and the patient is asked if he or she perceives any sensation; the same dermatome on the contralateral side is then tested. Care must be taken when using the sharp imple-

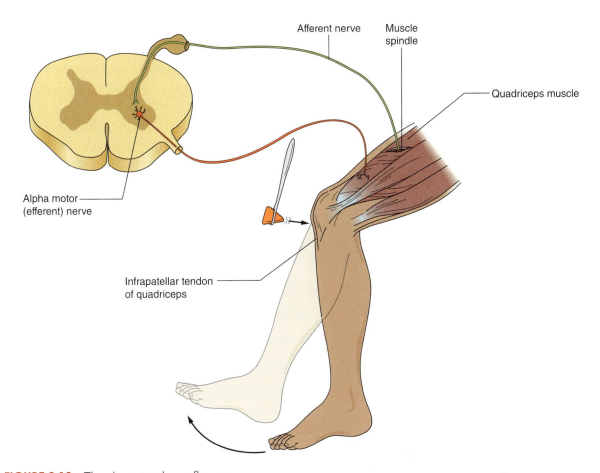

Afferent nerve   Muscle spindle

Quadriceps muscle

Alpha motor (efferent) nerve

Infrapatellar tendon of quadriceps

FIGURE 2.13   The deep tendon reflex arc.

ment to avoid puncturing the skin. Likewise, the brush is used to lightly brush a specific area and then test for the same sensation on the opposite limb. Other instruments that can provide a sharp, dull, and brushing effect can be used to conduct these sensory tests.

When assessing myotomes, the examiner asks the patient to actively move and then resist a given muscle group. The examiner then compares bilaterally. Tests of dermatomes and myotomes are common in orthopedic assessment and are used in many neurological assessments as well.

Cranial Nerve Assessment

Cranial nerve assessment is another valuable area of testing. When a patient has a suspected head injury, evaluation of these nerves is critical. Familiarity with their source and function is also important in evaluating many other neurological conditions. Table 2.4 provides an overview of these critical nerves, and chapter 11 covers the neurological system in depth.

Palpation

Palpation involves the use of the hands and fingers to gain information about a patient's condition through the sense of touch. The athletic trainer typically is proficient in palpation of orthopedic conditions and can gain valuable information about general medical conditions through

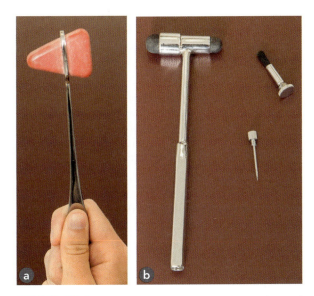

FIGURE 2.14   (a) Reflex hammer. (b) Neurological hammer.

TABLE 2.3   **Deep Tendon Reflex Grades**

Grade	Interpretation	Indication
0	Absent reflex	Complete loss of neuromuscular integrity (injury to nerve root or peripheral nerve)
+1	Diminished reflex	Reduced neurological function (incomplete injury to a nerve route or peripheral nerve)
+2	Normal reflex	Normal neurological integrity and function
+3	Exaggerated reflex	Upper motor neuron lesion (brain or spinal cord injury); hypersensitivity may also occur following brief, intense bouts of activity
+4	Clonus	Upper motor neuron lesion

Reprinted, by permission, from S. Shultz, P. Houglum, and D. Perrin, 2016, *Examination of musculoskeletal injuries*, 4th ed. (Champaign, IL: Human Kinetics), 118.

TABLE 2.4   **Cranial Nerve Function**

Source	Nerve	Sense	System
CNI	Olfactory nerve	Smell	Sensory
CNII	Optic nerve	Vision	Sensory
CNIII	Oculomotor nerve	Extraocular muscle movement Pupillary light reflex	Motor
CNIV	Trochlear nerve	Extraocular (upward) muscle movement	Motor
CNV	Trigeminal nerve	Muscles of mastication	Sensory/motor
CNVI	Abducens nerve	Extraocular (lateral) muscle movement	Motor
CNVII	Facial nerve	Muscles of facial expression Taste Tears and saliva	Sensory/motor
CNVIII	Vestibulocochlear nerve	Balance Hearing	Sensory
CNIX	Glossopharyngeal nerve	Taste sensation of the mouth	Sensory/motor
CNX	Vagus nerve	Swallowing Gag reflex	Motor Sensory
CNXI	Spinal accessory nerve	Sternocleidomastoid, trapezius movement	Motor
CNXII	Hypoglossal nerve	Tongue movement	Motor

the use of systematic palpation. The examiner uses the fingertips for palpation during the medical examination to feel for texture and quality of the skin as well as temperature, underlying masses, rigidity, fluid, or crepitus. The ulnar surface of the hand should be used to palpate vibrations during inspiration or expiration because it is more sensitive, whereas the dorsal surface of the hand is best for estimating temperature.

Palpation may be done with one or both hands. The examiner uses palpation with or after visual inspection, except when assessing the abdomen, where palpation is completed after auscultation. Light palpation is performed at a depth of approximately 1 cm and is useful for feeling skin and underlying tissue. Light palpation is always done before deep palpation. It helps the examiner to gain the patient's trust, identify areas of tenderness, and establish a systematic method of palpation from superficial to deep tissues. Deep palpation may approach 4 cm and must be done carefully because it may elicit tenderness or disrupt underlying tissue (figure 2.15). The patient should be relaxed during palpation because muscle guarding, especially of the abdominal region, will prevent the clinician from obtaining significant information from the examination. The patient is draped with consideration given to privacy and modesty, and only the area being palpated is exposed.

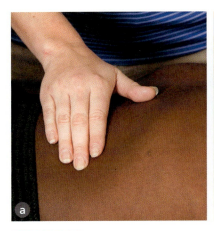
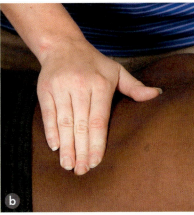
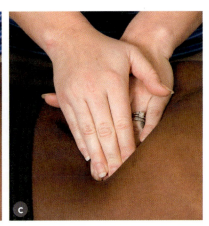

FIGURE 2.15   *(a)* Light palpation. *(b)* Deep palpation. *(c)* Bimanual palpation.

Percussion

Percussion is the process of assessing sounds transmitted through the organs and cavities of the body and is generated by tapping. It involves striking one object (fingers or hand) against another to produce vibrations and subsequent sound waves. The techniques of percussion are the same regardless of the structure being percussed and include either direct or indirect percussion.

Direct percussion involves lightly striking the chest or abdominal wall with the ulnar aspect of the fist. Indirect percussion involves the finger of one hand acting as the hammer, striking the finger of the other hand that is resting on the body part being percussed (figure 2.16). The striking action creates a vibration or resonance that with training and practice can be identified and quantified.

Practice is necessary to become proficient with percussion technique. The downward snap of the striking finger originates from the wrist and not the forearm or shoulder.

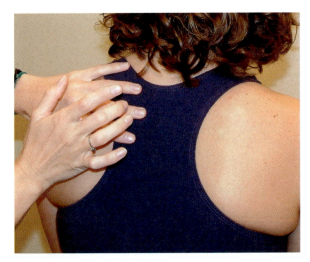

FIGURE 2.16   Indirect percussion.
© Micki Cuppett

The tap is sharp and rapid with the tip of the finger, not the pad. The ulnar surface of the fist may also be used for percussion and is generally used to elicit tenderness over solid organs, such as the liver or kidneys.

Percussion-generated sounds may be recognized on the basis of various characteristics, including intensity, pitch, and location. The general percussion tone over air is loud, over fluid it is less loud, and over solid areas it is soft (Ball et al. 2014; Perry, Potter, and Ostendorf 2014). It is often difficult to quantify percussion tones, especially for the novice examiner. The examiner should practice identifying tones from various parts of the body to learn how to quantify them, specifically noting the change from one tone to another when moving from percussing a known air-filled body part, such as the lungs, to the abdomen or a muscle.

Auscultation

Auscultation is the skilled listening by a trained ear for sounds produced by the body. Most body sounds, including the heart, lung, and bowel, are not audible without the use of a stethoscope. Auscultation takes practice so that the sounds can be identified and isolated from each other.

Certain basic principles apply to auscultation regardless of the system being examined:

- Perform auscultation after history, observation, and palpation in order to gather as much information as possible from other sources first.

- Perform auscultation in a quiet environment.

- Point the earpieces of the stethoscope toward the face.

- Make sure the earpieces of the stethoscope fit comfortably, following the angles of the ear canal.

- Listen for the presence or absence of sounds as well as their frequency, loudness, quality, and duration.

As mentioned previously, auscultation of the abdomen is done before palpation. The examiner uses the part of the stethoscope that best relays the pitch of the sound sought. The diaphragm is used for high-pitched sounds, such as bowel, lung, and normal heart sounds, whereas the bell is used for low-pitched sounds (Rakel and Rakel 2011). Abnormal heart and vascular sounds have a lower pitch and may be heard better with the bell (Potter and Perry 2011). Table 2.5 describes common characteristics of sounds heard during auscultation. Specific placement of the stethoscope for auscultation of lung, heart, and bowel sounds is discussed in chapters covering respiratory, cardiac, and gastrointestinal disorders.

TABLE 2.5   **Characteristics of Sound**

Characteristic	Description
Pitch	Number of sound wave cycles generated per second by a vibrating object. The higher the frequency, the higher the pitch of a sound and vice versa.
Loudness	Amplitude of a sound wave. Auscultated sounds are described as loud or *soft*.
Quality	Sounds of similar frequency and loudness from different sources. Terms such as *gurgling* describe quality of sound.
Duration	Length of time from when the sound is first heard to when the sound stops. Duration of sound is *short*, *medium*, or *long*.

Summary

The health care provider must be comfortable with general examination techniques in order to differentiate among the many disorders discussed in this text and to provide the best possible care for patients. The athletic trainer is often the first person the athlete approaches with a medical complaint and often serves as the "gatekeeper" to the medical community for the athlete. You should appreciate the differences between a focal orthopedic examination and the examination of a medical condition that may affect multiple organ systems. Many techniques discussed in this chapter, such as palpation, percussion, and auscultation, are important skills for the health professional to master but take considerable practice. Practice these techniques on a variety of people of varying ages and health statuses to appreciate the range of normal and abnormal findings.

 Apply It!   The case study for this chapter tests your knowledge related to completing a medical examination. Read the scenario and answer the questions at www.HumanKinetics.com/MedicalConditionsInTheAthlete.

Diagnostic Imaging and Testing

3

OBJECTIVES

At the completion of this chapter the reader should be able to do the following:

- Choose the appropriate diagnostic imaging and laboratory tests for a given medical condition.

- Explain test preparation and procedures to patients undergoing diagnostic evaluation.

- Describe the risks and side effects of specific procedures.

- Explain which medical conditions can be diagnosed by diagnostic imaging or laboratory testing.

- Apply appropriate pre-MRI testing health questions to patients.

- State normal values for urine and blood.

- Identify the radiation levels of assorted diagnostic tests.

- Describe the TNM cancer staging system.

Diagnostic imaging refers to special impressions usually produced by radiologists and radiology technicians to determine specific medical conditions. This type of diagnostics produces an image of internal structures to distinguish normal from abnormal anatomy and to view structures within the body that cannot be seen by the naked eye. Not all diagnostic imaging involves radiation; for example, an ultrasound uses sound waves and magnet resonance imaging uses magnets to create images of the internal structures. The specific type of imaging is typically ordered by a physician, and it is based on the patient's signs and symptoms and the location of those symptoms. The images ensure that an accurate diagnosis and treatment plan can be implemented. Radiologists are medical doctors who have completed residency training in radiology (often in a specific area of radiology). Radiologists read and interpret the images and provide the treating physician with a report of any abnormal findings.

Diagnostic testing refers to medical tests that are performed primarily in a laboratory setting; they include blood, urine, and cardiovascular tests. A medical technologist analyzes the blood and/or tissue and then sends a report to the provider. A cardiac technician or sometimes a nurse will administer special cardiac tests, which are read and interpreted by the physician or a cardiologist.

CLINICAL TIPS

Informed Consent

Before performing any diagnostic imaging or tests, patients must be made aware of the risks associated with the test and must agree to submit to testing.

Diagnostic Imaging

Radiography: X-Rays

An **X-ray** is a form of electromagnetic radiation that, when passed through a patient, allows viewing of internal structures. The X-ray beam is absorbed to different extents by the various body tissues. Less dense tissue appears darker because the radiation is not absorbed in these structures. For example, the lungs appear dark because air does not absorb radiation. Fat is gray, and bone and calcium are light or white (figure 3.1). Most of the X-ray beam is absorbed by the tissues or is scattered, while a small amount passes through the body part to the receptor, creating the image. The image may be developed on film or, in the case of digital radiographs, may be saved and viewed on a computer.

Because a radiograph is a two-dimensional picture of a three-dimensional body part, X-rays from several different angles may be administered in succession. Views are often named for the direction in which the X-ray beam passes through the body. For example, an image taken with the X-ray beam passing from the anterior to posterior aspects of the patient is called an **AP view**, whereas an image taken from back to front is called a posterior–anterior view (**PA view**). A view shot from the side is called a **lateral view**. Other views may be named for the person who first produced that view or perhaps for the place where it was first used.

During the procedure, the patient is asked to lie still and not move until the image has been taken. Depending on the type of radiograph taken, patients may be asked to hold their breath so that the image is not blurred by

movement of the rib cage. The test is painless and lasts only a few seconds, whereas an entire series of X-rays may last 10 min. More than one view may be taken of an area.

Radiographs are ordered when there is the possibility of a fracture, dislocation, bony abnormality or deformity, tumor, arthritis, bone cancer, foreign object, infection, or dental caries. For structures that cannot normally be imaged (blood vessels or hollow organs), a contrast medium (such as barium or iodine) may be introduced either by mouth or intravenously. These contrast agents will show up as white inside the hollow organ or blood vessel to allow the visualization of these structures on the image (Radiological Society of North America 2016). Because metal absorbs X-rays it shows up as white, obscuring anything behind it; for this reason, jewelry and even clothing in or near the area to be exposed to X-rays may need to be removed so that the image taken is clear and not distorted. Because the image is two-dimensional, remember that anything in the path of the X-ray beam, including items not necessarily in the patient, shows up on the image.

Risks or Side Effects

Radiographs should not be taken of women who are pregnant because the radiation may have an effect on the fetus. Pregnancy status must be determined by a blood or urine test before radiography is allowed. Any time that radiation is used there is a slight chance of developing certain types of cancer such as leukemia and melanomas. Physicians try to minimize exposure to X-rays by using the lowest amount of radiation necessary and by screening patients on the basis of criteria such as the Ottawa ankle rules. The Ottawa ankle rules are used to determine whether radiographs should be taken after an ankle injury. There are also criteria for the knee. Criteria for the ankle/foot are based on location of bone pain, tenderness, and weight-bearing ability. Criteria for the knee are slightly different, with consideration of age (over 55 yr), patella or fibular head tenderness, ability to flex the knee, and weight-bearing ability. Table 3.1 illustrates the amount of radiation introduced into the body for common diagnostic tests, including X-ray radiographs.

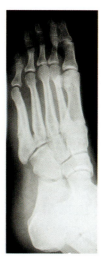

FIGURE 3.1   An anterior–posterior (AP) X-ray demonstrating a Jones fracture of the fifth metatarsal and a bipartite medial sesamoid in the left foot.
© Katie Walsh Flanagan

⚑ RED FLAGS FOR PREGNANCY AND DIAGNOSTIC IMAGING

Any female who has begun her menses must have her pregnancy status determined before being subjected to diagnostic imaging. A simple blood or urine test can verify the patient's status and prevent possible harm to a fetus.

Radionuclide Bone Scan

A **radionuclide bone scan** is a nuclear imaging test involving the injection of a short-lived radionuclide to assess abnormalities of the bones. Patients scheduled for such a scan will be asked to remove clothing and wear a gown for the procedure. A radionuclide tracer, which emits gamma rays, is injected into the brachial vein in the cubital fossa of the elbow. The tracer is attracted to increased metabolic activity. The patient may feel some warmth as the tracer circulates throughout the body. The technician providing the injection typically wears a radiation-protective lead vest and gloves when administering the injection. After a period of time (30 min to 2 h) to allow the isotope to circulate in the body, the patient is moved to the examination room and placed supine on a table. The patient lies still as a special camera moves around him or her. The camera identifies gamma radia-

TABLE 3.1 Comparison of Radiation from Imaging Versus Natural Radiation Exposure

Examination	Radiation dose (mSv)	Time to accumulate comparable natural background dose
Computed tomography		
Abdomen and pelvis	10.0	3 yr
Abdomen and pelvis, with and without repeated contrast	20.0	7 yr
Chest	7.0	2 yr
Chest (pulmonary embolism)	10.0	3 yr
Colonography	6.0	2 yr
Head	2.0	8 mo
Multiphase abdomen and pelvis	31.0	10 yr
Sinuses	0.6	2 mo
Fluoroscopy		
Barium swallow	1.5	6 mo
Coronary angiography	5.0-15.0	20 mo to 5 yr
Nuclear medicine		
Bone scan	4.2	1 y, 4 mo
Brain (PET)	1.0	4 mo
Cardiac perfusion (sestamibi)	12.5	4 yr
Lung ventilation/perfusion	2.0	8 mo
Tumor/infection	18.5	6 yr
Other		
Bone density (DEXA)	0.001	<1 d
Mammography	0.7	3 mo
Radiography		
Abdomen	1.2	5 mo
Chest	0.1	10 d
Extremity	0.001	<1 d
Lumbar spine	0.7	3 mo
X-rays, single exposure		
Dental (lateral)	0.02	<10 d
Dental (panoramic)	0.09	10 d
Hand or foot	0.005	<1 d
Hip	0.8	3 mo

tion, high levels of which indicate increased metabolic activity in bone, and the images are viewed on a computer or radiograph. Images are taken at various time intervals, revealing the rate at which the tracer is absorbed into the bone.

Areas of inflammation or injury to a bone will appear dark on a bone scan; these are called **hot spots**. Lighter areas on the bone scan show normal tissue and bone (Johns Hopkins Medicine 2016) (figure 3.2).

Bone scans are used to identify stress fractures, bone infections, bone cancer, and arthritis. The same nuclear technology may be applied to other structures such as the thyroid and heart, and it may be used to identify abscesses or tumors. Nuclear medicine may also be combined with computed tomography to allow visualization of the structure(s) in slices.

Risks or Side Effects

Patients are asked if they are allergic to red dye before the injection. If the patient is female, her pregnancy status should be determined before the test; patients who may be pregnant should not have a bone scan. Once the test is completed, the patient should drink plenty of water to flush out the radionuclide tracer. Most materials used in the test are not detectable even a day later, as most have a half-life of only a few hours.

Fluoroscopy

Fluoroscopy is a type of radiography that can be performed when the clinician wants to see a "live" image to determine the size, shape, and movement of tissue. It

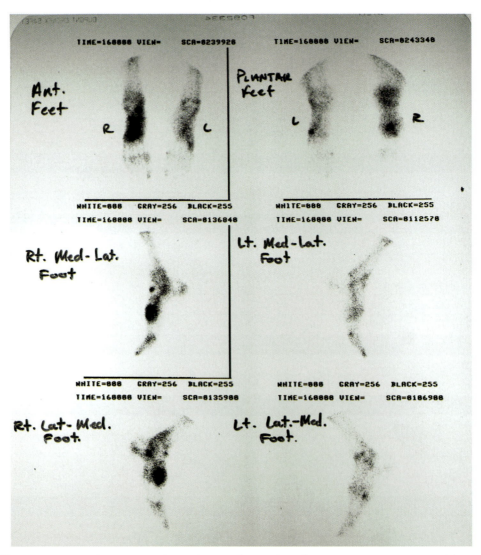

FIGURE 3.2 A bone scan showing uptake in the tarsal cuneiform bones, suggesting a possible stress reaction.
© Katie Walsh Flanagan

is not as detailed as an X-ray–based radiograph. Fluoroscopes are commonly found on-site at athletic venues of large universities and professional athletic venues; they are a quick and noninvasive means of determining whether a fracture has occurred or a joint is disarticulated, thereby warranting further studies. Fluoroscopic evaluation also assists in return-to-play decisions because the image can be taken with the patient in a weight-bearing position, thus allowing the diagnosis to be made immediately. Clothing should be removed from the area to be examined. Women should notify the technician if they might be pregnant, and they may be asked to undergo urinalysis or a blood test before fluoroscopy to rule out pregnancy.

The patient stands or sits next to the machine and the technician lines up the machine and the structure to be evaluated (figure 3.3). Radiation is allowed to pass through the skin, creating light and shadows that are viewed on a computer screen and can be printed. Dense areas such as bone will appear white on the film, and less dense areas such as the lungs will appear darker.

The fluoroscope can be used to look at blood flow, tumors, fractures, organs, foreign bodies, and some soft tissue. It can also be used to assist with biopsy, injections, catheter insertion, and even pacemaker insertion.

Risks or Side Effects

Any time that radiation is used there is a slight chance of developing certain types of cancer such as leukemia or skin cancer.

Computed Tomography Scan

A **computed tomography (CT) scan** (also computerized axial tomography [CAT] scan) combines specialized high-resolution radiographs with computers to give better visualization of internal structures in cross-section or three dimensions (3D). It works by passing rotating beams of X-rays through the patient and measuring the transmission at thousands of points. The images may be seen individually as a series of cross-sectional "slices," but 3D images can be produced by a computer. CTs

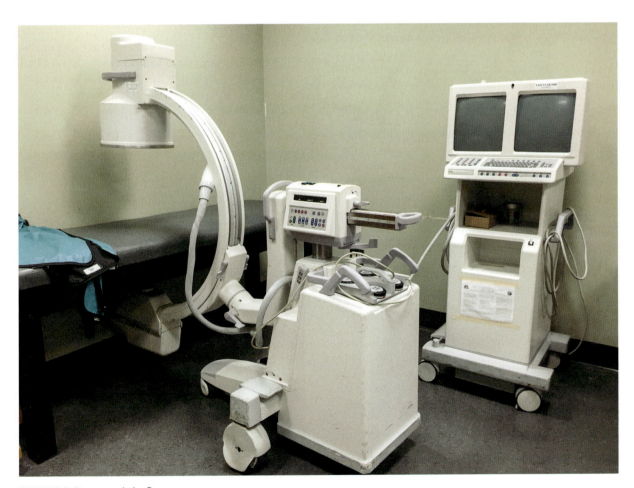

FIGURE 3.3 A mobile fluoroscope.
© Katie Walsh Flanagan

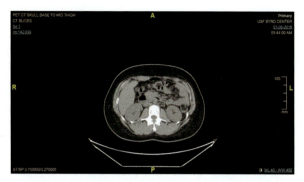

FIGURE 3.4 Computed tomography (CT) demonstrates the shoulders of a patient lying supine. The scapula, spine, and sternum are all visible in white.
© Lawrence Collins, PA-C, ATC

expose a patient to much greater levels of radiation than do X-rays (see table 3.1), and the risks of additional radiation exposure must outweigh the benefits of the definitive diagnosis. Depending on the structures to be examined, the patient may be injected with a contrast dye or asked to consume a barium or other contrast solution at various intervals before or during the CT scan. Contrast agents are usually the same iodinated agents used in other imaging studies. Patients may feel a warmth or cool sensation if the contrast dye is administered intravenously (emedicine 2016).

The patient must lie very still on a table that moves in and out of an open tube. At times the patient must hold his or her breath so that the images produced are clear. There is a whirring sound when the machine is operating, and it can sometimes be very noisy. The test is painless and lasts from 15 min to 1 h, depending on the structures to be examined.

CT scans are performed to look at cross-sections of internal organs, bone, soft tissue, and blood vessels (figure 3.4).

Risks or Side Effects

There is a slight risk, as with any radiation, of developing certain types of cancer such as leukemia or melanomas. On occasion, a patient will have an allergic reaction to the contrast dye. Every precaution is taken to avoid allergic reactions by taking an appropriate medical history, including allergies to food, medications, or dyes. Typically physicians require proof via serum blood test that a female of childbearing age (20 yr) is not pregnant before administering a CT scan.

Positron Emission Tomography Scan

A **positron emission tomography (PET) scan** is ordered to examine the cell metabolism and biochemistry of tissue and organs. PET scans can identify abnormal metabolic activity before it becomes apparent on a CT scan or by magnetic resonance imaging (MRI). The patient is administered a glucose-based radionuclide injection intravenously, or tablets by mouth, depending on the suspected condition. These radioactive materials (radiotracers) identify tissue changes at the cellular level and can indicate disease before more specific signs or symptoms appear (Radiological Society of North America 2015). The patient is placed on a table, and the imaging unit takes pictures of specific areas of the body. The patient needs to remain still at all times and may be asked not to breathe for short periods of time so that the image produced is clear. The table will move the patient in and out of the machine, similar to a CT scan. At times, the machine may move around the patient. The glucose-based radionuclide is absorbed by the area of abnormal metabolic activity and will appear dark on the body image view, similar to a bone scan, or as bright colors on 3D images (figure 3.5). This imaging mode is used to identify certain types of cancer, thyroid conditions, infections, and bleeding and to evaluate kidney function.

Risks or Side Effects

PET scans expose patients to a low dose of radiation, but the benefits outweigh the risks. Patients are asked if they are allergic to dyes before the injection or ingestion of radionuclide. Also, patients are asked to drink plenty of water after the scan to flush the radionuclide from their

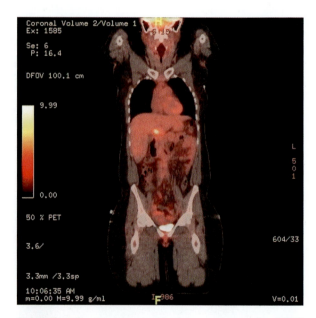

FIGURE 3.5 Positron emission tomography (PET) image demonstrating a healthy pelvis. The patient is in the supine position. The bright color at the bottom of the image is the bladder.
© Lawrence Collins, PA-C, ATC

systems. As with other imaging, women who could be pregnant should undergo a urinalysis or blood test; if the patient is pregnant or nursing, the test should not be performed.

Magnetic Resonance Imaging

An **MRI scan** (also termed an MR) is a test that applies a magnetic field to the body. The magnetic field aligns the body's atoms in such a way that, when released, they generate radio waves. The frequency of the emitted radio waves is related to the location and chemical environment of the atoms. A computer analyzes the data and creates an image. This image provides detailed information about organs, soft tissue, bones, tumors, bleeding, or infection. MRI scans are used to identify tumors, musculoskeletal injuries, soft-tissue conditions, fractures, and bleeding (figure 3.6).

The two most common imaging parameters are **T1** and **T2**. On a T1-weighted image, fat shows as a white or light signal, whereas water is dark. Conversely, on a T2-weighted image, fat shows as dark, whereas blood, edema, and cerebrospinal fluid (CSF) appear white. Calcium and bone do not show up well on MRI scans; however, the fat in bone marrow makes long bones appear white. At times, a contrast MRI scan is used to view structures such as the brain or cartilage more vividly. A contrast agent (gadolinium) can be introduced into the patient's body to better view structures as well as delineate a solid structure from a fluid one.

People who need MRIs will be asked a series of yes or no questions before the scan is scheduled. The results

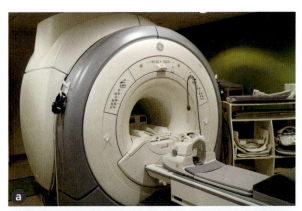

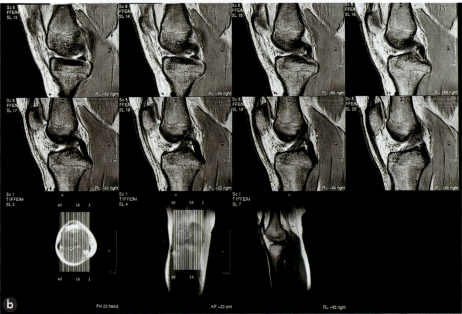

FIGURE 3.6   *(a)* A magnetic resonance imaging (MRI) machine. *(b)* MRI of the knee, clearly showing the posterior cruciate ligament (PCL) on the posterior aspect of the knee. Note the lower left aspect of the image. This displays the levels of "slices" this image portrays.

(a) © Micki Cuppett; *(b)* © Katie Walsh Flanagan

of this screening will be reviewed before the test is performed to determine whether they are at risk for injury if they undergo an MRI. Possible contraindications for MRI testing include the following:

- Cochlear implant
- Pacemaker
- Implantable cardio-verter–defibrillator (ICD)
- Heart or valve surgery
- Shunt, stent, filter, or intravascular coil
- Aneurysm clips
- Insulin pump (implanted)
- Pregnant
- Gunshot wounds/ shrapnel
- History of working with metal
- History of ocular injury involving metal or metal slivers
- Claustrophobia
- Allergies to dye
- Tattoos or permanent makeup
- Orthopedic clips, staples, plates, screws, and so on
- Implanted stimulator device (bone, neurological)
- Prosthesis

On arrival for the MRI, patients will be asked to wear a gown and to remove all metal jewelry, watches, body piercings, removable dental appliances, hearing aids, TENS (transcutaneous electrical nerve stimulator) units, glasses, hair accessories, and writing utensils. Metal items can interfere with the magnetic field of the MRI and alter the images. No metal or electronic devices are allowed in the room. The patient should also inform the technician of any metal implants before the test. MRI is safe for most patients with metal implants, screws, and pins, but there are a few exceptions (WebMD 2016). Patients will need to remain still throughout the entire test to avoid blurring of the image. There will be whirring, clicking, and knocking noises during the test, and the technician may provide earplugs or a headset for listening to music to eliminate some of the noise. If the patient receives a headset, the technician may use it to communicate with the patient during the test. The MRI may last 30 min to 1 h.

The patient must lie still on a movable table that slides into the magnetic area. The patient areas in older MRIs are very small tunnels that could be quite uncomfortable for the claustrophobic patient; however, newer models are more open, and the magnetic cylinder is much larger and thus more tolerable for patients. A series of images is taken while the patient is moved into the magnetic area. The signals are processed by a computer to show detailed "slices" or sections of tissue, or the data can be rendered as a 3D image.

Risks or Side Effects

MRI operates via magnets and has no documented side effects as long as the patient is honest and forthright in answering the preexamination questions. Patients who are claustrophobic should request an open MRI. If one is not available and a closed MRI will be used, patients may request a sedative so that they can be more comfortable. Women should notify the technician if they might be pregnant and should undergo a urinalysis or blood test before the test. The effects of magnetic imaging on a fetus have not been widely researched.

Diagnostic Ultrasound

Ultrasound consists of high-frequency sound waves that penetrate the body to produce images of internal structures in real time (figure 3.7). The images are produced by the magnitude and timing of returning echoes, which are the result of interfaces or changes in tissue density. An ultrasound examination is often thought of in the context of a woman having a sonogram to determine the developmental status (and gender) of her fetus. Gel is applied to the skin and a transducer is moved over the area to be examined. Sound waves are released through the transducer and transmitted into the tissue. Once the sound waves come in contact with internal organs, fluid, or tissue they bounce back, creating an image on the computer.

To prepare for this test, patients remove clothing and jewelry from the area to be examined so as not to distort the images, and they lie still during the test. The patient rarely feels anything except the transducer moving on the skin. The examination usually takes about 30 min. When used to examine the heart, this test is called an echocardiogram (ECHO) and is performed in conjunction with an ECG.

Ultrasound is used to identify tumors, enlarged lymph nodes, heart abnormalities, soft-tissue injury, bleeding, and fetal development. It is useful in the diagnosis

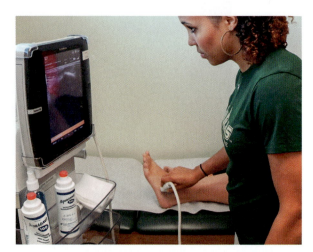

FIGURE 3.7   Diagnostic ultrasound of the ankle.
© Micki Cuppett

of tissue tears, blood clots, and deep vein thrombosis (DVT). In addition, a Doppler analysis can be performed, allowing the identification of moving blood. Diagnostic ultrasound is becoming more widely used to diagnose soft-tissue injuries to athletes, thus improving the promptness and safety of return-to-play decisions. Recent uses for non-therapeutic ultrasound in athletics include diagnosing muscular and tendon strains and inflammatory pathologies, as well as guided intraarticular injections.

Risks or Side Effects

Because this test uses sound waves, there are no documented side effects. Ultrasound is safe for pregnant women, and it is used to assess fetal development and gender.

Diagnostic Testing

Electromyography and Nerve Conduction Studies

Electromyography is done to measure the electrical activity in a muscle. The result is recorded on an **electromyogram (EMG)**. Taking an EMG involves inserting a needle into a muscle and recording the electrical activity. A normal muscle will have no electrical activity at rest. A **nerve conduction study (NCS)** is typically performed in conjunction with an electromyography. It measures the electrical signals of a nerve associated with a specific muscle. An NCS involves stimulating a nerve (via an electrical impulse delivered via a small needle inserted into the muscle) and recording the strength of the neurological reaction and the amount of time it takes to contract the muscle being tested (figure 3.8). Results

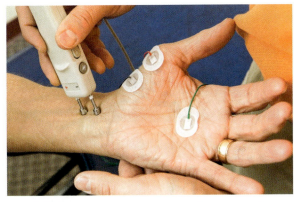

FIGURE 3.8 Electromyography and nerve conduction studies are traditionally evaluated at the same time by recording the electrical impulses in the muscle and the speed at which they travel when stimulated.

BanksPhotos/Getty Images

are displayed on an oscilloscope, as an audio signal, or both. Abnormal electrical activity will elicit an abnormal waveform (time of contraction) or sound.

EMGs are used to determine the cause of muscle weakness and abnormal nerve conduction, which may be due to medical conditions such as muscular dystrophy, myasthenia gravis, or amyotrophic lateral sclerosis (ALS). There may also be nerve irritation or injury to the carpal tunnel, cubital tunnel, brachial plexus, lumbar plexus, or other neuropathies that are the cause of abnormal electrical activity.

Preparation for an EMG involves cleaning the area to be evaluated and inserting a needle into the muscle to be tested. There is some discomfort, similar to having an injection, at the site. During the test the patient may be asked to contract the muscle. Typically, groups of muscles are assessed and compared with the muscles on the contralateral side. The only side effect associated with EMG testing is the possibility of slight soreness later in the muscle that was tested.

Electrocardiography

Electrocardiography is done to determine whether the electrical activity of the heart is normal. Electrodes are placed on the chest and extremities (if 12-lead electrocardiography is being done) to detect the electrical activity of the heart (figure 3.9). The electrical activity is charted on a graph (an **electrocardiogram**, or **ECG**) as waveforms. The waveforms are analyzed to determine whether there are any abnormalities. The number of leads that are used (ranging from 3 to 12) depends on the information that the physician is trying to access from different areas and structures of the heart.

An ECG is used to identify ischemia, heart attack, pericarditis, valvular disorders, electrolyte imbalances, palpitations, angina, and other related heart problems.

The patient will need to remove all jewelry and clothing in the chest area. The chest is cleaned and may be shaven. If the test is to use 12 lead, the wrists and ankles are also bared and cleaned. A gel is applied between the skin and the electrode. The patient should not feel anything during the test and may be asked to lie very still because movement may affect the results. The examiner should be informed if the patient is taking any medication or has a pacemaker. There are no known risks associated with ECG testing.

Holter Monitor

A **Holter monitor** is a device that is worn by a patient to monitor the heart's electrical activity. It is used to identify arrhythmias, ischemia, cardiomyopathies, and premature ventricular contractions and to monitor pacemakers. A

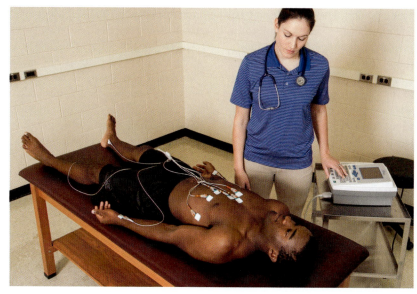

FIGURE 3.9   Twelve-lead electrocardiography is performed on some athletes as a baseline test in their preparticipation physical.

Holter monitor works in the same manner as an ECG. It traces the electrical activity of the heart, identifying any arrhythmias. The patient has two to five electrodes applied to the skin with a glue backing, and the leads are attached to a monitoring device (figure 3.10). The monitor is worn for between 24 h and 1 mo, depending on the suspected condition, and it records the heart rhythm. Patients must keep a diary of their activity and record any symptoms (skipped or racing heartbeat, or angina) they have had while wearing the Holter monitor. Those wearing the device longer than 24 h are given extra electrodes and taught how to apply them correctly. The electrodes may be removed daily for bathing. The typical Holter monitor is smaller than a deck of cards, with some about the size of a matchbook.

People prescribed Holter monitor testing undergo the same preparation as for an ECG. They should perform their normal activities, but they will not be able to bathe while wearing a Holter monitor. Female athletes can wear a Holter monitor in their sports bras. Patients are asked to provide a comprehensive history of prescribed medication, vitamins, supplements, and herbs routinely taken. For the most part, patients may continue their normal activities without interruption. As with ECG testing, there are no known risks associated with Holter monitor testing.

Interpretation of Results

The physician will review the information from the Holter monitor. Some units have a call-in number patients should use if they feel pain or cardiac arrhythmia. The Holter monitor then communicates with a computer or telephone

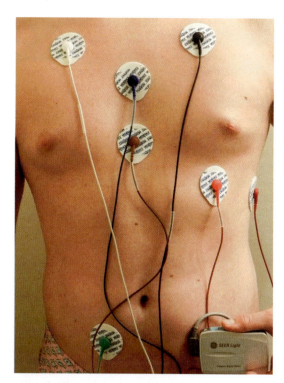

FIGURE 3.10   A Holter monitor is an excellent tool with which to evaluate a person's cardiac activity while performing acts of daily living.

Photo courtesy of Kathleen Knott / Johns Hopkins University

to deliver live cardiac readings. Otherwise, the data are downloaded on completion of the test and analyzed by a cardiologist or cardiovascular technician.

Cardiac Stress Test

A **cardiac stress test** is used to look at the heart's rhythm during exercise in a controlled environment. It is often used with patients who have several risk factors or are at medium risk of coronary heart disease. The patient is connected to an ECG machine, with a blood pressure cuff on the arm and a pulse oximeter on one finger to measure oxygen levels. A baseline ECG is taken for comparison. The cardiac stress test is done while the patient walks on a treadmill or pedals on a stationary bicycle (e.g., an Exercycle) (figure 3.11). At 3 min intervals the grade or intensity of the exercise increases. For a maximal stress test, the patient is asked to continue exercise until fatigued. In a submaximal stress test, the patient continues exercise to a predetermined level. During the cardiac stress test, heart rhythm, blood pressure, pulse, and oxygen levels are recorded.

A cardiac stress test is used to identify coronary artery disease, ischemia, and angina and to monitor the functional capacity of patients with heart disease. If radioactive nuclides are used in conjunction with the stress test, it is then called a **nuclear stress test**. This allows the cardiologist to detect regional areas of decreased blood

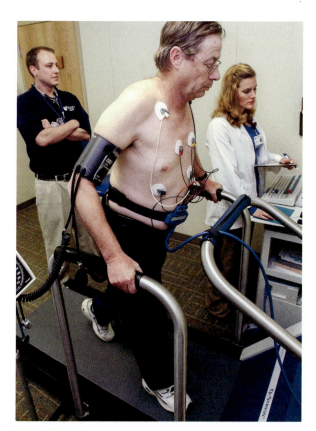

FIGURE 3.11 Cardiac stress tests can uncover a multitude of conditions associated with the cardiovascular system.

> ### 🚩 RED FLAGS FOR ENDING A CARDIAC STRESS TEST
>
> There are parameters for ending a cardiac stress test prior to a submaximal effort. These include the patient's desire to stop, signs of cyanosis or pallor, sustained ventricular tachycardia, patient dizziness, near syncope, moderate to severe angina, and hypertensive response (systolic blood pressure over 250 and diastolic blood pressure over 115), among other criteria (Akinpelu 2015).

flow. The risks are the same for a cardiac stress test as they are for exercise.

Laparoscopy

A **laparoscopy** is an invasive procedure in which a small incision is made in the abdomen and a scope is inserted into the incision to view the inside of the abdomen. Because the abdomen is distended with a gas before the scope is introduced, the abdominal organs are separated from the abdominal wall to allow for easier viewing. A laparoscopy allows the surgeon to see the internal structures of the abdomen and to determine any abnormalities.

Laparoscopy can be used to diagnose conditions of the abdomen; to provide a venue for surgical procedures for the gallbladder, appendix, uterus, and colon; and to perform biopsies.

General anesthesia is used for laparoscopy. A small incision is made in the abdomen and the laparoscope is inserted. The peritoneal cavity is distended with gas for better viewing. There is a camera on the scope that allows the physician to see the internal structures of the abdomen on a monitor. Other instruments may be introduced through another portal to facilitate moving the viscera for better viewing or to perform surgery.

The patient may be slightly sore for a few days, depending on the procedure performed. Because gas was introduced into the abdomen before the procedure, not all of it may have been released before the wound was closed. Gas-like abdominal discomfort is common, but it dissipates rapidly. If surgery was performed, the patient may be limited in terms of physical activity for a period of time. Each patient should be informed about signs of infection. If any symptoms of infection occur, the patient should call the physician immediately.

Colonoscopy

A **colonoscopy** is an invasive procedure done to examine the colon and rectum for abnormalities. A scope with a camera on the end, inserted through the rectum and into the colon, displays an image of these structures, allowing the physician to identify any abnormalities. It is recommended by the American Cancer Society that adults at age 50 undergo a colonoscopy for the detection and prevention of colorectal cancers or earlier if there is a history of colon cancer in the patient's immediate family. A colonoscopy is used to examine the patient for any early indication of colon cancer or polyps and to help explain bleeding or changes in normal bowel habits. Those without a trace of colon cancer are advised to undergo a colonoscopy every 10 yr following the initial one at age 50.

Preparation for the Test

The patient must eliminate all solid waste from the gastrointestinal tract. A liquid diet will be required, beginning 1 to 3 d before the procedure. The patient will be asked to take a laxative, to drink a special liquid and/or take tablets, and to consume only clear liquids. Clear liquids include bouillon or broth, flavored gelatin, water, coffee, tea, electrolyte drinks, or clear soft drinks. Patients taking any medication should inform the physician in advance of the procedure. On the day of the procedure the patient is given a sedative to be more comfortable. Air is introduced into the colon to make visualization of the colon clearer. The procedure usually takes 30 to 60 min.

Risks and Side Effects

Unlike the other diagnostic imaging covered in this chapter, the colonoscopy involves sedation and has risks associated with this. Typically, a person trained in anesthesiology is present to provide intubation, if necessary. Since biopsies can be obtained via the colonoscopy, bleeding and tears or perforation of the colon are risks of this procedure.

Side effects of a routine colonoscopy include temporary cramping or bloating after the procedure; because of the sedative, patients should not drive for 24 h. At times, there may be dizziness, weakness, and some blood in bowel movements after the procedure.

Laboratory Tests

Many common diagnostic tests are performed to confirm specific conditions. An athletic trainer needs to be familiar with these tests, what they are used for, and what the results indicate. Two of the most traditional laboratory examinations, urinalysis (UA) and complete blood count (CBC), as well as the lumbar puncture, are discussed next. Athletic trainers rarely perform laboratory tests, with the possible exception of urine test strips (such as Chemstrips), but they do need to appreciate the normal values of these examinations. Elsewhere in this text, the abnormal values of common tests and what they indicate in a specific condition or disease are discussed; here, emphasis is on the common normal values found in UA and CBC.

Urinalysis

A **urinalysis (UA)** is a urine test to determine pH, protein, glucose, ketone, bilirubin, hemoglobin, nitrite, leukocytes, urobilinogen, and specific gravity levels. The patient is asked to urinate into a clean plastic cup.

A UA may be ordered for various reasons. Results can indicate urinary tract infection, diabetes, starvation (including anorexia nervosa), liver problems, intravascular hemolysis, injury or bleeding in the renal system, and renal or glomerular damage. Illicit drugs, anabolic steroids, and alcohol can also be screened for in a urinalysis. A specific urinalysis can also confirm pregnancy.

If a "clean catch" specimen is ordered, then the external area of the urethra is cleaned with a disposable cloth before the patient voids into a cup. Collected urine should be refrigerated if it will not be assessed within 1 h.

CLINICAL TIPS

Conditions a Urinalysis May Reveal

- Blood in the urine (hematuria) can indicate a kidney injury or can occur benignly after an intense workout.
- The color of urine can reveal dehydration or may be the by-product of certain medications.
- Glucose is not normally present in urine unless high levels exist in the body; therefore glucose in the urine might indicate diabetes.
- Ketones also can reveal diabetes or a fasting athlete.
- pH is the acidity or alkalinity of the urine; a higher acid reading can be found with diabetes or dehydration, whereas an alkaline reading indicates infections of the kidney or urinary tract.
- Specific gravity of urine indicates its ion concentration and attests to the athlete's hydration level as well as the kidney's ability to process fluids.
- Urine tests can also indicate drug use, electrolyte levels, and the presence of infection.

In the athletic environment, the UA may consist of a simple dipstick placed in a container of urine. This is often used to determine the presence of hematuria to rule out trauma to the renal system. These dipsticks, or Chemstrips, are flexible, coated paper with multiple test components on each stick; they are dipped into collected urine and subsequently compared with a chart on the bottle's label to see if the color reaction matches a given component of urine. Common assessments include pH, red blood cells (if present, a sign of injury), white blood cells (if present, a sign of infection), glucose, specific gravity, and protein values. The bottle containing the sticks is dark to prevent light from penetrating and altering their reliability; the bottle must be tightly sealed to preserve the reactive chemicals on each stick. The side of the bottle is labeled with a chart for various parameters (e.g., blood or pH) and with associated color squares that indicate the presence or concentration of each (figure 3.12). Each value has a specific time frame for correct reaction response, typically from immediately to 2 min, and you must read the stick within the allotted time frame to obtain accurate results. Normal values for urine are found in table 3.2.

Complete Blood Count

A **complete blood count (CBC)** presents a microscopic review of a blood sample. It is used to examine specific components of whole blood and expresses those components in designated units (per volume of blood). Physicians often order a CBC as a basic screening test of overall health and to provide information about the ratios of cells per volume of blood. A CBC does not typically furnish information about cell shape or blood type.

TABLE 3.2 **Normal Values for Urine**

Aspect measured	Normal value
Color	Pale yellow to amber
pH	Tends to be acidic (4.6–8.0)
Specific gravity	1.003–1.030
Red blood cells	<5/HPF
White blood cells	<5/HPF
Protein	Negative
Glucose	Negative
Ketones	Negative
Nitrites	Negative
Crystals	None
Volume	800 to 2500 ml per 24 h

The CBC determines the number and types of white blood cells (WBCs) and red blood cells (RBCs), the hematocrit (Hct, volume of RBCs in whole blood), and hemoglobin (Hb) level. The number of platelets per unit is also estimated. Abnormal blood values can indicate a variety of conditions described in subsequent chapters. Common disorders such as anemia can be present when the hemoglobin level or hematocrit is low. High WBC counts can indicate infections ranging from a skin infection to mononucleosis to leukemia; low RBCs and platelets can be caused by internal bleeding. Table 3.3 shows normal CBC values for adults.

The cubital fossa of the arm is cleaned and a compression tourniquet is placed around the upper arm. The

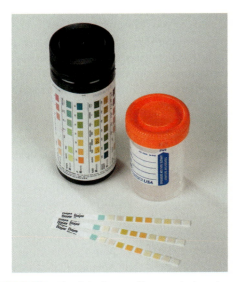

FIGURE 3.12 The label on a Chemstrip bottle can be used to assess strips for results of urinalysis.

CLINICAL TIPS
Components of Human Blood

- *Human blood* is composed of 52% to 62% plasma and 38% to 48% cells. A typical adult has about 5 L of blood, which is typed A, B, AB, or O, and has a positive or negative rhesus (Rh) factor.

- *Blood plasma* is largely water; the three chief cell components are erythrocytes (red blood cells [RBCs]), leukocytes (white blood cells [WBCs]), and thrombocytes (platelets). Leukocytes are further divided into five subtypes: neutrophils, basophils, lymphocytes, monocytes, and eosinophils. The function of RBCs is to carry oxygen to working tissues, whereas the WBCs primarily fight the invasion of unrecognized or foreign elements in the body.

TABLE 3.3 **Normal Adult Values for Complete Blood Count**

Parameter measured	Normal range
WBC count	$3.8–10.8 \times 10^3$ cells/µl
WBC differential: absolute neutrophils	1500–7800 cells/µl
WBC differential: absolute eosinophils	50–550 cells/µl
WBC differential: absolute basophils	0–200 cells/µl
WBC differential: absolute lymphocytes	850–4100 cells/µl
WBC differential: absolute monocytes	200–1100 cells/µl
RBC count	Males: $4.4–5.8 \times 10^6$ cells/µl Females: $3.9–5.2 \times 10^6$ cells/µl
RBC: MCV	78–102 fl
RBC: mean corpuscular Hb	27–33 pg/RBC
RBC: mean corpuscular Hb concentration	32–36 g/dl
RBC: distribution width	≤15%
Hb	Males: 13.8–17.2 g/dl Females: 12.0–15.6 g/dl
Hct	Males: 41%–50% Females: 35%–46%
Platelet	150,000–450,000/mcL

Hb = hemoglobin; Hct = hematocrit; MCV = mean corpuscular volume; RBC = red blood cell; WBC = white blood cell.

technician inserts a needle into a vein in the cleaned area of the patient's arm to remove some blood into a tube or syringe. The needle is removed and gauze is taped over the needle puncture site. The amount of blood removed depends on the type of blood test ordered, and the procedure is called a **venous puncture**. If multiple vials of blood are needed, the technician will collect them via the one venous puncture.

There are no risks or side effects when a CBC is performed under sterile conditions. There might be slight bleeding or bruising over the puncture site. The test results can be affected by stress, dehydration, or overhydration.

In addition to basic screening, a CBC is used to diagnose viral and bacterial infections, such as upper respiratory infections, mononucleosis, anemias, and leukemias. It is also typically ordered when determining cholesterol levels and vitamin and mineral deficiencies, as well as for drug testing.

Lumbar Puncture

A lumbar puncture can be used to withdraw cerebrospinal fluid (CSF) for examination. It can also be used to give injections to assist in radiographic imaging or to relieve the pain of a herniated disc. The diagnostic test of cerebrospinal fluid is performed when meningitis is suspected or when there is a need to measure the pressure of the CSF. In the case of diagnostic imaging, a radiopaque substance is injected into the subarachnoid space for clarification of structures in the radiographic image.

Lumbar puncture is performed by placing the patient in a side-lying position with knees pulled up to the chest and head fully flexed. This position helps to open the spaces between the vertebrae in the lumbar column. Lumbar puncture is performed under strict sterile conditions. A sterile hollow needle is inserted between two lumbar vertebrae (typically L3 and L4) and enters the subarachnoid space to draw out CSF for assessment (figure 3.13).

The CSF is assessed for pressure and color before being sent to the laboratory for evaluation of white blood cells, glucose, and protein. The lumbar puncture is a good diagnostic tool for meningitis, Lyme disease, Guillain-Barré syndrome, multiple sclerosis, tumors, and other neurological disorders. A physician will sometimes use this procedure to inject drugs or anesthetic for other medical procedures. After the puncture, the patient is typically kept prone for 4 to 6 h to reduce the risk of headache.

Pulse Oximeter

A pulse oximeter is a noninvasive device that quickly measures the amount of oxygen saturation in a person's blood. It is used to determine if a patient may benefit from supplemental oxygen. Most of these units operate via a pair of light-emitting diodes (LEDs) within a selected wavelength. The light passes through a translucent area, such as an earlobe or fingertip (figure 3.14) and is used to determine the amount of oxygen bound to hemoglobin. The signal vacillates with each heartbeat to display LED absorption in arterial blood. The instrument provides the value of the saturation of peripheral oxygen (SpO_2). Normal values are 95% to 100%. Values below 95% saturation identify hypoxia, and values below 85% are critical.

Limitations that may lead to inaccurate readings in oxygen saturation include external interference (motion, bright light), hypotension, hypothermia, carbon monoxide poisoning, and dark nail polish.

When recording results in a patient's chart, include the date, time, reading, patient position, and activity level. Also include the probe placement site and whether the reading was accompanied by supplemental oxygen.

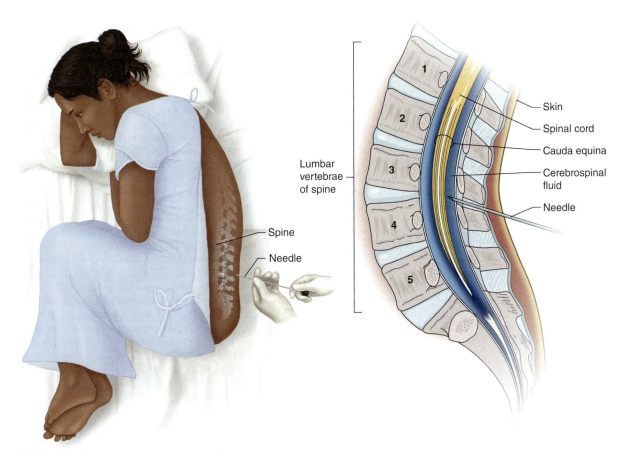

FIGURE 3.13 Proper setup for a lumbar puncture.

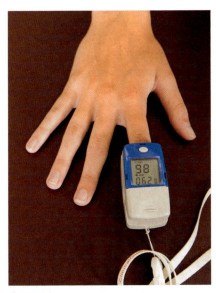

FIGURE 3.14 Pulse oximeter.

Reporting Cancer Diagnoses

Diagnostic imaging and testing are often used to diagnose and stage cancers. Although some cancers, such as melanoma skin cancer, have their own scale, the TNM scale is discussed here because it is a common and well-recognized method of determining the severity and spread of cancerous tissues.

Cancer is staged (categorized) in order to help determine prognoses in specific cases. The American Joint Committee on Cancer (AJCC) and the Union for International Cancer Control maintain the TNM system of staging. Many, but not all (for example, Hodgkin lymphoma), cancers use this system, where T indicates tumor, N represents nodes, and M is for metastasis. The cancer staging is accompanied by CT scans of the abdomen and pelvis to assess for spread of the disease (table 3.4). Other tests can be performed depending on the initial findings.

TABLE 3.4 **TNM System for Cancer Staging**

Stage	Characteristics
Primary tumor (T)	
T_x	No primary tumor can be assessed
T_0	No evidence of primary tumor
T_{is}	Carcinoma in situ (i.e., without spread)
T_1, T_2, T_3, T_4	Increasing size and extent of the primary tumor
Regional lymph nodes (N)	
N_x	Cannot be assessed
N_0	No regional lymph nodes involvement
N_1, N_2, N_3	Increasing involvement of regional lymph nodes
Distant metastasis (M)	
M_x	Presence of metastasis cannot be assessed
M_0	No distant metastasis
M_1	Distant metastasis

TNM = tumor, node, metastasis. The universally accepted TNM system for cancer staging helps to determine the extent or spread of the disease in order to establish treatment decisions and prognosis for recovery. It groups cancers into one of four stages (I to IV) or stage 0 for carcinoma *in situ*, which means without spread. Higher stages such as stage IV or M_4 represent distant metastasis and the worst prognosis.

Summary

Health care providers must understand the diagnostic imaging and laboratory tests available for active people. Being able to explain procedures and their expected results is important to help assuage patients' anxiety. Knowing how much radiation these procedures emit (see table 3.1) can help in determining which type of evaluation may be best for a given condition and patient. Athletic trainers can also explain the risks and side effects of the tests so patients can be informed and prepared.

 Apply It! The case study for this chapter evaluates your understanding of diagnostic imaging and testing for a 20-year-old field hockey player. Read the scenario and answer the questions at www.HumanKinetics.com/MedicalConditionsInTheAthlete.

PART II

Pharmacology and Interventions

Part II covers issues related to pharmacology, therapeutic drugs, and common procedures in athletic training. Chapter 4, "Basic Principles of Pharmacology," describes the principles of pharmacology, including pharmacokinetics and pharmacodynamics, and generalized pharmacologic science. It discusses the regulation of pharmaceuticals, including the roles of the DEA and FDA, and the differences between administering a drug and dispensing a drug. This information is important to athletic trainers because it offers guidance into which drugs may be permissible in sport as well as the legal issues involved in working with medications.

Chapter 5, "Drug Categories," discusses the categories of medications and their effects on the body. Mechanism of action and delivery, side effects, and adverse effects are discussed within each drug category. Therapeutic categories of drugs covered include anti-inflammatory agents, analgesics, antibiotics, antivirals, antifungals, bronchodilators, antihistamines, decongestants, and anti-diabetic agents. Their individual indications and contraindications and their effects on athletic participation are reviewed. Red Flags in this chapter include drugs that can have an adverse effect on participation. Also covered are medications that are banned by national and international organizations because they are considered dangerous or because they create unfair advantages for athletes.

Chapter 6 covers various common procedures in the athletic training clinic. It starts with a brief discussion on informed consent, preventing infection, and the importance of maintaining a sterile field. The chapter provides step-by-step photographic instructions for opening and donning sterile gloves, opening a sterile pack, and opening wrapped supplies. It also describes the use of adhesive skin tape, liquid skin adhesive, and sutures (including photographic demonstrations of various types of knot tying). Step-by-step photographic demonstrations (on pig skin) show simple interrupted sutures, vertical mattress sutures, and horizontal mattress sutures, as well as the removal of sutures and staples used for wound closure. Joint aspiration and injections are also discussed, and intravenous procedures are described and illustrated. The reader is reminded, once again, that some states' practice acts do not allow ATs to perform some of the procedures included in this chapter.

Basic Principles of Pharmacology

4

OBJECTIVES

At the completion of this chapter the reader should be able to do the following:

- Describe the basics of pharmaceutics and pharmacokinetics, including dosage forms, routes of administration, and drug storage.

- List the basic drug classifications, their indications, their contraindications, and their typical uses.

- Access various drug information resources to obtain more information about a drug.

This chapter provides an introduction to the regulatory, pharmacological, and pharmaceutical information that athletic trainers must be familiar with and understand. The role of the athletic trainer will invariably involve pharmaceutical agents and their use by athletes. Important regulatory agencies discussed in relation to athletic trainers include the Food and Drug Administration (FDA), the Drug Enforcement Administration (DEA), and the National Collegiate Athletic Association (NCAA). The basic principles of pharmacology cover pharmacokinetics, routes of administration, drug storage and resources, pharmacodynamics, indications and contraindications, and special considerations for athletes. Content about pharmaceuticals is organized by drug categories and identifies available drug forms and dosages, routes of administration, correct methods for storage of specific drugs, and side effects. Drug information resources also are reviewed. This chapter is designed as an overview and lists additional sources for continued reading and expanded content.

Regulation of Pharmaceuticals

Athletic trainers must understand the legal regulations that apply to the use of medications. Two entities of the U.S. federal government are charged with controlling the use of pharmaceutical products: the Food and Drug Administration (FDA) and the Drug Enforcement Administration (DEA). The equivalent agency in Canada to the FDA is Health Canada. Health Canada's various subdivisions are responsible for regulating food and health products, including pharmaceuticals, biological agents, and genetic therapies. The Health Products and Food Branch Inspectorate is responsible for compliance monitoring activities as well as industry inspection and product investigation (Health Canada 2016).

Drug Enforcement Administration

The DEA lays within the Department of Justice. Its function is to ensure compliance with the Controlled Substances Act of 1970 and to implement the regulations found in Title 21, Code of Federal Regulations, Part 1300 to the end. The DEA registers health care practitioners who will be prescribing or dispensing those drugs that are considered controlled substances and advises them on how to comply with controlled substance regulations.

Controlled substances are drugs that have a high potential for abuse (e.g., morphine, codeine). The DEA has established five categories or "schedules" of controlled substances (I–V). Table 4.1 lists drugs that are classified as controlled substances and are placed into one of these five categories on the basis of their likelihood for abuse.

Food and Drug Administration

The FDA is an agency of the Department of Health and Human Services. The FDA has three main responsibilities:

1. FDA is responsible for protecting the public health;
2. FDA is also responsible for advancing the public health; and
3. FDA plays a significant role in the nation's counterterrorism capability.

Its mission is to "promote and protect the public health by helping safe and effective products reach the market in a timely way and to monitor products for continued safety after they are in use" (FDA 2016). Through oversight of science-based information, the FDA seeks to speed innovations that make medicines more effective, safer, and more affordable for the public. In its role, in promoting the nation's counterterrorism capability, the FDA fulfills this responsibility by ensuring the security of the food supply and by fostering the development of medical products to respond to deliberate and naturally emerging public health threats (FDA 2016).

The FDA is responsible for approving and overseeing manufacturers who may produce medications for con-

TABLE 4.1 **Drug Enforcement Administration Schedules of Controlled Substances**

Schedule	Description	Examples of drugs*
I	Drugs with no accepted medical use in the United States High abuse potential	Opium Hallucinogens (heroin, LSD, mescaline) Marijuana**
II	Drugs with high abuse potential Severe psychic or physical dependence liability Tightly controlled prescribing requirements, including written prescription (*no* verbal orders) from physician No refills without additional prescription from physician	Morphine Cocaine Oxycodone Oxycodone combination products (Percocet) Methamphetamine
III	Drugs with less abuse potential than those in Schedule I or II	Benzphetamine Stimulants Depressants Clortermine Narcotic drugs Anabolic steroids
IV	Drugs with less abuse potential than those in Schedule III	Barbital Phenobarbital Oxazepam
V	Drugs with less abuse potential than those in Schedule IV Class consists of preparations containing limited quantities of certain narcotic ingredients generally for antitussive and antidiarrheal purposes	<200 mg of codeine or opium per 100 g

LSD = lysergic acid diethylamide.

*Examples of drugs in each schedule do not represent an all-inclusive list.

**As of May 2016, marijuana was still scheduled as Class I by the DEA; however, reports indicate that the status could change.

CLINICAL TIPS

Bioequivalence

Bioequivalence is the quality of having the same drug strength and providing an equivalent amount of drug to the target tissue in the same dosage form as another sample of a given drug substance. For example, for two drugs to be considered bioequivalent, they must meet the following criteria:

- Have the same dosage form (e.g., tablet, suspension)
- Have the same drug strength
- Provide equivalent blood levels or tissue levels of the drug

CLINICAL TIPS

Administration Versus Dispensing

- Administration is the direct application of a single dose of a drug.
- Dispensing includes packaging and labeling prescription medication (multiple doses).
- Facilities that dispense medications must have a Drug Enforcement Agency (DEA) certificate on file.

sumption, the approval of new chemical formulations for marketing and sale as either prescription or nonprescription, such as over-the-counter products, and the approval of generic drug products that must exhibit the bioequivalence of a brand-name product.

The FDA is also charged with determining how drugs may be marketed and sold in the United States, including the drug's indications, information contained in the product's package insert, and how the drug is manufactured. Pharmaceutical product manufacturers must meet very stringent manufacturing guidelines and pass FDA inspections. The drug products that they produce must consistently pass dissolution and bioequivalence tests. The FDA does not oversee the marketing or sale of food supplements and herbal products, many of which are used by athletes, and neither does any other government agency.

Administration Versus Dispensing

Most states regulate both the administration and the dispensing of drugs. The athletic trainer must understand the differences between these two actions. **Dispensing** is the act of delivering a medication to an ultimate user pursuant to a medical order issued by a practitioner authorized to prescribe (FDA 2016). This includes the packaging, labeling, or compounding necessary to prepare the medication for such delivery. A facility that dispenses prescription medication must have a separate DEA certification (Pedersen, Schneider, and Scheckelhoff 2011). **Administration** is the act of applying a medication by injection, inhalation, ingestion, or any other means to the body of a patient in a single dose.

Both dispensing and administration require a written prescription from a physician. In some states, verbal orders may be received from physicians, but the order must be properly documented and recorded when executing the order. The athletic training facility must comply with both state and federal regulations governing prescription medications. Most states require that an athletic training facility have a DEA certificate and a signed agreement with a physician in cases in which medical staff serve as an "agency" in the care of the physician's patients. In these situations, the athletic trainer is acting as an agent assigned by the DEA and is not acting under the scope of the state practice act for athletic trainers; at no time does the agent make any discretionary decisions about the administration or dosage of a medication. Different states have different laws for the administration and dispensing of medications. Studies conducted by the National Athletic Trainers' Association showed that among athletic trainers compliance with federal prescription drug regulations is improving overall (Kahanov, Roberts, and Wughalter 2010).

There is a growing emphasis on interprofessional training that will foster collaboration among health practitioners (Hajart et al. 2014; Morgan, Pullon, and McKinlay 2015; New et al. 2015). The athletic trainer, team physician, and team pharmacist must work together to ensure that state and federal regulations are being met.

Pharmacology

Pharmacology is the science of drugs and includes pharmacokinetics and pharmacodynamics. **Pharmacodynamics** is the study of the actions of a drug on the body, including mechanism of action and medicinal effect (the biochemical and physiological effects of the drug). This may involve a stimulatory or inhibitory reaction at the receptor. **Pharmacokinetics**, on the other hand, is the study of how the body acts on the drug. Pharmacokinetics includes the absorption, distribution, metabolism, and elimination of the drug in the body.

To better understand how drugs work within the body, it is important to know the process by which a drug gets into the body, is distributed, is metabolized, and finally is eliminated. The methods of absorption, distribution, metabolism, and elimination are discussed here.

Absorption is the process of getting the drug into the body. Drugs may be absorbed through various routes, including the rectal, intestinal, and dermal tissues. Which route is used depends on many different patient-related and drug-related factors. The age, level of consciousness, and disease being treated are patient-related considerations; drug-related factors include solubility and stability. The desired route of absorption will determine the formulation used; a rectal absorption will generally indicate using a suppository, but tablets, capsules, liquids, and suspensions may also be absorbed rectally.

Absorption has a major influence on the bioavailability of a drug. The bioavailability of a drug describes how much of the drug is available to the tissues after its administration. Bioavailability is an important concept in drug development, especially as it pertains to generic drugs. In order for any generic drug to be considered equivalent to a brand-name preparation, it must be shown to have bioavailability that is equal to the brand-name product.

Distribution refers to the process of moving the drug throughout the body. Most drugs are distributed throughout most or all of the body's tissues, but this distribution is not necessarily even. For example, many drugs do not cross the blood–brain barrier to enter the central nervous system (CNS). Factors such as the drug's pH, **hydrophilicity** (water solubility), and **lipophilicity** (fat solubility) will affect its distribution throughout the body (Brunton, Chabner, and Knollmann 2011). The concept of volume of distribution is used to describe the effective space in the body available to contain a drug. It

is the ratio of the total amount of drug in the body to the plasma concentration of drug. Drugs with a high volume of distribution have lower plasma concentrations and are more greatly distributed into extravascular tissues. Drugs with a lower volume of distribution have higher plasma concentration and less distribution into extravascular tissues.

Metabolism is the complex process by which a drug is changed into one or more chemical entities that differ from the parent drug. These entities may be active metabolites that have a pharmacological effect or inactive metabolites with no pharmacological effect (Clinical Pharmacology 2016). Drug metabolism occurs primarily in the liver through the action of various hepatic enzymes, although some metabolism does occur in a few other tissues in the body, such as the lungs.

Elimination is the process of getting the drug out of the body. A drug and its metabolites are eliminated through some combination of renal or fecal excretion. Although some drugs are completely eliminated either through renal or fecal excretion, most drugs and their metabolites undergo elimination through a combination of these two mechanisms. In persons with renal or hepatic impairment, the rate of drug elimination will be slowed to a degree dependent on the level of impairment. This means that the dose of a drug or the frequency of administration will often need to be adjusted in patients with renal or hepatic dysfunction.

Two concepts used to describe the elimination of a drug from the body are clearance and half-life. **Clearance** is the measure of the body's ability to eliminate a drug. It describes the volume of blood that is cleared of a drug over a given period of time, usually expressed in milliliters per minute. Drugs with a higher clearance rate will be removed from the body more quickly. Creatinine clearance is the rate of removal of creatinine from the serum into the urine. It is used as a measure of renal function. The normal creatinine clearance for men is 100 ml/min and for women it is 80 ml/min (Clinical Pharmacology 2016). In patients with impaired renal function, it is important to know the creatinine clearance. In pharmaceutical reference books, dosage adjustments for renal impairment are given on the basis of creatinine clearance.

Half-life is the length of time that it takes for blood levels or tissue levels of a drug to decrease by one-half. The clearance rate of a drug and the drug's volume of distribution will determine the half-life of the drug. The half-life is directly proportional to the volume of distribution and inversely proportional to the clearance. This means that a drug with a high clearance rate and a small volume of distribution will have a short half-life and be eliminated from the body very quickly. A drug with a large volume of distribution and a low clearance rate will have a long half-life (Brunton, Chabner, and Knollmann 2011).

A drug's half-life is one of the major determining factors in how often a drug will be given. As a rule, a drug with a long half-life will have a long dosage interval. A drug with a short half-life will have a short dosage interval. If the clearance rate of a drug is decreased by renal or hepatic dysfunction, this will increase the half-life of the drug and necessitate an increase in the dosage interval (Brunton, Chabner, and Knollmann 2011). Patients with an altered volume of distribution because of disease (e.g., ascites) also will have an altered drug half-life. It is important to know the disease's effect on a drug half-life so that changes in the dosage regimen may be made.

Routes of Administration

Drugs can enter the body through a variety of routes, and these paths of administration promote the drug's absorption. Following are the routes of administration:

Oral	Sublingual
Intravenous	Rectal
Intramuscular	Topical
Subcutaneous	Intravaginal
Inhalation	Intranasal
Intraarterial	Subarachnoid

The oral route is the most common, but often it is more appropriate to use a parenteral (nonoral) route of administration. The preferred route is determined by many factors, including ease of administration, patient adherence, desired onset of action, local versus systemic distribution, and properties of the drug itself. An example is the destruction of insulin in the gastrointestinal tract, which necessitates its administration through a nonoral route.

Oral

The oral route is a convenient, noninvasive way to deliver drugs that are distributed systemically. Tablets, capsules, solutions, and suspensions are dosage forms used to deliver drugs via the oral route. Tablets contain the drug compressed or embedded along with inert ingredients into a compact unit, and they may be either uncoated or coated. Enteric coatings are used to ensure that a tablet does not dissolve in the low pH of gastric acid but instead passes into the small intestine, where the tablet is dissolved and the drug absorbed. Drugs that are destroyed by gastric acid or drugs that may cause local irritation in the stomach, such as aspirin, are delivered in an enteric coating. Other coatings provide a controlled release of drug so that the drug is released from the tablet over an extended period of time, allowing for less frequent doses. Delayed release, extended release, and controlled release are all terms used to refer to dosage forms that are constructed to prolong the release of the drug from the tablet or capsule so that the drug may be given at extended dosage intervals.

Other mechanisms allow for controlled release of the drug from a tablet, such as an osmotic delivery system used to deliver the antihypertensive drug nifedipine (Procardia XL). In such systems, the drug is contained in an osmotically active core surrounded by a semipermeable membrane. When the tablet is exposed to the water in the gastrointestinal tract, water is drawn into the core at a controlled rate, resulting in a suspension of the drug that is pushed out through an orifice in the tablet.

Capsules are solid oral dosage forms that contain powdered, beaded, or liquid drug inside a gelatin shell. Some shells are formulated to dissolve in the stomach; others will dissolve in the intestines. Some capsule shells are designed to release the drug in a controlled fashion over an extended period.

Oral solutions, elixirs, and syrups contain drug completely dissolved in a liquid medium. Elixirs typically contain alcohol to aid in the dissolution of the drug. Syrups contain high concentrations of sugar to make them more palatable. Oral suspensions are also liquids, but they contain undissolved drug dispersed or suspended throughout the liquid. All suspensions must be shaken before administration to ensure that the drug is evenly dispersed throughout the liquid. Antibiotic suspensions often require refrigeration and may have a short expiration date after which they must be discarded.

Inhaled

Inhaled drugs are most often used for their local effect on the bronchial passages. Bronchodilators and corticosteroids are the drugs most often given via this route to treat bronchoconstriction from asthma. These drugs may be administered via metered-dose inhalers (mdis), dry-powder inhalers, or **nebulizers** (figure 4.1). Mdis and dry-powder inhalers deliver a set dose of the drug with each inhalation. Nebulizers are machines that use compressed air to cause aerosolization of a liquid drug,

---

CLINICAL TIPS

Dissolution

Dissolution is the process of dissolving a substance. In the context of pharmaceuticals, it is the process of a solid, oral dosage form (e.g., tablet or capsule) being dissolved in the gastrointestinal tract so that it can be absorbed. Poorly manufactured products may not dissolve at all and may be passed through the gastrointestinal tract and into the stool without allowing the expected dose of medication to be absorbed.

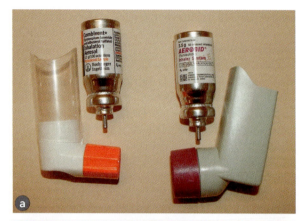

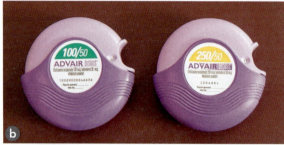

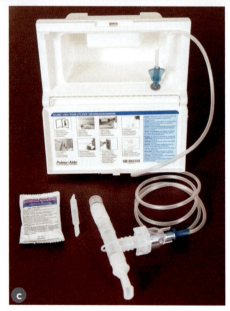

FIGURE 4.1 *(a)* Metered-dose inhalers, *(b)* dry-powder inhalers, and *(c)* nebulizers are commonly used to administer inhaled medications.

(a) © Micki Cuppett

which is then inhaled through a mask or a mouthpiece. Intranasal sprays and inhalers are used for a local effect on the intranasal passages. Corticosteroids and decongestants are the most common drugs delivered by the intranasal route to treat allergic rhinitis symptoms.

Ophthalmic

Ophthalmic administration of drugs may be used to treat eye infections, allergies, dryness, glaucoma, and other eye disorders. The droppers used to administer drugs into the eye must be kept sterile, and therefore the eyedropper must never touch the eye. Those who administer the drops must wash their hands thoroughly before and after administration of the drops. Warming the drops to body temperature by rolling the dropper bottle rapidly between the hands may increase the comfort of ophthalmic administration. Administration of the drops into the lateral area of the eye also increases comfort since the medial area, pupil, and iris are much more sensitive. Applying the drops laterally also helps bathe the eye since tears are produced laterally and flow medially to the nasolacrimal duct (figure 4.2).

Otic

Otic administration of drugs is used primarily to treat otitis, decrease pain from otitis, and prevent recurrence of otitis in athletes whose ear canals are often exposed to moisture, such as swimmers. The droppers used to administer drugs into the ear canal do not need to be sterile, but every attempt must be made to avoid touching the dropper to the ear during administration. As with ophthalmic administration, those who administer the drops must wash their hands before and after administration. Rolling the dropper bottle rapidly between the hands or running the bottle under warm water will bring the temperature of the drops closer to body temperature, which will make the administration of the drops more comfortable for the athlete. Administration of ear drops requires the patient to be in a sitting or side-lying position. The ear canal is straightened by pulling up and back on the pinna. The

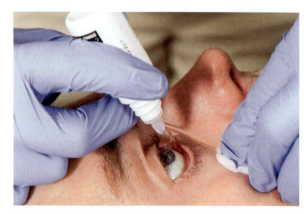

FIGURE 4.2 Ophthalmic solutions are applied by holding the eyedropper above the conjunctival sac laterally to allow the drops to flow toward the nasolacrimal duct.

dropper is held approximately one-half inch above the ear canal (figure 4.3). After the drops are administered, gently massage the tragus of the ear, and have the patient remain quiet for a few minutes so all the medication can work into the ear. Although it is not uncommon for ophthalmic drops to be prescribed for use in the ear, otic drops are never used in the eye.

Topical

Topical administration refers to the application of a drug to the outer areas of the body for a local effect rather than a systemic effect. Creams, ointments, gels, and solutions are the most common dosage forms used for topical administration. Topical drugs may be used for a number of purposes, such as treatment of infection, treatment of inflammatory skin disorders such as dermatitis, or treatment of acne. The drug and its intended use will determine the frequency of application, whether it should be applied in a thick layer or sparingly, and if a dressing or bandage should be used after application. The area where the drug is to be applied should be as clean and dry as possible. Those who apply topical preparations must wash their hands before and after application of the drug; some drugs necessitate the wearing of gloves.

Transdermal

Transdermal administration is the application of a drug to the skin, usually in the form of a patch. Once the drug is absorbed, it produces a systemic effect. Nitroglycerin, estrogen, testosterone, and fentanyl (a pain medication) are all available in patches for transdermal administration. The frequency with which old patches are removed and replaced with new patches will vary depending on the drug. Patches should be applied to hairless areas on the trunk, with the exception that estrogen patches should not be applied to the breasts. When an old patch is removed

and a new one applied, the new patch is put in a different area to minimize irritation. The old patch is then folded in on itself with the sticky side in and discarded in the trash so that the patch cannot be reapplied.

Intravenous

The intravenous (IV) injection of a drug directly into a vein (figure 4.4) is used in situations where immediate onset of drug action is required or where the use of other routes of administration is not possible because of patient condition or drug characteristics. The athletic trainer will see the IV route most often in situations where IV fluids (typically without medication added) are administered to achieve rapid hydration of an athlete who is experiencing heat-related illness. Athletic trainers must be aware of state practice laws to know the limits of their role in administering IV fluids. Some states allow athletic trainers to administer IV fluids under the supervision of a physician.

Intramuscular

The intramuscular (IM) route may be used for various reasons. In situations where a rapid, reliable onset of drug action is required but IV access is impractical, the IM route is the best alternative. Meperidine (Demerol) can be administered via IM injection for migraines. IM injection is also used for the injection of suspensions that will be slowly absorbed to deliver a drug over prolonged periods. Medroxyprogesterone (Depo-Provera), a birth control injection lasting for 3 mo, is given via the IM route. The IM route is used to administer nearly all vaccinations.

Subcutaneous, Intrasynovial, and Intraarticular Injections

Subcutaneous injection (SQ or SC) is the injection of a drug into the subcutaneous fat and is used for rapid, reliable

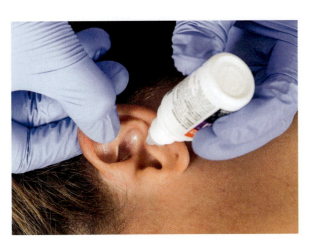

FIGURE 4.3 Otic administration drops.

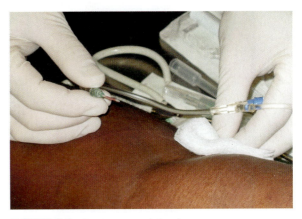

FIGURE 4.4 Intravenous injection.
© Micki Cuppett

onset of drug action when IV access is impractical. It is also preferred for medications that are self-injected (e.g., insulin, epinephrine in EpiPens, and some pain medications such as morphine). Pumps are now available that provide a continuous infusion of drug into a subcutaneous catheter (Rao et al. 2014). Athletes with diabetes using subcutaneous insulin pumps will adjust the insulin infusion rate on the basis of their current blood sugars, activity level, and food intake to achieve much better control of blood sugars than with conventional subcutaneous injections (figure 4.5). Epinephrine is often self-administered through an auto-injector or EpiPen for treatment of emergency anaphylaxis (figure 4.6). To use an EpiPen, take it out of the protective tube and remove the blue protective safety cap. Quickly jab the orange tip

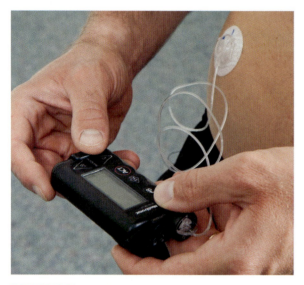

FIGURE 4.5 Insulin pump.

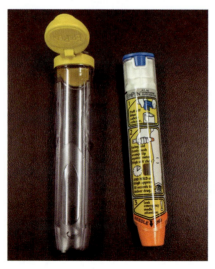

FIGURE 4.6 EpiPen.
© Katie Walsh Flanagan

into the thigh. The EpiPen will click so you will know that it worked. Hold the EpiPen against the thigh for 3 sec and then remove. The auto-injector is designed to go through clothing.

Intrasynovial injection is used to place a drug, usually an anti-inflammatory corticosteroid suspension, into the synovial cavity of a joint. The drug will not be systemically absorbed but will act locally to decrease inflammation.

Intraarticular injection refers to injection of the drug into the joint. As with intrasynovial injection, the drug will not be systemically absorbed but will act locally to decrease inflammation.

Iontophoresis and Phonophoresis

Drugs may also be introduced into the body through the use of electricity (iontophoresis) or ultrasound (phonophoresis). Both of these delivery methods "drive" ionized medication into the subcutaneous tissues. Iontophoresis uses low-voltage, high-amperage direct current (DC) and requires the use of customized electrodes (figure 4.7). Transdermal introduction has advantages over oral ingestion because it bypasses the liver, reducing metabolic breakdown of the medication, and can be concentrated in a local area. It provides advantages over injected medications because it is less painful and does not result in high concentrations in the soft tissue, which have been associated with tendon rupture (Raphael et al. 2015).

Iontophoresis also has disadvantages. It cannot reach deep tissue structures or areas of thick skin. Many medications may be used with iontophoresis, and they are usually dissolved in a carrier. Typical medications include acetic acid, dexamethasone, lidocaine, and epinephrine in varying combinations.

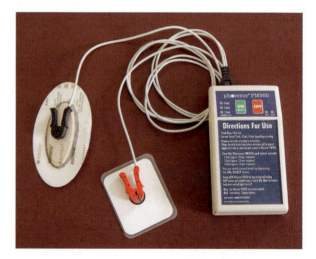

FIGURE 4.7 Iontophoresis delivers ionized medication using low-voltage, high-amperage direct current (DC).

Phonophoresis does not actually "drive" the ions of the medication through the skin but rather opens pathways that allow the medication to diffuse through the skin and pass deeper into the tissue. Some medications have been shown to be delivered up to 6 cm into the tissue with phonophoresis (Rigby et al. 2015). Medications typically administered this way include corticosteroids such as hydrocortisone and dexamethasone, salicylates, and anesthetics.

Additional research has produced significant breakthroughs for the delivery of topical medications (Lakshmanan et al. 2014; Roustit, Blaise, and Cracowski 2014). Athletic trainers will be expected to master new techniques as they are developed because they are the ones who provide most topical medications for athletes.

Drug Storage

The proper storage of drugs is essential to maintain drug potency. Temperature, humidity, and exposure to light must all be considered. Most drugs are best stored in a cool, dry, dark place. This means room temperatures of 65 °F to 80 °F, with a low humidity of less than 50% and limited exposure to sunlight (Brunton, Chabner, and Knollmann 2011). Drugs requiring refrigeration are typically oral antibiotic suspensions, immunizations, insulin, and injected drugs that have been reconstituted from powders.

Whereas some refrigerated drugs may be kept for limited times at room temperature, others will lose potency rapidly if left unrefrigerated. Many emergency drugs (e.g., epinephrine, phenylephrine) will degrade rapidly on exposure to sunlight or high temperatures. Other drugs cannot tolerate freezing.

It is particularly important to consider the storage needs of all drugs during transportation. Medical kits for use at outdoor athletic events must be inspected regularly to ensure the integrity of the drug products stocked in the kit. The security of the drugs must also be ensured. All prescription medications must be stored in a locked cabinet or a locked portable medical treatment kit. Protocols must be followed that do not violate state practice acts or federal DEA guidelines for dispensing prescription medication. Dispensing prescription medications is not within the scope of practice for athletic trainers in most states. However, some states may allow the athletic trainer to be licensed as an agent for the physician. The athletic trainer must only be assigned duties that are allowed by applicable state law (Kahanov, Roberts, and Wughalter 2010).

Pharmacodynamics

Pharmacodynamics is the study of how medications work in the body: the mechanisms of action, drug interactions, side effects, adverse reactions, and allergic reactions. Some concepts necessary for later discussion are reviewed here.

A drug's mechanism of action may be very simple. An example is the action of magnesium hydroxide in the stomach, where it neutralizes stomach acid through a simple acid–base reaction. Another simple mechanism of action is exhibited by bulk-forming laxatives, in which insoluble fibers cause increased stool volume in the large intestine.

Other drugs act through more complicated mechanisms. **Agonists** are drugs that exert their effect by attaching to cellular receptors in the body, causing stimulation of the receptors (figure 4.8). Agonists mimic the effects of endogenous chemicals, which normally target cellular receptors (Brunton, Chabner, and Knollmann 2011). Morphine, an opiate agonist, stimulates opiate receptors in the body that are normally the target of the body's own endorphins. Endorphins cause decreased sensitivity to pain and a sense of well-being or euphoria. Intense exercise causes the release of endorphins in the body, which explains the euphoria and pain tolerance that occur in many athletes during endurance events. Morphine is used for its therapeutic effect of decreasing one's sensitivity to pain. The euphoria produced by morphine is the reason for its high abuse potential.

Antagonists also act by binding to cellular receptors, but they do not cause stimulation of the receptor. An antagonist binds to the receptor and blocks other chemicals or agonists from binding to it. Antihistamines bind to histamine receptors in the body but cause no stimulation of the receptors. Rather, antihistamines block the binding of histamine-to-histamine receptors, thereby preventing the itching, rhinitis, and edema that histamine will cause when it is released by immune system cells in response to an allergen (Brunton, Chabner, and Knollmann 2011).

The inhibition of enzyme action is another important mechanism of action for several of the drugs discussed later in this chapter. Enzymes are proteins that act as biochemical catalysts for chemical reactions that occur in the body. Some drugs exert their effect by breaking down enzymes or blocking the effect of enzymes, thereby preventing or slowing down the reactions for which these enzymes are responsible. Cyclooxygenase-1 and -2 (COX-1 and COX-2) are enzymes that are involved in the biochemical transformation of arachidonic acid into prostaglandins. Prostaglandins are chemicals that cause pain and inflammation.

Anti-inflammatory drugs are cyclooxygenase inhibitors that prevent COX-1 or COX-2 from facilitating the production of prostaglandins. A drug's mechanism of action often is directly related to its side effects and drug interactions. For example, β-adrenergic agonists, which stimulate β-adrenergic receptors, cause bronchodilation

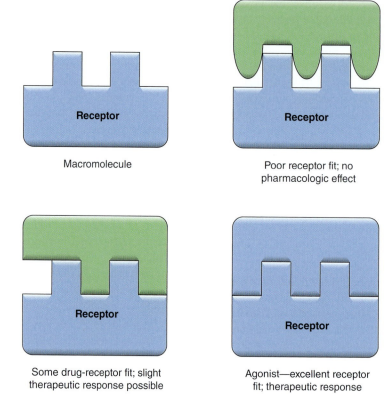

Macromolecule

Poor receptor fit; no pharmacologic effect

Some drug-receptor fit; slight therapeutic response possible

Agonist—excellent receptor fit; therapeutic response

FIGURE 4.8 Drug–receptor interaction can take place when agonists with shapes that match an endogenous chemical fit exactly into a cell receptor or when an antagonist binds to a receptor, thereby blocking the agonist and preventing it from stimulating the receptor.

and are used to treat asthmatic attacks. People who take β-blockers to treat hypertension may have a decreased response to β-agonists (Clinical Pharmacology 2016; Brunton, Chabner, and Knollmann 2011).

Indications

Drug **indications** outline conditions for which the drug shows a therapeutic effect. The indications are FDA approved, meaning the drug manufacturer has provided a body of research to the FDA supporting the use of the drug for a particular indication and the FDA has approved the use of the drug for that indication. FDA-approved indications are found on the drug package insert.

Contraindications

Contraindications are situations in which a drug must be avoided. Disease states, other medications, pregnancy, age, and gender may all be reasons for a particular drug to be contraindicated. For example, the use of tetracycline antibiotics is contraindicated in children under the age 7 because it will cause staining of the permanent teeth. Decongestants, which can cause profound, transient elevations in blood pressure, are contraindicated in people

> **CLINICAL TIPS**
>
> ## Indications and Contraindications
>
> - Indications: those conditions for which the drug has been found to have a therapeutic effect
> - Contraindications: situations where a drug should be absolutely avoided

with uncontrolled hypertension (Clinical Pharmacology 2016). Although athletic trainers do not prescribe or dispense medications, they need to be aware of contraindications to medications commonly used by athletes. They may know about an athlete's drug history. Working closely with the team physician and pharmacist will ensure the best health care for the athlete.

Warnings and precautions are statements that alert health care professionals to the serious adverse events associated with the use of a drug. Black box warnings are strong precautions that the FDA mandates be printed inside a black box at the very top of a product's package insert. As with contraindications, the athletic trainer must be familiar with the warnings and precautions for all drugs that are prescribed for the athletes.

Drug interactions most commonly refer to the interaction of one drug with another drug but may also refer to interactions between drugs and foods and drugs with disease states. Drug interactions with foods occur most commonly when the minerals in a particular food inhibit the absorption of a drug (table 4.2). For example, the administration of fluoroquinolone antibiotics with calcium-containing foods will decrease the absorption of the antibiotic because the calcium binds to the antibiotic and forms an insoluble complex.

Drug–disease interactions may occur for a variety of reasons. For example, the administration of drugs that block the β-adrenergic receptors, or β-blockers, is not recommended for people with diabetes because these drugs will mask the symptoms of hypoglycemia that are mediated by the sympathetic nervous system, such as tremors.

Drug–drug interactions occur when one drug affects the absorption, metabolism, distribution, receptor binding, or elimination of another drug. For example, many antibiotics, such as penicillin, change the bacterial composition of the intestine, which in turn alters the metabolism of oral contraceptives. The result is that the effectiveness of oral contraceptives may be decreased in women taking certain antibiotics. Although many drug interactions are undesirable, some interactions can be used for a beneficial therapeutic effect. Histamine$_2$ (H$_2$) receptor blockers, such as famotidine (Pepcid), interact with orally administered pancreatic enzymes (pancrease) in a way that is beneficial (Clinical Pharmacology 2016). Pancreatic enzymes are susceptible to acid–peptic enzyme degradation. The administration of an H$_2$ blocker raises the gastric pH and decreases the acid-peptic degradation of pancreatic enzymes, thereby decreasing the dose of pancreatic enzymes required.

Drug allergies occur when the medicine produces a response different from what is expected. Symptoms

TABLE 4.2 Selected Drug–Food Interactions

Drug	Food	Interaction
Analgesics/antipyretics	Alcohol	Increased risk of liver damage
Antihistamines	Alcohol	Can add to drowsiness caused by these medications
Benzodiazepines	Caffeine	Antagonism of antianxiety action
Bronchodilators	Caffeine Alcohol	Can cause increased excitability, nervousness, and rapid heartbeat Increased chance of nausea, vomiting, headache, and irritability
Griseofulvin	Fatty foods	Increased blood levels of griseofulvin
MAO inhibitors	Coffee, tea, chocolate (caffeine-containing)	Excessive consumption can lead to hypertensive crises or dangerous cardiac arrhythmias
Quinolone antibacterials (ciprofloxacin, moxifloxacin)	Dairy products Caffeine	Dairy products can interfere with absorption May increase the effects of caffeine
Statins	Grapefruit juice	Increased bioavailability, inhibition of first-pass metabolism, increased toxicity*
Tetracyclines	Dairy products high in calcium, ferrous sulfate, antacids	Impaired absorption of tetracycline
Thiamine	Blueberries, fish, alcohol	Foods containing thiaminases; decreased intake, absorption, utilization
Timed-release drug preparations	Alcoholic beverages	Increased rate of release for some

*Grapefruit interaction pertains to statins metabolized through cytochrome P450-3A4, including lovastatin, simvastatin, and atorvastatin.

RED FLAGS FOR DRUG ALLERGIES

- Severe itching
- Hives or other signs of allergic response
- Bronchospasm
- Shock

may include severe itching and hives, signs of an allergic response. Some allergic reactions may be anaphylactic and may include bronchospasm and shock. It is important to distinguish drug allergies from drug side effects. Drug side effects are conditions reported by the majority of people who take a particular medication, but a drug allergy is an unusual presentation seen in approximately 6% to 10% of the patients who take that medication (Lexicomp Online 2016). Because of the potential severity of drug allergy reactions, it is important to know if the athlete is allergic to any medications. Allergy to a medication is obviously a contraindication for taking that medication.

The side effects or adverse reactions to a drug are the drug's nontherapeutic actions. Usually drugs of the same class will have similar side effect profiles. For example, ibuprofen (Advil, Motrin) and naproxen (Naprosyn, Aleve), both nonsteroidal anti-inflammatory drugs (NSAIDs), have nearly identical side effects (Kanbayashi and Konishi 2015). Serious adverse effects of a drug should be reported to the FDA's MedWatch program at www.fda.gov. This includes any adverse effect that results in death, disability, hospitalization, life-threatening condition, or congenital anomaly. Adverse drug effects that require medical or surgical intervention to prevent permanent impairment should also be reported. The pharmacy that dispensed the medication or the office of the prescribing physician may help to produce the report. Reporting of adverse reactions is extremely important, especially in the case of newly approved drugs, because it is used to identify potentially serious adverse effects of

 RED FLAGS FOR COX-2 ANTI-INFLAMMATORY AGENTS

In 2004, a COX-2 anti-inflammatory medication called rofecoxib (Vioxx) was voluntarily pulled from the market by its manufacturer amid concerns that it increased the risk of cardiovascular problems (Bavry et al. 2014). As with any medication, potential benefits must be weighed against the drug's adverse side effects. The athletic trainer must remain current on drug cautions and recalls.

a drug that may lead to changes in the product's labeling or even withdrawal of the drug from the market.

Many drugs are being given expedited, fast-tracked FDA approval. Thus, compared with other drugs that are not fast tracked, fewer people will have used these drugs before they are approved. Serious adverse reactions or serious drug interactions may not be discovered until after the drug has received FDA approval. The FDA and the drug manufacturers rely on post-marketing surveillance, including the MedWatch program, for reports of these adverse incidents.

Dosages

Drug dosages take many factors into consideration. The first consideration is age. Children over age 12 may generally be given dosages using guidelines for adults. For children under age 12, many dosages are simply based on age. This approach presumes that a child is of normal weight. For premature infants and underweight or overweight children, determining doses by age range is not optimal.

On the opposite end of the age spectrum, many drugs must be used at a decreased dose in older adults. The two main reasons for this are (1) advanced age causes an increased sensitivity to many drugs such as central nervous system depressants, and (2) aging also is associated with diminished hepatic and renal function, which decreases the rate at which drugs are eliminated from the body and necessitates the use of smaller doses.

Dosages based on weight or body surface area are a preferable method to use when children need medications. The *Harriet Lane Handbook*, *Micromedex*, and *The Pediatric and Neonatal Dosage Handbook* are all excellent resources on pediatric dosages. Also, a few drugs used in adults have dosages based on weight or body surface area, such as cancer chemotherapy drugs or certain antibiotics. In children and adults who are obese, it may be necessary to use an ideal body weight or adjusted body weight to calculate an appropriate drug dose.

For some drugs given by weight, the dose will be expressed in terms of milligrams, grams, or units per kilogram per dose (e.g., acetaminophen, 10 mg/kg/dose given every 4 to 6 h). For other drugs, the dose will be published as milligrams, grams, or units per kilogram per day (Lexicomp Online 2016) followed by the recommended number of divided doses per day (e.g., amoxicillin, 40 mg/kg/d divided every 8 h, or in three divided doses). It is important to make the distinction between whether the dose is being expressed as the total daily dose or as the quantity to be given in a single dose. Physicians typically express dosages on prescription pads or orders as abbreviations. Therefore, the athletic trainer must be familiar with common medical abbreviations used in prescribing.

Special Considerations for Athletes

Sometimes the drug of choice for an athlete with a particular condition is not viable because it may be banned during competition or is ergolytic and negatively affects athletic performance. Therefore, a particular drug may not be the drug of choice but rather the most viable drug choice. Athletes, athletic trainers, coaches, and compliance officers are expected to know the most current list of prohibited agents. The list is published by the World Anti-Doping Agency (WADA), with the United States Anti-Doping Agency (USADA) being a signatory of the WADA published list (United States Anti-Doping Agency 2015; United States Anti-Doping Agency (USADA) 2016; World Anti-Doping Agency (WADA) 2016). The National Collegiate Athletic Association (NCAA) maintains a similar list of banned and monitored substances (National Collegiate Athletic Association (NCAA) 2015b). The WADA specifies which medicinal agents are permanently banned, as opposed to specific cases when an agent may be banned. There may be instances when an athlete has a medically diagnosed illness or condition that requires the use of medication(s) listed on the WADA prohibited list. In these cases, the athlete may apply for a therapeutic use exemption (TUE) from the WADA. Adequate documentation will be required, and the athlete must comply with all testing requirements. NCAA collegiate athletes have a similar process for requesting medical exceptions (National Collegiate Athletic Association (NCAA) 2015a). Because the lists of the WADA, USADA, and NCAA are subject to change, consult the agency websites when questions arise.

Potential Drug Misuse

We often think that if some of a thing is good, more is better. This is extremely problematic when dealing with medication. Athletes will often self-medicate with over-the-counter drugs using prescription-strength dosages. Warner and colleagues found that 75% of high school football players surveyed were daily users of over-the-counter drugs and took NSAIDs independently without supervision (Warner et al. 2002). The athletic trainer must help to educate athletes about the dangers of self-medicating or taking medications in dosages other than what is indicated on the prescription or on the over-the-counter label.

Athletes may also be tempted to use medications in ways other than intended or indicated in hopes of improving their performance. Educating athletes about the dangers of using drugs for purposes other than those prescribed is paramount for their continued safety. Although drug testing may be a deterrent for some athletes, the technology used to circumvent drug tests is typically years ahead of the technology for detecting the drugs.

Resources

The number of pharmaceutical products on the market, among generic, brand, and biologic medications, continues to grow at a very steady rate each year. With the continued emphasis on biomedical research, and the vast volume of research being published, it is essential that anyone involved in health care have up-to-date resources available. The best options are electronic references that are updated frequently, such as Lexicomp or Micromedex, but subscriptions to these services can be quite costly. Those who work at universities may have access to online drug information resources through their library's subscription. There are also free services online that are sufficient for most practitioners.

Drug information programs are also available for use with mobile applications on smartphones or tablets. Both desktop and mobile app versions are available for many online drug information programs. The advantages of electronic drug references over printed references are that the medical professional may easily select two or more drugs and access comparative information, including drug interactions. In addition, the electronic drug references are updated on a regular basis and do not rely on publication schedules to be updated.

Printed references are still a viable option as long as they are replaced annually. The *Physician's Desk Reference (PDR)* is published annually and remains popular. The *PDR* contains a collection of package inserts from all prescription products available in the United States. There is a companion volume that contains information for over-the-counter products. The *PDR* is limited, however, because comparative information among various drugs and information on a drug's off-label uses (indications that are not approved by the FDA) are not included.

Popular printed drug information references include *Drug Facts and Comparisons*, which receives monthly updates; the *American Hospital Formulary Service*, which is published by the American Society of Health System Pharmacists with a new edition annually; and the *United States Pharmacopoeia Drug Information*, which contains information for the patient in nontechnical language. Information about pediatric patients is available in *The Harriet Lane Handbook*. When foreign medications need to be used, the health professional may refer to Martindale's, which provides information in print and online. The ability to synthesize the drug information available and apply it to real situations requires an advanced level of training.

Summary

The athletic trainer's responsibility is to monitor for and prevent allergic reactions when possible, recognize and report adverse drug reactions, and recognize situations in which drug interactions may occur. The athletic trainer is often asked by athletes to recommend over-the-counter or herbal supplements. In complex situations, where multiple medications or supplements are involved, it is advisable to seek an opinion from either a physician or a pharmacist.

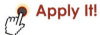 **Apply It!** The case study for this chapter tests your knowledge of common pharmacology terms. Read the scenario and answer the questions at www.HumanKinetics.com/MedicalConditionsInTheAthlete.

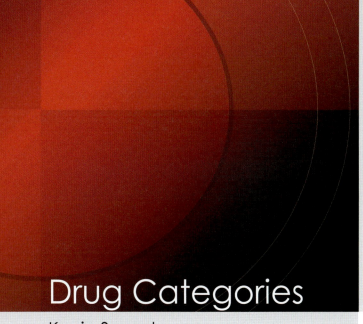

Drug Categories

Kevin Sneed

OBJECTIVES

At the completion of this chapter the reader should be able to do the following:

- List the basic drug categories in which drugs are classified, including mechanism of action, side effects, and adverse effects.
- Describe the inflammatory process, and discuss appropriate pharmacological management of inflammation.
- Describe the key points for using a metered-dose inhaler (MDI) and the medications commonly administered with an MDI.
- Describe the indications, contraindications, dosage, and side effects of antihistamines and decongestants and their implications for athletic participation.
- List common narcotic analgesics, and understand the federal restrictions for administration of the drugs and their potential for addiction.
- Appreciate the risks to the athlete who participates in athletics while using local anesthetics.
- Understand the actions of antibiotics, including bactericidal and bacteriostatic actions.
- List the common antivirals and antifungals, their indications, contraindications, dosage, and side effects.
- Describe the basic use of anticoagulants in athletics and their mechanism of action, as well as precautions to be observed with the use of this class of drugs.

This chapter discusses various categories in which drugs are classified. Within each category, the mechanism of action in the body for various drugs is discussed. Side effects and adverse effects of drugs are also discussed. For information about pharmacodynamics and pharmacokinetics, please see chapter 4.

Anti-Inflammatory Agents

One of the most common conditions that athletic trainers encounter is inflammation. Following injury, irritation, or overuse, inflammation occurs to limit the spread of the damage to adjacent tissue. It is both a chemical and a vascular response at the site of injury or exposure to the injurious agent. The process is nonspecific and is the same regardless of whether the injury or irritation is mechanical or is caused by a noxious foreign substance.

Initially, a vasoconstriction occurs to prevent the loss of blood. This is followed by the release of chemical mediators such as prostaglandin, histamine, leukotrienes, and bradykinins. These mediators cause vasodilation and an increase in cell wall permeability, which results in fluid escaping from the cells into the interstitial spaces in the quickly progressing inflammatory cascade. Inflammation results in pain, redness, warmth, swelling, and loss of function. The inflammatory process is covered in detail in many therapeutic modality texts for athletic trainers.

The physician may prescribe anti-inflammatory medication to limit the extent of the inflammatory process or cascade. Anti-inflammatory medications are classified as steroidal or nonsteroidal anti-inflammatory agents.

Steroidal Anti-Inflammatory Agents: Corticosteroids

Corticosteroids are defined as hormones that are secreted by the adrenal cortex or synthetic analogs of these hormones. Although corticosteroids and anabolic steroids, which are analogs of testosterone, both contain a steroid ring, corticosteroids have very different pharmacological actions from anabolic steroids. The actions of corticosteroids can be classified as either mineralocorticoid or glucocorticoid. Mineralocorticoid actions are those that affect electrolytes, fluid balance (with the net effect being sodium and fluid retention), and potassium and hydrogen excretion. Glucocorticoid actions decrease inflammation, cause immune system suppression, and stimulate gluconeogenesis. They also promote protein catabolism, redistribute peripheral fat to central areas, decrease intestinal absorption of calcium, and increase renal excretion of calcium. The pharmacological effects of the corticosteroids are most likely caused by their complex influence on various enzyme systems. For the athletic trainer, the most important effects of corticosteroids are their anti-inflammatory properties, which are beneficial in the treatment of inflammatory joint disorders and environmental allergies (table 5.1).

Most corticosteroids used to treat joint disorders are administered in one of three ways: intrasynovial injection, intraarticular injection, or iontophoresis. It is not unusual for these injections to be accompanied by a short-acting anesthetic such as lidocaine (Xylocaine) (Soriano-Maldonado et al. 2016). Injectable corticosteroids are typically used after more conservative treatments have failed and the inflammatory process can be localized to a small area.

The immunosuppressive properties of corticosteroids make them invaluable in the treatment of allergies and inflammatory joint conditions. Prednisone (Deltasone) and methylprednisolone (Medrol) are the oral agents used most often in the treatment of allergic reactions and acute joint inflammation. Typically, a large dose, equivalent to 30 mg of prednisone, will be given on the first day of treatment and then the dose will be reduced by 5 mg/d until the drug is completely tapered off. The initial dose and subsequent doses may be given as a single daily dose or in divided doses. The very popular Medrol Dosepak contains 4 mg methylprednisolone tablets in a six-row blister pack with complete instructions for how the drug is to be started and tapered off over the course of 6 d. For inflammatory conditions of a joint, the steroid taper will be followed by a course of a nonsteroidal anti-inflammatory

TABLE 5.1 Corticosteroids

Trade Name(s)	Generic Name	Route	Usual Dose/Dosage
Cortef, Solu-Cortef	Hydrocortisone	Intraarticular or intralesional IM or IV PO Rectal	5–75 mg 15–240 mg/d 20–240 mg/d 100 mg/d
Deltasone, Liquid Pred, Orasone	Prednisone	PO	5–60 mg/d
Various	Prednisolone	IM IV Intraarticular or soft tissue PO	4–60 mg 5–60 mg/d
Medrol, Solu-Medrol	Methylprednisolone	IM Intraarticular or soft tissue Dermatological IV PO	80–120 mg 4–80 mg 40–120 mg/wk 10–40 mg 4–48 mg/d
Kenalog, Kenacort, Aristocort	Triamcinolone	IM Intraarticular or intrabursal Intradermal Intralesional or sublesional PO	25–60 mg/d 2.5–40 mg/d 1 mg per site 5–48 mg 8–16 mg/d
Decadron	Dexamethasone	IM Intraarticular or soft tissue PO	4–8 mg 4–16 mg 0.75–9 mg/d

IM = intramuscular; IV = intravenous; PO = oral (per os).

Data from Clinical Pharmacology 2016; Lexicomp Online 2016.

drug, such as ibuprofen or a COX-2 inhibitor. If the condition being treated is exacerbated during the taper, then the dose of steroid will be increased and maintained for a short time before the taper is restarted.

Inhaled Corticosteroids

Intranasal steroids are also used in the treatment of allergic rhinitis or allergies. They include beclomethasone dipropionate (Beconase AQ, Vancenase AQ), flunisolide (Nasalide), fluticasone propionate (Flonase), and mometasone furoate (Nasonex). These steroids are manufactured as intranasal metered-dose sprays, which provide a local anti-inflammatory effect and reduce the effects of environmental allergens through immunosuppressive mechanisms.

Inhaled corticosteroids are used in the treatment of asthma. Beclomethasone dipropionate (Beconase AQ, Vancenase AQ), fluticasone (Flovent), and triamcinolone (Azmacort) are dispensed from metered-dose inhalers (MDIs); the dry powder inhaler ADVAIR DISKUS dispenses a combination of two drugs: fluticasone propionate and salmeterol. Inhaled corticosteroids provide a local anti-inflammatory effect in the airways. They should never be used for acute exacerbations of asthma because they do not cause immediate bronchodilation.

Side Effects

The side effects of corticosteroids depend on the dose and the route of administration. They are minimal with intrasynovial injection, intraarticular injection, intranasal application, inhalation, or short-term therapy. However, tendon ruptures have occurred in patients receiving corticosteroid injections (Maffulli et al. 2013). The Achilles tendon is especially susceptible to this effect (Soriano-Maldonado et al. 2016). Research supports the position that repeated short courses, intranasal corticosteroids, and inhaled corticosteroids may also cause decreased bone density and osteoporosis and increased risk of pneumonia (Bavry et al. 2014; Iannella, Luna, and Waterer 2013; Skoner 2016).

For orally administered short-course tapers, the most common side effects are increased appetite, restlessness, insomnia, fluid retention, gastrointestinal disturbances, and decreased glucose tolerance. Gastrointestinal effects are diminished if doses are taken along with food. Less common but serious effects of corticosteroids are the development of and the impaired healing of peptic ulcers.

In addition, high doses or the prolonged use of corticosteroids to treat systemic inflammatory or autoimmune diseases, such as lupus, multiple sclerosis, or inflammatory bowel syndromes (e.g., Crohn's disease), may produce devastating side effects. These may include changes in physical appearance caused by changes in fat deposition, adrenal suppression, cataracts, or peptic ulcers. Long-term use of corticosteroids causes decreased bone density and osteoporosis (van Vollenhoven et al. 2016).

In the diabetic athlete, corticosteroids, even in short courses, must be used with caution because of their effects on glucose tolerance. Changes in insulin doses or diet may be required in diabetic patients during treatment with corticosteroids.

Corticosteroids, including those administered intranasally, may reduce growth velocity in pediatric patients but have no impact on final adult height (Allen 2002). The growth of pediatric patients receiving corticosteroids should be monitored routinely. In addition, in order to prevent decreases in bone density, children older than 11 yr should receive calcium, 1500 mg/d, and vitamin D, 800 IU/d, throughout the course of treatment with corticosteroids (Skoner 2016).

Repeated intrasynovial or intraarticular injection will not result in any systemic effects but will cause damage to the joint. Intraarticular injections in major weight-bearing joints are not recommended because of the potential softening of joint cartilage. Even after a single injection, if the joint is not allowed proper time to heal, damage may occur. Iontophoresis is a much less invasive way to administer corticosteroids superficially since it uses direct electrical current to introduce ions into the body. Often ionized medications can be introduced through iontophoresis; however, the most common are the corticosteroids in combination with a topical anesthetic such as lidocaine (Rigby et al. 2015). There have been questions whether iontophoresis is as effective as intraarticular injection (Bello and Kuwornu 2014).

Intranasal corticosteroids are generally very well tolerated. The most common side effects are nasal irritation, pharyngeal irritation, and dryness. Similarly, the most common side effects of inhaled corticosteroids are hoarseness, dry mouth, sore throat, and oropharyngeal fungal infections, such as *Candida albicans* or *Aspergillus niger*. After the use of an inhaled corticosteroid, the mouth is always rinsed to prevent oral fungal infections.

Nonsteroidal Anti-Inflammatory Agents

Among the most common medications used in the athletic setting are the NSAIDs (table 5.2). NSAIDs decrease pain, inflammation, and fever (that is, they have an **antipyretic** effect). Many of these drugs are available over the counter, so their use is common.

CLINICAL TIPS

Inhaled Corticosteroids

The anti-inflammatory benefits of inhaled corticosteroids are not realized until after 1 to 4 wk of therapy.

TABLE 5.2 **Nonsteroidal Anti-Inflammatory Drugs (NSAIDs)**

Trade name(s)	Generic name	Usual dose	Maximum dose per day
Advil, Motrin	Ibuprofen	400 mg every 4–6 h	3200 mg
Aleve, Anaprox, Naprosyn	Naproxen	250 mg every 6–8 h	1250 mg
Cataflam, Voltaren	Diclofenac	50 mg 3 times daily	200 mg
Lodine	Etodolac	200–400 mg every 6–8 h	1200 mg
Indocin	Indomethacin	25–50 mg PO or rectally 2 or 3 times daily	200 mg
Orudis, Orudis KT	Ketoprofen	25–50 mg every 6–8 h	300 mg
Toradol	Ketorolac	IV: 30 mg × 1 dose or 30 mg every 6 h IM: 60 mg × 1 dose or 60 mg every 6 h PO: 20 mg initially, then 10 mg every 4–6 h	120 mg 120 mg 40 mg
Mobic	Meloxicam	7.5 mg every day	15 mg
Relafen	Nabumetone	1000–2000 mg every day or twice daily	2000 mg
Daypro	Oxaprozin	1200 mg every day	1800 mg
Feldene	Piroxicam	20 mg every day or twice daily	40 mg
Celebrex	Celecoxib	100–200 mg twice daily	400 mg
Bextra*	Valdecoxib	10–20 mg once or twice daily	40 mg
Vioxx*	Rofecoxib	12.5–50 mg every day	N/A

IM = intramuscular; IV = intravenous; N/A = not applicable; PO = oral (*per os*).

*Bextra and Vioxx were taken off the U.S. market in 2005.

Data from Clinical Pharmacology 2016; Lexicomp Online 2016.

Drugs in this class exert their pharmacological effects through the inhibition of prostaglandin synthesis. The NSAIDs inactivate the COX-1 and COX-2 enzymes and the prostaglandin G/H synthase 1 and 2 enzymes that catalyze the formation of prostaglandins from arachidonic acid (figure 5.1). The COX-2 inhibitors (e.g., celecoxib [Celebrex], valdecoxib [Bextra]) are selective for the COX-2 enzyme. NSAIDs are given primarily by the oral route, although ketorolac (Toradol) may be given orally (PO), IM, or IV. Lower doses are adequate for treating pain and fever (200 to 400 mg of ibuprofen or 5 to 10 mg/kg/dose in children 6 months to 12 years of age), whereas higher doses are required for anti-inflammatory effects (Lexicomp Online 2016). The best results in inflammatory conditions are obtained when scheduled doses of 600 to 800 mg every 6 to 8 h around the clock are given for several weeks (Dieu-Donne et al. 2016).

Side Effects

The major side effects of NSAIDs are gastrointestinal and include dyspepsia, heartburn, nausea, vomiting, abdominal pain, peptic ulcer, and gastrointestinal bleeding. Prostaglandins stimulate the secretion of a protective mucosal layer in the gastrointestinal tract.

Inhibition of these prostaglandins leads to a breakdown in this mucosal layer, which leads to ulceration.

Aspirin, when administered without an enteric coating, buffers, or antacids, causes increased entry of acid into the gastric mucosa, leading to cellular damage at the site of dissolution. As mentioned previously, enteric-coated aspirin will undergo dissolution in the small intestine, therefore avoiding the direct effect on the gastric lining. The administration of NSAIDs with food or milk will minimize gastrointestinal adverse effects (Kanbayashi and Konishi 2015). Coadministration of aspirin and other NSAIDs along with corticosteroids increases the risk of gastrointestinal lesions. People who drink alcohol or alcoholics who are taking aspirin or NSAIDs are at higher risk of upper gastrointestinal bleeding, a risk that is elevated by increased alcohol consumption (Pelletier et al. 2016).

Aspirin, salicylates, and to a much lesser extent NSAIDs, have hematological effects that must be considered in the athlete. Aspirin inhibits platelet aggregation and decreases hepatic synthesis of blood coagulation factors. At normal doses of up to 6 g/d, aspirin rarely increases **prothrombin time (PT)**, the time it takes blood to clot, by more than 2 to 3 s. Higher doses, fever, and increased metabolic rate may cause larger increases in PT (Hamilton et al. 2015). For athletes in contact sports, (Hamilton et al. 2015), especially where the likelihood of head trauma is high, aspirin may not be a good ther-

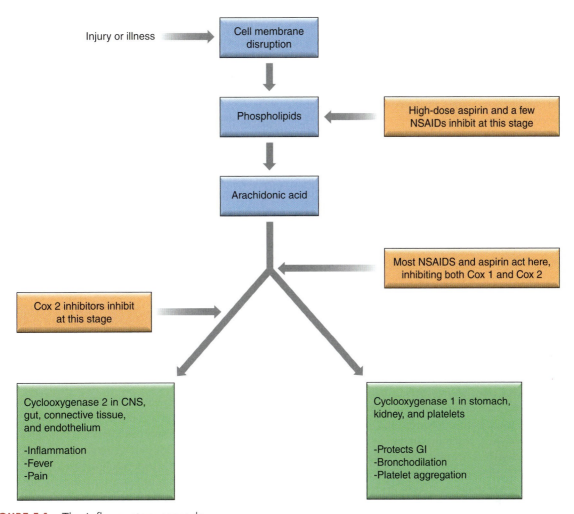

FIGURE 5.1   The inflammatory cascade.

apeutic choice. Head trauma occurring in an athlete in an anticoagulated state might increase the risk or extent of intracranial bleeding. Research is mixed on whether aspirin causes increased intracranial bleeding following head trauma for the patient who is receiving low-dose aspirin therapy.

Other NSAIDs, such as ibuprofen, do inhibit platelet aggregation but to a lesser extent than aspirin. This has raised some concern that NSAIDs not be used by athletes in sports that may put them at risk for head trauma. Physicians have varying views on this subject. Athletic trainers must know and uphold the views of the team physicians on this subject.

CLINICAL TIPS
Anti-Inflammatory Agents
It will typically take 2 wk for the maximum anti-inflammatory response to occur, although some decrease of inflammation will occur after 2 to 7 d.

The renal effects of NSAIDs are also of concern. Prostaglandins play a role in maintaining renal perfusion in people with certain renal conditions (e.g., decreased extracellular fluid depletion). An athlete receiving long-term NSAID therapy who becomes dehydrated may be at risk for renal impairment and needs to be monitored for symptoms of azotemia, such as malaise, fatigue, or loss of appetite.

Other adverse effects of NSAIDs include rashes, dermatitis, photosensitivity (use sun block), dizziness, headache, nervousness, fatigue, drowsiness, fluid retention, anaphylaxis, bronchospasm, tinnitus, and visual disturbances.

Previously the safety of the COX-2 NSAIDs had been questioned with the voluntary recall of rofecoxib (Vioxx), which was shown to increase the risk of cardiovascular events. Studies involving the COX-2 inhibitor celecoxib (Celebrex) have had conflicting results. Many clinical reviews have determined that there is at least a moderately increased risk of cardiovascular events associated with COX-2 inhibitors (Bavry et al. 2014; Bhosale et al.

2015; Cannon and Cannon 2012). The athletic trainer and general consumer must remember that along with benefits, potential adverse effects occur with any drug. Individual patient needs and risk factors must be considered to make the best drug therapy choices. The lowest possible effective dose should always be used to minimize the chance of adverse drug events.

Contraindications

NSAIDs are contraindicated for those who have had a previous hypersensitivity reaction or other severe allergic reaction to aspirin or any other NSAID and for those who have experienced bronchospasm, angioedema, or nasal polyps when taking aspirin or other NSAIDs. Extreme caution is needed when giving aspirin or other NSAIDs to individuals with a history of gastrointestinal lesions (such as peptic ulcer), athletes who have sickle cell anemia, and those taking blood thinners such as enoxaparin (Lovenox) or warfarin (Coumadin) (Díaz-González and Sánchez-Madrid 2015).

Interactions

Because many NSAIDs are readily available over the counter, athletes may be tempted to take them with acetaminophen (Tscholl et al. 2015). These two drugs have different mechanisms of action, and therefore it is safe to combine them if the maximum dosage of over-the-counter NSAIDs is not providing enough analgesia. However, better prescription medications are probably available, and if the athlete's discomfort is not relieved with over-the-counter medications, the team physician should be consulted about the condition. The athletic trainer must also teach athletes that many products contain the same active ingredients, and therefore care must be taken when combining over-the-counter medications of any kind (Ussai et al. 2015).

Narcotic Analgesics

Narcotic analgesics affect pain by stimulating the opiate receptors (table 5.3). Some of these agents are derived from opium, such as morphine, codeine, and oxycodone. Others, including meperidine (Demerol), sufentanil, and fentanyl, are synthetic opiate agonists that share structural similarities. A third group of related opiate agonists includes methadone.

These agents stimulate opiate receptors, causing analgesia, sedation, and euphoria. The analgesia is produced not by an actual decrease in the level of pain but rather by altering the way that pain is perceived. Opiate agonists cause dissociation from the pain. A person who takes an opiate agonist still has pain but does not care about it. Because these drugs also cause a feeling of euphoria, there is significant potential for addiction.

Opiates are found in combination with aspirin, ibuprofen, or most commonly acetaminophen. This is very effective because the aspirin and ibuprofen decrease the production of pain mediators (e.g., prostaglandins), and the opiate agonist minimizes the perception of pain.

Side Effects

The side effects of opiate agonists are constipation, physical dependence or addiction, sedation, drowsiness, dry mouth, blurred vision, urinary retention, nausea, vomiting, histamine release, respiratory depression, and allergic reactions. The athlete taking these medications must avoid alcohol and use caution if taking other drugs that cause CNS sedation. These sedating effects are additive and can be very dangerous. Athletes taking opiate agonists also should avoid operating any machinery that could be dangerous, such as an automobile (Lexicomp Online 2016). Obviously the athlete who is in enough pain to warrant narcotic analgesics should not participate in sports. The use of patient-controlled infusion pumps allows the hospitalized patient to self-administer the narcotic analgesic as needed to control pain.

To minimize opiate agonists' constipating effects, fluid and fiber intake can be increased. It may be necessary for the athlete to take a stool softener such as docusate sodium (Colace) to alleviate the constipation. To minimize nausea and vomiting, opiate agonists are taken with food rather than on an empty stomach.

Opiate agonists can also cause the release of histamine, which may result in mild to severe itching, especially in the facial area. This itching can be alleviated by antihistamines, such as diphenhydramine (Benadryl); again, caution is needed because of the additional sedative effects. The itching is sometimes confused with an allergic reaction, but itching alone in the absence of a rash or hives is an irritating but harmless side effect. An allergic reaction to opiate agonists will manifest itself through hives, difficulty breathing, and facial or tongue swelling. Allergic reactions to opiates are a contraindication to prescribing these medications. There will be cross-allergenicity between those agents sharing structural similarities (e.g., codeine and morphine or methadone

> ## 🚩 RED FLAGS FOR NARCOTIC ANALGESICS
>
> - Alcohol and other sedating drugs must be avoided when taking narcotic analgesics because their additive effects may be dangerous.
> - Athletes should not operate motor vehicles while taking narcotic analgesics.

TABLE 5.3 Narcotic Analgesics

Trade name(s) (opioid, ASA, or APAP)	Combination	Dosage
Percodan, Roxiprin (4.88/325 mg)	Oxycodone with aspirin	1 every 6 h
Vicoprofen (7.5/200 mg)	Hydrocodone with ibuprofen	1 every 4–6 h up to 5 times/d
Tylox (5/500 mg)	Oxycodone with acetaminophen	1 every 6 h*
Roxicet (5/325, 5/500 mg)	Oxycodone with acetaminophen	1 every 6 h*
Endocet (5/325, 7.5/325, 7.5/500, 10/325, 10/650 mg)	Oxycodone with acetaminophen	1 every 6 h*
Percocet (2.5/325, 5/325, 7.5/325, 7.5/500, 10/325, 10/650 mg)	Oxycodone with acetaminophen	1 every 6 h*
Vicodin (5/500, Vicodin ES, 7.5/750, Vicodin HP 10/660 mg)	Hydrocodone with acetaminophen	1–2 tablets every 4–6 h*†
Lorcet (HD 5/500, Lorcet 7.5/650, Lorcet Plus 10/650 mg)	Hydrocodone with acetaminophen	1–2 tablets every 4–6 h*†
Lortab (2.5/500, 5/500, 7.5/500, 10/500 mg)	Hydrocodone with acetaminophen	1–2 tablets every 4–6 h*†
Anexsia (5/325, 5/500, 7.5/325, 7.5/650, 10/660 mg)	Hydrocodone with acetaminophen	1–2 tablets every 4–6 h*†
Norco (5/325, 7.5/325, 10/325 mg)	Hydrocodone with acetaminophen	1–2 tablets every 4–6 h*†
Zydone (5/400, 7.5/400, 10/400 mg)	Hydrocodone with acetaminophen	1–2 tablets every 4–6 h*†
Maxidone (10/750 mg)	Hydrocodone with acetaminophen	1–2 tablets every 4–6 h*†
Darvocet (50/325, 100/650 mg)	Propoxyphene‡ with acetaminophen	1–2 tablets every 4 h*
MSIR (15, 30 mg), MS	Morphine sulfate	PO: 5–30 mg every 4 h
Contin, Avinza, Kadian	Morphine sulfate	200 mg 30 mg/24 h (maximum, 1600 mg) SC/IM, 10 mg every 4 h IV, 2–10 mg/70 kg over 4–5 min
Tylenol with codeine (15/300, 30/300, 60/300 mg)	Codeine with acetaminophen	1/2–4 every 4 h*
Dolophine, Methadose	Methadone	2.5–10 mg IM, SC, or PO every 3–4 h
Demerol	Meperidine	50–150 mg IM, SC, or PO every 3–4 h

APAP = acetaminophen; ASA = aspirin; IM = intramuscular; IV = intravenous; PO = oral (per os); SC = subcutaneous.

*Daily dose of acetaminophen should not exceed 4000 mg.

†Daily dose of hydrocodone should not exceed 60 mg.

‡Daily dose of propoxyphene should not exceed 600 mg. The FDA has new requirements for labeling of propoxyphene-containing products to address the risk of overdose and the potential for cardiovascular events, including life-threatening arrhythmias associated with the use of propoxyphene products (www.fda.gov/Safety/MedWatch/SafetyInformation; accessed May 2010).

Data from Clinical Pharmacology 2016; Lexicomp Online 2016.

and propoxyphene). If an athlete reports an allergy to opiates, the athletic trainer must determine whether or not the reaction is just itching caused by histamine release.

Narcotic analgesics have a very high potential for misuse. The use of tramadol in individuals with a history of dependence on opioids may cause this dependence to reemerge. Although the athletic trainer must be alert for signs of dependence, such as drug-seeking behavior, the vast majority of those who take opioids for legitimate pain never experience a physical dependence.

Local Anesthetics

Local anesthetics produce their effects by reversibly blocking nerve conduction near the site of administration (table 5.4). Blocked nerve conduction is caused by a decrease in the permeability of the nerve cell membrane to sodium ions. Small nerve fibers (e.g., C- and A-delta) are affected more than large fibers (e.g., A-α and A-β). Autonomic activity is affected first, then loss of sensory

functions, and finally loss of motor activity. The anesthetic effects regress in the reverse order.

Although allergic reactions occur rarely, there is cross-allergenicity between agents having the same type of linkage. There is no cross-allergenicity between agents having different linkages. Therefore, a person who is allergic to procaine (Novocain) will also be allergic to benzocaine but will not be allergic to lidocaine.

As the name implies, local anesthetics are used to produce a temporary, localized loss of sensory function. In some cases, these drugs may be used for a therapeutic effect in treating pain. In other cases, the anesthetic effect is desired for dental and surgical procedures or sutures. Local anesthetics may be administered in several ways. Topical administration, ophthalmic administration, infiltration, and nerve block are the most common methods of administration seen by the athletic trainer.

Infiltration anesthesia involves the injection of the local anesthetic intradermally, subcutaneously, or submucosally across the nerves that supply the area being anesthetized. Nerve block is the injection of the anesthetic agent into or around the nerve trunks or ganglia that supply the area being anesthetized. Local anesthetics for injection will often be combined with vasoconstrictors, usually epinephrine, to decrease the systemic absorption of the anesthetic and to decrease bleeding. Epinephrine is especially useful when the athlete needs sutures because it helps control bleeding, but it is contraindicated in areas that have poor blood supply, such as the tips of the fingers or the nose (Clinical Pharmacology 2016).

Topically administered agents, such as lidocaine or EMLA cream, may be used to numb the skin before certain procedures. Benzocaine and dibucaine are used

> ### CLINICAL TIPS
>
> ## Narcotic Analgesics
>
> Almost all narcotic analgesics are banned by the U.S. Anti-Doping Agency (USADA) and the National Collegiate Athletic Association (NCAA). See www.usada.org for the latest information (National Collegiate Athletic Association 2015; United States Anti-Doping Agency 2015; World Anti-Doping Agency [WADA] 2016).

TABLE 5.4   Local Anesthetics

Type	Trade name(s)	Generic name	Route of administration	Duration of action
Ester	Americaine, Ora-Jel	Benzocaine	Topical	Short (oral gels have longer duration)
	Nesacaine	Chloroprocaine	Parenteral	Short
	Novocain	Cocaine	Topical	Short
	Alcaine, AK-Taine	Procaine	Parenteral	Short
	Pontocaine	Proparacaine	Topical	Short
	Cetacaine	Tetracaine	Parenteral, topical	Long
		Tetracaine, benzocaine	Topical	Long
Amide	Marcaine, Sensorcaine	Bupivacaine	Parenteral	Long
	Nupercainal	Dibucaine	Topical	Long
	Duranest	Etidocaine	Parenteral	Long
	Chirocaine	Levobupivacaine	Parenteral	Long
	Xylocaine	Lidocaine	Parenteral, topical	Intermediate
	Carbocaine, Polocaine	Mepivacaine	Parenteral	Intermediate
	Citanest	Prilocaine	Parenteral, topical	Intermediate
	EMLA	Lidocaine, prilocaine	Topical	Intermediate

Data from Clinical Pharmacology 2016; Lexicomp Online 2016.

in topical preparations for the relief of sunburn pain. Benzocaine is also found in otic preparations for the relief of ear pain associated with otitis. Other topical anesthetics, such as benzocaine-containing oral gels or throat lozenges, are formulated for application to the oral mucosa to relieve minor irritations of the mouth or throat. These agents are for short-term use only. Any persistent pain in the ears, mouth, or throat should be evaluated by a physician.

Proparacaine and tetracaine are examples of topical ophthalmic anesthetic agents. Topical anesthetics should be used in the eye only to desensitize or anesthetize the eye before ophthalmic procedures such as corneal scraping or foreign body removal. They should never be used for pain control because prolonged use of topical ophthalmic anesthetics has been associated with severe keratitis and permanent corneal opacity and scarring.

Side Effects

The adverse effects associated with local anesthetics vary with the site of application. The most common adverse effect is a burning or stinging sensation associated with an application or injection. For the injected agents, adverse reactions usually result from high concentrations of the local anesthetic in the blood, either from inadvertent IV injection or from high doses (Reurink et al. 2014). These adverse reactions will affect the central nervous and cardiovascular systems. When anesthetic agents are combined with epinephrine, adverse effects of the epinephrine must be considered. Table 5.5 lists side effects of local

TABLE 5.5 Side Effects of Local Anesthetics

System	Effect
CNS (initial)	Anxiety Restlessness Confusion Tremors Seizures
CNS (delayed)	Drowsiness Respiratory arrest
Cardiovascular	Bradycardia Cardiac arrhythmias Hypotension Cardiovascular collapse Cardiac arrest
Integumentary	Vasoconstriction occurs when coupled with epinephrine; problematic when used as local anesthetic in fingers, toes, ears, and tip of nose

CNS = central nervous system.

anesthetics. Anxiety, palpitation, dizziness, headache, restlessness, tremors, tachycardia, and hypertension may result from high blood levels of epinephrine.

The use of local anesthetics often presents difficult decisions for the team physician. Athletes may want to receive anesthetics so they can participate; however, such use must be strictly monitored to prevent further harm to athletes (Stevens et al. 2010). Local anesthetics should only be administered when medically justifiable. The risks of participation need to be fully explained to the athlete and only allowed when there is no increased chance for injury in the anesthetized body part.

Antibiotics

Antibiotics are drugs used to treat bacterial infections. The discussion of antibiotic medications or antimicrobial therapy is a very broad and complex topic. Although the coverage in this text is neither comprehensive nor exhaustive, it does include the most commonly used agents that will be encountered by the athletic trainer.

Antibiotics may be classified in many different ways on the basis of their chemical structure, mechanism of action, or the spectrum of bacteria for which they are used. The four primary mechanisms of action are disruption of the cell wall, disruption of cytoplasmic metabolism, disruption of deoxyribonucleic acid (DNA) replication, and disruption of protein synthesis. Tables for each class of antibiotic, along with common indications, dosages, and adverse reactions, are listed within each section that follows.

Antibiotics that disrupt cell wall synthesis are **bactericidal**. They bind to enzymes in the cytoplasmic membrane that are essential to cell wall synthesis. β-lactam antibiotics (cephalosporins, penicillins, carbapenems, vancomycin) act through this mechanism. Polymyxin B, which is found in many topical antibiotic creams and ointments, exerts its bactericidal effect through cell wall disruption.

A few antibiotics exert their effect by interfering with cellular metabolism. Sulfonamides, such as sulfamethoxazole, a component of co-trimoxazole (Bactrim, Septra), interfere with the early stages of folic acid production in organisms that synthesize their own folic acid.

Antibiotics that disrupt protein synthesis do so by binding irreversibly to ribosomal subunits. Aminoglycosides, macrolides, clindamycin, and tetracyclines fall into this category. Aminoglycosides are bactericidal. Macrolides and tetracyclines are **bacteriostatic**.

The physician determines which antibiotic is appropriate to use in a particular situation, ideally on the basis of a culture of body fluids or tissues from the infected area. For practical reasons, culture is reserved for those situations when the infection is serious or resistant to empirical therapy. In most cases, choosing an antibiotic empirically will suffice.

Patient age, history of allergic reactions, and adverse reactions to previous antibiotic therapy must be considered. Antibiotics with a broad spectrum of action are reserved for infections where resistant organisms or multiple organisms may be the cause of the infection. Antibiotics must be used appropriately to achieve complete eradication of the infecting organisms. Incomplete courses of antibiotic therapy, inappropriate use of broad-spectrum antibiotics, and the use of antibiotics to treat viral infections all contribute to bacterial resistance.

If antibiotic therapy is discontinued prematurely, then not only is there a chance the infection will reoccur but also the infecting organisms are likely to show resistance to the antibiotic used. This resistance arises because the bacteria most susceptible to the antibiotic will be eradicated first, while the bacteria with some resistance to the antibiotic will linger for longer; the latter organisms will be those that cause a recurrence of the infection.

When antibiotic therapy is initiated unnecessarily (e.g., to treat viral infections), then bacteria in the body are being exposed to antibiotics unnecessarily. Exposure of bacteria to any antibiotic gives the organism an opportunity to develop adaptive resistance mechanisms to the agent. The more often that bacteria are exposed to an antimicrobial agent, the greater the likelihood that resistance will develop. Antibiotic use must be minimized in order to prevent the development of resistant bacteria.

The use of broad-spectrum antibiotics is reserved for those situations in which the infecting bacteria have exhibited resistance to other antimicrobials either through culture results or treatment failure. Broad-spectrum antibiotics are the most powerful tools in the antimicrobial arsenal. They should be used only when no other agents will work.

Side Effects

Adverse reactions associated with antibiotics include nausea, vomiting, diarrhea, and abdominal pain (table 5.6). Specific side effects for various antibiotics are also discussed individually with common uses and dosages. A more serious gastrointestinal adverse effect associated with the use of certain antibiotics is antibiotic-associated pseudomembranous colitis and diarrhea. The seriousness of this infection ranges from mild to life threatening (Ferri 2016). Pseudomembranous colitis may respond to discontinuation of the antibiotic or may require additional antibiotic therapy and supportive treatment to resolve.

Antibiotic therapy commonly contributes to the overgrowth of nonsusceptible bacteria or fungi, often described as a superinfection. It is common for women taking antibiotics to develop vaginal fungal infections as a result of the disruption of normal vaginal flora. The physician may choose to prescribe an antifungal agent for use as needed whenever antibiotic therapy is prescribed in women who commonly experience such infections.

Rashes, pruritus, urticaria, and other dermatological reactions are also common with various antibiotics. These rashes may or may not be associated with a hypersensitivity or allergic reaction. Amoxicillin often causes rashes in the presence of certain viral infections, but these rashes are not due to an allergic reaction to the drug. A very serious, sometimes fatal dermatological reaction

TABLE 5.6   **Common Adverse Effects of Antibiotics**

Gastrointestinal	Dermatological	Central nervous system	Systemic	Gynecological	Cardiovascular	Metabolic
Nausea	Rash	Headache	Fever	Vaginal candidiasis	Tachycardia	Hepatic dysfunction
Vomiting	Pruritus	Behavioral changes	Chills	Decreased effectiveness of birth control pills	Hypotension	
Diarrhea	Urticaria	Hallucinations	Arthralgia			
Abdominal pain		Insomnia	Lymphade-nopathy			
Cramping		Tremor				
Heartburn		Vertigo				
Anorexia		Tinnitus				

Data from Clinical Pharmacology 2016; Lexicomp Online 2016.

to antibiotics is **Stevens-Johnson syndrome**, which is a severe form of erythema multiforme that includes involvement of the oronasal mucosa, eyes, and viscera; malaise; headache; fever; and arthralgia (Ferri 2016).

Aminoglycosides

Aminoglycoside antibiotics are used primarily via the IV, topical, and ophthalmic routes (table 5.7). They are active against aerobic gram-negative and aerobic gram-positive bacteria. The athletic trainer will see these drugs used most often for the treatment of eye infections and some-

times for skin infections. When used for eye infections, the most common adverse effects are transient burning or stinging.

Macrolides

Macrolide antibiotics are administered primarily via the PO, IV, and topical routes. Athletic trainers will see these drugs used most often as oral preparations for the treatment of infection. Some athletes may be using erythromycin topical preparations (A/T/S, Benzamycin) for the treatment of acne.

TABLE 5.7   **Aminoglycosides**

Medication	Common indication(s)	Usual adult dosage	Adverse reactions
Gentamicin (Garamycin) 0.3% ophthalmic ointment 0.3% ophthalmic solution 0.1% topical cream 0.1% topical ointment	Ocular bacterial infections Dermatological infections	Ointment: 1/2 in. to affected eye(s), 2–3 times daily Solution: 1–2 drops into affected eye(s) every 4 h Topical cream and ointment should be applied 3–4 times daily to affected area(s)	Ointment: stinging, blurred vision Solution: stinging
Tobramycin (Nebcin, Tobrex) 0.3% ophthalmic ointment 0.3% ophthalmic solution	Ocular bacterial infections Dermatological infections	Ointment: 1/2 in. to affected eye(s), 2–3 times daily Solution: 1–2 drops into affected eye(s) every 4 h	Ointment: stinging, blurred vision, hypersensitivity (tearing, itching, edema, conjunctival erythema) Solution: stinging, hypersensitivity (tearing, itching, edema, conjunctival erythema)

Data from Clinical Pharmacology 2016; Lexicomp Online 2016.

Erythromycin is used in the treatment of several sexually transmitted diseases, Lyme disease, diphtheria, pertussis, Legionnaire's disease, and penicillin-sensitive infections in individuals with penicillin allergy. Clarithromycin (Biaxin) is used in the treatment of upper and lower respiratory tract infections, skin and skin structure infections, otitis media, *Helicobacter pylori* infections associated with peptic ulcer disease, pharyngitis, tonsillitis, and Lyme disease (Lexicomp Online 2016). Azithromycin (Zithromax) is used in the treatment of mild to moderate upper and lower respiratory tract infections, uncomplicated skin and skin structure infections, sexually transmitted diseases, acute otitis media, pharyngitis, tonsillitis, and pelvic inflammatory disease. The major advantage of azithromycin over other antibiotics is its once-daily dosage frequency and 5 d duration of therapy. Several sexually transmitted diseases may be treated with a single, 1 g dose of azithromycin (Clinical Pharmacology 2016).

Table 5.8 gives the most common adverse effects of macrolides. Less common are heartburn, anorexia, melena, pruritus ani, and reversible mild acute pancreatitis. Prolonged or repeated erythromycin therapy has been associated with pseudomembranous colitis. These adverse gastrointestinal effects occur less often with clarithromycin and azithromycin than with erythromycin.

TABLE 5.8 **Macrolides**

Medication	Common indication(s)	Usual adult dosage	Adverse reactions
Erythromycin (E-mycin, Erythrocin)	Sexually transmitted diseases Lyme disease Diphtheria, pertussis Legionnaire's disease Penicillin-sensitive infections in individuals with penicillin allergy	250 mg PO 4 times daily 333 mg PO 3 times daily 500 mg PO 2 times daily	Nausea, vomiting, diarrhea, abdominal pain, cramping, stomatitis, heartburn, anorexia, melena, pruritus ani, reversible mild acute pancreatitis, pseudomembranous colitis Hepatic dysfunction, reversible cholestatic hepatitis (estolate) Mild allergic reaction: rash, urticaria
Clarithromycin (Biaxin)	Upper and lower respiratory tract infections Skin and skin structure infections Otitis media *Helicobacter pylori* infections (peptic ulcer) Pharyngitis, tonsillitis Lyme disease	250–500 mg PO 2 times daily	Nausea, vomiting, diarrhea, abdominal pain, cramping, stomatitis, heartburn, anorexia, melena, pruritus ani, reversible mild acute pancreatitis, pseudomembranous colitis Mild allergic reaction: rash, urticaria Abnormal taste, headache, behavioral changes, hallucinations, insomnia, tinnitus, tremor, vertigo
Azithromycin (Zithromax)	Mild to moderate upper and lower respiratory tract infections Uncomplicated skin and skin structure infections Sexually transmitted diseases Acute otitis media Pharyngitis, tonsillitis Pelvic inflammatory disease	500 mg on the first day of treatment followed by 250 mg daily for 4 d A single 1 g dose may be used in the treatment of sexually transmitted diseases	Nausea, vomiting, diarrhea, abdominal pain, cramping, stomatitis, heartburn, anorexia, melena, pruritus ani, reversible mild acute pancreatitis, pseudomembranous colitis

PO = oral (*per os*).

Data from Clinical Pharmacology 2016; Lexicomp Online 2016.

Azithromycin does interact with aluminum- and magnesium-containing antacids, which decrease the rate of absorption of azithromycin.

Erythromycin and clarithromycin also have a significant interaction with warfarin (similar to heparin). Patients stabilized on warfarin have experienced prolonged prothrombin time and bleeding when erythromycin or clarithromycin therapy was initiated. Prothrombin time needs to be monitored closely in patients receiving warfarin and one of these macrolides simultaneously. Hepatic dysfunction may occur in patients receiving erythromycin. Erythromycin estolate can cause hepatotoxicity or reversible cholestatic hepatitis in adults who have received the drug for 10 d or longer. The estolate salt of erythromycin should not be used in adults.

Penicillins

Penicillins may be administered by PO, IM, or IV routes (table 5.9). These drugs were the magic bullet against bacterial infection in the early 20th century but can be rendered ineffective by some enzymes. The athletic trainer most often will see these agents being given via the PO route. The penicillins that will be addressed here are the orally administered agents penicillin V, dicloxacillin, ampicillin, and amoxicillin. Penicillin V is classified as a natural penicillin exhibiting activity against *Strepto-*

TABLE 5.9 **Penicillins**

Medication	Common indication(s)	Usual adult dosage	Adverse reactions
Natural penicillins (penicillin VK)	Upper and lower respiratory tract infections	250–500 mg every 6 h for 7–14 d	Mild to severe allergic reactions: rash, urticaria, pruritus, Stevens-Johnson syndrome, fever, chills, malaise, arthralgia, myalgia, lymphadenopathy, splenomegaly, angioedema, anaphylaxis Gastrointestinal disturbances: nausea, vomiting, diarrhea
Aminopenicillins (ampicillin)	Upper and lower respiratory tract infections Gastrointestinal tract infections Skin and skin structure infections, genitourinary tract infections Otitis media	250–500 mg PO every 6 h	Same as for the natural penicillins Mild, nonallergic maculopapular rash (especially in viral infection) Candidal or bacterial superinfections
Aminopenicillins (amoxicillin)	Upper and lower respiratory tract infections Gastrointestinal tract infections Skin and skin structure infections, genitourinary tract infections Otitis media	250–500 mg PO every 8 h	Same as for the natural penicillins Mild, nonallergic maculopapular rash (especially in viral infection) Candidal or bacterial superinfections
Penicillinase-resistant penicillins (dicloxacillin)	Skin and skin structure infections Acute or chronic osteomyelitis	250–500 mg PO every 6 h for at least 14 d Osteomyelitis may require up to 2 mo of oral therapy after initial course of therapy with an IV penicillinase-resistant penicillin	Same as for the natural penicillins Prolonged therapy: hematological, renal, and hepatic adverse events

PO = oral (*per os*).

Data from Clinical Pharmacology 2016; Lexicomp Online 2016.

coccus pneumoniae; group A, B, C, G, H, K, L, and M streptococci; nonenterococcal group D streptococci; and many other bacteria as well.

Penicillin V is used principally for the treatment of upper and lower respiratory tract infections and skin and skin structure infections caused by susceptible organisms (e.g., group A β-hemolytic streptococci) and Lyme disease. It may also be used for the treatment of upper and lower respiratory tract infections caused by susceptible strains of *Streptococcus pneumoniae*. The prevalence of *Streptococcus pneumoniae* resistance to penicillin ranges between 24% and 28% (ASHP 2004). For this reason, the prevalence and pattern of penicillin resistance of *Streptococcus pneumoniae* in the local community must be considered before using penicillin for empirical therapy. Penicillin G or some other form of IM penicillin may be used in the treatment of sexually transmitted diseases caused by susceptible organisms such as syphilis.

The most common adverse reaction to penicillins is an allergic reaction ranging from mild to severe (see table 5.9). The most serious reaction to penicillins, occurring in 0.05% of people receiving the drug, is anaphylaxis, which is fatal in 5% to 10% of cases. Anaphylactic reactions usually occur within 30 min of administration of the drug (Clinical Pharmacology 2016).

A highly significant drug interaction with penicillins and many other antibiotics is an interaction with oral contraceptive agents. The use of penicillins and many other antibiotics concomitantly with estrogen-containing oral contraceptives may decrease the efficacy of the contraceptive and increase the incidence of breakthrough bleeding.

Dicloxacillin is classified as penicillinase-resistant penicillin. It is used mainly in the treatment of skin and skin structure infections, such as cellulitis, that are caused by staphylococci. Dicloxacillin may also be used in the treatment of acute or chronic osteomyelitis after an initial course of IV therapy with penicillinase-resistant penicillin (e.g., nafcillin).

The adverse reactions associated with the use of dicloxacillin are the same as for the natural penicillins. Prolonged therapy with penicillinase-resistant penicillins,

such as therapy for osteomyelitis, has been associated with adverse hematological, renal, and hepatic events.

Amoxicillin and ampicillin are classified as aminopenicillins. Aminopenicillins have the same spectrum of antimicrobial activity as the natural penicillins with enhanced activity against gram-negative bacteria. Aminopenicillins are used in the treatment of upper and lower respiratory tract infections, gastrointestinal tract infections, skin and skin structure infections, genitourinary tract infections, and otitis media caused by susceptible organisms.

The aminopenicillins exhibit the same adverse reactions as the natural penicillins (see table 5.9). In addition to hypersensitivity reactions, ampicillin and amoxicillin often cause a mild maculopapular rash, more intense at pressure areas (e.g., knees, elbows), that resolves in 1 to 2 wk even if drug therapy continues. This rash, which is not an allergic reaction, occurs more often when aminopenicillins are used in patients with viral disease and will resolve in 1 to 7 d if the drug is discontinued. This amoxicillin rash must be differentiated from a true allergic reaction, and those experiencing it must not be labeled as penicillin allergic. Prolonged therapy with aminopenicillins needs to be accompanied by periodic monitoring of renal, hepatic, and hematological function. The drug interactions of the aminopenicillins are the same as those for the natural penicillins.

Cephalosporins

Cephalosporin antibiotics may be administered by PO, IV, or IM routes. The agents in this class that will be discussed are cephalexin (Keflex), cefadroxil (Duricef), cefuroxime (Ceftin), cefdinir (Omnicef), and cefixime (Suprax) (table 5.10).

Cefadroxil (Duricef) and cephalexin (Keflex) are classified as first-generation cephalosporins. First-generation cephalosporins are active against gram-positive cocci including *Staphylococcus aureus, Staphylococcus epidermidis*, group A β-hemolytic streptococci, group B streptococci, and *Streptococcus pneumoniae*. Cefadroxil and cephalexin are used in the treatment of mild to moderate respiratory tract infections, skin and skin structure infections, acute bacterial otitis, pharyngitis, and tonsillitis caused by susceptible bacteria. They also are used in the treatment of mild to moderate urinary tract infections caused by susceptible gram-negative organisms.

Cefuroxime (Ceftin) is classified as a second-generation cephalosporin and is used in the treatment of mild to moderate respiratory tract infections caused by susceptible bacteria, acute otitis media, uncomplicated urinary tract infections, uncomplicated gonorrhea, and early Lyme disease.

Cephalosporins should be used with caution in patients with a history of penicillin hypersensitivity because there is a partial cross-allergenicity between penicillins and

RED FLAGS FOR CONTRACEPTIVES

Many antibiotics interact with oral contraceptives and decrease the efficacy of the contraceptive. This can increase the incidence of breakthrough bleeding. The female athlete taking oral contraceptives and receiving antibiotic therapy should use a second form of birth control during sexual intercourse to prevent pregnancy.

TABLE 5.10 **Cephalosporins**

Medication	Common indication(s)	Usual adult dosage	Adverse reactions
First Generation			
Cephalexin (Keflex)	Mild to moderate respiratory tract infections Skin and skin structure infections Acute bacterial otitis Pharyngitis, tonsillitis Mild to moderate urinary tract infections	250–500 mg every 6 h Uncomplicated urinary tract infections: 500 mg every 12 h	Gastrointestinal reactions (including pseudomembranous colitis) Headache Hypersensitivity reactions: rash, urticaria, pruritus, fever, chills, arthralgia, edema, hypotension, Stevens-Johnson syndrome, and rarely anaphylaxis Renal dysfunction, nephropathy, increases in serum hepatic enzyme concentrations, increased serum bilirubin, hepatic dysfunction, dizziness, malaise, fatigue, cough, rhinitis, superinfections
Cefadroxil (Duricef)	Mild to moderate respiratory tract infections Skin and skin structure infections Acute bacterial colitis Pharyngitis, tonsillitis Mild to moderate urinary tract infections	500 mg twice daily Uncomplicated urinary tract infections: 1 or 2 g single dose Other urinary tract infections: 1 g twice daily	Same as above
Second Generation			
Cefuroxime (Ceftin)	Mild to moderate respiratory tract infections Acute otitis media Uncomplicated UTIs Uncomplicated gonorrhea Early Lyme disease	250–500 mg every 12 h Uncomplicated UTIs: 125–250 mg every 12 h Uncomplicated urethral, endocervical, or rectal gonorrhea: single 1 g dose	Same as above Decreased hemoglobin and hematocrit in 10% of individuals
Third Generation			
Cefdinir (Omnicef)	Mild to moderate upper and lower respiratory tract infections Acute otitis media Streptococcal pharyngitis and tonsillitis Uncomplicated skin and skin structure infections	600 mg once daily or 300 mg twice daily	Gastrointestinal reactions (including pseudomembranous colitis) Headache Hypersensitivity reactions: rash, urticaria, pruritus, fever, chills, arthralgia, edema, hypotension, Stevens-Johnson syndrome, and rarely anaphylaxis Renal dysfunction, nephropathy, increases in serum hepatic enzyme concentrations, increased serum bilirubin, hepatic dysfunction, dizziness, malaise, fatigue, cough, rhinitis, superinfections
Cefixime (Suprax)	Uncomplicated UTIs Acute otitis media Streptococcal pharyngitis and tonsillitis Respiratory tract infections	400 mg once daily or 200 mg twice daily	Same as above

UTI = urinary tract infection.

Data from Clinical Pharmacology 2016; Lexicomp Online 2016.

cephalosporins. Hypersensitivity reactions occurring with cephalosporins are rash, urticaria, pruritus, fever, chills, arthralgia, edema, hypotension, Stevens-Johnson syndrome, and rarely anaphylaxis. Other adverse reactions reported with cephalosporins include renal dysfunction, nephropathy, hepatic dysfunction, dizziness, headache, malaise, fatigue, cough, rhinitis, and superinfections. Cefixime causes adverse events in 50% of individuals, most commonly gastrointestinal (30%), headache (15%), and hypersensitivity reactions (up to 7%). Cefuroxime use has been associated with decreased hemoglobin and hematocrit in 10% of patients (Clinical Pharmacology 2016).

Fluoroquinolones

Ciprofloxacin (Cipro) is a broad-spectrum fluoroquinolone antibiotic active against most gram-negative aerobic bacteria and many gram-positive aerobic bacteria with the exception of streptococci.

Ciprofloxacin is used orally in the treatment of urinary tract infections, acute sinusitis, lower respiratory tract infections, skin and skin structure infections, or bone and joint infections. Oral ciprofloxacin has also been used in the treatment of salmonella infections, uncomplicated gonorrhea, and infectious diarrhea and in the prevention or empirical treatment of travelers' diarrhea. Ciprofloxacin and hydrocortisone otic drops (Cipro HC) are used in the treatment of otitis externa and chronic otitis media. Ciloxan, ophthalmic ciprofloxacin, is used in the treatment of bacterial conjunctivitis and corneal ulcers caused by susceptible bacteria.

Levofloxacin (Levaquin) is a fluoroquinolone with a similar antimicrobial spectrum to ciprofloxacin but with increased activity against gram-positive organisms, including *Streptococcus pneumoniae*. Levofloxacin is used in the treatment of acute sinusitis, lower respiratory tract infections (e.g., community-acquired pneumonia), skin and skin structure infections, and urinary tract infections. Oral levofloxacin has also been used in the treatment of traveler's diarrhea.

The adverse reactions for ciprofloxacin and levofloxacin are similar to those that occur with other antibiotics (see table 5.11). Tendon ruptures have been reported in patients receiving fluoroquinolones (Lewis and Cook

2014); however, in the athlete, this is of particular concern. Any athlete taking a fluoroquinolone who experiences pain or inflammation of a tendon needs to discontinue use of the drug immediately. The risk of rupture may increase in athletes taking fluoroquinolones and corticosteroids simultaneously.

The safe use of fluoroquinolones in children under the age of 18 has not been established. Although altered skeletal growth in human children has not been reported, fluoroquinolones cause arthropathy in young animals. Therefore, fluoroquinolones are avoided in children and adolescents whose skeletal growth is incomplete.

Aluminum, magnesium, calcium, iron, and zinc decrease the absorption of orally administered fluoroquinolones; therefore, antacids and multivitamin or mineral supplements containing these minerals should be avoided during fluoroquinolone therapy. If concomitant use is unavoidable, then the minerals or antacids should not be ingested within 2 to 4 h of the fluoroquinolone.

Fluoroquinolones cause blood glucose disturbances, both hypoglycemia and hyperglycemia, in individuals taking either oral antidiabetic agents or insulin. These agents must be used with caution in athletes receiving oral hypoglycemic agents or insulin to treat diabetes. Ciprofloxacin may cause adverse events including nausea, vomiting, dizziness, headache, tremor, agitation, confusion, seizures, tachycardia, and respiratory failure. Levofloxacin occasionally causes anemia, leukopenia, thrombocytopenia, eosinophilia, fever, chills, rash, and itching. Levofloxacin, whose use has been associated with seizures, may lower the seizure threshold and must be used with caution in persons with a history of seizure. The risk of seizure is increased if NSAIDs and levofloxacin are being used concomitantly.

Tetracyclines

Tetracyclines are antibiotics with activity against most *Rickettsia, Chlamydia, Mycoplasma,* and spirochetes. Many gram-negative bacteria are susceptible to tetracyclines. Most gram-positive bacteria are susceptible to the tetracyclines, although staphylococci and streptococci are becoming increasingly resistant. Tetracyclines are used in the treatment of rickettsial infections, including Rocky Mountain spotted fever and Q fever; urogenital chlamydial infections; psittacosis; *Mycoplasma pneumoniae*; nongonococcal urethritis; infections caused by uncommon gram-negative bacteria (e.g., brucellosis); gonorrhea; anthrax; acne; syphilis; Lyme disease; *Helicobacter pylori* gastrointestinal infections; cholera; and leprosy (Clinical Pharmacology 2016). Tetracyclines may also be used for the prevention of malaria. The athletic trainer most often will see the oral tetracyclines doxycycline (Vibramycin), minocycline (Minocin), and tetracycline (Sumycin) used for the treatment of acne.

🚩 RED FLAGS FOR MINERALS AND ANTACIDS

The athlete should avoid minerals and antacids when taking fluoroquinolones, if possible. They decrease absorption of orally administered fluoroquinolones. If minerals and antacids cannot be avoided, they should be taken 2 to 4 h after the antibiotic.

TABLE 5.11 Fluoroquinolones

Medication	Common indication(s)	Usual adult dosage	Adverse reactions
Ciprofloxacin (oral, Cipro; ophthalmic, Ciloxan; otic, Cipro HC)	UTIs Acute sinusitis, lower respiratory tract infections Skin and skin structure infections Bone and joint infections Salmonella Uncomplicated gonorrhea Infectious diarrhea, traveler's diarrhea Otic: otitis externa, chronic otitis media Ophthalmic: bacterial conjunctivitis, corneal ulcers	Oral: 250–750 mg every 12 h Ophthalmic: 1–2 drops every 2–4 h Otic: 3–5 drops twice daily	Bone marrow depression, eosinophilia, hemolysis in individuals with G6PD deficiency, ECG changes, CNS disturbances, nausea, vomiting, diarrhea, taste disturbances, tendon rupture
Levofloxacin (oral, Levaquin; ophthalmic, Quixin)	Acute sinusitis, lower respiratory tract infections (e.g., community-acquired pneumonia) Skin and skin structure infections Urinary tract infections, acute pyelonephritis Traveler's diarrhea Ophthalmic: bacterial conjunctivitis, corneal ulcers	Oral: 250–500 mg once daily; single-dose therapy may be used for STDs Ophthalmic: 1–2 drops every 2–4 h	Bone marrow depression, eosinophilia, hemolysis in individuals with G6PD deficiency, ECG changes, CNS disturbances, blood glucose disturbances, nausea, diarrhea, taste disturbances, nephrotoxicity; rash, hypersensitivity reactions, Stevens-Johnson syndrome, arthralgias, tendon rupture Ophthalmic: ocular pain, burning, dryness, transient decreased vision
Ofloxacin (oral and otic, Floxin; ophthalmic, Ocuflox)		Oral: 300–400 mg twice daily; 400 mg single dose used for STDs Ophthalmic: 1–2 drops every 2–4 h Otic: 10 drops 1–2 times daily	Blood dyscrasias, hemolysis in individuals with G6PD deficiency, CNS disturbances, nausea, vomiting, diarrhea, taste disturbances, vaginitis, dysuria, skin eruptions, rash, eczema, photosensitivity, arthralgia, myalgia, tendon rupture, hypersensitivity Otic: dizziness or vertigo Ophthalmic: burning, redness, itching, blurred vision, dryness

CNS = central nervous system; ECG = electrocardiogram.

Data from Clinical Pharmacology 2016; Lexicomp Online 2016.

Common adverse reactions associated with tetracyclines are similar to other antibiotics (see table 5.12). Dysphagia, sore throat, and black, hairy tongue have also been reported. Photosensitivity reactions can be striking; they can appear almost immediately or within a few hours after ingestion. Other dermatological reactions, such as rash and discoloration of the nails, may occur occasionally. A Jarisch-Herxheimer reaction occurred in some cases when tetracyclines were used to treat spirochetal infections, Lyme disease, or brucellosis. This reaction consists of headache, fever, malaise, myalgia, and arthralgia, and it typically occurs within 12 to 24 h after initiation of tetracycline therapy. Minocycline use is associated with a high incidence of vestibular symptoms (up to 90%) (Lexicomp Online 2016). These symptoms include lightheadedness, dizziness, vertigo, ataxia, drowsiness, headache, fatigue, nausea, and vomiting.

> ⚑ **RED FLAG FOR PHOTOSENSITIVITY**
>
> - Photosensitivity can occur with tetracycline antibiotics. This reaction appears as a severe sunburn that can develop a few minutes to a few hours after sun exposure and may last 1 to 2 d after discontinuing the offending antibiotic.
> - Sunblock is of little value in preventing the reaction.
> - Because minocycline is a tetracycline antibiotic that rarely causes this reaction, it may be the best choice in this case for sun-exposed athletes.

Tetracyclines will bind to orally administered aluminum, calcium, and magnesium ions, resulting in decreased gastrointestinal absorption of the tetracyclines. Antacids containing these minerals should not be taken within 2 h of the tetracycline. Iron more significantly decreases the absorption of tetracyclines and should not be ingested within 3 h of tetracyclines. Antidiarrheals containing kaolin, pectin, or bismuth subsalicylate also impair the absorption of tetracyclines and should not be used concurrently.

Oral tetracyclines can reduce the effectiveness of oral contraceptives. Concurrent use has resulted in pregnancy and breakthrough bleeding. Women taking oral contraceptives and tetracyclines need to use a second form of birth control during sexual intercourse to avoid pregnancy.

Antivirals

The agents discussed here are used to treat herpes and influenza infections, but antivirals used in the treatment of human immunodeficiency virus (HIV) infection are not covered. Acyclovir and valacyclovir (a prodrug of acyclovir) are used in the treatment of herpesvirus, which causes infections of the skin and mucous membranes. Genital herpes infections are contracted through sexual contact, but there are many ways in which herpesvirus may be spread through nonsexual contact. Wrestlers may experience herpes infections of the skin that are contracted through skin-to-skin contact with infected wrestlers (see chapter 16 for a discussion on viral skin infections).

Acyclovir (Zovirax) is most often administered as a topical agent that is applied five or six times per

TABLE 5.12 Tetracyclines

Therapeutic use	Usual adult dosage	Adverse effects
Rocky Mountain spotted fever Q fever Urogenital chlamydial infections Psittacosis *Mycoplasma* ("walking") pneumonia Nongonococcal urethritis, gonorrhea, syphilis Anthrax Acne Lyme disease, *Helicobacter pylori* gastrointestinal infections, cholera, leprosy	Doxycycline: 100 mg twice daily Minocycline: 100 mg twice daily Tetracycline: 250–500 mg orally 1 or 2 times daily	Gastrointestinal reactions: nausea, vomiting, diarrhea, anorexia, abdominal discomfort Rash, discoloration of the nails Jarisch-Herxheimer reaction: headache, fever, malaise, myalgia Tetracycline and doxycycline: photosensitivity Minocycline: lightheadedness, dizziness, vertigo, ataxia, drowsiness, headache, fatigue, nausea, vomiting

Data from Clinical Pharmacology 2016; Lexicomp Online 2016.

day directly on the herpes lesions. Before valacyclovir became available, oral acyclovir was the only oral drug that could treat herpes infections. Unfortunately, oral acyclovir must be administered five or six times per day, which makes it extremely inconvenient. Valacyclovir (Valtrex) oral tablets are administered only one to three times daily. For treatment of acute, localized herpes lesions, the dose of valacyclovir is 1 g every 8 h for 7 d (Lexicomp Online 2016; Clinical Pharmacology 2016).

Wrestlers are often given valacyclovir prophylaxis throughout the wrestling season to prevent the occurrence of cutaneous herpes infections. The dose for prophylaxis is 500 mg twice daily.

For athletes with genital herpes, the treatment dose of valacyclovir is 1 g twice daily for 10 d. For the treatment of cold sores, two 2 g doses are given separated by an interval of 12 h. Regardless of the condition, treatment is most effective if it is started within 48 h of the onset of symptoms.

Side Effects

Oral acyclovir and valacyclovir are generally well tolerated. The most common adverse effects are gastrointestinal in nature and include nausea, vomiting, or diarrhea. Malaise and headache also occur in around 10% of patients. Occasionally, dermatological reactions such as rash, pruritus, or urticaria may be seen. It is extremely rare to see any adverse reaction from topical acyclovir, although 30% of patients using topical acyclovir in the treatment of genital lesions will experience burning and pain on application.

Antifungals

Discussion of antifungal agents is limited to agents that are used in the treatment of dermatological and vaginal fungal infections. The most common fungal conditions are tinea pedis, tinea corporis, and tinea cruris, which are generally caused by *Trichophyton* species or *Epidermophyton floccosum* (see chapter 16 for descriptions of these conditions).

Antifungal agents exert their fungicidal effects through a variety of mechanisms: alteration of the fungal cell wall permeability, inhibition of transmembrane transport, interference with fungal cellular metabolism, and growth inhibition. Topical fungal infections are common, and the athlete can often safely self-medicate with over-the-counter agents. These products include miconazole products, such as Desenex and Micatin, or clotrimazole products, such as Lotrimin. Terbinafine creams, such as Lamisil, and tolnaftate-containing products, such as Tinactin, are also popular. Over-the-counter antifungal medications are available in sprays, powders, and creams.

The typical rule of thumb is that sprays and powders are used prophylactically, and the creams are used for active fungal infection. Topical antifungal agents are sometimes combined with corticosteroids (e.g., Lotrisone), which relieve the itching and burning that may be caused by the fungal infection. Caution is necessary when using these combination products because the corticosteroid may inhibit the activity of some antifungal agents against certain pathogens.

If the infection has not resolved by the end of the duration of therapy recommended for the antifungal being used, if the infection is recurring, or if a hastier recovery is needed, such as in returning a wrestler to competition, then oral antifungals may be prescribed by the physician.

Vaginal fungal infections are caused by *Candida albicans* or other species of *Candida*. Many women experience vaginal candidiasis during antibiotic therapy because of a suppression of the normal vaginal flora that allows for overgrowth of *Candida*. These infections may be safely self-medicated in otherwise healthy individuals. Any athlete who is diabetic or immunocompromised should consult a physician rather than self-medicate. If vaginal candidiasis occurs during a woman's menstrual period, she should either delay therapy until after the flow has stopped or begin treatment but avoid the use of tampons. Several products for the treatment of vaginal candidiasis have a petroleum base that may interact with the rubber or latex used in condoms or contraceptive diaphragms (Clinical Pharmacology 2016; Lexicomp Online 2016). Condoms or diaphragms should not be used within 72 h of a dose of these products. As with topical fungal infections, if relief of vaginal candidiasis is not achieved by the end of the recommended duration of therapy, then the advice of a physician is needed.

Oral candidal infections, which may also occur during antibiotic therapy, should be treated under the advice of a physician using either clotrimazole or nystatin. Table 5.13 lists various antifungal agents, their uses, and the adverse effects associated with each. Two oral antifungal agents, griseofulvin and ketoconazole, are used in the prevention and treatment of topical fungal infections in wrestlers. These athletes are at risk for developing fungal infections from skin-to-skin contact with other wrestlers or contact with wrestling mats (Estes 2015). Griseofulvin (Fulvicin, GrisPEG) comes in two different forms: microsize and ultramicrosize. The difference between these two is the particle size in the drug, which affects absorption. The microsize drug has a particle size of 4 mm; anywhere from 25% to 70% of an oral dose is absorbed (Clinical Pharmacology 2016; Lexicomp Online 2016). Absorption is increased by administering the drug with a high-fat meal. The ultramicrosize drug has a particle size of 1 mm and is almost completely absorbed. The griseofulvin microsize is given as a 500 to 1000 mg dose once daily.

TABLE 5.13 Antifungal Agents

Antifungal agent	Trade name(s)	Use(s)	Duration of therapy	Adverse effects
Butenafine 1% cream	Mentax	Tinea pedis, tinea corporis, tinea cruris, tinea versicolor	Tinea pedis: 4 wk Tine corporis, tinea cruris, tinea versicolor: 2 wk	Burning, stinging, local irritation
Butoconazole 2% vaginal cream*	Femstat-3, Myclex-3	Vulvovaginal candidiasis	3 d	Burning, itching
Ciclopirox 0.77% gel, cream, lotion	Loprox	Tinea pedis, tinea cruris, tinea corporis, tinea versicolor	Tinea versicolor: 2 wk All other conditions: 4 wk	Pruritus, transient burning
Clotrimazole 1% cream, solution, lotion, lozenges	Mycelex, Lotrimin, Gyne-Lotrimin, Lotrisone (with betamethasone)	Tinea pedis, tinea cruris, tinea corporis Vulvovaginal and oral candidiasis	Tinea cruris: 2 wk Tinea corporis and tinea pedis: 4 wk Vulvovaginal candidiasis: 7 d Oral candidiasis: 14 d	Erythema, pruritus, burning, stinging, peeling, contact dermatitis
Econazole 1% cream	Spectazole	Tinea corporis, tinea cruris, tinea pedis, tinea versicolor	Tinea cruris, tinea corporis, tinea versicolor: 2 wk Tinea pedis: 1 mo	Burning, stinging, pruritus, erythema
Ketoconazole 2% cream and shampoo	Nizoral	Tinea corporis, tinea cruris, tinea pedis, tinea versicolor	Tinea corporis, tinea cruris, tinea versicolor: 2 wk Tinea pedis: 6 wk	Irritation, pruritus, stinging, contact dermatitis
Miconazole 1% and 2% aerosol, cream, lotion, powder, solution, vaginal cream, vaginal suppositories (100 mg and 200 mg)*	Desenex, Lotrimin AF, Micatin, Ting, Monistat, Femizol-M, Nystat-Rx	Tinea pedis, tinea cruris, tinea corporis, tinea versicolor Vulvovaginal candidiasis	Tinea cruris, tinea corporis, tinea versicolor: 2 wk Tinea pedis: 1 mo Vulvovaginal candidiasis: 3–7 d	Irritation, burning, contact dermatitis
Nystatin Oral suspension, tablets, lozenges, cream, ointment, powder	Mycostatin, Nystex, Nystop, Mycolog with triamcinolone, Mycogen with triamcinolone	Vulvovaginal and oral candidiasis	Vulvovaginal candidiasis: 14 d Oral candidiasis: 14 d	Irritation
Oxiconazole 1% cream and lotion	Oxistat	Tinea corporis, tinea cruris, tinea pedis, tinea versicolor	Tinea corporis, tinea cruris, tinea pedis: 2–4 wk Tinea versicolor: 2 wk	Pruritus, burning, contact dermatitis
Sulconazole 1% cream or solution	Exelderm	Tinea corporis, tinea cruris, tinea pedis, tinea versicolor	Tinea corporis, tinea cruris, tinea pedis: 2–4 wk Tinea versicolor: 2 wk	Pruritus, erythema, burning, irritation, stinging, tingling
Terbinafine 1% cream or solution	Lamisil	Tinea corporis, tinea cruris, tinea pedis, tinea versicolor	Tinea corporis, tinea cruris, tinea versicolor: 1 wk Tinea pedis: 2 wk	Burning, pruritus, erythema, skin discoloration

Antifungal agent	Trade name(s)	Use(s)	Duration of therapy	Adverse effects
Terconazole 0.4% and 0.8% cream, suppositories (80 mg)*	Terazol	Vulvovaginal candidiasis	Vulvovaginal candidiasis: 3–7 d	Itching, burning, pruritus, irritation, abdominal pain, dysmenorrhea, fever, chills, headache
Tioconazole 6.5% ointment*	Monistat-1, Vagistat-1	Vulvovaginal candidiasis	Vulvovaginal candidiasis: single dose, improvement in 3 d	Burning, vaginitis, pruritus, headache, abdominal pain, dysuria, nocturia, pharyngitis, rhinitis
Tolnaftate 1% powder, cream, solution	Tinactin, Aftate, Zeasorb-AF	Tinea corporis, tinea cruris, tinea pedis, tinea versicolor	Tinea corporis, tinea cruris, tinea pedis, tinea versicolor: 4–6 wk	Slight local irritation

*These products contain a petroleum base that may interact with the latex or rubber of condoms or contraceptive diaphragms. Do not use condoms or a contraceptive diaphragm within 72 h following a dose of these products.

Data from Clinical Pharmacology 2016; Lexicomp Online 2016.

The griseofulvin ultramicrosize is given as a 330 to 750 mg dose once daily.

The most common side effects of griseofulvin therapy are headache, which often resolves with continued therapy, fatigue, dizziness, insomnia, gastrointestinal disturbances, rash, urticaria, and photosensitivity. Griseofulvin rarely causes proteinuria, hepatotoxicity, and leukopenia, but because of the serious nature of these disorders, it is recommended that hepatic function, renal function, and white blood cell (WBC) counts be monitored periodically throughout the course of therapy.

Griseofulvin may cause tachycardia and flushing when taken concurrently with alcoholic beverages. Griseofulvin may also potentiate the effects of alcohol; therefore, it may be wise to advise athletes to avoid ingestion of alcohol during treatment. Griseofulvin may also decrease the effectiveness of warfarin. In athletes taking warfarin and griseofulvin concurrently, prothrombin time (PT) and **international normalized ratio (INR)** should be monitored. The dose of warfarin also may need to be adjusted during therapy with griseofulvin (American Hospital Formulary Service 2016). Griseofulvin is known to decrease the effectiveness of oral contraceptives and cause amenorrhea or breakthrough bleeding. A form of contraception other than birth control pills must be used during therapy. Griseofulvin also has significant teratogenic potential, which makes the requirement for an alternative form of birth control even more urgent. Because griseofulvin has caused sperm abnormalities in mice studies, it is recommended that men wait at least 6 mo after the discontinuation of griseofulvin therapy before fathering a child.

Ketoconazole (Nizoral) is prescribed in a 200 to 400 mg single daily dose. The most common side effect of ketoconazole is gastrointestinal disturbance, which may be lessened by administration with food. Gynecomastia with breast tenderness has also been reported in males taking ketoconazole (Svetaz et al. 2016). This condition may resolve with continued therapy, but some cases may require discontinuation of the drug. Because of the unusual nature of this reaction, all men receiving ketoconazole should be advised of this reaction and encouraged to continue therapy.

Rarely, ketoconazole can cause hepatotoxicity. More frequently, increases in liver function tests (LFTs) will be transient. The hepatotoxicity usually resolves on discontinuation of the drug and usually occurs very early in the course of therapy. Athletes receiving ketoconazole should have LFTs performed before the initiation of therapy, every 2 wk thereafter for the first 2 mo of therapy, and then every month until therapy is discontinued.

Ingestion of alcohol during treatment with ketoconazole may result in an Antabuse-like reaction consisting of flushing, rash, nausea, vomiting, and headache. Although this reaction is not dangerous, it is quite uncomfortable. Athletes receiving ketoconazole therapy are cautioned not to ingest alcohol within 48 h of a dose of ketoconazole.

The absorption of ketoconazole is significantly decreased by drugs that decrease gastric acidity. For this reason, ketoconazole should not be administered within 2 h of antacids, H$_2$ antagonists (Zantac, Pepcid), or proton pump inhibitors (Prilosec, Prevacid).

Ketoconazole may increase the anticoagulant effect of warfarin. PT and INR should be monitored when the two drugs are used together and the dose of warfarin adjusted accordingly. When ketoconazole is administered with phenytoin or theophylline, metabolism of the latter two drugs may be altered. Serum levels need to be monitored and doses adjusted accordingly.

Ketoconazole may cause increased plasma concentrations of systemically administered corticosteroids. In addition, ketoconazole may potentiate the adrenal suppression caused by corticosteroids. For these reasons, the dose of corticosteroids may need to be decreased when they are administered with ketoconazole.

Bronchodilators

Bronchodilators are β-adrenergic agonists (table 5.14). These agents stimulate the β-adrenergic receptors in the bronchi and bronchioles to cause a widening of these airways and allow for improved airflow. In the athlete, exercise-induced asthma is the most common cause of airway constriction requiring treatment with bronchodilators. Albuterol is the agent used to treat exercise-induced bronchospasm. Albuterol is available as a metered-dose inhaler (MDI), which offers the most convenient dosing, but proper technique must be used for the drug to be maximally effective (see figure 5.2).

Proper technique for using an inhaler is essential to ensure that the medication reaches the target.

1. Remove the mouthpiece cover from the MDI and the mouthpiece of the spacer device.
2. Have the patient take a deep breath and exhale completely.
3. Shake the inhaler well for 2 to 5 s (five or six shakes).
4. The patient opens his or her lips and places the inhaler mouthpiece in the mouth with the opening of the MDI toward the back of the throat (figure 5.2).

Another appropriate technique is described here:

1. With the inhaler properly positioned, have the patient hold the inhaler with his or her thumb at the mouthpiece and the index finger and middle

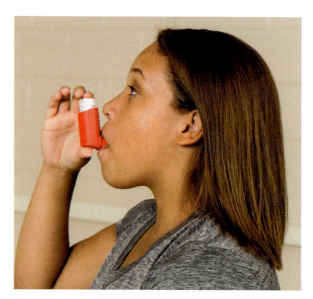

FIGURE 5.2   Proper technique for MDI use.

finger at the top. This is a three-point or bilateral hand position.
2. Instruct the patient to tilt his or her head back slightly, inhale slowly and deeply through the mouth for 3 to 5 s, and then depress the medication canister fully.
3. Have the patient hold his or her breath for approximately 10 s.
4. Remove the MDI from the mouth before exhaling; then exhale slowly through the nose or pursed lips.

A spacer that holds the puff of medicine between the inhaler device and the athlete can increase the ease of use. When a spacer is used, the actuation of the inhaler does not have to be timed to the inhalation of the drug; the inhaler delivers the drug into the spacer (figure 5.3). The athlete then inhales the drug slowly and often more completely through the spacer as a separate step.

Nebulizers are machines that use air pressure to aerosolize the drug and then deliver the quickest onset and maximized amount of drug. They are expensive and bulky to transport, but the drug can be delivered simply by placing a tube inside the mouth or a mask over the mouth and nose (figure 5.4).

TABLE 5.14   **Bronchodilators**

Drug	Administration
Albuterol (Ventolin, Proventil)	Metered-dose inhaler, oral tablets, oral solution, solution for nebulization
Levalbuterol (Xopenex)	Solution for nebulization
Racemic epinephrine (S2 inhalant)	Solution for nebulization

Data from Clinical Pharmacology 2016; Lexicomp Online 2016.

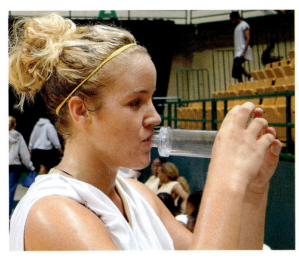

FIGURE 5.3 An athlete demonstrates the use of a metered-dose inhaler with a spacer.

© Micki Cuppett

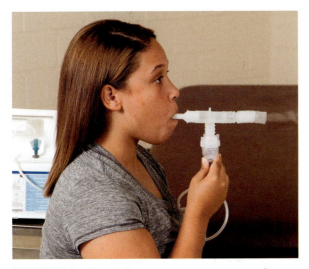

FIGURE 5.4 A nebulizer contains a pump and compressor that deliver a mist of medication through a face mask or tube.

Side Effects

The main adverse effects of bronchodilators are tremor, nervousness, dizziness, headache, nausea, and tachycardia. A paradoxical bronchospasm also has been reported in 8% of individuals using bronchodilators. It is usually associated with the first use of a new MDI canister and may be related to exposure to the propellant. To avoid this reaction, a new MDI can be actuated into the air a few times before its first use. Nebulized albuterol caused coughing in 4% of individuals in various clinical trials. Side effects that occurred in less than 3% of individuals but that may be significant in the athlete include muscle

cramping, muscle spasm, and dilated pupils (Parsons 2014).

Levalbuterol (Xopenex) is the R-enantiomer of albuterol. It is only available as a solution for nebulization. Levalbuterol is considerably more expensive than albuterol, but it is associated with a lower rate of adverse effects. For treating exercise-induced asthma in the athlete, albuterol, the less expensive alternative, is adequate (Allen 2002).

Antihistamines

Antihistamines are drugs used to treat allergies. When the body's immune system reacts to an allergen, histamine is released by the mast cells and basophils. Histamine binds to histamine receptors in the nose, eyes, respiratory tract, and skin, causing the classic allergic signs (e.g., rhinitis, sneezing, watery eyes, itching, dermatitis). Antihistamines are antagonists that block the histamine receptors and prevent histamine from binding to the cell's receptors.

The histamine antagonists are classified into two groups on the basis of their likelihood of causing sedation. The first-generation, or sedating, antihistamines are older agents with a much higher incidence of anticholinergic adverse effects, including sedation (table 5.15). They are used in the treatment of seasonal allergies and some cold symptoms. The sedating properties associated with these drugs also make them useful in the short-term treatment of insomnia. In addition, some antihistamines, such as meclizine (Antivert) and hydroxyzine (Atarax, Vistaril), are used in the treatment of nausea, vertigo, motion sickness, and hives. Sedating antihistamines are commonly used to treat allergy symptoms associated with seasonal allergies and are usually formulated in combination with decongestants.

Nonsedating, or second-generation, antihistamines are used to treat and prevent seasonal allergies and to treat chronic idiopathic urticaria. These antihistamines are often the drug of choice for the athlete because they are nonsedating (table 5.16). In recent years, these nonsedating antihistamines have become available without a prescription. Many are also formulated in combination with the decongestant pseudoephedrine (Zyrtec-D, Allegra-D).

The adverse effects most often associated with the first-generation sedating antihistamines are those caused by CNS depression, such as drowsiness, muscular weakness, and dizziness. Therefore, antihistamines should be used with caution by athletes participating in events where coordination and alertness are needed to prevent injury. Even mild sedation may increase the incidence of injury and decrease performance. Anyone taking antihistamines should avoid alcohol intake because of the additive effect on CNS depression.

TABLE 5.15 **Sedating Antihistamines**

Antihistamine	Trade name(s)	Usual adult dosage
Azatadine	Optimine, 1 mg Rynatan and Trinalin, 1 mg; Pseudoephedrine, 120 mg	1–2 mg twice daily
Brompheniramine	Numerous	4 mg every 4 h or 6–12 mg every 12 h (extended release)
Dexbrompheniramine with pseudoephedrine	Drixoral	6 mg every 12 h (extended release)
Carbinoxamine with pseudoephedrine	Rondec, Cardec	4 mg 4 times daily or 8 mg every 12 h (extended release)
Chlorpheniramine	Chlor-Trimeton, numerous others	4 mg every 4–6 h or 8–12 mg twice daily (extended release) or 16 mg once daily (extended release)
Clemastine	Tavist	1.34 mg every 12 h
Diphenhydramine	Benadryl, numerous others	25–50 mg every 4–6 h
Promethazine	Phenergan	6.25 mg every 4–6 h
Triprolidine	Actifed	2.5 mg every 4–6 h

Data from Clinical Pharmacology 2016; Lexicomp Online 2016.

TABLE 5.16 **Nonsedating Antihistamines**

Antihistamine	Trade name(s)	Usual adult dosage	Drug interactions	Adverse effects
Cetirizine*	Zyrtec	5–10 mg once daily		Somnolence, fatigue, dizziness, dry mouth
Desloratadine*	Clarinex, Clarinex RediTabs	5 mg daily		
Fexofenadine*	Allegra	60 mg twice daily or 180 mg once daily	Aluminum- and magnesium-containing antacids decrease absorption and peak plasma levels; do not take fexofenadine within 2 h of antacids	Headache, insomnia, dizziness, back pain
Loratadine*	Claritin, Alavert	10 mg once daily		Headache, sedation, insomnia, nervousness, dry mouth, abdominal pain

*Available over the counter.

Data from Clinical Pharmacology 2016; Lexicomp Online 2016.

Additional adverse effects seen with first-generation antihistamines are gastrointestinal and include nausea, vomiting, diarrhea, or constipation. These antihistamines also cause anticholinergic side effects, such as dry mouth, blurred vision, urinary retention, impotence, nervousness, and irritability.

Antihistamines must be used with caution in people with hyperthyroidism and hypertension (see chapter 8). Although there is some controversy over the potential for antihistamines to induce asthma attacks by virtue of their drying effect on bronchial tissues, antihistamines are contraindicated in those who experience acute asthmatic attacks. The drug interactions of the sedating antihistamines are primarily with other CNS depressants, which will cause an additive CNS depressant effect.

Decongestants

Decongestants are drugs that primarily stimulate the α-adrenergic receptors and to a lesser extent the β-adrenergic receptors (table 5.17). The beneficial result of this α-adrenergic stimulation is vasoconstriction in the nasal mucosa that shrinks swollen nasal passages, thereby relieving nasal congestion. The decongestants are used orally either alone or in combination with other agents used to treat cold and allergy symptoms, such as antihistamines. Topical decongestants such as Afrin can also be applied directly to the nasal mucosa to provide relief from congestion without systemic side effects. Ophthalmic decongestants like Visine are applied to the eyes to produce vasoconstriction of the conjunctival vasculature, reducing redness of the eyes.

Pseudoephedrine (Sudafed) is the oral decongestant most commonly used alone or in combination products. Pseudoephedrine is a naturally occurring substance found in plants of the genus *Ephedra* and is an isomer of ephedrine. The usual adult dose of pseudoephedrine is 30 to 60 mg every 4 to 6 h. Sustained-release products of pseudoephedrine are available as 120 mg tablets given every 12 h and 240 mg tablets given every 24 h. The side effects associated with the use of pseudoephedrine include mild CNS stimulation such as nervousness, dizziness, weakness, insomnia, and headache. Because pseudoephedrine causes minimal blood pressure changes in patients with normal blood pressure, it should be used with caution by those with high blood pressure because α-adrenergic stimulation causes vasoconstriction and may raise blood pressure.

Pseudoephedrine can be used to make methamphetamine, a CNS stimulant with high addictive potential. For this reason, federal law limits the quantity of pseudoephedrine that can be sold by retail distributors. It is also vital that the athletic trainer be aware that as CNS stimulants, oral decongestants are listed in the NCAA bylaws as banned drugs. So, for athletes subject to drug testing, the drug of choice for allergic rhinitis should not contain pseudoephedrine (Trinh, Kim, and Ritsma 2015).

Phenylephrine (Neo-Synephrine) is used as a topical decongestant in nasal drops and sprays. It is also listed on the NCAA list of banned drugs because of its stimulant properties. Phenylephrine nasal drops or sprays for adults are available as 0.25% or 0.5% solutions that are applied to the nasal mucosa every 4 to 6 h (American Hospital Formulary Service 2016). Adverse effects of phenylephrine nasal solutions include transient burning, stinging, sneezing, rhinitis, and nasal dryness. Prolonged use of phenylephrine nasal solutions should be avoided because it may result in chronic or rebound swelling of the nasal mucosa, which resolves within 1 wk of discontinuing the drug.

Oxymetazoline (Afrin, Dristan) and xylometazoline (Otrivin) are long-acting topical decongestants found in nasal sprays and drops. These long-acting agents should not be used for more than 3 d because significant rebound congestion often occurs and may promote overuse of these drugs.

Ophthalmic decongestants, such as tetrahydrozoline (Visine), provide relief of conjunctival redness and minor eye irritation. Prolonged use of ophthalmic decongestant solutions must be avoided, however, because rebound **hyperemia** may result and promote overuse of the products. It is also important that the use of ophthalmic decongestants not mask an underlying condition that may need medical attention. If ocular pain, redness, or irritation occurs or if visual changes are experienced during the use of these products (Trevor, Katzung, and Knuidering-Hall 2015), the athlete must immediately stop using them and seek medical attention.

Athletes with glaucoma should not use ophthalmic decongestants without consulting a physician or optometrist. Also, most manufacturers recommend that contact lenses be removed before using any ophthalmic decongestant product. Allergic reactions to the ophthalmic decongestants themselves are extremely rare, whereas allergic reactions to the preservatives used in these products are common.

Antidiabetic Agents

With the increase in the prevalence of diabetes mellitus worldwide, athletic trainers are likely to encounter athletes who are diabetic. There are also well-recognized genetic risk factors for diabetes. There are two types of diabetes mellitus, type 1 and type 2. Type 1 diabetes is associated with autoimmune-mediated destruction of B-cells of the pancreatic islets. This results in a total (or near-total) lack of insulin production by the pancreas. Type 2 diabetes is now believed to be a combination of complex metabolic conditions that ultimately results in impaired insulin secretion and insulin action (Ferri 2016). It is increasingly important for athletic trainers to understand diabetes, to be familiar with the pharmacological treatments that athletes may be using, and to understand the impact that these medications may have on training and rehabilitation.

There are now many medications to treat diabetes mellitus. For patients who have diabetes mellitus type 1, the most prevalent treatment is insulin. Insulin is available

TABLE 5.17 Decongestants

Generic name	Trade name(s)	Usual adult dosage	Adverse effects
Naphazoline	Privine	2 drops every 3–6 h	Rebound congestion, burning, stinging, nasal dryness, sneezing, headache, hypertension, palpitations, tachycardia, reflex bradycardia, nervousness, nausea, dizziness, weakness, sweating
Oxymetazoline	Afrin Allerest Cheracol Dristan Genasal Neo-Synephrine Maximum Strength	2–3 drops/sprays every 10–12 h for no more than 3 d	Rebound congestion, burning, stinging, rhinorrhea, nasal dryness, sneezing, hypertension, nervousness, nausea, dizziness, headache, insomnia, palpitations, tachycardia, reflex bradycardia
Phenylephrine	Neo-Synephrine Alconefrin Vicks Sinex	2–3 drops or 1–3 sprays every 4 h	Rebound congestion, burning, stinging, sneezing, rhinorrhea, nasal dryness, palpitation, tachycardia, PVCs, headache, pallor, tremors, sweating, hypertension, nausea, dizziness, nervousness
Propylhexedrine	Benzedrex	2 inhalations every 2 h	Rebound congestion, burning, stinging, nasal dryness, sneezing, headache, hypertension, nervousness, tachycardia
Tetrahydrozoline	Tyzine	2–4 drops/sprays every 4–6 h	Rebound congestion, burning, stinging, nasal dryness, sneezing, headache, hypertension, weakness, sweating, palpitations, tremor
Xylometazoline	Otrivin	2–3 drops/sprays every 8–10 h for no more than 3–5 d	Rebound congestion, burning, stinging, nasal dryness, sneezing, hypertension, nervousness, nausea, dizziness, headache, insomnia, palpitations, tachycardia, arrhythmias
Ophthalmic decongestants			
Naphazoline	Allerest Clear Eyes Naphcon VasoClear Comfort Vasocon	1–3 drops every 3–4 h	Blurred vision, mild stinging or irritation, pupil dilation, headache, hypertension, palpitations, tachycardia, reflex bradycardia, nervousness, nausea, dizziness, weakness, sweating
Oxymetazoline	OcuClear Visine LR	1–2 drops every 6 h	
Phenylephrine	Isopto Frin Ocu-Phrin Prefrin Relief Zincfrin Vasosulf	1–2 drops every 3–4 h	Headache, blurred vision, irritation, pupil dilation, palpitations, tachycardia, PVCs, headache, pallor, tremors, sweating, hypertension, nausea, dizziness, nervousness
Tetrahydrozoline	Collyrium Fresh Geneye Extra Murine Plus Visine	1–2 drops up to 4 times daily	Irritation, blurred vision, pupil dilation, rebound congestion, headache, hypertension, weakness, sweating, palpitations, tremor

PVC = premature ventricular contraction.

Data from Clinical Pharmacology 2016; Lexicomp Online 2016.

in various forms and delivery methods, including insulin pens, pumps, and injectors, in addition to traditional needle injections.

Patients with diabetes mellitus type 2 have multiple pharmacological options, all designed to work on different organ systems. Our coverage here will be neither comprehensive nor exhaustive; we will simply focus on the diabetes medications most likely to be encountered by the athletic trainer.

Insulin Secretagogues and Oral Hypoglycemic Agents

There are a number of medications that are designed to stimulate the secretion of insulin from the pancreas (table 5.18). Some are referred to as hypoglycemic agents because of their ability to induce low blood glucose levels in patients once introduced to the body. Other medications are called insulin secretagogues because they can promote insulin secretion without necessarily producing low glucose levels. These medications are for patients with diabetes mellitus type 2.

Sulfonylureas and Meglitinides

These two classes are hypoglycemic agents that work by stimulating the sodium–potassium channels in pancreatic beta cells. The sulfonylureas are separated into first generation and second generation, the latter of which are by far the more commonly used. Most of them are taken once daily, but they may be twice daily depending on the tablet formulation. The meglitinides have a similar mechanism of action to the sulfonylureas, but their duration of activity is much less. Therefore, they must be taken more often, up to three times daily, usually with meals. For these classes, it is important to monitor for signs and symptoms of hypoglycemia (sweating, shaking, chills, rapid heartbeat).

Dipeptidyl Peptidase-4 Inhibitors (DPP-IV Inhibitors)

This class of diabetes medications is commonly called the "gliptins." They raise incretin levels in the body by preventing their degradation. This in turn results in

TABLE 5.18 Diabetes Medication Classes

Diabetes medication class	Glycemic action	Generic name	Brand name
Sulfonylureas	Hypoglycemic	Glyburide Glipizide Glimepiride	Diabeta Glucotrol Amaryl
Meglitinides	Hypoglycemic	Repaglinide Nateglinide	Prandin Starlix
Biguinides	Anti-hyperglycemic	Metformin	Glucophage
Thiazolidinediones	Anti-hyperglycemic	Pioglitazone Rosiglitazone	Actos Avandia
Alpha glucosidase inhibitors	Anti-hyperglycemic	Acarbose Miglitol	Precose Glyset
Incretin mimetic	Anti-hyperglycemic	Albiglutide Dulaglutide Exenatide Liraglutide	Tanzeum Trulicity Byetta Saxenda
DPP-IV inhibitors	Anti-hyperglycemic	Alogliptin Sitagliptin Linagliptin Saxagliptin	Nesina Januvia Tradjenta Onglyza
SGLT2 inhibitors	Anti-hyperglycemic	Dapagliflozin Empagliflozin Canagliflozin	Farxiga Jardiance Invokana

DDP-IV = dipeptidyl peptidase-4; SGLT2 = sodium-glucose cotransporter 2.

Hypoglycemic agents can produce hypoglycemia as a result of facilitated insulin secretion from the pancreas.

Anti-hyperglycemic agents control elevations in blood glucose levels; they usually do not promote hypoglycemia.

Data from Clinical Pharmacology 2016; Lexicomp Online 2016.

increased insulin secretion when the secretion is stimulated by a meal. The gliptins have few adverse effects, but one adverse effect is a risk of hypoglycemia. At present, all of the gliptins are orally administered.

GLP-1 Agonists

This class of diabetes medications works by stimulating GLP-1 receptor activity, which results in insulin secretion. The GLP-1 receptor, when activated, has multiple actions in the body, including insulin secretion, inhibiting glucagon release, delaying gastric emptying, and reducing food intake by actions of the satiety center of the brain (Dejgaard et al. 2016). This class of medications may cause moderate weight loss in patients. Adverse effects commonly seen include gastric cramping and nausea. Hypoglycemia associated with the GLP-1 agonist is rare. In recent years, post-marketing surveillance data have shown possible associations with pancreatitis, although the prevalence is not common (Minze et al. 2013; Lando, Alattar, and Dua 2012; Anderson and Trujillo 2010).

Antihyperglycemic Medications

As the name implies, these are medications that try to prevent significant increases in glucose levels in patients through means other than pancreatic insulin secretion. The most common medication in this category is metformin. This medication has multiple mechanisms of action to control glucose levels in patients. The primary action in the body is decreasing liver glucose production and increasing peripheral glucose uptake in target cells. Metformin has very minimal effect on glucose levels in patients with normal levels, and it does not promote insulin secretion. This results in very rare instances of hypoglycemia being reported. Adverse effects for metformin include gastrointestinal effects (e.g., nausea,

cramping, diarrhea) and rare association with lactic acidosis. Because of the potential for lactic acidosis, renal function should be monitored periodically (Pasquel et al. 2015; Decker et al. 2015). Other classes of antihyperglycemic medications include the thiazolidinediones, α-glucosidase inhibitors, and the newest class called sodium-glucose cotransporter 2 (SGLT2) inhibitors.

Insulin

When oral medications have not succeeded in controlling a patient's glucose levels, insulin is the next level of medication to be used. There is wide variability in the prescribing and administration of insulin because of the need to individualize insulin therapy for each patient. Patients with diabetes mellitus type 1 require insulin as their primary source of glucose control; type 2 patients may be prescribed insulin after all other forms have failed to produce desired glucose control. The specific nature of the diabetes may also affect insulin therapy. Experienced clinicians should be in control of the type of insulin regimen recommended for each patient.

Insulin is primarily categorized according to its duration of action: short-acting versus long-acting (see table 5.19). Short-acting insulin is administered to quickly control and reduce glucose levels in patients. This rapid control may be used in response to meals to prevent postprandial glucose increases, in response to very significant elevations in glucose levels, or as a feature of insulin pumps that release very small amounts of insulin in a very controlled manner. Long-acting insulin is administered to provide continuous control of glucose levels over a span of 10 to 24 h in single or multiple administrations. Patients should be taught the proper administration techniques for insulin injections and how to monitor for both positive glucose control and possible adverse effects.

TABLE 5.19 **Types of Insulin**

Insulin	Onset	Peak	Duration
Ins. lispro, aspart	<15 min	1–2 h	3 h
Regular	0.5–1 h	2–3 h	2–5 h
NPH/Lente	2–4 h	6–10 h	10–12 h
70/30, 50/50	0.5–1 h	2–10 h	10–12 h
H'LOG 75/25, N'LOG 70/30	<15 min	1–8 h	10–12 h
Ins. Glargine	1–2 h	Flat	24 h
Ins. Detemir	1–2 h	Flat	12–24 h
Ins. Degludec	1–2 h	Flat	24 h
Afreeza (inhaled)	<15 min	1–2 h	3 h

NPH = neutral protamine Hagedorn.

Data from Clinical Pharmacology 2016; Lexicomp Online 2016.

Because insulin can cause hypoglycemia, patients should also know how to manage these episodes if they should occur. Athletic trainers may also benefit greatly from understanding how to manage hypoglycemic episodes should they occur in their presence.

Supplements

No U.S. federal agency, not even the FDA, regulates the content of food supplements and herbal products. The assumption is that these products contain the ingredients or the quantities of each ingredient that are listed on the label and that the ingredients listed are safe. This puts the person using these products at risk because there has been no regulatory follow-up to make sure the products actually provide what is listed and, further, are safe for human consumption. In Canada, however, the Natural Health Products Directorate enforces the natural health products regulations, ensuring all Canadians ready access to natural products that are safe, effective, and of high quality.

Ephedra (ma huang) and ephedrine, substances closely related to pseudoephedrine, are used in weight-loss products, "thermogenics," and other products sold for their "energy-producing" properties. Many products sold as nutritional supplements and herbal products for weight loss or energy may contain ephedra or ephedrine. These two substances are also stimulants on the USADA and NCAA banned drug lists (National Collegiate Athletic Association [NCAA] 2015; United States Anti-Doping Agency 2015).

Both ephedra and ephedrine can cause hypertension, increased cardiac workload, and arrhythmias, especially in high doses (>150 mg per 24 h). The use of these agents has been associated with hemorrhagic stroke (Trinh, Kim, and Ritsma 2015). Other problems associated with the use of food supplements or herbal products containing ephedra or ephedrine include the lack of consistency and reliability of active ingredient content in these products (Buell et al. 2013).

Caffeine is another CNS stimulant that is banned in high doses from international competitions. A concentration of caffeine in the urine of greater than 12 mg/ml of urine is banned. The athlete electing to have a couple of cups of coffee before competition will not be at risk for such high urinary concentrations, but the athlete who takes a supplement containing guarana or a caffeine pill may be over the limit because these supplements do not metabolize at the same rate, and they produce higher urine concentrations of caffeine than coffee or soft drinks.

Other supplements, such as anabolic steroids, are typically not used therapeutically and are not covered in this chapter. The NCAA and USADA are good sources of information on additional banned substances in athletes.

Summary

This chapter describes several commonly used classes of medications prescribed to athletes to treat various medical conditions. Although dispensing medications is not within the scope of practice of the certified athletic trainer, the athletic trainer must understand the range of common medications that athletes may be using as well as potential interactions with other medications or foods and possible adverse reactions (Burns et al. 2004). It is also important for the athletic trainer to be familiar with the basic drug classifications used in the athletic population along with their indications, contraindications, and typical patterns of use.

In addition, the athletic trainer must know how to access current drug information and should have a good working relationship with the team physician and pharmacist to ensure the best treatment for athletes.

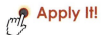 **Apply It!**   The case study for this chapter evaluates your knowledge about drug categories and treatment advice for a 19-year-old lacrosse player. Read the scenario and answer the questions at www.HumanKinetics.com/MedicalConditionsInTheAthlete.

Common Procedures in the Athletic Training Clinic

6

OBJECTIVES

At the completion of this chapter the reader should be able to do the following:

- Name the limitations of the practice act pertaining to invasive procedures.
- Demonstrate the use of an appropriate informed consent before performing any of the procedures described in this chapter.
- Employ fundamental aseptic procedures, including the use of sterile gloves and the creation of a sterile field.
- Properly unpack a sterile package and prepare for a sterile procedure.
- Compare the various types of sutures and suture needles and their specific applications.
- Describe the difference among interrupted, running, and mattress sutures and the advantages and disadvantages of each.
- Prepare the patient for injection and aspiration.

This chapter begins with a disclaimer about state practice acts. At present 49 states regulate the practice of athletic training in some fashion, whether it be by certification, licensure, or other regulation (Board of Certification 2016). What is important to remember is that the practice acts for athletic trainers as well as other health care professionals vary widely by state. Clinicians must be familiar with their own states' practice acts. Recognizing the limitations of one's own practice act will allow the athletic trainer to fully use his or her skills and knowledge base to provide appropriate health care to patients and athletes.

The techniques and procedures outlined in this chapter may be prohibited or not addressed in particular state rules and regulations. Despite this, learning new techniques will allow the practitioner to evolve with changes in the profession and revisions in state practice acts, or to practice to the full scope of the profession, if he or she moves to a state with a different set of guidelines. With the growing number of athletic trainers working in physicians' offices and other health care settings, many are now performing the procedures described in this chapter in their daily practice. Even if they do not perform the procedures themselves, many athletic trainers are asked to help prepare patients and the environment for invasive procedures in the athletic training clinic.

Informed Consent

Informed consent ensures one's right to participate in decisions about their own health care. Everyone should receive enough information to make an informed decision about whether to consent to a treatment or procedure. Legally, it is the physician who must obtain informed consent, but the physician may delegate this responsibility to another health care provider. A health care provider who is substantially involved with the patient's care must obtain the informed consent. Figure 6.1 shows an example of an informed consent form. Informed consent should include, at a minimum, a thorough discussion of the following:

- The patient's diagnosis
- The nature and purpose of a proposed treatment or procedure
- The risks and benefits of a proposed treatment or procedure
- Alternatives to the proposed treatment or procedure (regardless of the cost or the extent to which the treatment options are covered by health insurance)
- The risks and benefits of the alternative treatment or procedure
- The risks and benefits of not receiving or undergoing a treatment or procedure

Preventing Infection

As indicated in detail in chapter 1 of this textbook, OSHA and the Centers for Disease Control and Prevention

CLINICAL TIPS

Preventing Sharps Injuries

Use the following best practices for handling sharps in the medical clinic:

- Use standardized sterile field setups.
- Keep all sharps on instrument tables or trays with the points away from staff members.
- The hands-free or neutral zone method should be used for passing all sharps.
- Dedicate the neutral zone for sharps only (these include suture and hypodermic needles, scalpels, and other sharp instruments).
- Only one sharp at a time should be in the neutral zone.
- Use a needle holder or forceps to handle suture needles. Avoid manually handling needles. Do not hold a sharp and any other instrument simultaneously.
- Don't multitask when using sharps. Focus on making safe passes and exchanges and nothing else.
- Look before you reach.
- Confine and contain all sharps in a disposable, puncture-resistant needle container.

(CDC) define *universal precautions* as a simple set of effective practices designed to protect health care workers and patients from infection by a range of pathogens, including bloodborne viruses. These practices are used when caring for all patients regardless of diagnosis (Centers for Disease Control and Prevention 2016).

Universal precautions apply to blood and to other body fluids that contain visible blood, semen, and vaginal secretions. Universal precautions also apply to tissues and to cerebrospinal, synovial, pleural, peritoneal, pericardial, and amniotic fluids. Universal precautions do not apply to feces, nasal secretions, sputum, sweat, tears, urine, and vomitus unless they contain visible blood. Universal precautions do not apply to saliva except when visibly contaminated with blood or in the dental setting where blood contamination of saliva is predictable.

Universal precautions provide for the use of protective barriers such as gloves, gowns, aprons, masks, and protective eyewear, which can reduce the risk of exposing the health care worker's skin or mucous membranes to potentially infective materials. It is also recommended that all health care workers take precautions to prevent injuries caused by needles, scalpels, and other sharp instruments or devices (Centers for Disease Control and Prevention 2016).

Asepsis and Aseptic Technique

Preventing infection and maximizing healing should be the primary goals when performing any invasive procedure. The term **asepsis** means the absence of infectious organisms, and the goal of **aseptic technique** is to prevent the transfer of microorganisms into the wound (Association of periOperative Registered Nurses 2014; Longo et al. 2013; Phillips 2013; Rothrock 2016). Preventing site contamination requires all team members to use their knowledge and experience in aseptic practices.

Whenever an invasive procedure is performed, aseptic practices *must* be followed:

- Assess the patient for any risk factors.
- Assess any environmental concerns.
- Ensure proper disinfection and sterilization of instruments.
- Observe the use of universal precautions.

Sterile Versus Nonsterile Individuals

Aseptic technique can include both sterile and nonsterile individuals. Once a person dons sterile equipment (gown, gloves, etc.) he or she must pay particular attention to maintaining sterility. Nonsterile personnel must be careful not to contaminate the sterile person or

Assumption of Risk and Release: Asthma

State of _____

This release, executed by _____, a resident of (city), (state) and a student at (university), is given to the (university), its Board of Governors, administrative staff, agents and employees, and to (university), (state), its Board of Trustees, administrative staff, physicians, including those physicians who provide services to the University pursuant to a contract, and all agents and employees of the University having any connection with the athletic program at (university), and particularly the _____ program.

Statement of Facts and Intent

The student is a _____ (freshman, sophomore, junior, senior) at (university), and is a member of the University's _____ team.

As a result of a preexisting asthmatic condition, the student has been determined to be at risk when involved in strenuous physical activities including conditioning exercises and playing and practicing college _____.

Dr. XXXX, who is designated as the (university) team physician, has conferred with (student) and advised him/her as to the risk of participating in intercollegiate _____ and has further recommended that if (student) elects to participate in intercollegiate _____ despite these risks, he/she should take certain precautions.

Based on the foregoing statement of facts, and in consideration of (university) permitting (student) to participate in intercollegiate _____, the (student) (and parents if student is a minor) execute the following assumption of risk and release:

Operative Provisions

1. (Student) acknowledges that he/she is fully aware that playing or practicing in any sport can be a dangerous activity involving many risks of injuries. Further, that the dangers and risks of playing or practicing in _____ include, but are not limited to, death or serious injury resulting from an asthmatic attack or an exercise induced asthma attack.

2. (Student) acknowledges that he/she has been fully advised by the team physician and (university) that because of his/her preexisting asthmatic condition, his/her participation in intercollegiate _____ could result in death or serious injury secondary to bronchospasm following an asthmatic attack or exercise induced asthmatic attack.

3. (Student) understands that if he/she elects to play _____ despite the risks noted herein, the team physician and (university) officials have advised him/her to use a short acting bronchodilator inhaler. Specifically, the team physician and these University officials have advised him/her to administer two puffs ten to fifteen minutes prior to any strenuous activity and two puffs every four hours as needed.

4. (Student) agrees to inform a member of the (university's) athletic training staff whenever he/she experiences any symptoms related to his/her asthmatic condition including wheezing, cough, shortness of breath, and tightness in the chest during exercise.

5. By execution of this assumption of risk and release and in consideration of (university) permitting him/her to engage in intercollegiate _____, (student) acknowledges and assumes the risk of serious injury or death that could result from an asthmatic attack or exercise induced asthmatic attack.

6. (Student) agrees that no representation has been made to him/her by (university) except as set forth in this assumption of risk and having had the risks explained to him/her, he/she wishes to continue his/her participation in intercollegiate _____ despite these risks.

This is the _____ day of _____ 20_____.

_____   _____
Signature of student-athlete   Signature of parent (if student-athlete is a minor)

_____   _____
Witness   Witness

FIGURE 6.1 An informed consent form for asthma should outline the responsibilities of each party as well as the risks and benefits of participating in athletics with the condition.

Proper Technique for Opening and Donning Sterile Gloves

1. Peel away the packaging, exposing the sterile gloves *(a)*.

2. Hold opened package horizontal to the table *(b)*.

3. Flip the contents onto the table without releasing either end of the packaging *(c)*.

4. While keeping the package flat on the table, pinch the bottom corners and open *(d)*.

5. Pinch the bottom corners inside the package and unfold *(e)*.

6. Pinch the top corners inside the package and unfold *(f)*.

7. Without touching the fingertips of the gloves, gently unfold the packaging, leaving it flat on the table *(g)*.

8. Pick up the right glove and gently slide your fingertips inside, using your left hand for guidance and assistance *(h, i)*. Make sure not to touch the fingertips of the glove.

9. Properly applied sterile glove *(j)*.

10. With your gloved right hand, place your fingertips inside the pocket of the left glove, while sliding your left hand into the gloves *(k, l)*.

11. Properly applied sterile gloves *(m)*.

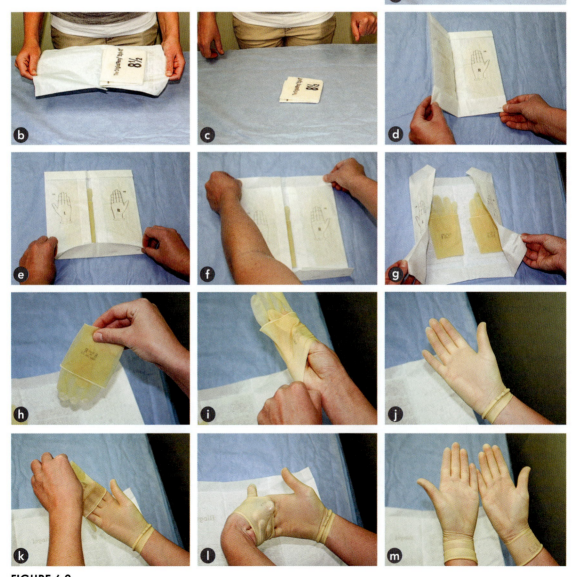

FIGURE 6.2

© Micki Cuppett

the sterile field. Before performing a sterile procedure, the clinician must don sterile gloves. This procedure is very different from the use of latex gloves under normal universal precautions.

Before donning sterile gloves the clinician must perform a thorough hand scrub with antibiotic soap. If close contact with body fluids or tissue is likely, or in the event of potential splash, a surgical mask and protective eyewear should also be worn.

Sterile Field

Sterile drapes are used to create a sterile field. The sterile field may be thought of as an imaginary "box" that also encompasses the space above the person. Sterile drapes should be placed on the patient to leave only the procedural area exposed. Sterile drapes are used to establish an aseptic barrier between nonsterile and sterile areas.

All items placed within the sterile field must be sterile. Only sterile packages, instruments, and materials should be placed in the sterile field. Under no circumstances should sterile and nonsterile items be mixed. Nonsterile persons (such as a student who is observing) should

CLINICAL TIPS

Sterile Field

Keep in mind that after draping, only the top surface of the draped area is considered sterile.

never reach across or into the sterile field. To ensure sterility, all sterile items should be inspected for package integrity. If a package has been compromised, it should be considered contaminated and should not be used. When a sterile packaged item is dropped on the floor, air can penetrate the sterile package. The force that is created when the package contacts the floor can cause the sterile barrier to be penetrated by forcing sterile air out and allowing contaminated air and particles into the package (Rothrock 2016; Potter and Perry 2011; Perry, Potter, and Ostendorf 2014). Nonsterile personnel must use good judgment when dispensing sterile items onto the sterile field either by presenting them directly to the sterile person or by placing them securely on the sterile field. Proper technique must be used when opening wrapped supplies.

Proper Technique for a Nonsterile Person Opening a Sterile Pack

1. Grasp the tip of folded paper and open *away* from the pack *(a)*.
2. Unfold each flap individually *away* from the pack *(b, c)*.
3. *Do not* reach under the folds or flaps *(d)*.

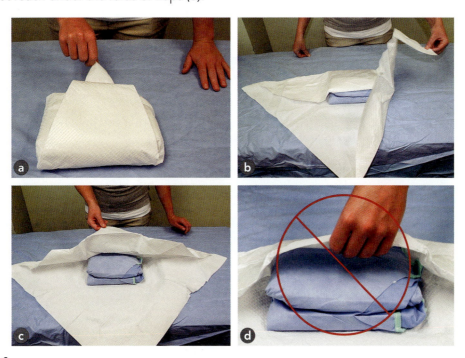

FIGURE 6.3
© Micki Cuppett

A sterile field should be maintained throughout the procedure and monitored constantly. Sterility can never be guaranteed, but every reasonable effort to reduce the likelihood of contamination should be taken, and personnel should be vigilant to avoid breaches in sterility.

When a breach of sterility occurs, team members must take immediate and appropriate action to correct the break in technique to reduce further risk of contamination. If there is doubt about an item's sterility, consider it not sterile. The sterile field should be prepared as close as possible to the time of use. Once set up, the sterile field needs to be monitored constantly (Association of periOperative Registered Nurses 2014).

Everyone moving near or in a sterile field should do so in a manner that maintains the sterile field. Once gloved, personnel should remain in or close to the sterile field without wandering around the room. Gloved personnel should keep their arms and hands within the sterile field at all times to avoid any accidental contact with nonsterile items or areas. Just as the sterile person must maintain a safe distance from nonsterile areas and persons, nonsterile personnel must always be aware of and maintain a "margin of safety" when approaching sterile fields and scrubbed personnel. And finally, when delivering sterile supplies to the sterile field, nonsterile team members must always maintain a margin of safety between themselves and the sterile field, never contacting or reaching over any portion of the sterile area. This margin of safety is considered to be a minimum of 12 in. (30 cm) (Rothrock 2016).

Policies and procedures for maintaining a sterile field should be written, reviewed annually, and readily available within the practice setting. These recommended practices for aseptic technique should be used as guidelines for developing policies and procedures within the practice setting. Training in aseptic technique requires experienced surgical team members to demonstrate these skills to new and inexperienced personnel. New personnel should be assigned an experienced mentor who will be a good role model and teacher in perioperative practice.

Maintaining Asepsis

All medical team members must practice aseptic technique to help prevent the transfer of microorganisms into the wound during the procedure. Team members must develop a strong conscience, adhering to the principles of asepsis and rectifying any improper technique they see during the procedure. In addition, proper surgical attire plays an important role in the reduction of site infections by reducing the amount of hair and skin contaminants reaching the sterile field (Association of periOperative Registered Nurses 2014).

Procedures Used to Close Lacerations

Caring for a laceration is a common occurrence in the athletic training clinic. Often simply cleaning the wound and applying an antibiotic ointment and an adhesive bandage are sufficient. Sometimes, however, more aggressive measures must be used to close the laceration to achieve good healing and cosmetic results. This section discusses common skin closure materials and techniques.

Proper Technique for Opening Wrapped Supplies

1. Nonsterile person opening sterile packs for a person wearing sterile gloves (a).
2. Peel packs are opened by peeling back the wrapping at the corner and holding the package open for a sterile person to reach in and remove sterile items (b, c).

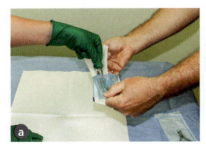 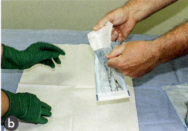 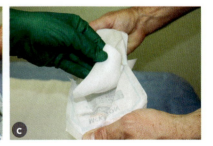

FIGURE 6.4
© Micki Cuppett

Adhesive Skin Tape

Adhesive skin tape is used to close small, superficial, low-tension wounds and to reinforce larger wounds closed with sutures or after removing sutures to protect the wound during the proliferation and early remodeling periods of healing (figure 6.5).

Adhesive skin tape is designed to facilitate quick, simple closure of minor wounds with minimal risk. The noninvasive application technique reduces tissue trauma and is relatively pain free. In an athletic setting, it is also used to temporarily close wounds during competition before more definitive wound closure after the competition.

Topical Liquid Skin Adhesives

Tissue adhesives are polymers that are formulated to be used in place of nonabsorbable sutures for primary closure of skin wounds. Commercially available tissue adhesives include Histoacryl (B. Braun, Melsungen, Germany), Dermabond (Ethicon, Somerville, NJ), and Indermil (Syneture brand; Covidien, Dublin, Ireland). These products are approved for closing skin wounds and forming barriers against certain bacterial infections (figure 6.7). The products have shown a lower incidence of wound infection and wound **dehiscence** than other wound closure techniques (Grimaldi et al. 2015).

Skin tissue adhesives may be used in place of nonabsorbable sutures for primary closure of skin wounds. For wounds that are under tension, deep sutures are recommended. These products should not be used on the oral mucosa or across joints, where repetitive movement may cause the adhesives to slough prematurely. These adhesives do not replace the necessity for appropriate wound care. Wounds still need careful examination and

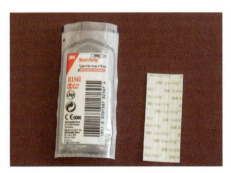

FIGURE 6.5 Adhesive closures can be used to close minor wounds, or they can be used after sutures have been removed.

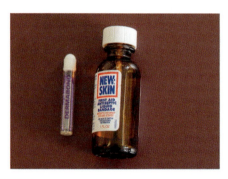

FIGURE 6.7 Tissue adhesive has become more commonplace and can be used instead of adhesive skin tape or sutures on lacerations or incisions with clean, well opposed edges.

Application Technique for Adhesive Skin Tape

1. Clean the wound.
2. Inspect the wound.
3. Dry the edges and surrounding skin.
4. Consider an adhesive application such as tincture of benzoin or Mastisol (Ferndale Laboratories, Ferndale, MI). Both may be applied to the skin with a cotton-tipped applicator before applying tape. They may offer some degree of protection from allergy to the adhesive in the tape, and they improve the adherence of the tape. Mastisol does appear to have superior adhesion and fewer adverse reactions. If significant swelling is anticipated, it is probably best not to apply an adhesive. Elastic tape may be used, but it should be used with caution if swelling is anticipated as it may also cause blistering of the skin.

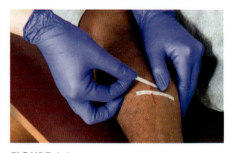

FIGURE 6.6

5. Ensure that the wound edges are nicely aligned. Starting at the center of the wound, apply strips in an evenly spaced manner opposing gravity until the edges of the wound are approximated.
6. Do not apply too much tension across a wound that may swell, or the tape may cause blisters.

exploration with irrigation and debridement when appropriate (Brolmann et al. 2012; Grimaldi et al. 2015; Levy and Tang 2014; Singer, Perry, and Allen 2008; Skelhorne and Munro 2002). These tissue adhesives polymerize to form a firm, pliable film that bridges the edges of the wound and binds to the epithelium. The adhesives are water resistant enough to permit showering after 48 h, and the material typically sloughs off with keratinized epithelium about 5 to 10 d after application (Brolmann et al. 2012).

If used appropriately, the adhesive will act as a strong bridge to hold well-apposed wound edges together (Levy and Tang 2014). When necessary, deep dermal sutures (vertical mattress stitches) are used to bring the skin edges into everted apposition. Everted edges are extremely important to successful closure with tissue adhesives because they prevent scar broadening and improve the cosmetic result. Everted skin apposition should be maintained with forceps or fingers during the application of adhesive.

The adhesive should be applied to dry tissue that is under very little tension. For best results, a thin layer should be applied over the epidermis and allowed to dry for approximately 20 to 30 s (Levy and Tang 2014). This method prevents pooling and running of the tissue adhesive, and it also provides a layer of protection from the heat generated by the exothermic polymerization. Subsequent layers of the adhesive are then applied over this initial layer.

When applying tissue adhesives, it is important to ensure that the adhesive does not leak into the wound. If leakage into the wound occurs, the adhesive acts as a barrier to epithelialization (Brolmann et al. 2012). The adhesive may also cause a foreign-body reaction and potentially increase the risk of infection if it enters the wound. It is also important to remember to use proper sterile technique and to minimize tissue trauma while applying these products. Always reduce skin tension at the site of the laceration and ensure that no dead space is present before sealing with a tissue adhesive.

Sutures

It is essential to understand the principles of wound healing before learning and mastering suturing techniques. We assume that you are well versed in these principles. Sutures are used to approximate wound edges in good apposition to facilitate the healing process, and they should be left in place long enough to allow healing to proceed to a sufficient degree that the natural properties of the skin can hold the wound together. Remove facial sutures after 3 to 5 d. (The physician may give instructions to remove every other suture on day 3 and the rest on day 5.) For extremities and trunk, sutures should remain in place for 5 to 7 d. On the scalp, back, feet, hands, and over the joints, sutures may need to be left in place for 10 to 14 d. Leaving sutures in place for an extended period may increase the risk of leaving permanent marks in the skin. Although an athletic trainer may not perform the actual suturing, depending on the state practice act or the direction of the physician, he or she may often be asked to assist in the preparation of materials and preparation of the patient to expedite the suturing process. Athletic trainers should be familiar with the materials and techniques used in suturing. Suture materials are made of various materials with various tensile strengths and degradability. Suture materials can be categorized according to the following characteristics:

- Absorbable versus nonabsorbable
- Natural versus synthetic
- Monofilament versus multifilament

Absorbable Sutures
Absorbable sutures degrade and are eventually eliminated either by inflammatory reactions caused by enzymes in the body or by hydrolysis. Absorbable sutures include the following:

- Purified collagen (catgut, chromic; see their description below)
- Polyglycolic acid (Vicryl, Monocryl)
- Polydioxanone (PDS II)

Nonabsorbable Sutures
Nonabsorbable sutures, although they do weaken, are permanent and do not dissolve in the body. Examples of nonabsorbable sutures include the following:

- Polyester (Ethibond)
- Polypropylene (Prolene)
- Nylon (Ethilon)
- Stainless steel
- Silk (not a truly permanent material; silk eventually degrades over a prolonged period of time, i.e., years)

Natural Sutures
Natural sutures are biological in origin and typically cause a more intense inflammatory reaction in tissue. Examples of natural sutures include the following:

- Catgut: purified collagen fibers from the intestines of healthy sheep or cows

---

CLINICAL TIPS

Tissue Adhesives

Everted edges are extremely important to successful closure with tissue adhesives because they prevent scar broadening and improve the cosmetic result.

- Chromic: treated with chromium salts, resists enzymes, prolongs time to degradation
- Silk

Synthetic Sutures

Synthetic sutures are made from various polymers and do not cause as intense an inflammatory reaction as that seen with natural sutures. Examples include the following:

- Polyglycolic acid (Vicryl, Monocryl)
- Polydioxanone (PDS II)
- Polyester (Ethibond)
- Polypropylene (Prolene)
- Nylon (Ethilon)

Monofilament

Suture material may also be characterized as being *monofilament* (a single strand of suture material) or *multifilament* (multiple fibers are twisted or braided together). Monofilament sutures generally cause less tissue trauma and have better resistance to microorganisms. Monofilament sutures do require more knots than multifilament sutures because there is more "memory" in these sutures.

- Polyglycolic acid (Monocryl)
- Polydioxanone (PDS II)
- Polypropylene (Prolene)
- Nylon (Ethilon)

Multifilament

Multifilament sutures may have greater resistance in tissue, although they do require fewer knots and may be significantly stronger. Examples are as follows:

- Polyglycolic acid (Vicryl, braided)
- Chromic (twisted)
- Silk (braided)
- Ultrahigh molecular weight polyethylene ("super") sutures (Orthocord [DePuy Mitek, Raynham, MA], FiberWire [Arthrex, Naples, FL])

Suture Sizes

Sutures are sized according to diameter, with 0 as the reference size. Numbers alone indicate progressively larger sutures (1, 2, 3, and so on), whereas numbers followed by a 0 indicate progressively smaller sutures (2-0, 4-0, 6-0, and so on). A human hair is roughly the size of a 6-0 suture.

Needles

Needles are classified according to shape (curved or straight), the type of point (taper point, cutting, reverse cutting, etc.), and the degree of curvature. Cutting needles are typically used for tougher tissue such as skin. Taper point needles, which are used when tearing through tissue, such as tendon, may be a risk.

Technique

The goals for suturing or closing any wound should be to optimize the potential for a good outcome by adhering to the principles of wound healing and by appropriately approximating the tissues. Proper wound preparation and assessment should include the evaluation and stabilization of deep tissues and copious irrigation to remove dirt, foreign bodies, and loose nonviable tissue. On occasion, debridement of wound edges may be needed to eliminate nonviable tissue.

Here are some tips to improve and facilitate the ease of suture placement:

- A proper grip on the needle with the needle holder should be ensured from the beginning. The needle may be inserted directly into the needle holder, or it may be loaded directly from the suture packet (figure 6.8).
- Introduce the needle perpendicular to the tissue surface (figure 6.9).
- Supinate the forearm—do not push the needle.
- If the needle is inserted inappropriately, then remove the needle from the wound and reinsert to ensure entrance into the skin.
- The sutures should be placed deeper rather than wider, to help ensure everted edges.

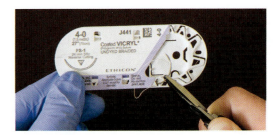

FIGURE 6.8 Load the needle holder: Clamp the needle holder approximately one-third the distance from the swage or eye to the point of the needle.

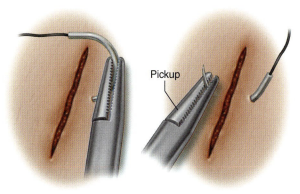

Pickup

FIGURE 6.9 Correct way to introduce a suture needle into the skin.

Note: A colored rope is used to clearly represent the two ends of the "suture" being tied.

1. The purple strand is held in the left hand, with the index finger supporting the strand *(a)*.
2. Bring the white strand (held in the right hand) forward, crossing the purple strand on the index finger *(b)*.
3. The white strand is then looped over and under the purple strand *(c)*.
4. The right hand pulls the white strand away from the body, and the left hand pulls the purple strand toward the body *(d)*.
5. Completed first throw (the term used to describe the first part of the knot) *(e)*.
6. With the purple strand held in the left hand, loop the purple strand *behind* the left thumb. The white strand is held away *(f)*.
7. The right hand pulls the white strand toward the body, crossing the purple strand over the thumb *(g)*.
8. The white strand is then looped under the purple strand *(h)*.
9. The white strand is grasped with the right hand *(i)*.
10. The right hand pulls the white strand toward the body, while the left hand pulls the purple strand away from the body *(j)*.
11. Finished square knot. Be sure the knot lies flat *(k)*.

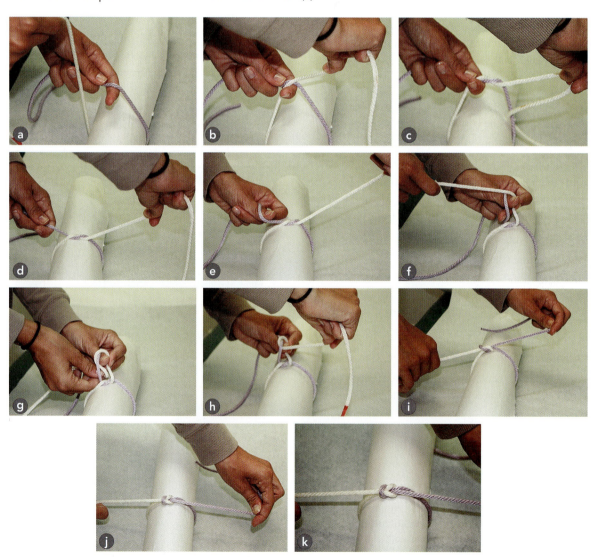

FIGURE 6.10
© Miki Cuppett

- Use the rule of halves: Insert the first suture at the wound's midpoint, the next two sutures at the midpoints of the two halves created by the first suture, and so on.
- Bridge the gaps of the wound to avoid "dog ears" or flaps of skin protruding from the wound.

Knot Tying   Sutures need to be tied off to make them secure and to keep the suture from sliding through the skin during the healing process. The *two-hand square knot* is the easiest and most reliable knot. It is used to tie most suture material.

The *instrument tie* is the most common technique used for laceration repair (see "Simple Interrupted Suture" later in this chapter). It is useful when one or both ends of the suture material are short. Techniques for suturing should include closing the wound in layers if needed. Proceed from deep to superficial, while obtaining adequate hemostasis, ensuring good skin apposition with minimal tension and everting skin edges.

Basic Suturing Techniques   There are several suturing techniques that may be used depending on the type of wound, the area to be sutured, and the preference and experience of the person suturing (figure 6.11). This section describes some of the more common techniques as well as the advantages and disadvantages of each.

Simple Interrupted

- Quick, easy
- Single stitches, individually knotted
- Used for uncomplicated laceration repair and wound closure
- Often done poorly—may result in poor cosmetic outcome

Continuous (Running)

- Good for hemostasis

Vertical Mattress

- Better eversion with precise approximation of skin edges
- It is a two-step stitch:
  - Simple stitch made "far, far" relative to wound edge (large bite)
  - Needle reversed and second simple stitch made inside the first "near, near" (small bite)
- Increased "crosshatching": poor **cosmesis**

Horizontal Mattress

- Better for thicker tissues
- Provides added strength in fascial closure
- Useful in callused skin (such as palms and soles)

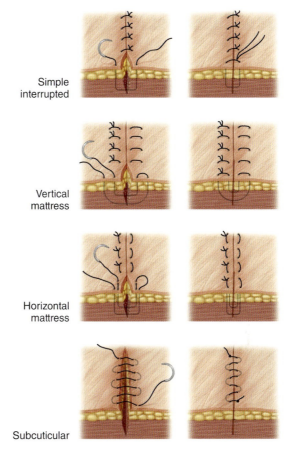

Simple interrupted

Vertical mattress

Horizontal mattress

Subcuticular

FIGURE 6.11   Types of sutures.

- It is a two-step stitch:
  - Simple stitch made
  - Needle reversed and second simple stitch made adjacent to first (same size bite as first stitch)
- Increased ischemia possible if too tight

Subcuticular (Intradermal)

- Best cosmetic results
- Fast, easy
- Requires good approximation of underlying dermis
- Usually a running stitch but can be interrupted
- Intradermal horizontal bites
- Ability to allow the suture to remain in the tissue for a longer period of time without the development of crosshatch scarring

After Suture Care and Complications   Wound infections can be minimized with meticulous attention to wound debridement and irrigation, strict aseptic technique, and antibiotics if indicated. The sutured area should be kept clean and dry for 24 to 48 h and should

Simple Interrupted Suture

1. With Adson forceps everting the skin, and with the needle perpendicular to the skin on the opposite side of the incision, supinate the wrist, allowing the needle to penetrate the skin (a).

2. With Adson forceps holding the skin, the needle should now be perpendicular to the subcutaneous tissue (b).

3. Supinate the wrist, allowing the needle to penetrate through the skin. Grasp the needle with Adson forceps (c).

4. Pull the suture through, leaving some excess with which to tie a knot (d).

5. With the hand holding the forceps, wrap the suture around the needle holder twice (e).

6. Once the suture is wrapped around twice, use the tip of the forceps to grasp the end left in excess (f).

7. Exert tension on both ends until the knot lies flat; this completes the first throw (g).

8. Wrap the suture around the needle holder once; be sure it is in the opposite direction from which the suture was initially wrapped around, and exert tension (h). The direction in which the needle holder is being pulled should not be the same direction pulled after the first throw (i).

9. Continue these alternating throws two more times.

10. Cut the suture, leaving approximately one-half inch for tails (j).

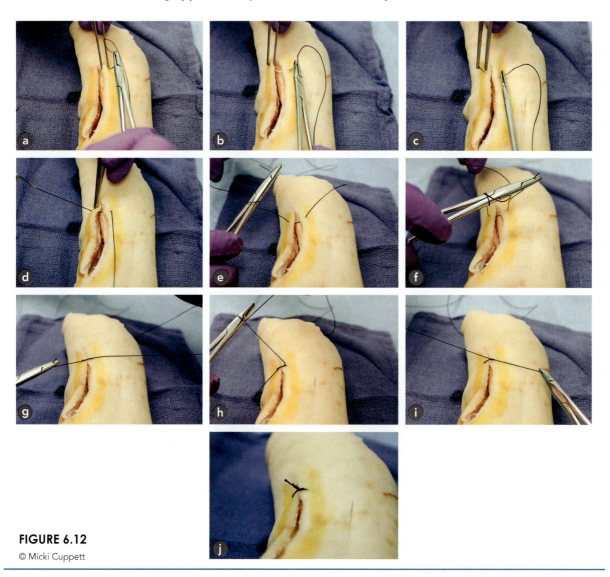

FIGURE 6.12
© Micki Cuppett

Vertical Mattress Suture

An easy way to remember this type of suture: it's called a "far-far, near-near" stitch.

1. Holding the skin with forceps, insert the needle perpendicular to the skin at point A *(a)*.
2. Holding the other side of the incision with forceps, insert the needle through the subcutaneous tissue and skin at point B *(b)*.
3. Holding the same side of the incision with forceps, insert the needle perpendicular to the skin at point C *(c)*.
4. Holding the opposite side of the incision with forceps, insert the needle through the subcutaneous tissue and skin at point D *(d)*.
5. After pulling the excess suture through, leaving a small tail, wrap the suture around the needle holder twice *(e)*.
6. Exert tension on both ends of the suture, allowing the knot to lie flat *(f)*.
7. Wrap the suture around the needle holder once *(g)*. Exert tension on both ends of the suture, locking the knot. This completes one throw knot *(h)*.
8. Repeat single throws two more times, in opposite directions (for a total of four throws).
9. A completed vertical mattress suture *(i)*.

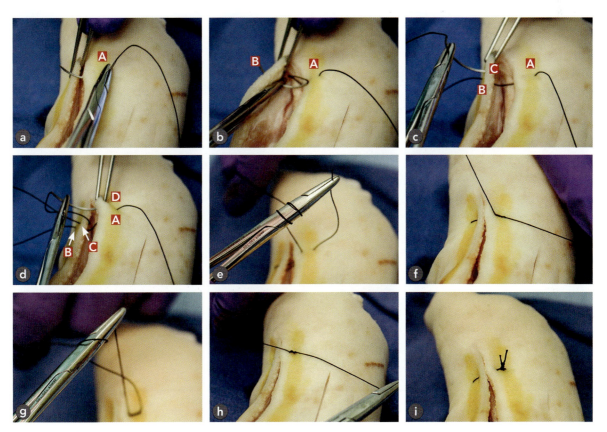

FIGURE 6.13
© Micki Cuppett

Horizontal Mattress Suture

1. With the needle perpendicular to the skin, supinate the wrist, allowing the needle to penetrate from the skin to the subcutaneous tissue at point A *(a)*.

2. The needle then penetrates from the subcutaneous tissue to the skin at point B *(b)*.

3. Either just distally to point A, or just proximally to the previous suture at point B, to the point at which the needle exits the skin, reinsert the needle, penetrating skin to subcutaneous tissue at point C *(c)*. Cross the wound and reinsert the needle, penetrating from subcutaneous tissue at point D.

4. Exert tension on the suture, keeping some excess suture for knot tying *(d)*.

5. Wrap the suture around the needle holder twice *(e)*.

6. Grasp the end of the suture with the tip of the needle holder and exert tension. The suture should lay flat *(f)*.

7. A completed horizontal mattress suture. Snip the ends, leaving approximately one-half inch for tails *(g)*.

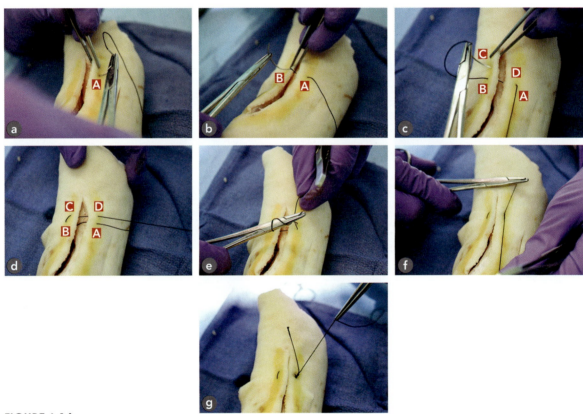

FIGURE 6.14

© Micki Cuppett

be inspected for signs of infection. The sutured wound is typically covered with a bandage. Wound tattooing or discoloration may occur if dyed sutures are used too close to the skin and if dirt or grit is left superficially in the wound. Wound scarring can be minimized by decreasing the tension across the closed wound and by ensuring that the tension is unidirectional and that the skin edges are everted (Rothrock 2016). The risk of wound dehiscence can be reduced by using appropriate techniques and proper suture placement and knot tying.

Suture Removal   Many athletic trainers may not be in a position to suture, but most will have the opportunity to remove sutures. To remove sutures, the clinician should open the sterile suture removal kit per previous instruction in this chapter. Put on gloves, and then remove and discard the dressing on the wound. Inspect the wound for healing and/or signs of infection. With forceps, lift the suture. Snip the suture as close to the skin as possible (figure 6.15*a*). Grasp the knotted end with forceps and slowly pull the suture through from the other side (figure 6.15*b*). Place the removed suture on gauze for disposal. Cover the healing wound with appropriate dressing or Band-Aid.

Staples

Metal skin staples are quite commonly used to approximate skin after surgery or for wound closure. Staples have been shown to be similar to sutures in their mechanical and histological characteristics, and contaminated wounds often demonstrate lower infection rates when stapling is employed (Smith et al. 2010; Phillips 2013). Staples also provide other advantages including decreased inflammatory response, wound width, and wound closure times, as well as promotion of wound edge eversion, formation of an incomplete loop with decreased tissue strangulation, and a lack of residual cross marks when compared with sutures. Studies have also demonstrated that total costs and patient satisfaction can be improved with the use of skin staples compared with sutures (Smith et al. 2010).

Using a Skin Stapler

To use a skin stapler, approximate and evert the skin edges with forceps. The stapler is held at 90° to the skin while applying gentle pressure (figure 6.16*a*). The staple is then ejected from the device, typically by gently squeezing the handle and then releasing it. Move the device to position the next staple and repeat the procedure. Staples are typically placed ¼ to ½ in (6 to 13 mm) apart. Each staple should hold the edges of the wound slightly everted with the edges nicely opposed (figure 6.16*b*).

Staple Removal

Staple removal requires a special staple extractor kit. As in suture removal, open the sterile staple removal kit and put on the sterile gloves provided. Inspect the wound and

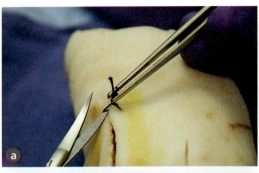
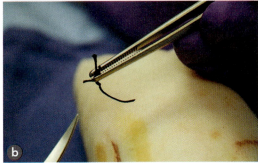

FIGURE 6.15 Removing sutures. *(a)* Seize the knot with needle holders and gently pull upward. With suture-cutting scissors, snip the suture. Make sure to leave the knot intact. *(b)* Complete suture removed.

© Micki Cuppett

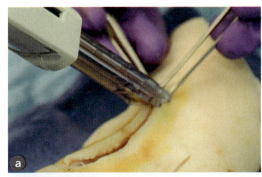
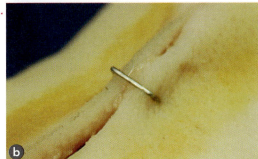

FIGURE 6.16 Using a skin stapler. *(a)* Have an assistant evert the skin edges while staples are applied. The stapler is held at 90° to the skin with gentle pressure. *(b)* Once the staple is ejected from the stapler, it should hold the edges of the wound slightly everted with the edges nicely opposed.

© Micki Cuppett

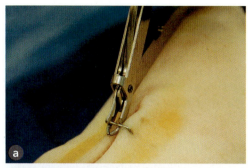

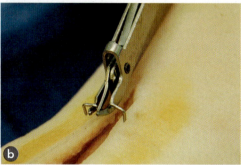

FIGURE 6.17 Staple removal. *(a)* Place the lower tip of the staple extractor under the first staple. *(b)* Close the handle of the extractor, depressing the center of the staple, causing it to bend and be released from the skin.

© Micki Cuppett

suture line for healing and/or signs of infection. Cleanse the suture line and staples with antiseptic swabs. Place the lower tip of the staple extractor under the first staple (figure 6.17*a*). Close the handle on the extractor to depress the center of the staple, causing the outer edges to bend upward simultaneously, away from the skin (Perry, Potter, and Ostendorf 2014) (figure 6.17*b*). Apply appropriate dressing if necessary.

Joint Aspiration and Injection

Joint aspirations (**arthrocentesis**) and injections are performed for a variety of reasons, most commonly for diagnostic or therapeutic purposes. Aspirations are typically performed to evaluate joint fluids for the presence of crystals, white blood cells, or bacteria; to confirm an acute hemarthrosis; and to relieve pressure due to an abnormal amount of fluid. Joint injections are usually performed to provide pain relief for arthritic or painful inflammatory conditions. Contraindications to joint aspirations or injections include the following:

- Local osteomyelitis
- Bacteremia
- Infectious arthritis
- Periarticular cellulitis
- Poorly controlled diabetes mellitus
- Uncontrolled coagulopathy

The most commonly injected joints are the knees and the shoulder. Common medications used for joint injections include a combination of a local anesthetic and a corticosteroid or hyaluronic acid (e.g., Synvisc). Other substances are also occasionally used. See figure 6.18 for typical supplies and equipment necessary for joint injections and aspirations.

Corticosteroid injections are relatively safe and have few systemic side effects. Common side effects include allergic reactions, steroid flare, or temporary exacerbation of underlying diabetes. Hyaluronic acid injections also have proven to be safe with few side effects. As with suturing, some athletic trainers may not be in a position to perform injections or aspirations, but they may be asked to assist the physician in the preparation of the patient and the supplies. Those athletic trainers who are employed as physician extenders may be asked to perform these techniques on a regular basis.

After diagnostic arthrocentesis, interventions will be dictated by the results of the fluid analysis. Large effusions can recur and may require repeat aspiration. It is helpful to inform the patient that the immediate relief from the local anesthetic may wear off after 4 to 6 h and that the joint may be sore until the corticosteroid effects begin, which may take a day or so. Applying ice several times for 20 to 30 min will help relieve some of the soreness. Resting the joint will also help.

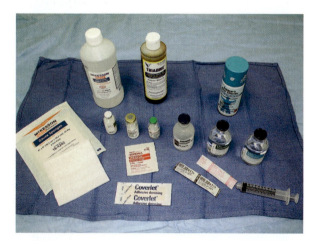

FIGURE 6.18 Supplies for joint injections and aspirations are alcohol, povidone-iodine solution, ethyl chloride spray, sterile gauze, alcohol wipe, bandage, and 10 cm³ syringe. Also needed but not shown are an 18-gauge needle (to draw up injection) and 22-gauge needle (for injection).

© Micki Cuppett

Technique for Knee Aspiration and Injection

The lateral approach is the most functional and is outlined here. Sterile gloves should be worn for asepsis and universal precautions, but there is no consensus as to whether gloves are necessary.

1. The patient lies supine on the table with the knee extended.

2. The superior lateral aspect of the patella is palpated. The skin is marked with a pen, one finger-breadth above and one fingerbreadth lateral to this site. This location provides the most direct access to the suprapatellar pouch. The most distal aspect of the vastus lateralis also is a good landmark in many patients.

3. The skin is washed with povidone-iodine (or alcohol) solution *(a)*. An 18-gauge, 1- or 1½-in. needle is attached to a 20- or 60-ml syringe, depending on the anticipated amount of fluid present for removal. The barrel of the syringe should be slid in and out once or twice before the procedure in order to remove air and reduce friction in the syringe.

4. Ethyl chloride spray may be applied topically to the skin after preparation and immediately before needle insertion. Stretching the skin with the opposite hand can also reduce needle insertion discomfort by stretching the pain fibers in the skin. The needle is directed at a 45° angle distally, with the needle held just below parallel to the table *(b)*.

5. Pay particular attention as the needle is inserted, to sense when the needle penetrates the joint capsule—there is usually a subtle but palpable "pop." Maintain slight backpressure on the syringe while inserting the needle, and once the needle has entered the joint aspirate should begin filling the syringe *(c)*. It is not necessary to fully insert the needle, although in obese patients the entire needle (or occasionally a 3 in. spinal needle) may be needed. Continue to draw back on the plunger with steady pressure, holding the syringe and needle still. Using the nondominant hand, or employing an assistant, to compress the opposite side of the joint and the patella may aid in arthrocentesis.

6. Once the aspirate is completely removed, a sterile hemostat may be placed on the hub of the needle and used to hold the needle steady while the syringe is removed (unscrewed) *(d)*, and the injection syringe is attached to the needle or another syringe for aspirate is used *(e)*.

7. Various mixtures are used for injection, based on the provider's experience. The author prefers betamethasone (Celestone, 6 mg/ml), 3 ml, mixed with 7 ml of 0.25% bupivacaine for injection alone or 3 ml of betamethasone and 2 ml of bupivacaine after aspiration. After injection of the medication, the needle and syringe are withdrawn.

8. The skin is cleansed with alcohol and a bandage is applied over the puncture site. Apply compression wrap.

Note: If no aspiration is being performed—that is, for an injection only—a 22-gauge, 1½-in. needle may be used instead of an 18-gauge needle. The clinician may choose to have the patient sitting with the knee at a 90° angle.

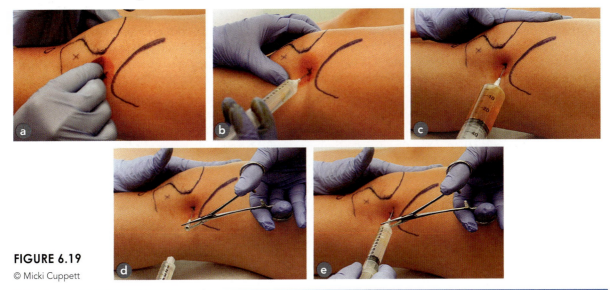

FIGURE 6.19
© Micki Cuppett

Technique for Knee Injection Only

If no aspiration is needed, the clinician can more easily do a joint injection of the knee with the patient in a seated position.

1. Cleanse the injection area with Betadine *(a)*.
2. Insert the needle into the anterolateral side of the joint, keeping it parallel to the ground *(b)*.
3. Keep one hand in contact with the skin surface while keeping the other hand on the syringe. This will help with proprioception of the syringe *(c)*.

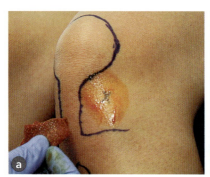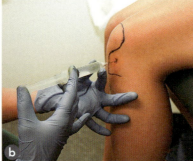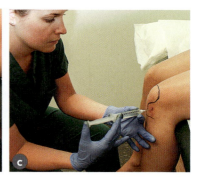

FIGURE 6.20
© Micki Cuppett

Subacromial Injection Technique

1. The patient should be seated in a chair with the affected shoulder exposed. The arm is resting in the lap or next to the body. The posterolateral approach is direct and avoids having the patient observe the procedure. After taking the appropriate medical history, performing a physical examination, and discussing with the patient the procedure and obtaining informed consent, complete the following steps.
2. The acromial border is palpated and the posterolateral corner is marked with a pen, one finger-breadth below the acromion on the posterior aspect of the shoulder. A soft area will be able to be palpated at that location.
3. The skin is washed with povidone-iodine (or alcohol) solution *(a)*. Sterile gloves should be worn for asepsis and universal precautions, but there is no consensus as to whether gloves are necessary.
4. A 22-gauge, 1½ in. needle is attached to a 10 ml syringe. Slide the barrel of the syringe in and out once or twice before the procedure in order to remove air and to reduce friction in the syringe. Ethyl chloride spray may be used topically on the skin after the preparation and immediately before needle insertion. Stretching the skin with the opposite hand may also reduce needle insertion discomfort by stretching the pain fibers in the skin *(b)*.
5. The needle is directed at an angle corresponding to the slope of the acromion. The acromion may be palpated with the opposite hand, which is also useful for proprioception of the needle. There should be almost no resistance when injecting *(c)*. Pay attention as the needle is inserted; it is possible to sense when the needle penetrates the subacromial space. Maintain slight back-pressure on the syringe while inserting it and, once the needle has entered the space, begin injecting the solution. A common subacromial injection is betamethasone (Celestone, 6 mg/ml), 3 ml, mixed with 7 ml of 0.25% bupivacaine. After injection of the medication, the needle and syringe are withdrawn.
6. The skin is cleansed with alcohol and a bandage is applied over the puncture site.

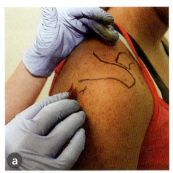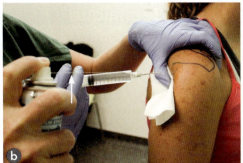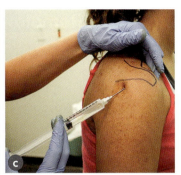

FIGURE 6.21
© Micki Cuppett

Intraarticular Injection Technique

1. Cleanse the injection area with povidone-iodine (Betadine).
2. Insert the needle from the posterolateral aspect of the shoulder, below the acromion. The needle should be parallel to the floor. There should be almost no resistance when injecting.

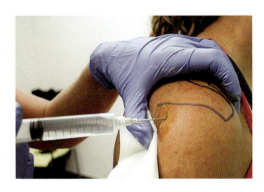

FIGURE 6.22
© Micki Cuppett

Acromioclavicular Injection Technique

1. Cleanse the injection area with povidone-iodine (Betadine).
2. Palpate the distal end of the clavicle and the acromion. Insert the needle perpendicular to the joint. There should be almost no resistance when injecting.

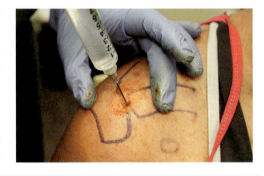

FIGURE 6.23
© Micki Cuppett

Subungual Hematoma Drilling and Drainage

Nail **trephination** usually can be performed up to 36 h after injury or recognition of hematoma. Before performing the procedure, appropriate physical examination should be performed and informed consent obtained.

There are several ways to drain the nail bed. Melting a small hole in the nail by means of a heated paper clip or a surgical electrocautery device is an effective and simple technique. There are also several commercially available devices specifically designed for this purpose. Another method is to use an 18-gauge needle as a handheld drill. This method is quick, inexpensive, and easy to learn.

Antibiotics are not usually necessary unless there is gross contamination of the wound. Instruct the patient to elevate the hand for several days to prevent swelling. Soaking the digit in warm water with povidone-iodine

Subungual Hematoma Drilling Technique

1. Cleanse the digit with povidone-iodine solution or alcohol. Local anesthesia is usually not necessary for isolated nail trephination.
2. Position an 18-gauge needle with the tip in the center of the hematoma.
3. Hold the hub of the needle between the thumb and index finger.
4. Roll the needle back and forth quickly and observe as it begins to bore into the nail.
5. Blood should soon begin to emerge from the hole—be careful, the blood may be under pressure and may spray from the hole.
6. You will not need to press any deeper, but slowly enlarge the hole by drilling. Be careful not to press too deeply or you will violate the nail bed, and this will be painful.
7. Cleanse the nail again, and apply a sterile dressing.
8. If possible, allow a small portion of the gauze to enter the hole as a wick to keep it from clotting.

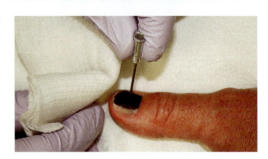

FIGURE 6.24
© Micki Cuppett

solution for 15 min, three or four times a day, will help prevent infection. Make sure that the patient understands that the nail may be lost (although it will often regrow), and that there is a small risk of permanent nail deformity as a result of the initial injury to the nail bed.

Paronychial Incision and Drainage

A paronychia is a tender, inflamed infection of the hand (most commonly) or foot, where the nail and skin meet. It is usually caused by a bacterial infection, but it may also be fungal or viral. Paronychia are often associated with trimming of the nails. If the infection is noticed early, antibiotics and soaking in warm water and povidone-iodine solution may be effective. Incision and drainage are indicated to control pain, speed healing, and prevent the spread of infection.

Drainage is usually sufficient to clear up the infection. Topical antibiotics are typically used, and oral antibiotics may also be considered.

Instruct the patient to elevate the hand or foot for several days to prevent swelling. Follow-up should be performed within 2 to 3 d, at which time the packing

Paronychial Incision Technique

1. Cleanse the digit with povidone-iodine solution. *Note:*
   ◦ A cutaneous nerve block is usually tolerated much better than local infiltration of anesthetic.
   ◦ The digital cutaneous nerves run along the medial and lateral aspects of each finger.
   ◦ These nerves can be blocked at any point above the distal phalanx.
2. Use a 25-gauge needle to raise a skin wheal by administering approximately 0.25 ml of lidocaine directly over the lateral and medial cutaneous nerve.
3. Advance the needle perpendicular to the digit (nerve) until you reach the bone.
4. Inject about 1 ml of lidocaine, sliding the needle up and down on the dorsal and volar sides of the finger.

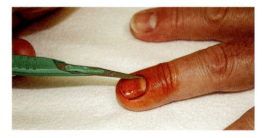

FIGURE 6.25
© Micki Cuppett

5. Allow 5 to 10 min for the block to develop.
6. Cleanse the entire digit again with povidone-iodine solution.
7. Using a #11 scalpel, make an incision parallel to the axis of the finger. *Note:*
   ◦ The incision should be an extension of the lateral and medial nail groove and deep enough to enter the abscess being treated.
   ◦ Do not direct the scalpel toward the bone.
8. Using scissors, debride necrotic tissue if needed. *Note:*
   ◦ If the infection has progressed under the nail, the proximal nail must be removed as well.
9. Use mosquito forceps to lever up and hold the nail.
10. Cut the nail off in a straight line, using the scissors.
11. Place gauze packing under the flap of overhanging tissue and the cuticle.
12. Culture the infected material removed from under the nail to determine the exact pathogen causing the infection.

should be removed. After the packing is removed, the digit should be soaked in warm water with povidone-iodine solution for 15 min, three or four times a day. After each soaking, a dry, nonstick dressing should be applied. Inform the patient that the nail must be protected from being torn away from the nail bed until it completely regrows. This process may take several months. After the healing process is complete, the nail and cuticle may be deformed.

Inserting an Intravenous Catheter

The intravenous (IV) route involves the injection of a drug directly into a vein. It is used when drug action must begin immediately or when other routes of administration cannot be used because of patient condition or drug characteristics (Potter and Perry, 2011). This is a common occurrence in the hospital or surgical center. The athletic trainer will see the IV route used most often when IV fluids (typically without medication added) are administered to achieve rapid rehydration of an athlete who is experiencing heat-related illness. Athletic trainers must be aware of state practice laws that address their potential role in administering IV fluids. Some states allow athletic trainers who have gone through IV training and certification to administer IV fluids under the supervision of a physician. In other situations, the athletic trainer may be asked to assist the physician in preparing the patient and the materials for IV administration. It is up to the athletic trainer to know the laws and to work only under the authorized scope of practice. In addition, before starting an IV, the practitioner must make certain that an order for the IV line has been given and is noted in the patient's chart.

Equipment

The following equipment is required for starting an IV line:

- Towel
- Alcohol wipes (Povidone-iodine wipes may also be used)
- Tourniquet
- Angiocatheter
- IV tubing
- IV fluid
- Sterile transparent dressing or tape
- Gloves
- Gauze

Anatomy

There are many acceptable sites for performing an IV. The antecubital fossa and the dorsal veins of the hand are probably the most common due to the presence and easy accessibility of several large veins (cephalic, basilic, and median cubital) (figure 6.26).

Preparing the IV Tubing

Remove the sterile cover from the IV bag and portal and open the IV tubing set. Maintain aseptic technique when opening sterile packages and IV solution. Clamp the tubing; then uncap the spike on the tubing and insert the spike into the entry portal on the IV bag (figure 6.27*a*). Squeeze the drip chamber on the tubing set (figure 6.27*b*), and allow it to fill at least halfway (figure 6.27*c*). Open the clamp and allow enough fluid to flow until all air bubbles have disappeared from the tubing (figure 6.27*d*). Reclamp the tubing and maintain sterility of setup.

Catheter Selection

Selecting an appropriate-sized catheter is very important. A catheter that is too large will make it more difficult to enter the vein, increase the likelihood of rupturing the vein, and be likely to increase discomfort. A catheter that is too small will limit the amount of fluid that can be given

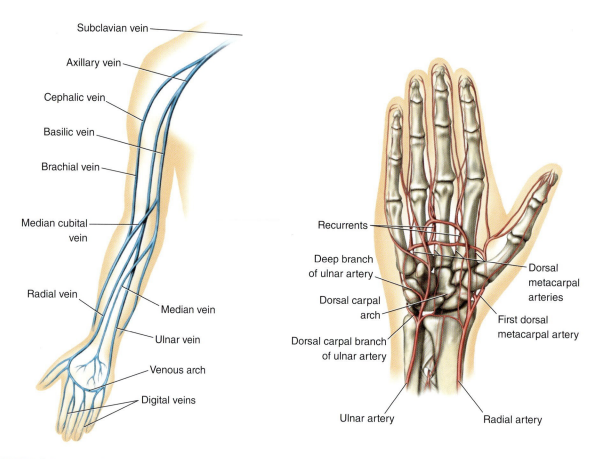

FIGURE 6.26 Superficial veins of the antecubital fossa typically are used for starting an IV. The dorsal veins in the hand may also be used.

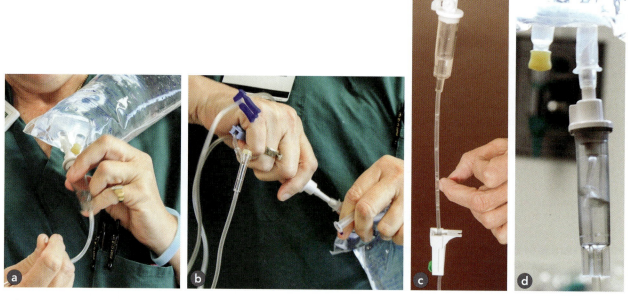

FIGURE 6.27 Preparing IV tubing for use.
© Micki Cuppett

over a period of time. Sometimes it is necessary to use a smaller-than-desired catheter to begin an IV treatment; later, if it is needed, another IV line can be installed at a different site once the patient is better hydrated. An 18- or 20-gauge catheter is typically used; occasionally a larger 16-gauge or a smaller 22-gauge catheter may be needed (figure 6.28).

Failed Attempt

If the first attempt is unsuccessful in entering the vein (or there is no flashback or the flashback disappears), slowly withdraw the catheter without pulling all the way out. Watch for the flashback to occur. If the vein has still not been entered, advance the catheter again in another attempt to enter the vein. If several attempts at entering the vein fail, the tourniquet should be released, gauze placed over the puncture site, the catheter withdrawn, and tape placed to hold the gauze. Identify another site for another attempt.

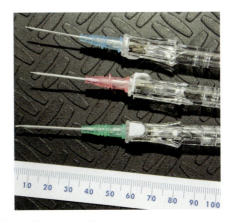

FIGURE 6.28 Typically an 18- or 20-gauge catheter is used to administer IV fluids; however, occasionally a large-bore (16-gauge or above) is used for rapid infusion. A smaller needle may be used for comfort when rapid infusion is not needed.

© Micki Cuppett

Technique for Inserting a Catheter

Preparing the Arm

1. Identify and palpate the selected site. For the antecubital area, apply a tourniquet high on the upper arm (a). The tourniquet should be tight enough to restrict blood flow. One way to help increase venous engorgement is to ask the patient to squeeze his or her hand into a fist several times.
2. Reidentify the selected vein and palpate for patency (b).
3. Clean the area by wiping several times with alcohol swabs. Some health care providers prefer to prep the area by wiping with povidone-iodine swabs and then a final wipe with alcohol.
4. Don gloves if not already wearing them.

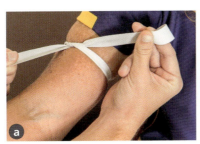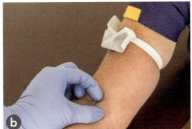

Inserting the Catheter

1. Remove catheter from sterile package. It may be helpful to slide the catheter in and out of the metal stylet once or twice to feel how much force is needed.
2. Use one hand to apply distal tension to the skin, toward the wrist in the opposite direction from that in which the needle will be advancing (c). Be careful not to compress the vein and prevent flow, which may cause the vein to collapse.
3. Using a deliberate—but not too forceful—motion, advance the catheter through the skin and into the vein. Aim the catheter along the direction of the vein so as not to poke through the vein (d). Slowly advance the catheter into the vein and look for the flashback of blood at the catheter hub (e). This will indicate that the catheter is within the vein.

4. With the catheter positioned in the vein, slide the plastic catheter forward into the vein over the top of the metal stylet. The catheter should slide forward easily until the hub is all the way to the skin. Do not force it or the vein may rupture.

5. With the catheter advanced to the hub, release the tourniquet while simultaneously applying pressure over the vein to collapse it. This will prevent blood from flowing out of the catheter when the stylet is removed (Perry, Potter, and Ostendorf 2014).

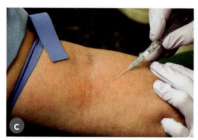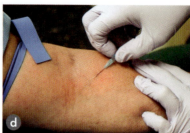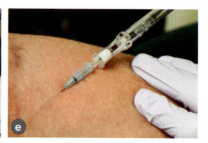

Attaching IV Tubing

1. Remove the stylet and set it aside to be disposed of in a sharps container, or drop it immediately into the sharps container.

2. Attach the IV tubing to the catheter (f). This is usually done with a rotating "Luer-lock" mechanism, and successful locking is signaled by a click.

3. Release pressure from the vein; there should be a small amount of blood backflow into the tubing.

4. Open the clamp on the tubing and allow the IV fluid to flow into the catheter.

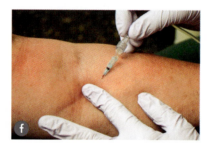

Securing the IV

1. Secure the catheter in place with the transparent sterile dressing and tape the IV in place using several strips of tape. This will prevent movement of the tubing. Another method is to place gauze over and under the tubing near the catheter to protect the skin and to soak up any blood droplets.

2. Place tape over the puncture site and over loops of tubing so there is less pressure on the tubing (g, h).

3. Make sure the tubing is secure to prevent any accidental removal of the catheter.

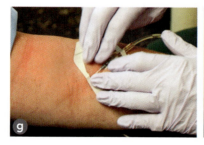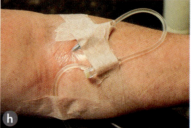

FIGURE 6.29
© Micki Cuppett

Adjusting Flow

In an emergency situation with an athlete suffering from heat illness, the roller clamp is opened completely to allow for rapid rehydration with the IV fluid, and the flow rate is not determined. There may be situations in which the physician will want to determine the rate of infusion, and the roller clamp can be adjusted to increase or decrease the flow rate. The flow rate is determined by counting drops in the drip chamber for 1 min. There are many conversion charts and calculators available either in print or electronic format to assist the health care professional in translating the drips for 1 min into ml/h.

Summary

Many of the techniques outlined in this chapter may be new even to practicing athletic trainers or other health care professionals. It is crucial to know which procedures are allowed under your state practice acts. Even if you are not directly involved in the actual procedure, it is imperative for you to understand asepsis and aseptic technique so as not to contaminate a procedure when in close proximity to the patient and to the sterile person performing the procedure.

Many of these procedures take considerable practice to master. There are simulators available to allow clinicians to practice many of the techniques. There are injection models that realistically simulate the feeling of a correctly placed needle as it is inserted into the joint capsule. Similarly, there are models available for suture practice. Clinicians may also practice suturing on pigs' feet, as was done in this chapter for illustration purposes.

 Apply It! The case study for this chapter looks at a collegiate hockey player who needs sutures after being hit with a player's stick. Read the scenario and answer the questions at www.HumanKinetics.com/MedicalConditionsInTheAthlete.

PART III

Medical Conditions by System

Chapters 7 through 16 follow a systematic approach as they address common conditions and diseases by body system. Most chapters follow a simple template, beginning with an overview of the relevant anatomy and physiology as they relate to the body system; then identifying specific conditions; explaining signs and symptoms and differential diagnoses, referral and diagnostic tests, and finally, discussing prognoses, treatment, and implications for sport participation. If a condition has age- or gender-specific considerations, those issues are also discussed. If relevant, implications for pediatric and mature athletes are also included. The systems covered are as follows:

- "Respiratory System" (chapter 7) covers conditions such as asthma, chronic obstructive pulmonary disease, upper respiratory infections, and pneumonia. All conditions discussed can occur in an otherwise healthy person. Knowing the early signs and symptoms of respiratory conditions and the evaluation techniques unique to this system can help prevent a situation from becoming worse, or in cases of pneumothorax or hemothorax, can save a life.

- "Cardiovascular System" (chapter 8) includes conditions such as causes of sudden cardiac death, Marfan syndrome, arrhythmias, and hypertension. Anemias and sickle cell trait are also discussed. Medical standards for safe athletic participation for athletes with cardiac conditions are discussed throughout the chapter.

- "Gastrointestinal System" (chapter 9) covers the stomach, abdomen, and digestive system, including the appendix and gallbladder. In addition to common conditions, such as nausea, vomiting, and diarrhea, it covers food poisoning and parasitic infections. These conditions are especially critical to recognize in athletes, for they

travel quite often, and they can be subjected to a variety of food that may cause these ailments. Gastroesophageal reflux disease and ulcers, irritable bowel syndrome, celiac disease, and inflammatory bowel conditions are all discussed, as are their implications for athletes who need to have proper nutrition to perform at optimal levels.

- "Genitourinary and Gynecological Systems" (chapter 10) covers conditions found in both genders such as kidney stones, sports hematuria, urinary tract infection, and sexually transmitted infections. Specific to males, testicular torsion and testicular and prostate cancers are among the conditions discussed. Vaginitis, pelvic inflammatory disease, conditions related to the menstrual cycle, ovarian and cervical cancers, and pregnancy are covered for the female athlete.

- "Neurological System" (chapter 11) discusses concussions (traumatic brain injury), migraine, stroke, and chronic conditions such as Guillain-Barré syndrome, multiple sclerosis, and epilepsy. Also reviewed are amyotrophic lateral sclerosis (ALS) and complex regional pain syndrome (CRPS).

- "The Eye" (chapter 12) covers infectious conditions such as conjunctivitis and acute traumatic injuries such as hyphema, orbital fracture, and lacerations to the eyelid. Protective eyewear is also addressed, as there are national safety guidelines that govern eyewear in certain sports.

- "Ear, Nose, Throat, and Mouth" (chapter 13) discusses conditions unique to the systems of hearing, smelling, and taste. It begins with a very common issue, especially in swimmers, otitis externa (swimmer's ear), but it also addresses traumatic ruptured eardrum. Conditions that can be related to allergies, rhinitis and sinusitis are covered, as is epistaxis (nosebleed). Mouth and throat ailments include tonsillitis, laryngitis, and lesions of the mouth, including oral cancers.

- "Systemic Disorders" (chapter 14) describes conditions that cross body systems or present to more than one system, such as malignancies involving the lymphatic system and blood, diabetes, and Lyme disease. Systemic lupus erythematosus, fibromyalgia, chronic fatigue syndrome, and endocrine disorders are also discussed.

- "Infectious Diseases" (chapter 15) discusses conditions that are infectious and can be transmitted. Some of these infectious conditions are covered in chapter 16 on dermatological conditions. In chapter 15 we cover infection transmission and prevention. Conditions discussed include influenza, infectious mononucleosis, childhood conditions (e.g., mumps, measles, chicken pox), and hepatitis. Streptococcal and staphylococcal infections and the danger they present are reported. Life-changing or threatening infections such as encephalitis, meningitis, and the Zika virus are discussed, as are prevention of the spread and treatment of these diseases.

- "Dermatological Conditions" (chapter 16) discusses common viral, fungal, and bacterial skin disorders that can be found in the physically active population, including skin cancers and insect bites.

Chapter 17 covers psychological issues and substance use disorders. These topics are important because many active people have these conditions and recognizing them is critical. Mood, anxiety, eating, and attention deficit hyperactivity disorders are discussed. Drug and alcohol abuse are also discussed.

Chapter 18 looks at working with special populations, specifically the medical concerns about specific pathological conditions. Issues concerning paraplegia, including boosting, hyperthermia, pressure sores, and spasms are discussed. Other conditions covered are cerebral palsy, amputations, and sensory disabilities. These topics are important because of the increasing number of athletes who have genetic disabilities or who compete after sustaining traumatic injuries. These athletes participate in local events, national trials, and the Paralympics. They should have appropriate medical care that may be outside the realm of the primary physicians who treat them.

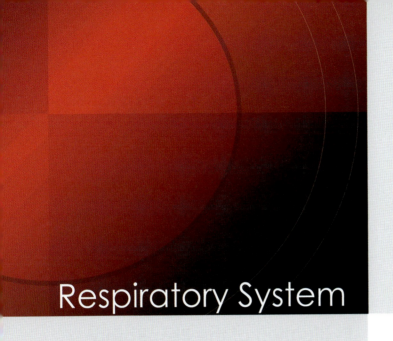

Respiratory System

OBJECTIVES

At the completion of this chapter the reader should be able to do the following:

- Describe the basic anatomy and physiology of the respiratory system.
- Define common, normal, and abnormal respiratory patterns.
- Perform a basic evaluation of the respiratory system, including auscultation and percussion.
- Identify characteristics of normal and abnormal breath sounds.
- Recognize common pathological conditions including signs and symptoms, differential assessment, referral, standard medical treatment, and implications for participation in athletics.

Respiratory disorders can be very alarming to the athlete and the medical professional. Not only do respiratory conditions affect athletic performance, but also acute respiratory distress can be life-threatening. Great strides have been made in the recognition and treatment of common airway disease. Only a few years ago, it was uncommon for an athlete with airway disease to be able to compete at the highest level. Advances in the management of these disorders in both the athletic and nonathletic populations have allowed affected patients to participate in activities they love even at competitive levels. Because so many more people with respiratory conditions are participating in physical activity, the athletic trainer must be able to recognize, evaluate, and refer patients with these conditions.

This chapter describes the evaluation techniques, including percussion and auscultation, that are used with a person who exhibits a respiratory condition. Normal and abnormal breathing patterns are reviewed to identify potential problems of the respiratory system. Common respiratory disorders such as asthma, influenza, pneumonia, bronchitis, and other viral upper respiratory infections are discussed. Signs and symptoms of these conditions, as well as the need for medical attention, are presented. Respiratory health is integral to physical activity and must be properly assessed, with referral of the athlete to a physician if warranted.

Overview of Anatomy and Physiology

The pulmonary system is primarily involved in the exchange of oxygen and carbon dioxide, which are vital in the production of the energy needed for metabolism at the cellular level. This process, known as respiration, can be divided into two distinct but simultaneous steps: ventilation and oxygenation. During **ventilation**, air moves through the respiratory tract. **Oxygenation** describes the actual exchange of gases in the alveolar–capillary beds.

The organs of respiration are divided into the upper and lower respiratory tracts. The upper respiratory tract consists of the following:

- Nasal passages
- Paranasal sinuses
- Pharynx, including nasopharynx and oropharynx
- Larynx or voice box

The upper respiratory tract is mainly responsible for warming, humidifying, and filtering the air as it reaches the lower respiratory tract (Ball et al. 2014). As air is pulled from the external environment into the nasal passages, secretions from the paranasal sinuses add moisture. Cilia, which are tiny hairlike projections that line the upper airway, filter out fine particles of debris as the air moves into the lower respiratory tract. The lower respiratory tract is composed of the following:

- Trachea
- Right and left bronchi
- Lung parenchyma

In the lungs, each mainstem bronchus is further divided into bronchioles and terminal alveoli (figure 7.1). The tracheobronchial tree is a tubular system supported by cartilaginous rings that divide from the trachea into the right and left bronchi at approximately T4 or T5. These main bronchi then divide further into three branches on the right and two on the left. This tubular system serves as a passageway for air as it reaches the bronchioles and, finally, the terminal alveoli, where the exchange of oxygen and carbon dioxide from the surrounding capillary beds takes place. The right lung is divided into three separate lobes: upper, middle, and lower. The left lung has only an upper lobe and a lower lobe.

Evaluation of the Respiratory System

A considerable amount of information can be gleaned from a physical examination of the respiratory system. The patient's history can provide telltale clues about the frequency, intensity, and triggers for respiratory issues. General observations of the patient's demeanor will give the clinician clues if there is any respiratory distress or

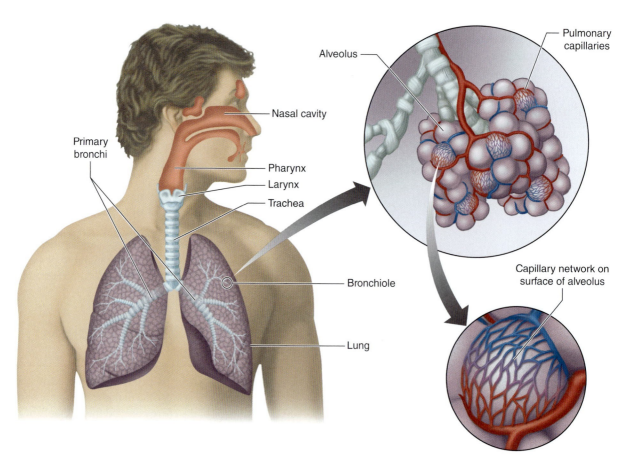

FIGURE 7.1 Organs of the respiratory system, with a detailed view of the alveolar sac.

discomfort with breathing. Breath sounds themselves give clues as to the nature of the condition.

History and Inspection

An athlete may present with an acute or chronic respiratory condition while complaining of shortness of breath, abnormal breathing pattern, or cough. Respiratory pathologies often present with nonspecific symptoms that can make initial diagnosis difficult. The first step in evaluation is to take a thorough history, which includes questions about how long the problem has existed, what exacerbates the condition, and the severity of the symptoms. In an athlete experiencing an acute respiratory attack, the history is abbreviated to only those questions needed to determine the immediate course of action. A more thorough history is taken once the immediate emergency is under control. If the patient complains of a cough, the examiner asks the patient to describe the characteristics of the cough. Is it "dry" or "barking," or is it productive of sputum? Attention should also be paid to any discoloration of the sputum with the cough. Timing of the cough is also important: Is the cough worse at night, as is often the case with asthma or gastroesophageal reflux disease (GERD) (see chapter 9), or does it occur shortly after exertion as in exercise-induced bronchospasm? If shortness of breath or dyspnea is the complaint, the examiner tries to discover its severity (e.g., how long the athlete has felt short of breath, what activity precipitated it, and whether it occurs at rest or only with activity). Does the patient struggle with inhalation, exhalation, or both? Was there any trauma to the chest or abdomen? Associated chest pain is another important symptom to ascertain to consider cardiac causes for dyspnea. Tightness in the chest or the throat? Throat tightness may indicate exercise-induced laryngeal obstruction (EILO) (Backer 2010; Nielsen, Hull, and Back 2013). Also, the examiner asks the athlete about any past history of respiratory infections, smoking, and environmental exposure to potential allergens.

The chest is inspected after the history is taken. In the athletic training clinic, a chest examination is usually performed on a male athlete who has removed his shirt and on a female athlete dressed in a sports bra and shorts. The examiner inspects the chest for shape and configuration, including any skeletal deformities. Congenital deformities, such as scoliosis or kyphosis, as well as other chest deformities may be present and may affect not only the shape of the chest but also the efficiency of respiration. In a normal adult, the thorax is elliptical in shape and is narrower anterior to posterior than it is across the transverse axis (figure 7.2a). A barrel chest presents as a rounded shape that is the same diameter from anterior to posterior as it is transversely (figure 7.2b). Barrel chest is associated with chronic emphysema and asthma but may also be present in the normal, older adult. Pectus excavatum, a congenital shape, is usually not symptomatic but presents as a depression at the junction of the xiphoid with the sternum (figure 7.2c). Pectus carinatum presents as a forward protrusion of the sternum (figure 7.2d). It is less common than pectus excavatum, and minor conditions require no treatment.

The clinician also inspects the chest for potential bruising of the ribs or chest wall, with special attention to the effort and posture of the athlete when breathing, and notes the rate and rhythm of respirations (Intravia and DeBeradino 2013). Symmetry of chest wall movement with breathing is also important.

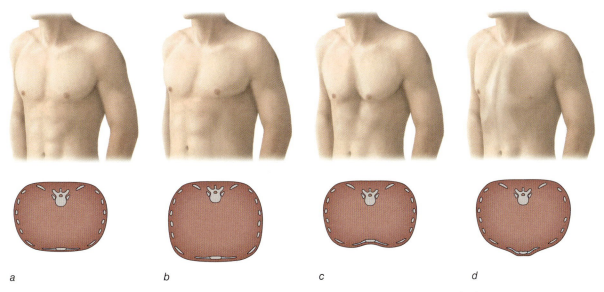

a   b   c   d

FIGURE 7.2 Common chest shapes: (a) normal, (b) barrel, (c) pectus excavatum, and (d) pectus carinatum.

Respiratory Patterns

Breathing involves several simultaneous processes. Chemoreceptors in the medulla oblongata of the brain sense changes in pH and carbon dioxide levels. Decreases in pH, as well as corresponding increases in carbon dioxide, result from normal cellular metabolism and stimulate an increase in ventilation to remove these by-products. Neural control of breathing comes from the phrenic nerve, which arises from cervical nerve roots C3, C4, and C5 and innervates the diaphragm, as well as the nerves that innervate the intercostal muscles. As the diaphragm and intercostal muscles contract, the thoracic cavity expands. This generates negative pressure, which causes movement of air into the lungs during inspiration. When alveolar pressure equalizes with atmospheric pressure, intercostal stretch receptors fire and inspiration ceases. The elastic recoil of the thoracic cage results in the passive process of expiration. Accessory muscles of breathing, which include the abdominal, sternocleidomastoid, and scalene muscles, are relatively quiet during normal breathing but become active as the work of normal breathing increases.

Normal respiration is unlabored, with 12 to 20 breaths/min. When breathing becomes disordered, several patterns can emerge. The term **dyspnea** refers to the subjective sensation of difficulty in breathing or shortness of breath. When patients have dyspnea, it is important to determine its severity. For example, does the difficulty occur at rest or only with exertion? Certain situations may produce dyspnea, such as eating, being exposed to cold **ambient temperatures**, or lying down at night. A condition known as **paroxysmal nocturnal dyspnea** is found in patients with underlying congestive heart failure and causes the individual to be short of breath when lying down at night. Dyspnea may accompany other symptoms in various disease processes, such as fever in lung infections, wheezing in asthma, or chest pain in acute myocardial infarction.

Tachypnea refers to breathing that has become more rapid than 24 breaths/min. This can be seen in a number of respiratory conditions that require the body to increase ventilation. Pulmonary embolism will cause tachypnea. Conditions that limit diaphragmatic excursion, such as an enlarged liver or spleen, also cause tachypnea. **Hyper-**

CLINICAL TIPS

Neural Control of Breathing

Neural control of breathing comes from the phrenic nerve, which arises from cervical nerve roots C3, C4, and C5 and innervates the diaphragm, and from the nerves that innervate the intercostal muscles.

CLINICAL TIPS

Classification of Breathing Terms

- tachypnea—Rapid breathing: >24 breaths/min
- hyperpnea—Tachypnea with very large breaths
- bradypnea—Slow breathing: <12 breaths/min
- hypopnea—Shallow, slow breaths
- orthopnea—Shortness of breath when lying down

pnea refers to a type of tachypnea in which breaths are unusually large and deep, resulting in hyperventilation. This can be seen after normal exercise and in anxiety but is also associated with certain metabolic and central nervous system disorders. One example of hyperpnea is known as **Kussmaul breathing** and is found in patients with **diabetic ketoacidosis (DKA)**.

When breathing slows to fewer than 12 breaths/min, it is called **bradypnea**. Electrolyte and acid–base disturbances can produce this pattern, but well-conditioned athletes with higher levels of cardiorespiratory fitness can develop this slowed breathing pattern as well. When breathing becomes slow and shallow, it is called **hypopnea** and is seen as an adaptive response to pleuritic pain situations such as rib fractures. The absence of spontaneous respiration is known as **apnea**. A condition called obstructive sleep apnea occurs primarily in obese patients during rapid-eye-movement sleep. Periods of apnea can also be found in a respiratory pattern called **Cheyne-Stokes respiration**, or periodic breathing. This breathing pattern can be normal in children and infants during sleep, but it also occurs pathologically in brain-damaged individuals. Figure 7.3 is a visual representation of the respiratory patterns.

As mentioned earlier, disordered breathing may have a cardiac origin. The symptom of **orthopnea**, which describes a type of dyspnea that begins or increases as the patient lies down, results from the pulmonary edema of congestive heart failure. The severity of orthopnea is often gauged by the number of pillows needed for the patient to sleep. Dyspnea that reliably occurs with exertion may be attributed to cardiac **angina** rather than to a respiratory condition. The athletic trainer should consider the possibility of cardiac involvement when abnormal breathing or chest pain occurs.

Palpation and Percussion of the Chest

The next step of the evaluation is to palpate the chest for symmetrical expansion. The examiner places the hands

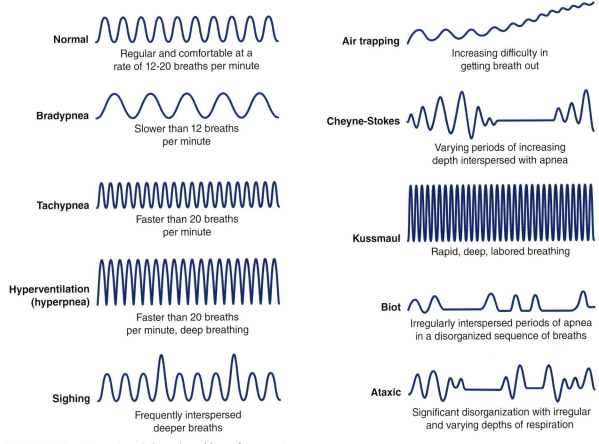

FIGURE 7.3 Normal and disordered breathing patterns.

on the posterior chest wall with the thumbs placed on either side of the spine at the level of thoracic vertebra 9 (T9) or T10 (figure 7.4*a*). The examiner asks the athlete to inhale deeply and then watches the hands move apart symmetrically with the chest wall. Next, one feels for **tactile fremitus**. This is a palpable vibration that is generated from the larynx and transmitted through the patient's bronchi and lungs to the chest wall. Use the palmar or ulnar surface of the hand to feel the vibrations over the posterior chest wall while the patient speaks the words "ninety-nine" (figure 7.4*b*). The intensity of the fremitus is not as important as the symmetry between lungs. Fremitus will decrease over the scapulae and will also decrease as the hand is moved distally to the lower posterior chest. Fremitus is increased when there is consolidation of the lung tissue such as in pneumonia. Decreased fremitus occurs when anything obstructs the transmission of the vibrations to the chest wall (Jarvis 2012). Examples of obstructions include pleural effusion, pneumothorax, or emphysema, which are all discussed in detail later in this chapter.

Percussion

Percussion is the process of assessing sounds transmitted through the organs and cavities of the body and is gener-

ated by tapping. It involves striking one object (fingers or hand) against another to produce vibrations and subsequent sound waves. The techniques of percussion are the same regardless of the structure being percussed and include either direct or indirect percussion.

Direct percussion involves lightly striking the chest with the ulnar aspect of the fist. Indirect percussion involves the finger of one hand acting as the hammer, striking the finger of the other hand that is resting on the area of the chest being percussed. The striking action creates a vibration or resonance that, with training and practice, can be identified and quantified.

Practice is necessary to become proficient with percussion technique. The downward snap of the striking finger originates from the wrist and not the forearm or shoulder. The tap is sharp and rapid with the tip of the finger, not the pad. The ulnar surface of the fist may also be used for percussion and is generally used to elicit tenderness over solid organs such as the liver or kidneys. Percussion-generated sounds may be recognized by different characteristics, including intensity, pitch, and location. The general percussion tone over air is loud, over fluid it is less loud, and over solid areas it is soft. Common sounds produced by percussion are listed in table 7.1. It is often difficult to quantify percussion tones, especially

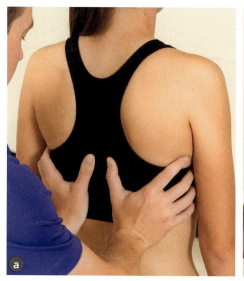
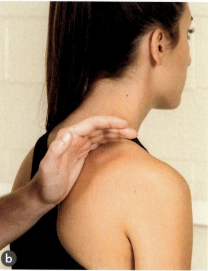

FIGURE 7.4 *(a)* Palpation of the chest for symmetrical expansion. *(b)* Tactile fremitus.

TABLE 7.1 **Sounds Produced by Percussion**

Sound	Pitch	Intensity	Quality	Duration	Common location
Tympany	High	Loud	Drumlike	Moderate	Gastric bubble or intestine
Resonance	Low	Moderate to loud	Hollow	Long	Normal lung tissue
Hyperresonance	Very low	Very loud	Booming	Longer than resonance	Emphysematous lung
Dull	High	Soft to moderate	Thudlike	Moderate	Dense organs (liver, spleen)
Flat	High	Soft	Flat	Short	Muscle, bone

for the novice examiner. The examiner should practice identifying tones from various parts of the body to learn how to quantify them, specifically noting the change from one tone to another when moving from percussing a known air-filled body part, such as the lungs, to the abdomen or a muscle or over a bone.

The examiner uses a systematic sequence of percussion, alternating from one side of the chest to the other to compare sounds (figure 7.5) and starting at the apices of the lungs at the top of the shoulders. The predominant sound found at the top of the shoulders will be resonant. Progressing inferiorly, the examiner percusses the chest at approximately 5 cm intervals in the intercostal spaces. In a healthy adult lung, resonance will be the predominant sound. Hyperresonance is found when too much air is present, such as in pneumothorax or emphysema. A flat note will occur over bone (e.g., over the scapula) or where there is abnormal density in the lungs, which is seen in pneumonia or pleural effusion (Jarvis 2012). Dullness will also be found when percussing the inferior

posterior chest wall over the liver and abdominal viscera (figure 7.6).

Auscultation

Auscultation is the skilled listening by a trained ear for sounds produced by the body. Most body sounds, including those of the heart, lung, and bowel, are not typically audible without the use of a stethoscope. Auscultation takes practice so that the sounds can be identified and isolated from each other.

Certain basic principles apply to auscultation regardless of the system being examined:

- Perform auscultation after history, observation, and palpation in order to gather as much information as possible from other sources first.

- Perform auscultation in a quiet environment.

- Listen for the presence or absence of sounds as well as their frequency, loudness, quality, and duration.

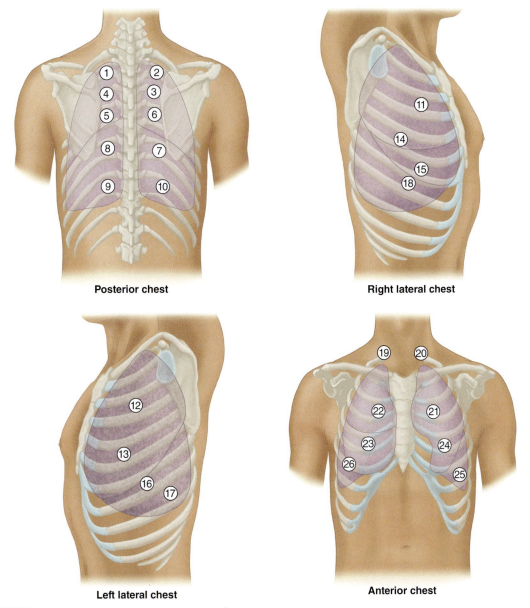

Posterior chest

Right lateral chest

Left lateral chest

Anterior chest

FIGURE 7.5 Suggested percussion and auscultation sequence.

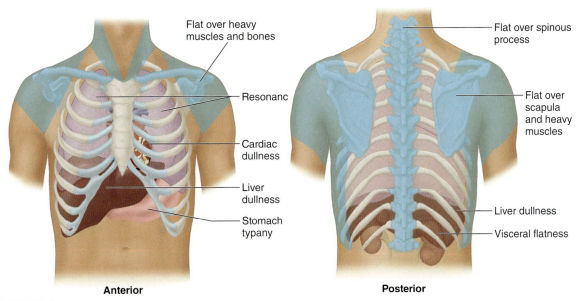

Flat over heavy muscles and bones

Resonanc

Cardiac dullness

Liver dullness

Stomach typany

Flat over spinous process

Flat over scapula and heavy muscles

Liver dullness

Visceral flatness

Anterior

Posterior

FIGURE 7.6 Percussion tones throughout the chest.

- Make sure the earpieces of the stethoscope fit comfortably, following the angles of the ear canal.
- Point the earpieces of the stethoscope toward the face.

The examiner uses the part of the stethoscope that best relays the pitch of the sound sought. The diaphragm is used for high-pitched sounds, such as bowel, lung, and normal heart sounds, whereas the bell is used for low-pitched sounds. Abnormal heart and vascular sounds have a lower pitch and may be heard better with the bell (Jarvis 2012). Common characteristics of sounds heard during auscultation are listed here:

- Frequency: Number of sound wave cycles generated per second by a vibrating object. The higher the frequency, the higher the pitch of a sound and vice versa.
- Loudness: Amplitude of a sound wave. Auscultated sounds are described as *loud* or *soft*.
- Quality: Sounds of similar frequency and loudness from different sources. Terms such as *blowing* or *gurgling* describe quality of sound.
- Duration: Length of time sound vibrations last. Duration of sound is *short*, *medium*, or *long*.

Characteristics of Normal and Abnormal Breath Sounds

Characteristic qualities, such as intensity, pitch, quality, and duration in both inspiration and expiration, help the medical professional assess breath sounds.

The diaphragm of the stethoscope is used on bare skin to auscultate the lungs. The examiner must listen systematically at each position throughout inspiration and expiration (Ball et al. 2014; Jarvis 2012) and evaluate lungs in the anterior, posterior, and lateral aspects to ensure that each lobe of the lungs is properly examined. Figure 7.7 shows the surface markings of the lobes of the lung. The examiner is always mindful of which lobe is being examined: The front of the chest primarily provides access to the upper lobes, whereas auscultation of the back mainly exposes the lower lobes of the lungs.

One useful technique involves listening in the same sequence that is used in percussion from left side to right at symmetrical locations to make comparisons as the examiner moves downward from the apex to the base of the lungs. When the athletic trainer listens to the lungs, three different sounds can be appreciated in normal individuals, depending on the position of the stethoscope (figure 7.8):

- **Bronchial breath sounds** are loud, high pitched, and predominantly expiratory. These sounds represent air moving through large airways and

sound more tubular. They are normally heard only over the trachea in the anterior chest midline.
- **Bronchovesicular breath sounds** are heard when air moves through medium-sized airways such as the mainstem bronchi, and they can be heard both anteriorly and posteriorly, toward the center of the thorax. These sounds are of medium pitch and moderate intensity. Inspiratory and expiratory phases are approximately equal.
- **Vesicular breath sounds** predominate in most of the peripheral lung tissue and represent the air as it moves into the smaller airways, such as the bronchioles and lung **parenchyma**. These sounds are soft, low-pitched noises that involve mostly inspiration.

When disease affects the lungs, normal breath sounds are altered, depending on the condition (table 7.2). Fluid in the pleural space may make breath sounds distant or even absent; however, fluid within the lung parenchyma, such as in pulmonary edema or pneumonia, may accentuate breath sounds because sound is transmitted more quickly through liquids than through air. Similarly, consolidated masses within the lungs, such as those caused by pneumonia, will transmit louder sounds. Most of the abnormal breath sounds will be superimposed on normal breath sounds and are called **adventitious breath sounds**.

Crackles, or rales, are adventitious sounds that occur as a result of disruption of airflow in the smaller airways, usually by fluid. They are brief, discontinuous noises that can be either low or high pitched depending on the location within the respiratory tree. They commonly resemble the noise made when several strands of hair are rubbed together between the thumb and index finger held close to the ear.

Wheezes are also adventitious sounds that represent airway obstruction from mucus, spasm, or even a foreign body. These sounds are usually more pronounced during expiration and can be either high-pitched, musical noises in the smaller airways (e.g., asthma) or low pitched in the larger airways (e.g., bronchitis). Such low-pitched, sonorous wheezes are also referred to as **rhonchi**. The **stridor** sound is also caused by airway obstruction and can often be confused with wheezes. The obstruction in stridor generally occurs in the central airways, such as

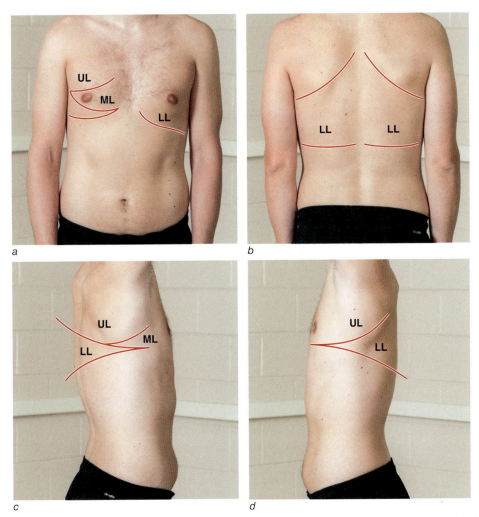

FIGURE 7.7 Surface markings of the lobes of the lung. *(a)* Anterior. *(b)* Posterior. *(c)* Right lateral. *(d)* Left lateral. LL = lower lobe; ML = middle lobe; UL = upper lobe.

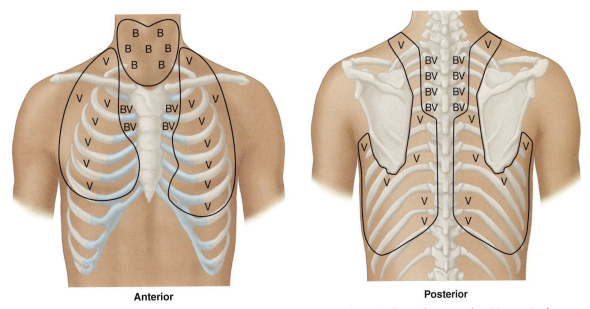

FIGURE 7.8 Normal auscultation sounds. B = bronchial (tracheal); BV = bronchovesicular; V = vesicular.

TABLE 7.2 **Physical Findings Associated With Common Respiratory Conditions**

Condition	Inspection	Palpation	Percussion	Auscultation
Asthma	Tachypnea Dyspnea	Tachycardia	Occasional hyperresonance	Prolonged expiration Wheezes Diminished lung sounds
Bronchitis	Occasional tachypnea Occasional shallow breathing Often no deviation from normal	Tactile fremitus	Resonance	Occasional crackles Occasional expiratory wheezes
Pneumonia	Tachypnea	Increased fremitus in presence of consolidation	Dullness if consolidation is great	Variety of crackles Bronchial breath sounds Egophony, bronchophony
Pneumothorax	Tachycardia Cyanosis Respiratory distress Tracheal deviation	Diminished to absent fremitus Tachycardia	Hyperresonance	Diminished to absent breath sounds Sternal and precordial clicks and crackling Diminished to absent whispered voice sounds

Adapted from H.M. Seidel et al., 2003, *Mosby's guide to physical examination*, 5th ed. (St. Louis: Mosby), 397-398.

the trachea or larynx, and is more pronounced during inspiration as opposed to the expiratory-predominant wheeze (Ball et al. 2014; Jarvis 2012). **Croup** is a condition that classically can produce stridor. **Pleural rubs** are sounds that occur outside the respiratory tree and result from friction between visceral and parietal pleura in conditions that cause inflammation of the pleura, such as pleurisy, or pleuritis. Usually low pitched, they can be heard in both inspiration and expiration and can resemble the sound made when two balloons are rubbed together.

Abnormalities can also be detected by listening to the transmission of speech while auscultating the lungs. Transmitted speech is normally muffled and is best heard toward the midline. In pneumonia, when there is consolidation, changes in vocal resonance occur. **Bronchophony**

occurs when speech becomes clearer and louder. In the extreme, namely, **whispered pectoriloquy**, whispered speech can be heard clearly through the stethoscope. Consolidation of lung tissue will also produce **egophony**, in which a spoken "e" is heard as "a." Conversely, any obstruction of the respiratory tree causes diminished vocal resonance.

The athletic trainer must become familiar with normal breath sounds through auscultation, thus better realizing when adventitious sounds are present in the lungs. Here is a summary of the steps in the evaluation of an athlete's respiratory system:

History

- Determine onset and duration of symptoms.
- Ask about cough, shortness of breath, and chest pain.
- Obtain history of previous respiratory infections.
- Obtain smoking and environmental exposure history.
- Obtain family history.

Inspection

- Check rate, rhythm, and effort of respirations.
- Assess skin color and condition.
- Check posture associated with breathing (note use of accessory muscles).

Palpation

- Palpate any point tenderness or masses.

RED FLAGS FOR RESPIRATORY DISORDERS

- Labored breathing with the use of accessory muscles (not associated with exercise)
- Adventitious breath sounds
- Hemoptysis
- Orthopnea
- Dyspnea of rapid onset
- Prolonged cough
- Deviated trachea

- Confirm symmetrical expansion.
- Palpate for tactile fremitus.

Percussion

- Percuss over lungs, starting at the apex.

Auscultation

- Assess breath sounds, comparing side to side over all lobes of lung.
- Auscultate both anterior and posterior chest.
- Listen for normal breath sounds, and note any abnormal breath sounds.
- Listen for sounds with speaking, such as egophony and bronchophony.

In addition, the athletic trainer needs to be vigilant in recognizing the signs and symptoms of respiratory disorders.

The following sections discuss the pathological conditions of the respiratory system, beginning with the signs and symptoms of each disorder and including differential diagnosis, referral and diagnostic tests, treatment, implications for return to participation, and prevention.

Asthma

Airway disease is the most frequently encountered chronic respiratory condition in athletes (Hull et al. 2012). Several terms are often used to describe airway disease, especially if a definitive diagnosis has not yet been determined. Asthma, exercise-induced asthma (EIA), and exercise-induced bronchoconstriction (EIB) are the most common of the airway diseases (Krafczyk and Asplund 2011; Simpson, Romer, and Kippelen 2015). Many sources use these terms interchangeably because they clinically present with many of the same signs and symptoms. Specifically, however, EIB is used to describe an exercise-induced, transient, and reversible narrowing of the airways, and it may occur in persons with or without underlying asthma. Exercise triggers bronchoconstriction but does not induce the clinical syndrome of asthma (Krafczyk and Asplund 2011). Asthma is a pulmonary disorder characterized by reversible airway obstruction that results from hyperreactivity; it is also referred to as "twitchy" airways (Boulet 2012). Allergens, stress or anxiety, smoke or other environmental pollutants, cold ambient temperatures, and even exercise commonly trigger this hyperreactivity (Carey, Aase and Pliego 2010).

The rule of thumb is that asthma occurs outside of exercise or strenuous activity and generally has two components that lead to the obstruction: inflammation and spasm. Inflammation, characterized by mucosal edema and increased secretions, along with bronchospasm of smooth muscle, results in an increase in airway resistance and impeded airflow.

Asthma often begins in childhood and has various degrees of severity and progression. Some people need daily oral or inhaled medicines, whereas others need only sporadic or intermittent treatment. Many patients do not have asthmatic symptoms except during strenuous exercise. Despite the various presentations of asthma, it can be life-threatening if not treated promptly and adequately.

Signs and Symptoms

Patients with airway disease (asthma, EIA, and EIB) experience episodic, paroxysmal attacks of shortness of breath and wheezing as well as other symptoms, such as chest tightness and a dry cough. These episodes can be transient, lasting a few minutes to hours, or prolonged over several days. Severe attacks can be associated with much respiratory distress and tachypnea. Wheezing may be audible to the unaided ear in some cases. Mild cases may present as only a chronic cough (cough variant asthma).

Asthma should be differentiated from other upper and lower respiratory diseases, including laryngeal dysfunction, croup, infiltrative lung disease, and even foreign body aspiration. Determining whether the condition is asthma (occurs at rest) or only occurs with exercise (EIB, EIA) is helpful (Parsons et al. 2012; Krafczyk and Asplund 2011). The examiner must always consider cardiac failure, chronic obstructive pulmonary disease, or airway tumors as differential diagnoses in older patients, especially smokers.

On examination, both the respiratory rate and heart rate may be elevated, depending on the severity of the condition. In particular, the use of accessory muscles of respiration may be seen during respiratory distress. The sternocleidomastoid, trapezius, and levator muscles will contract during respiratory distress, giving patients the appearance of lifting their shoulders as they breathe (Millward et al. 2009). On auscultation, wheezes are usually present, particularly during expiration. There is also prolongation of the expiratory phase as airway resistance is increased. Breath sounds can be diminished.

Referral and Diagnostic Tests

If the patient history and examination suggest asthma, response to empirical treatment with β-agonist medications such as albuterol is often diagnostic. A decrease in the predicted forced expiratory volume within the first second (FEV_1) measured by spirometry, particularly in response to **cholinergics** such as methacholine (i.e., methacholine challenge test), is considered the "gold standard" for diagnosis (Millward et al. 2009; Morris 2010; Ostrom et al. 2011). A peak flow meter provides a quick record of pulmonary function and can be used to help assess the severity of the asthma or the effectiveness of medication. Here is how a patient should use a peak flow meter:

1. Stand or sit up straight.
2. Place the mouthpiece onto the peak flow meter.
3. Slide the indicator to the base of the meter.
4. Exhale completely.
5. Take a deep breath.
6. Place the mouthpiece in mouth and seal lips tightly around the mouthpiece.
7. Blow out as hard and fast as you can one time.
8. Reset the indicator.
9. Repeat steps 4 through 7.
10. Record the higher of the two numbers.
11. Assess forced expiratory volume.

Treatment and Return to Participation

Inhaled β-agonist medications, both long- and short-acting, are the mainstays in the treatment of asthma (Hull et al. 2012; Boulet, Hancox, and Fitch 2010; Boulet 2012). Other medications used to treat asthma include oral and inhaled steroids, mast cell stabilizers such as cromolyn, leukotriene modifiers, and theophylline (Morris 2010; Barros, Prinzivalli, and Christi 2016). Treatment recommendations generally follow a stepwise approach in the use of both "rescue" and maintenance medications as the severity of the disease dictates (Stack and Hakemi 2011). Refer to chapter 5 for a complete description of asthma medications and indications. In addition to pharmacotherapy, attention needs to be given to the avoidance of known triggers and the treatment of concomitant allergies. Although strenuous exercise can provoke airway disease, several studies have shown that regular exercise and improvement in physical fitness (specifically pulmonary function) may reduce the symptoms and irritability of the airways (Stack and Hakemi 2011; Parsons et al. 2012).

In general, athletes with mild asthma may participate in most sports. However, because cold ambient temperatures are known to exacerbate the symptoms of asthma, many athletes with asthma prefer sports that involve competition in warm, temperate climates, such as track and field. Individuals with moderate to severe asthma are unlikely to be involved in vigorous athletic activities because the disease often will limit performance. Athletes with acute exacerbations of the disease should refrain from activity until the acute attack resolves and they no longer need rescue medications, such as albuterol, on a regular basis.

Exercise-Induced Bronchospasm

The terms EIA and EIB are often used interchangeably, but EIB specifically denotes the reduction in lung function that occurs after a standardized exercise test (Carver 2009). More recently, the term exercise-induced bronchoconstriction has been introduced as actual spasm of the airways does not always occur. Some clinicians use EIA to describe individuals with known asthma who have bronchoconstriction during exercise. However, some use EIA to describe patients who have bronchoconstriction only during exercise, and they use EIB to describe patients with asthma who have bronchoconstriction with exercise. Generally, EIB is used to indicate bronchospasm with decreased pulmonary function testing following exercise, and EIA is used to indicate those patients with asthma difficulties associated with exercise.

Symptoms of EIB usually occur 10 to 15 min after the onset of strenuous exercise and are defined by a fall in FEV_1 of 15% or more during exercise spirometry. EIB is more common in winter sport athletes who compete in cold ambient temperatures (Carey, Aase, and Pliego 2010).

Signs and Symptoms

EIB should be suspected in any athlete who complains of shortness of breath, dyspnea, cough, chest congestion, or tightness with exertion. These symptoms usually occur during strenuous exercise and peak about 5 to 10 min after exercise (Hull 2012; Krafczyk and Asplund 2011; Simpson, Romer, and Kippelen 2015). Other subtle clues might be a dry cough that develops after practice or exercise (i.e., locker-room cough) or simply unusual fatigue compared with similarly trained athletes. Athletes will often complain that they feel out of shape despite regular training. Self-reported symptoms have been shown to be poor predictors of EIB because other conditions can cause similar symptoms. Symptoms alone should not be used to diagnose EIB.

In athletes suspected of having EIB, other etiologies, such as acute sinusitis, otitis media (middle ear infection), bronchitis, or even pneumonia, need to be excluded, particularly in the context of other constitutional symptoms, such as fever, chills, or night sweats. If fatigue is the only presenting symptom, deconditioning may also be a cause. In addition, environmental allergies can account for many of the nonspecific symptoms that mimic EIB (Backer 2010; Hull et al. 2012; Stack and Hakemi 2011). More serious cardiac causes, such as arrhythmias and pericarditis, might also need to be excluded. Another important differential is **exercise-induced laryngeal obstruction (EILO)**, where the wheezing and dyspnea are caused by transient obstruction of the upper airways during exercise (Nielsen 2013; Backer 2010).

Referral and Diagnostic Tests

The physical examination is usually normal. Some athletes with EIB may experience symptoms that develop several hours after exercise. This late-phase response is due to the activity of inflammatory mediators. Most commonly, a bronchial provocation challenge is used to determine the diagnosis of EIB (Parsons et al. 2011; Hayden et al. 2011; Morris 2010). Figure 7.9 shows a decision tree commonly used for the diagnosis of EIB. Alternatively, many physicians choose to just evaluate the patient's response to an empirical trial of a β-agonist medication before exercise.

Treatment and Return to Participation

The treatment of choice in EIB is an inhaled β_2-agonist from a metered-dose inhaler (e.g., albuterol) taken 15 to 30 min before the onset of exercise. An athlete who has asthma symptoms outside the exercise setting or who is using a β_2-agonist more than three times per week should be treated with a regular inhaled corticosteroid. Here is how to properly use an inhaler:

1. Remove dust cap and shake the inhaler system before each use.
2. Inspect mouthpiece for contamination or foreign objects.
3. Breathe out through the mouth, exhaling as completely as possible.
4. Hold the inhaler system upright with mouthpiece in mouth and lips closed tightly around mouthpiece.
5. Breathe in slowly while pressing down on the metal cartridge.
6. Hold breath as long as possible.
7. Release pressure while still holding breath.
8. Remove mouthpiece.
9. Wait for the container to repressurize, shake, and then repeat steps 3 through 8 when more than one inhalation is prescribed.
10. Rinse mouth with water after prescribed number of inhalations.
11. Clean the inhaler system every few days by removing metal cartridge and rinsing the plastic inhaler and cap with running warm water. Replace cartridge and cap.

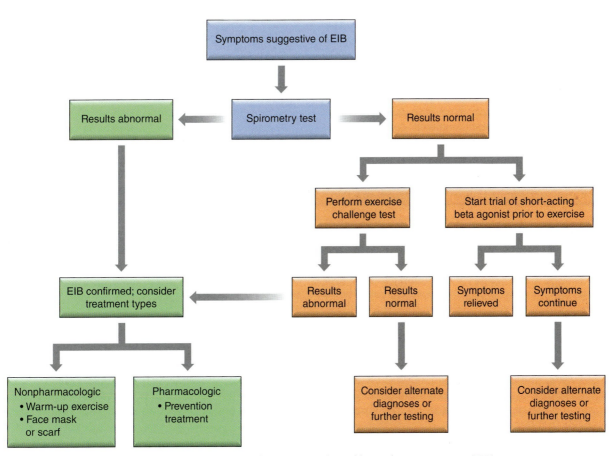

FIGURE 7.9 Decision tree for the diagnosis of exercise-induced bronchoconstriction (EIB).

Emerging studies show promise using long-acting β_2-agonists such as salmeterol and leukotriene inhibitors such as montelukast (Singulair) (Parsons 2010). Other nonpharmacological strategies include pre–warm-up bursts of physical activity at 80% to 90% of the individual's maximal workload to induce a refractory period that lasts up to 3 h after the initial attack of EIB (Hull et al. 2012; Millward et al. 2009; Boulet, Hancox, and Fitch 2010). Strategies to humidify inspired air and dietary interventions may also prove to be beneficial (Carey, Aase, and Pliego 2010; Bussotti, Di Marco, and Marchese 2014).

For an athlete experiencing a severe asthma attack or when an inhaler is ineffective, a nebulizer may be used. A nebulizer, also known as an *atomizer*, is a machine that vaporizes liquid medication into a fine mist to be inhaled into the lungs via a mouthpiece or mask. Although studies have shown that both inhalers and nebulizers tend to be equally effective in delivering medications, nebulizers are preferred for use in more serious rescue situations when the patient is experiencing a severe asthma attack. Nebulizers can administer a higher dose of medication, but inhalers are easier to use, preferred for their portability and low cost, and good for everyday use. Medications typically administered with a nebulizer include albuterol and ipratropium (Atrovent).

Athletes with controlled EIB need not be excluded or discouraged from participating in sports. Effective strategies, both pharmacological and nonpharmacological, exist that can allow an athlete to compete even at an elite level.

Bronchitis

Bronchitis refers to any inflammatory condition of the bronchial passages. In general, it can present in one of two ways: acute or chronic. The chronic condition is discussed later, in the section "Chronic Obstructive Pulmonary Disease." In acute bronchitis, the inflammation most commonly results from self-limited viral infections. Acute bronchitis is rarely caused by bacterial infections in healthy people. Bacterial infections occur more commonly in smokers and in patients with chronic obstructive pulmonary disease (see discussion later in this chapter) who have underlying impairment of bronchial ciliary motility. Acute bronchitis can also occur as a noninfectious condition in response to environmental allergens.

Signs and Symptoms

The most common sign seen in a person who presents with acute bronchitis is a productive cough. Sputum is usually clear but can have a yellowish tinge. Chest congestion or tightness may be present along with some mild shortness of breath. If the cause is infectious, constitutional symptoms, such as fever, chills, or night sweats, may be present although transient. Because most cases (90%) (Albert 2010, Gonzales, Bartlett, and Besser 2001; Braman 2006) are viral in origin, acute bronchitis commonly presents with an upper respiratory infection with its associated symptoms of runny nose, nasal congestion, and sore throat. The common cold typically lasts 7 to 10 d while symptoms of acute bronchitis typically persist for longer. The causative pathogen for bronchitis is rarely identified. The physical examination of the chest is often normal, but occasionally rhonchi and crackles can be heard.

Bronchitis must be differentiated from underlying pneumonia, which can present similarly. The respiratory symptoms tend to be more severe with pneumonia, and the constitutional symptoms, such as chills and fever, are less severe and more self-limited in cases of acute infectious bronchitis. Underlying allergic rhinitis, as well

---

CONDITION HIGHLIGHT

Exercise-Induced Bronchospasm

Research shows that the prevalence of EIB in athletes varies from 10% to 50% depending on the population studied and occurs in about 80% to 90% of patients with intrinsic asthma (Hull et al. 2012; Krafczyk and Asplund 2011). Exercise-induced cough is particularly prevalent in swimmers and winter sports athletes, and it occurs more often during winter training (Boulet 2012). Studies consistently demonstrate a higher prevalence of EIB in athletes (up to 50–70%) than in the general population (Hull et al. 2012).

The differential diagnosis is often broad, and the patient may not present with any "asthma-like" symptoms but may only complain of a decline in performance and endurance or a "locker-room cough." Figure 7.9 shows an algorithm commonly used for the diagnosis of EIB. Pharmacological and nonpharmacological interventions should be considered, including strategies to humidify inspired air, the use of intensive warm-up to invoke a refractory period, and short-acting β_2-agonist treatment prior to exercise.

as sinusitis, may also present with a persistent cough secondary to postnasal drainage. In athletes with intermittent bouts of bronchitis, the diagnosis of asthma, either intrinsic or exercise induced, needs to be considered.

Referral and Diagnostic Tests

Although no diagnostic tests other than the clinical examination are used to diagnose bronchitis, specific tests may help to exclude other causes. Chest radiographs, as well as a complete blood count (CBC) to look for elevations in white blood cells (WBCs), are useful in diagnosing pneumonia (Boulet 2012). Computerized tomography (CT) of the sinuses may reveal an underlying sinusitis, and an empirical trial of an antihistamine can help distinguish allergic causes. Testing for influenza may be considered when risk is thought to be intermediate and the patient presents within 36 h of symptom onset. Because most cases of bronchitis are self-limited, if symptoms do not resolve, referral for medical evaluation is indicated.

Treatment and Return to Participation

Treatment in most cases is supportive. Mucolytics, cough suppressants, and nonsteroidal anti-inflammatory drugs (NSAIDs) are helpful in reducing the severity of symptoms. Fluids to keep secretions loose are also essential. Because of the risk of antibiotic resistance, antibiotics should not be routinely used in the treatment of acute bronchitis. Clinical data support the view that antibiotics do not significantly change the course of acute bronchitis, and they may provide only minimal benefit compared with the risk of antibiotic use itself (Braman 2006; Little et al. 2005).

Acute viral cases of bronchitis may last 7 to 10 d. Athletes with acute bronchitis may be allowed to play as tolerated so long as the fever has resolved. Because a small increase in expectorated secretions is possible, attention to fluid status and adequate hydration are essential in minimizing the risk for dehydration.

Chronic Obstructive Pulmonary Disease

Closely related to asthma, which is a type of reversible obstructive pulmonary disease, chronic obstructive pulmonary disease (COPD) is characterized by nonreversible airway obstruction. It is typically found in long-term smokers, and this diagnosis is broadly divided into two main categories: emphysema and chronic bronchitis.

Emphysema is characterized by destruction of the alveoli and pulmonary capillary bed. As a result, there is a decreased ability to oxygenate blood as the lung loses its elastic recoil properties. The body also compensates with lowered cardiac output and hyperventilation. Chronic bronchitis, on the other hand, is defined by excessive mucus production with upper airway obstruction. Damage to the lining of the airways impairs the mucociliary response that clears bacteria and mucus. Because of the severity of respiratory impairment associated with COPD, it is rarely seen in the athletic population.

Signs and Symptoms

Patients with COPD tend to be older with a long-standing history of cigarette smoking. Patients with emphysema have high respiratory rates and a ruddy skin tone due to muscle wasting, which makes peripheral capillaries more visible. As a result, they are said to have the "pink puffer" variant of COPD. On examination, their chests are more rounded or "barrel" shaped due to hyperinflation. Diffuse wheezing and decreased breath sounds can be heard on auscultation. In contrast, patients with chronic bronchitis have the typical productive "smoker's cough." Because they often present with signs of right heart failure, such as edema and cyanosis, they are said to have the "blue bloater" variant of COPD. Coarse rhonchi and wheezing are noted on physical examination as well as a markedly prolonged expiratory phase of breathing.

Early in the course of the disease, COPD may present similarly to asthma, with wheezing and shortness of breath. Also, acute bronchitis can occur in the setting of COPD, that is, the "acute on chronic" condition. Patients with COPD, particularly those with emphysema, are at risk for developing a pneumothorax. Those with chronic bronchitis are more prone to developing pneumonia, which distinguishes itself by persistent constitutional symptoms such as fever. In the advanced stages of chronic bronchitis, symptoms are similar to those of congestive heart failure.

Referral and Diagnostic Tests

COPD is generally diagnosed clinically in patients who have long-standing airway obstruction and tobacco abuse. Chest X-rays and CT scans can also be suggestive. The diagnosis can be confirmed by pulmonary function testing and the absence of reversibility (Johnson-Warrington et al. 2014). In those patients who have clinical findings consistent with COPD in the absence of a history of cigarette smoking, a workup should include investigation for other environmental exposure that may be toxic to the lungs, as well as for autoimmune causes and metabolic disorders such as α_1-antitrypsin deficiency. Although unlikely, any athlete with COPD who has significant shortness of breath at rest or with minimal activity needs to be referred to and evaluated by the team physician immediately.

Treatment and Return to Participation

The treatment of COPD focuses on addressing the two main processes involved: spasm and inflammation. In more advanced cases, typically not seen in the athletic population, oxygen therapy may be needed (Spielmanns et al. 2015). Agonist medications, either short- or long-acting, are used to control bronchospasm. Similarly, inhaled anticholinergic medications such as ipratropium (Atrovent) help with bronchospasm but also help to control the copious secretion production seen with chronic bronchitis. Glucocorticosteroids, either inhaled or taken orally, are used primarily to treat the chronic inflammation of the airways. Holland et al. (2012) recommend breathing exercise therapy for the treatment and control of COPD. Focusing on smoking cessation, of course, is paramount to the successful treatment of COPD.

Given that patients with COPD typically do not have the pulmonary reserve to compete in sports, athletic participation is rare. For those with mild disease, participation in sports is permitted as tolerated. Klign et al. (2012) found that varying exercise modes improves overall endurance in patients with COPD over traditional endurance and resistance training. It is recommended that those athletes have their disease under control and be compliant with maintenance medications (Holland et al. 2012). Precautions need to be taken to address any acute flare-up of the disease, such as in asthma, by having a short-acting β-agonist (albuterol) readily available.

Pneumonia

Pneumonia is a diagnosis given to any condition that results in inflammation of the lung parenchyma. Usually the cause is infectious and can result from a viral, bacterial, or fungal pathogen. By far, the more common forms are viral or bacterial. Fungal infections typically occur in the immunocompromised patient. Patients with pneumonia generally appear ill, although some forms of "walking pneumonia" caused by atypical bacteria such as *Mycoplasma pneumoniae* may not be severe. In general, community-acquired pneumonia is easily treatable once properly identified, although hospitalization is sometimes needed in severe cases.

Signs and Symptoms

Patients with pneumonia often have constitutional symptoms that persist if not treated adequately. They may complain of shortness of breath or pleuritic chest pain. A productive cough with dark, discolored sputum is not unusual. If the pneumonia affects the lower lobes of the lungs, diaphragmatic irritation and abdominal pain may be the presenting symptoms.

At physical examination, the respiratory rate may be mildly elevated and breathing may be labored. If there is consolidation, dullness to percussion over the affected lung field may be detected as well as changes in vocal resonance, such as bronchophony or egophony, on auscultation of the involved areas. Pooling of secretions in the lower lobe can produce adventitious rales at the lung bases along with an occasional wheeze.

Pneumonia can present similarly to other infections of the upper respiratory tract, such as bronchitis and sinusitis. Bronchitis is often confused with pneumonia, particularly when the pneumonia is not severe (Smoote and Hosey 2015). Tuberculosis is also a possibility in a patient who presents with pneumonia of the upper lung lobes. On occasion, pneumonia results from an obstruction by a foreign body or mass in the airway.

Referral and Diagnostic Tests

It is virtually impossible to distinguish viral from bacterial pneumonia on the basis of the clinical examination. Because of the morbidity associated with pneumonia, it is often treated empirically with antibiotics. The athletic trainer refers to a physician any febrile athlete who exhibits resting labored breathing with chest pain or cough and presents with signs of consolidation. Additional diagnostic tests, such as a chest radiograph, are often ordered by the physician and can aid in confirming the diagnosis. Certain microorganisms, such as viruses and atypical bacteria, may not consolidate, and a normal chest radiograph will result. Sputum cultures taken to isolate specific organisms are usually done when empirical treatment fails. In general, athletes should be referred as soon as possible for further evaluation when they are suspected of having pneumonia.

Treatment and Return to Participation

Treatment for pneumonia with first-line antibiotics such as azithromycin (Zithromax) or clarithromycin (Biaxin) is usually successful. Attention to proper hydration and supportive care with mucolytics and cough suppressants (Robitussin DM liquid [guaifenesin and dextromethorphan]) are also helpful. Athletes who do not improve within 2 to 3 d after initiating therapy should be referred to a physician for reevaluation. Older adult and high-risk patients should be encouraged to ask their physicians about the pneumococcal vaccine, which provides protection against the most common strains of pneumonia.

As with any acute infection, participation is restricted until the athlete is no longer febrile and vital signs return to normal. In addition, in cases of bacterial pneumonia it is recommended that definitive treatment with antibiotics be initiated before an athlete returns to activity. Because of the respiratory compromise that often accompanies acute pneumonia, athletes may not feel well enough to return to sport for about 7 to 10 d.

Pleurisy

Pleurisy is a descriptive term for any inflammation of the pleura (i.e., the lining of the lungs) that causes subsequent pain. It is also known as *pleuritis* or *pleuritic chest pain.* Pleurisy may develop in the presence of lung inflammation, such as pneumonia or tuberculosis, but it can also develop in association with rheumatic diseases, chest trauma, cancer, and asbestos-related diseases. This condition often results in fluid accumulation at the site of pleural inflammation, known as a pleural effusion. The fluid that collects between the lining of the lung and the chest wall may alleviate the chest pain despite worsening of the illness. Large accumulations of fluid can compromise breathing and cause coughing, dyspnea, tachypnea, cyanosis, and intercostal **retractions**.

Signs and Symptoms

The hallmark of pleurisy is chest pain at the site of inflammation; the pain occurs in association with breathing or any movement of the chest wall, such as coughing, sneezing, or laughing. Pain may be referred to the shoulder, and symptoms of coexisting respiratory infection, such as fever, cough, and malaise, may occur (Domino et al. 2016). The normally smooth pleural surfaces, now roughened by inflammation, rub together with each breath and can produce a rough, grating sound called a *friction rub.* This can be heard easily with a stethoscope or an unassisted ear held to the patient's chest. Other physical examination findings include rales or rhonchi if there is an accompanying pneumonia or bronchitic condition. If a pleural effusion is present, the examiner also can appreciate decreased breath sounds.

When the diagnosis of pleurisy is possible, the health care professional should always consider primary processes, such as pneumonia, tuberculosis, malignancies including mesothelioma, and autoimmune conditions, in particular systemic lupus erythematosus.

Referral and Diagnostic Tests

A diagnosis of pleurisy is based primarily on the clinical examination. Patients with nontraumatic chest pain associated with breathing should be referred to a physician for the evaluation of secondary causes and underlying pathology that is necessary to initiate adequate treatment. Laboratory tests, including a CBC, can help differentiate bacterial from viral infections. A chest radiograph may reveal an underlying pneumonia or mass, which may or may not be a malignancy. Chest CT can also be useful to further clarify underlying lung disease, and an ultrasound of the chest can detect fluid associated with pleurisy. If fluid is present, an invasive procedure called a **thoracentesis** may be performed diagnostically to analyze the fluid or therapeutically to alleviate the symptoms associated with a pleural effusion.

Treatment and Return to Participation

Treatment of pleurisy is directed at the underlying illness. Bacterial infections are treated with appropriate antibiotics. Viral infections normally run their course without medications. NSAIDs are helpful in alleviating pain and inflammation associated with pleurisy. Recovery depends on the nature of the underlying illness but is generally good with treatment. Recuperation from pleurisy caused by malignant disease depends on the type and extent of the illness. Early treatment of bacterial respiratory infections can prevent pleurisy. No treatments are available for viral respiratory infections with the exception of several drugs for influenza type A.

An athlete with pleurisy may return to activity once a workup has been completed to rule out a primary condition such as pneumonia and once the athlete remains **afebrile**. In addition, the athlete refrains from activity if there continues to be any evidence of respiratory compromise at rest or with exertion. When an athlete returns to activity, workloads should be increased gradually over a period of weeks to ensure safe return to competition.

Influenza

Generally known as the "flu," influenza is a common viral infection. Outbreaks in the United States usually occur during the fall and winter months. Various strains of the influenza virus can cause outbreaks in epidemic proportions and lead to thousands of hospitalizations each year. More information about the spread and impact of influenza may be found in chapter 15. People most susceptible to severe complications are considered high risk and include older adults, those who live in close quarters (e.g., students), and people with compromised immune systems, diabetes, or chronic heart, lung, or kidney disease. Influenza is transmitted from person to person via contagious droplets that are spread when an infected person sneezes or coughs (figure 7.10).

Signs and Symptoms

Whereas milder forms of influenza can be confused with other viral upper respiratory infections, such as the common cold, patients with influenza are generally sicker than those with a regular cold. The onset of symptoms is rapid and can include high fever, headache, muscle aches,

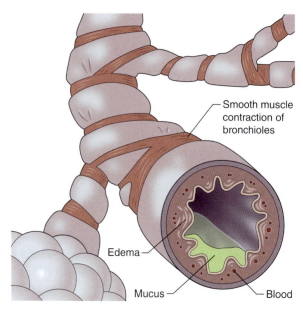

Smooth muscle
contraction of
bronchioles

Edema

Mucus

Blood

FIGURE 7.10 Influenza causes interstitial inflammation of the bronchiolar and alveolar tissues.

cough, chest pain, shortness of breath, fatigue, loss of appetite, nasal congestion, and sore throat. One clue that aids diagnosis is the reported contact with others who have been diagnosed with influenza. Complications may include secondary bacterial infections, such as sinusitis or pneumonia. The influenza virus also can cause pneumonia and encephalitis, an infection of the brain.

Influenza must be differentiated from sinusitis, bronchitis, upper respiratory infection, and pneumonia. Fever is a hallmark of influenza, whereas the patient with sinusitis is typically afebrile.

Referral and Diagnostic Tests

The athletic trainer should refer athletes who have had close contact with a person diagnosed with influenza and are symptomatic to the team physician for further evaluation and diagnosis. Diagnosis is usually made on clinical grounds, but occasionally antigen testing on secretions from a nasopharyngeal swab is used for definitive results. These tests are called rapid influenza diagnostic tests (RIDTs) and are immunoassays that can identify the presence of influenza A and B viral nucleoprotein antigens in respiratory fluids. They have limited sensitivity, however, and may be only marginally useful in determining whether antivirals should be prescribed (Havers et al. 2015; Korownyk, Garrison, and Kolber 2015; Viets 2015). Laboratory tests, including CBCs, can be used to delineate viral versus bacterial infection, and blood and sputum cultures obtained in severe illness can isolate pathogens and determine the presence of bacteremia (Havers et al. 2015). Chest radiographs will be ordered if pneumonia is suspected on the clinical examination.

Treatment and Return to Participation

Treatment for influenza is often supportive and includes bed rest, analgesics for muscle aches and pains, and increased intake of fluids for mild illness in generally healthy people. The athlete should be sent home to rest and, if possible, should avoid contact with teammates to limit the spread of the disease. If influenza is diagnosed within 48 h of symptom onset, in particular among high-risk groups, several antiviral medications are available that may shorten the duration of symptoms by approximately 1 d. These medications include amantadine or rimantadine (active against influenza A only) and oseltamivir (Tamiflu) or zanamivir (active against influenza A and B) (Havers et al. 2015; Korownyk, Garrison, and Kolber 2015). In most individuals who are otherwise healthy, influenza fully resolves within 7 to 10 d. Among individuals in high-risk groups, influenza may be quite severe and can lead to complications. Athletes recovering from the flu are usually fit to return to activity in 1 to 2 wk and must be afebrile and have no respiratory compromise at rest, such as shortness of breath or pleuritic chest pain.

Prevention

The best approach in the management of influenza is prevention. Depending on the supply of vaccine, the athletic trainer should encourage all athletes to be immunized yearly against the common strains of the influenza virus. Immunization typically begins in late October and early November. Those at high risk are generally immunized first. The vaccine has a variable success rate from season to season, generally ranging from 60% to 70% in preventing influenza in people with normal immune systems. The vaccinations are available for intramuscular or intradermal injection or a nasal spray that can be given to children as young as 6 mo (Centers for Disease Control and Prevention 2015). Other means of prevention, especially for the athletic population, include hand washing and not sharing drinking receptacles or bench towels.

Upper Respiratory Infections

Upper respiratory infection (URI) is a diagnosis typically given to any number of self-limited viral infections affecting the upper respiratory tract, including the nasopharynx, trachea, and bronchi. Common pathogens include **rhinovirus**, which produces the "common cold," adenovirus, and parainfluenza virus. These viruses are highly transmissible through contact with infected respiratory

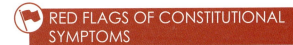

RED FLAGS OF CONSTITUTIONAL SYMPTOMS

- Fever greater than 100 °F
- Chills
- Night sweats

droplets expelled by coughing or sneezing, and therefore whole households are usually affected.

Signs and Symptoms

URI symptoms are generally mild; although the symptoms are an annoyance, patients can go about their normal daily activities. These symptoms may include fever, which usually resolves in 24 to 48 h, cough, nasal congestion, sore throat, and runny nose. The sore throat and fever are usually the first presenting symptoms, with cough usually the last to resolve. Secondary bacterial infections such as otitis media (i.e., middle ear infection) and sinusitis may result if mucosal inflammation persists. Viral URI symptoms often last 7 to 10 d.

Viral URIs are diagnosed clinically and many times to the exclusion of other, more severe infections such as influenza and bacterial infections. Diagnostic testing is usually not indicated or useful (Hull et al. 2012).

Referral and Diagnostic Tests

When symptoms include high fever, dark, purulent nasal discharge, or duration longer than 7 to 10 d, athletes should be referred to the team physician for evaluation of other potential causes, including a secondary bacterial infection.

Treatment and Return to Participation

The athletic trainer should assure athletes with a URI that the condition is self-limited. Treatment is mainly supportive. Medicines such as over-the-counter cough suppressants, decongestants, antihistamines, and expectorants can alleviate symptoms. Patients should be encouraged to keep hydrated so that secretions remain loose. This is particularly important for athletes, where fluid losses associated with exertion may exacerbate symptoms. Hand washing and not sharing drinking containers and towels are particularly important in preventing URI transmission. Athletes may participate in sport as long as they are afebrile and able to drink plenty of fluids.

Tuberculosis

Pulmonary tuberculosis (TB) is a highly contagious bacterial infection caused by the organism *Mycobacterium tuberculosis*. The infection involves primarily the lungs, but it can spread to other organs. TB can develop after inhaling droplets sprayed into the air from a cough or sneeze by someone infected by the disease. It is characterized by the development of granulomas (granular tumors) in the infected tissues (CDC 2015; Smoote and Hosey 2015). The primary stage of the infection is usually asymptomatic and is otherwise known as latent TB. The CDC reports that in 2014, 9.6 million people around the world contracted TB. There were 1.5 million deaths worldwide.

In the United States, a total of 9,421 TB cases were reported. Those most at risk for developing active TB have compromised immune systems. Among individuals with human immunodeficiency virus (HIV) infection, for example, the rate of progression to TB may be as high as 162 per 1,000 person-years of observation. Individuals recently infected with *M. tuberculosis* are also at high risk; for them, the rate is 12.9 cases per 1,000 person-years within the first year (CDC 2015). TB may occur within weeks after the primary infection, or it may lie dormant for years before causing active disease. The risk of contracting TB increases with the frequency of contact with people who have the disease, when living in crowded or unsanitary conditions, and under conditions of poor nutrition.

Signs and Symptoms

Patients are asymptomatic in cases of latent TB. For those with active pulmonary TB, the symptoms may be mild and insidious. Fatigue, fever, weight loss, and cough are common (Tierney and Nardell 2011). The cough may produce sputum containing blood (i.e., **hemoptysis**). Other symptoms include chest pain, shortness of breath, and wheezing. Auscultation of the lungs may reveal crackles or wheezing. A pleural effusion may also be found. Enlarged or tender lymph nodes may be present in the neck and other areas. Often, active TB produces some degree of hypoxia and, if present for some time, results in clubbing of the fingers or toes.

Differential diagnoses include community-acquired bacterial pneumonia, fungal pneumonias, primary as well as metastatic lung malignancies, interstitial lung disease, and opportunistic infections of HIV disease. Any athlete with a persistent cough and constitutional symptoms should be referred to the team physician for follow-up evaluation.

Referral and Diagnostic Tests

Latent TB infections are identified solely on the basis of a positive skin test involving a subcuticular injection of a purified protein derivative (PPD), which causes local induration and erythema of the skin when an infection with *Mycobacterium tuberculosis* is present (Coitinho et al. 2014; Tierney and Nardell 2011). Active TB is diagnosed when patients with a positive PPD test have symptoms consistent with pulmonary TB and radiographic evidence of infection. A chest radiograph typically demonstrates granulomatous disease with a predilection for the upper lung fields. Definitive diagnosis of active disease is made with sputum cultures demonstrating acid-fast bacilli.

Treatment and Return to Participation

Despite the low conversion rate to active TB, latent TB is usually treated by **chemoprophylaxis** with medications such as isoniazid and rifampin for several months under the supervision of a physician. Because of the emerging multidrug-resistant strains of *Mycobacterium tuberculosis,* the treatment of active TB involves the concomitant use of several antibiotics (up to four) to treat the infection (CDC 2015; Tierney and Nardell 2011).

Anyone suspected of having TB must be suspended from activity and referred to a physician immediately. All active cases of tuberculosis need to be reported to the local health department for tracking and surveillance. Hospitalization may be indicated to prevent the spread of the disease to others until the contagious period has resolved through the patient's receiving drug therapy. Normal activity can be continued after the contagious period has passed.

Lung Cancer

Lung cancer is by far one of the most common cancers in the United States and is the leading cause of death from cancer. This disease primarily affects smokers, although there is increased risk among those exposed to secondhand smoke. Physical activity has been shown to decrease the risk of certain cancers (Sormunen et al. 2014). Each of the various types of lung cancer affects different types of cells within the lung. Some are more aggressive than others, and some are more responsive to therapy. In general, the prognosis is poor for all types because most lung cancers are not detected until the later stages, usually after there is involvement of or spread to other organs, including the brain.

Signs and Symptoms

Symptoms of lung cancer develop slowly over time and are often overlooked until the later stages of the disease. Constitutional symptoms predominate and include fever, fatigue, weight loss, and loss of appetite. A cough is usually present with or without bloody sputum. There may be chest pain and shortness of breath. Pneumonia can develop as a secondary consequence. The physical examination is usually nonspecific; however, a pleural effusion can sometimes be detected.

The primary diagnostic dilemma in lung cancer is to determine whether the malignancy is primary or has metastasized from another site. Histological analysis of tissue biopsies can usually reveal the source. Clinical presentation of lung cancer can be similar to that of many chronic lung diseases, including tuberculosis, interstitial lung disease, and COPD. On radiographs, lung cancers may resemble benign granulomas, consolidated pneumonias, or even lung abscesses.

Referral and Diagnostic Tests

Chest radiographs can detect possible malignancies that can be more clearly visualized by CT scans if necessary. Definitive diagnosis is made when cells obtained by bronchoscopy or biopsy are found to be malignant. Other laboratory test abnormalities that may suggest lung cancer include elevated serum (blood) calcium and alkaline phosphatase, decreased serum sodium (i.e., hyponatremia), and abnormal serum levels of carcinoembryonic antigen (CEA) (Cabry et al. 2013).

Treatment and Return to Participation

Treatment of lung cancer depends on its type and stage at diagnosis. (For more information about the staging of cancer, refer to chapter 14.) Options to treat lung cancer may include radiation therapy, chemotherapy, or surgical excision. In the most advanced cases, **palliative therapy** is the only viable option. Overall survival depends on the stage of the disease. For limited disease, cure rates may be as high as 25%, whereas cure rates for advanced stages are less than 5%.

Spontaneous Pneumothorax and Hemothorax

A **pneumothorax** is a condition that results when gas or air is trapped in the chest wall between the parietal and visceral pleura and causes the lung to collapse (figure 7.11). It is deemed spontaneous if the pneumothorax

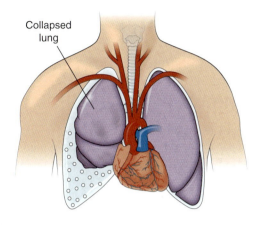

Pneumothorax

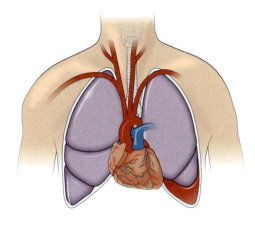

Hemothorax

FIGURE 7.11 Pneumothorax and hemothorax.

occurs in the absence of a traumatic injury to the chest or lungs (Feden 2013). Pneumothorax tends to be more common in tall, thin men in the second and third decades of life and is usually the result of the rupture of a small **bleb** or an air- or fluid-filled sac called a **bulla** (Light 2015). Other lung diseases commonly associated with spontaneous pneumothorax include tuberculosis, pneumonia, asthma, cystic fibrosis, lung cancer, and certain forms of interstitial lung disease.

A more serious condition, known as a **hemothorax**, occurs when blood collects in the pleural space. This condition usually is a result of trauma to the chest wall. In athletes, rib fractures that bleed into the plural space are a common cause (Feden 2013). Hemothorax may also result from malignancies.

Signs and Symptoms

A spontaneous pneumothorax is characterized by the sudden onset of pleuritic chest pain and shortness of breath. Patients are usually tachypneic and have a cough that exacerbates the chest pain (Mensinger 2013). Mild respiratory distress may be apparent, and there may be little chest wall motion on the affected side with breathing (Light 2015). A common sign of pneumothorax is a shift of the trachea away from the affected lung as air pressure pushes the lung toward the midline (figure 7.12). Physical examination of the lungs with a stethoscope reveals decreased or absent breath sounds over the pneumothorax. A hemothorax is also characterized by pleuritic chest pain and dyspnea that worsen rapidly as the chest wall fills with blood. Dullness to percussion in dependent areas can also be appreciated on examination.

A small pneumothorax can easily be missed clinically and sometimes is overlooked as pleurisy, EIA, bronchitis,

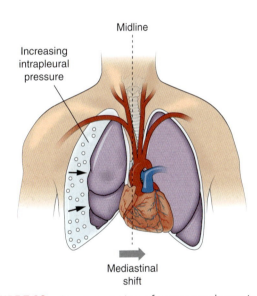

FIGURE 7.12 A common sign of a pneumothorax is a shift of the trachea away from the affected lung as air pressure pushes the lung toward the midline.

or a simple URI. Larger pneumothoraces are associated with some degree of respiratory compromise and can present a clinical picture similar to conditions such as a pulmonary embolism or foreign body aspiration.

Referral and Diagnostic Tests

Any athlete suspected of a pneumothorax or hemothorax should be immediately referred to a medical facility. In general, a chest radiograph is conclusive in the diagnosis of a pneumothorax, although small pneumothoraces may be overlooked without clinical suspicion. In some cases, air continues to be trapped in the chest cavity through a one-way valve mechanism and can result in a dangerous, life-threatening condition known as a **tension pneumothorax**. This condition requires immediate attention and needle decompression of the chest. The diagnosis of a hemothorax is definitively made when blood is aspirated by thoracentesis.

Treatment and Return to Participation

The physician's treatment objective is to remove the air from the pleural space, allowing the lung to reexpand. Small pneumothoraces may resolve without treatment. Aspiration of air, using a catheter linked to a vacuum bottle, may reexpand the lung. The placement of a chest tube between the ribs into the pleural space allows the evacuation of air from the pleural space when simple aspiration is not successful or the pneumothorax is large (Light 2015). Reexpansion of the lung may take several days with the chest tube left in place. Hospitalization is required for chest tube management. Surgery may be indicated for recurrent episodes.

If a hemothorax is suspected, immediate hospitalization for decompression and drainage of blood is required. Exploration for an active bleeding site is mandatory, and other coexisting traumatic injuries to the chest are possible.

Individuals diagnosed with a pneumothorax or hemothorax cannot participate in athletics until the condition has resolved radiographically and the athlete is clinically asymptomatic. Because the recurrence rate of a spontaneous pneumothorax can be as high as 50% (Uramoto, Shimokawa, and Tanaka 2012), the physician will encourage patients to discontinue smoking and avoid flying in unpressurized aircraft. Moreover, those with increased risks, such as scuba divers and athletes competing at high elevation, need to be counseled carefully and possibly encouraged to discontinue their activities.

Summary

The athletic health care provider must remember that chest pain and dyspnea may indicate a respiratory condition but also can point to a cardiovascular problem. The ability of clinicians to perform a thorough examination of the respiratory system will help them to distinguish less serious conditions from those that need immediate attention. It takes considerable practice to recognize characteristics of normal and abnormal breath sounds. There are many websites and other resources that include both audio and animated replication of normal and abnormal breath sounds.

In addition, being familiar with the signs and symptoms, differential diagnoses, and common treatments of respiratory conditions such as asthma, bronchitis, pneumonia, upper respiratory infections, and influenza is paramount. Understanding common treatments, the implications of illness and treatment on participation in sports, and prevention techniques enables athletic trainers to provide the best medical care and follow-up for their athletes. Awareness of conditions that less commonly affect athletes, such as hemothorax or pneumothorax, emphysema, tuberculosis, and lung cancer, is important because the athletic trainer is often the first person an athlete seeks help from when experiencing respiratory system problems. Recognizing an abnormal respiratory condition can facilitate quick referral for an athlete who otherwise might not seek further medical assistance.

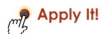 **Apply It!**   The case study for this chapter looks at a 19-year-old football player with a history of fatigue, tightness in his chest, and difficulty catching his breath. Read the scenario and answer the questions at www.HumanKinetics.com/MedicalConditionsInTheAthlete.

Cardiovascular System

OBJECTIVES

At the completion of this chapter the reader should be able to do the following:

- Understand the anatomy and physiology of the cardiovascular system.
- Understand cardiovascular adaptations to exercise.
- Identify various cardiac arrhythmias.
- Identify signs and symptoms of cardiovascular abnormalities.
- Know when to refer an athlete to a physician for further cardiovascular evaluation.

Cardiovascular disorders in the athlete have taken on particular importance because of their potential for catastrophic consequences during exercise. Although these tragedies bring notable publicity, many people with cardiac conditions can safely participate in myriad physical activities. The athletic trainer must be knowledgeable about and able to distinguish between the normal physiological changes of the heart seen with exercise training and the pathological cardiac conditions that can result in exercise-related sudden death.

Vascular conditions, such as hypertension and deep vein thrombosis (DVT), result in and can precipitate potentially fatal conditions such as myocardial infarction (MI—heart attack) and pulmonary embolus. Early referral for diagnosis and treatment can limit harmful complications. Hematological conditions ranging from anemia to sickle cell trait are also discussed in this chapter. Promptly referring athletes to a physician for these conditions can enhance athletic performance and might even save a life.

Overview of Anatomy and Physiology

The heart is a strong, muscular organ made up of four chambers, two atria and two ventricles, which are responsible for pumping the blood that circulates through the body. Blood from the right side of the heart flows to the lungs, and simultaneously blood from the left side of the heart is pumped into the body. The two sides of this muscular pump are separated by the septum and work in a parallel manner. The right side atrium and ventricle pump the pulmonary circuit. The left side atrium and ventricle pump the systemic circuit.

Four valves help to direct the flow. The tricuspid valve separates the right atrium and ventricle; the mitral valve lies between the left atrium and left ventricle. Another set of valves connects the ventricles to the distal circulation.

On the right side of the heart, the pulmonary valve is connected to the pulmonary artery, whereas on the left side, the aortic valve controls flow to the aorta (figure 8.1). Blood flow returning to the heart from the body enters the right atrium: pulmonic blood into the left atrium via the pulmonary vein and systemic blood into the right atrium via the superior and inferior vena cava.

The heart is positioned in the chest like an acorn, pointing inferiorly and to the left. The anterior surface of the heart consists primarily of the right ventricle. A sliver of the left ventricle makes up the left border and the apex or inferior end of the anterior cardiac surface. Many times the heartbeat can be palpated at this apical end located on the left side (the fifth rib interspace at the nipple line).

The systemic vasculature is a pipeline that delivers blood to the organs and tissues throughout the body. Arteries carry blood to the tissues via a high-pressure system, and veins return blood to the atria under much lower pressure. With each contraction of the ventricle, a pressure wave (i.e., the pulse) is created, moving through the arteries.

Pulse palpation can provide much useful clinical information. The intensity, contour, and regularity of the pulse are just as important as the rate. The pulse diminishes with inspiration, but this may not be perceptible. Weak, decreased pulses may indicate shock, heart failure, or a mechanical obstruction such as **aortic stenosis**. Strong, bounding pulses are common after exercise but at rest may be a sign of anemia, **hyperthyroidism**, or anxiety. A double-peak pulse is called a **bisferiens pulse** and can be detected in hypertrophic cardiomyopathy or aortic regurgitation.

CLINICAL TIPS

Measuring Heart Rate

Heart rate can be measured by counting the pulse for 15 s and multiplying by 4. A heart rate at rest that is less than 60 beats/min (common in athletes) is termed *bradycardia*.

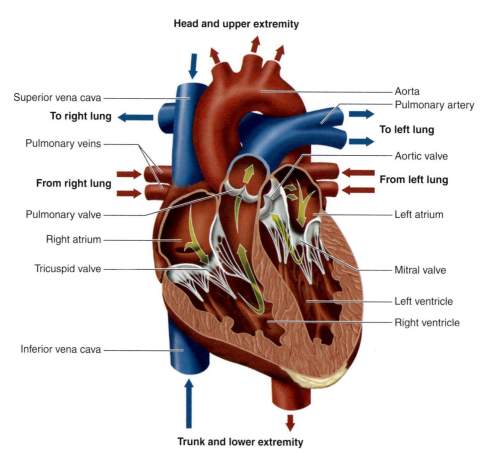

FIGURE 8.1 Anatomy of the cardiac chambers and the course of blood flow through the chambers.

Understanding how the cardiovascular system responds to exercise requires an understanding of basic cardiovascular physiology at rest. The right and left sides of the heart work together, pumping 5 to 6 L of blood per minute at rest (i.e., cardiac output). The heart pumps in a rhythmic cycle. Both ventricles contract during systole and relax during diastole. During the relaxed stage, they are passively filled with blood by atrial contraction. Pressures are rising and falling during this cardiac cycle, which permits the heart valves to open and close.

Cardiac muscle is unique because it can contract within itself and operates on a serial electrical system, free from stimuli external to the heart. An electrical impulse begins at the sinoatrial (SA) node within the upper walls of the right atrium. This impulse travels through both atria to the atrioventricular (AV) node in the atrial septum. After a brief delay, the electrical impulse is promulgated to the bundle of His along the ventricular septum to the Purkinje fibers through the inferior and lateral ventricles (figure 8.2).

An electrocardiogram (ECG) records this electrical activity as two phenomena: depolarization (the spread of electricity through the cardiac muscle) and repolarization (the return of the stimulated heart to rest) (figure 8.3) (Ball et al. 2015). The basic components of the ECG represent important aspects of cardiac function:

- P wave: electrical stimulus through the atria (atrial depolarization)
- PR interval: time between stimuli of atria and ventricles
- QRS complex: stimuli traveling through ventricles (ventricular depolarization)
- ST segment and T wave: ventricular repolarization (relaxing)
- U wave: final stage of ventricular repolarization

When the ventricles begin to contract, the pressure increases, closing the mitral and tricuspid valves. A sound is produced, which is called the first heart sound, or S1. As the pressure continues to rise, it forces the aortic and pulmonic valves to open. Once the blood is expelled, the ventricular pressure drops and the aortic and pulmonic valves close. The sound of this closure is the second heart sound, or S2. Because of pressure differences between the right and left sides of the heart, this sound splits into two components during inspiration but is one sound during expiration.

As the ventricles relax, the pressure drops and allows the mitral and tricuspid valves to open. The rush of blood into the ventricles can cause a sound in children and young adults that is called S3. There is a fourth heart sound, or S4, that marks atrial contraction and

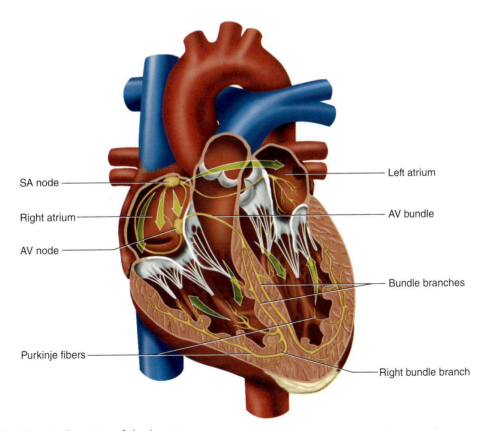

SA node
Right atrium
AV node
Purkinje fibers
Left atrium
AV bundle
Bundle branches
Right bundle branch

FIGURE 8.2 Electrical activity of the heart.

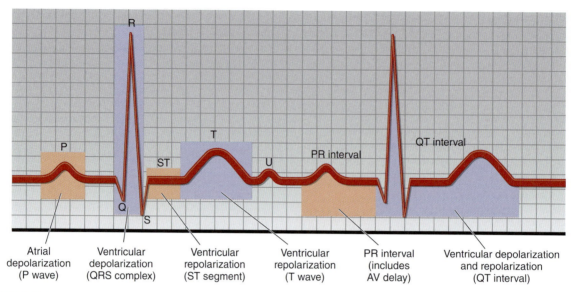

Atrial depolarization (P wave)

Ventricular depolarization (QRS complex)

Ventricular repolarization (ST segment)

Ventricular repolarization (T wave)

PR interval (includes AV delay)

Ventricular depolarization and repolarization (QT interval)

FIGURE 8.3   A graphic illustration of the phases of the resting electrocardiogram.

immediately precedes S1 of the next cardiac cycle. In older adults, S3 and S4 can be pathological heart sounds. *Pathological* is a term used to indicate a condition that involves or is caused by a disease or condition (O'Toole 2013). Other pathological sounds, such as snaps and clicks, may also be heard via auscultation.

Another sound that is often heard is a murmur caused by turbulent blood flow or valvular vibration. Heart murmurs can be benign or pathological. Pathological conditions include leaky (i.e., regurgitation) or stiff (i.e., stenosis) valves, holes between chambers (i.e., septal defects), and metabolic conditions, such as anemia. Murmurs can occur during or throughout systole, diastole, or both. They can be localized to a particular valvular area, or they may be diffuse. The sound, called a **bruit**, can transmit into the carotid vasculature. Besides location and radiation, murmurs can vary in intensity, pitch, and quality. They can be loud or soft, harsh or blowing, and high or low pitched in character. Respiration or positioning of the patient can alter the murmur.

Benign murmurs are common in children and young adults. A common cause of a benign murmur is increased venous return and subsequent flow through the pulmonic valve. These types of murmurs are most commonly heard at the upper left sternal border or pulmonic area and vary with position (i.e., the loudest when supine, the quietest when standing). Quite often they are found incidentally on examination. Over time, they may disappear.

When the left ventricle contracts, a volume of blood called the stroke volume is ejected into the aorta and through peripheral circulation. *Blood pressure* describes the pressure that the blood is subjected to with each contraction. It has a peak, which is the systolic measurement, and a trough, which is the diastolic measurement. The

difference between the systolic and diastolic pressures is known as the pulse pressure. The average blood pressure in adults is 120/80 mmHg.

High blood pressure, or *hypertension,* is defined as either systolic or diastolic pressure at or above 140/90 mmHg. Conversely, *hypotension,* or *low blood pressure,* is defined as either systolic or diastolic pressure at or below 90/60 mmHg. Children have lower blood pressure than adults. In fact, a blood pressure of 120/80 in an 8-year-old child would suggest hypertension (Ball et al. 2015). During dehydration from illness or heat, a drop in blood pressure caused by the decreased plasma volume can occur. A fall in systolic blood pressure of 20 mmHg or more when accompanied by symptoms such as light-headedness or fainting is called orthostatic hypotension. When this happens, the patient's blood pressure should be checked in the supine, sitting, and standing positions.

Blood volume is just one factor that influences blood pressure. Cardiac output, peripheral resistance, blood viscosity, and the elasticity of the large arteries can cause variations in systolic pressure, diastolic pressure, or both. Because of the potential variability in blood pressure, proper measurement is important. Making sure the patient is calm and relaxed, using the proper size cuff, supporting the patient's arm, and keeping the blood pressure cuff level with the heart are all important points to remember when measuring blood pressure. Chapter 2 gives instructions on how to take blood pressure.

Cardiovascular Adaptations to Exercise

The heart and cardiovascular system adjust to activity, and well-trained individuals gain tremendous health benefits from the adaptations. Resting heart rate and blood pressure drop with aerobic training and return more quickly to preactivity rates after exercise at a high intensity. The cardiac muscle enlarges with training, but it will return to pretraining size when athletes decondition.

Review of Exercise Physiology

Exercise is usually defined in terms of metabolic characteristics: dynamic or aerobic exercise versus static or anaerobic exercise (Booher and Smith 2003). Most exercise is a composite of both types. Endurance running and swimming are examples of dynamic exercise, whereas sprint running and power weightlifting are examples of static exercise.

In immediate outcomes, dynamic exercise results in increased cardiac output. Both components of cardiac output, stroke volume and heart rate, are increased. Enhanced cardiac contractility and increased venous return to the heart increase stroke volume. Blood flow is redistributed to the heart and skeletal muscles at the expense of the viscera while remaining constant to the brain. Vascular resistance is decreased because of vasodilation in the skeletal muscle, but blood pressure does not decrease because of the increased cardiac output (Booher and Smith 2003; Charlton and Crawford 1997). Pulse pressure is widened during dynamic exercise. Maximal dynamic exercise results in a four- to sixfold increase in cardiac output, a threefold increase in heart rate, and a twofold increase in stroke volume (Booher and Smith 2003).

Heart rate and blood pressure increase in static exercise. The pressure increase can be dramatic, with systolic pressure exceeding 250 mmHg (Booher and Smith 2003). High blood pressure is required to maintain blood flow to exercising muscles whose vessels are being occluded because of the intense muscle contraction. Stroke volume, ejection fraction, and systemic vascular resistance remain unchanged. The higher pressures result in a higher cardiac workload compared with dynamic exercise.

Over the long term, dynamic exercise training results in increased cardiac output. The maximal heart rate cannot change with training, so increased cardiac output is the result of increased stroke volume. The heart adapts to the dynamic work by increasing in size, called *hypertrophy*. With this hypertrophy comes ventricular cavity dilation caused by the chronic volume loading. The increased diastolic volume permits greater stroke volume for less work. These changes can occur in athletes across the life span, including master-level athletes (Booher and Smith 2003).

Because stroke volume is increased at rest while cardiac output is maintained, a decreased resting heart rate occurs. This decrease in heart rate also occurs at submaximal workloads. Therefore, highly aerobically trained athletes have decreased resting heart rates, or bradycardia, when compared with their less trained counterparts.

Blood pressure during ongoing dynamic exercise training in elite athletes has been commonly thought to decrease. This has not been supported in many research studies (Booher and Smith 2003). Scientific evidence, however, supports lowered blood pressure in sedentary adults after they engage in dynamic exercise training (Pescatello and Kulikowich 2001).

Long-term, static exercise training also causes cardiovascular adaptations. In untrained subjects, small decreases are found in heart rate and blood pressure (Booher and Smith 2003). Heavy weight training has been commonly believed to cause hypertension, but this has not been shown in body builders (Booher and Smith 2003). In individuals with hypertension, however, chronic heavy weight training is not recommended. Pressure overload from chronic resistance training can cause cardiac hypertrophy without the chamber enlargement seen with dynamic exercise. Septal and posterior left ventricular wall thickening may also be seen.

Athlete's Heart

The term **athlete's heart** refers to the physiological and morphological adaptations mentioned previously, which an athlete's cardiovascular system may undergo as a result of ongoing exercise training (Charlton and Crawford 1997). Some of these adaptations can be confused with pathological cardiac conditions. It is important to allow healthy individuals the privilege of sport participation; it is even more important to distinguish athlete's heart from pathological disease and to minimize the risk of sudden cardiac death.

Both long-term dynamic and static exercise training can result in cardiac hypertrophy; these changes can occur after just a few weeks of training. Because heart wall thickness can be quite variable, sometimes as thick as 19 mm (Nagashima et al. 2003), one way to evaluate whether the cardiac changes are pathological is to detrain the athlete. If the wall thickness shrinks, the previous hypertrophy was probably due to the benign effects of athlete's heart. A hypertrophic ventricle that does not diminish in size with detraining indicates possible cardiac disease or an idiopathic anomaly.

Preparticipation Examination

As discussed in chapter 1, the preparticipation examination (PPE) sheds light on any medical problems that may affect athletic participation. The American Academy of Family Physicians (AAFP) recommends an initial evaluation for first-time participation in school or college athletics, with annual follow-up questions in certain areas. One of the areas of concern on both the initial and subsequent annual evaluation is cardiac health. Recommended questions for PPEs, including those related to potential cardiac problems, are listed here:

- Have you ever passed out during or after exercise?
- Have you ever been dizzy during or after exercise?
- Have you ever had chest pain during or after exercise?
- Do you get tired more quickly than your friends do during exercise?
- Have you ever had racing of your heart or skipped heartbeats?
- Have you had high blood pressure or high cholesterol?
- Have you ever been told you have a heart murmur?
- Has any family member or relative died of heart problems or sudden cardiac death before the age of 50 years?
- Have you had a severe viral infection (e.g., myocarditis or mononucleosis) within the past month?
- Has a physician ever denied or restricted your participation in sports for any heart problems?

These questions are designed to alert the physician to potential life-threatening anomalies related to the heart and especially sudden death events. Any athlete who complains of symptoms consistent with these questions should be referred to a physician, preferably a cardiologist, before continuing activity, regardless of whether the athlete has already passed a PPE screening.

General Evaluation of the Cardiovascular System

When assessing an athlete for cardiac sounds, the patient needs to be in a still and quiet environment. The most important aspect of cardiac auscultation is to develop a routine and listen to five specific areas of the chest (figure 8.4) while the athlete is in one position (e.g., sitting) and then repeat the sequence of auscultation while the athlete is supine (figure 8.5) and again with the athlete lying in a lateral recumbent position. The five auscultatory areas are as follows:

1. Aortic valve: second right intercostal space at right sternal border
2. Pulmonic valve: second left intercostal space at left sternal border
3. Second pulmonic valve: third intercostal space at left sternal border
4. Tricuspid valve: fourth intercostal space along lower left sternal border
5. Mitral valve: fifth intercostal space at apex of heart (midclavicular line)

The diaphragm of the stethoscope is warmed before being placed on the athlete's bare chest if the examination is not caused by an emergent situation. When auscultating, the clinician explains what is being done before placing the stethoscope and always follows proper draping protocol when working with female athletes. Cardiac sounds can be assessed on a woman wearing a sports bra if the stethoscope is placed on the skin under the clothing.

Accurate cardiac auscultation takes time. The examiner pauses at each auscultatory area to completely hear

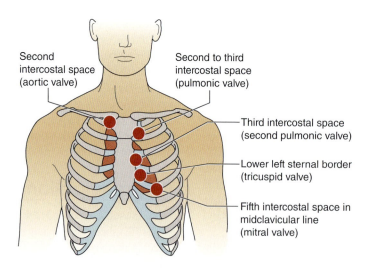

Second intercostal space (aortic valve)

Second to third intercostal space (pulmonic valve)

Third intercostal space (second pulmonic valve)

Lower left sternal border (tricuspid valve)

Fifth intercostal space in midclavicular line (mitral valve)

FIGURE 8.4 Frontal view showing the five traditional designated areas for auscultation of the heart.

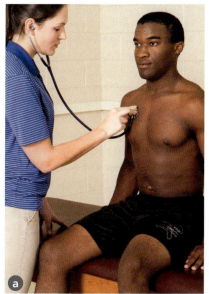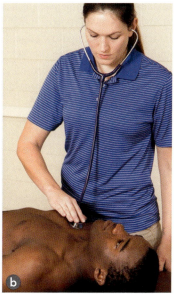

FIGURE 8.5   Cardiac auscultation with *(a)* the athlete sitting and *(b)* the athlete supine.

and isolate the sounds of each valve opening and closing. This skill requires patience, practice, and a quiet area. The examiner listens for the normal rate and rhythm of the heart in each auscultatory area and then specifically listens for the sounds associated with systole (i.e., contraction of the ventricles) followed by diastole (i.e., relaxation of the ventricles). Diastole is a longer interval than systole (Ball et al. 2015). When auscultating in each area, the examiner should also make sure to listen for adventitious or extra sounds or noises. The examiner should be aware that if athletes are asked to hold their breath during expiration, S1 may be more predominant; holding their breath on inspiration will cause S2 to be more distinct.

The physical examination of the athlete can be variable and nonspecific. In many high-performance athletes, particularly those who practice endurance sports, an increase in parasympathetic tone may cause a resting bradycardia. Resting heart rates have been recorded as low as 25 beats/min in elite endurance athletes. Resting blood pressure usually is not changed, but it may be lowered. Third and fourth heart sounds may be present and are of no clinical significance as an isolated finding. Palpation may reveal a left ventricular impulse that is displaced to the left and prolonged. Because of the cardiac hypertrophy, 3% to 50% of high-performance athletes may have a mild mid-systolic heart murmur (Pelliccia et al. 1991). These benign flow murmurs are best heard in the supine position and often disappear on standing.

The ECG in an individual with athlete's heart can mimic many pathological conditions. The increased vagal tone and resultant bradycardia seen in trained athletes are associated with a greater incidence of benign arrhythmias, such as **premature atrial contraction (PAC)** and **premature ventricular contraction (PVC)**, than in the general population (Smith and Ciocca 2002). Complete, or third-degree, **atrioventricular (AV) blocks**, however, are rare and need to be investigated for pathology. High voltage on the ECG is common and can skew the determination of hypertrophy. The most common change seen in the athletic heart is early repolarization of the ventricles. On the ECG, this is evidenced by characteristic ST- and T-wave changes (Huston, Puffer, and Rodney 1985).

Pathological Conditions of the Cardiac System

This section reviews various pathological cardiac conditions that may be seen in athletes. Rare congenital cardiac conditions are beyond the scope of this chapter. The most recent recommendations for determining eligibility for competition by athletes with cardiovascular abnormalities were published from the 36th Bethesda Conference in April 2005.

Sudden Cardiac Death

Death by sudden cardiac arrest (SCA) is a rare event in the young athlete. In the United States, elite athletes are viewed as near invincible because of their incredible physical feats. Nevertheless, it is reported that the rate of collegiate athlete death due to SCA is higher than that of high school athletes, with a suspected 110 SCA deaths annually in the United States among young athletes (Casa et al. 2012). Any time a tragedy of this proportion occurs, the public reacts with disbelief, and medical knowledge is called into question. Studies that have tracked these deaths during sports used the National Federation of State High School Associations (NFHS), the National Collegiate Athletic Association (NCAA) governing organizations, and state and federally funded research groups for data collection, such as the National Center for Catastrophic Sport Injury Research (NCCSIR), based in Chapel Hill, North Carolina. Approximately 90% of the data collected involved male athletes, with an equal distribution between Caucasians and African-Americans (Borjesson and Pelliccia 2009). According to the NCCSIR, there were 10 indirect (due to exertion) fatalities in middle school through college football athletes in 2014, and six were attributed to a cardiac event (Kucera et al. 2015). An additional five football athletes died of suspected cardiac conditions due to nonexertional factors in the same year (Kucera et al. 2015). Sudden death cases in young women are rare, and the most common cause of sudden cardiac death was congenital cardiac disease.

The prevalence of sudden cardiac death in young athletes (those less than 35-year-old) is estimated to be between 1 and 3 in 100,000 (Borjesson and Pelliccia 2009). This is much higher than statistics reported in a more general population of active individuals (Harmon, Klossner, and Drezner 2011). These data indicate that active people are not immune to cardiovascular events that may result in death.

Causes

The most common cause of sudden cardiac death in the young athlete is hypertrophic cardiomyopathy, which accounts for up to 50% of the cases. Other significant causes of sudden cardiac death in a young athlete are coronary artery anomalies, increased cardiac mass, aortic rupture, myocarditis, and aortic stenosis (Borjesson and Pelliccia 2009). Rare causes include dilated cardiomyopathy, atherosclerotic coronary artery disease, mitral valve prolapse, isolated arrhythmias such as long QT syndrome and Wolff-Parkinson-White syndrome, and

CLINICAL TIPS

Potential Causes of Sudden Death

Sudden collapse in athletes could be caused by heatstroke, a cardiac event, sickle cell collapse, or injury. Understanding the presentation of each will facilitate rapid response and the appropriate disposition.

arrhythmogenic right ventricular dysplasia (ARVD) (Harmon, Klossner, and Drezner 2011). In the Veneto region of Italy, researchers have found ARVD to be the most common cause of sudden cardiac death in the athlete (Thiene et al. 1988). This research suggests that a specific population may have different genetic subtraits.

In the older athlete, coronary artery disease is by far the most common cause of sudden death. Rarely is sudden death in the older athlete caused by hypertrophic cardiomyopathy, mitral valve prolapse, or acquired valvular conditions (Maron et al. 2014; Nagashima et al. 2003; Semsarian, Sweeting, and Ackerman 2015; Marijon et al. 2015).

Traumatic sudden cardiac death has not captured as much attention because its epidemiology is more difficult to track. However, it is a growing problem that strikes without warning. Between 1996 and 2007, a reported 180 cases of blunt-force death in the United States were attributed to commotio cordis (Maron et al. 2006). Most cases involved children with a mean age of 13, with 95% of the deaths occurring in males (Maron et al. 2013).

Commotio cordis refers to trauma to the chest wall that interrupts the electrical impulse in the heart. If the cardiac rhythm is not promptly normalized, the individual dies. Typically the ribs or sternum is not broken, although some contusions may be found. Research has found that a chest blow occurring during the vulnerable phase of repolarization, just prior to the T-wave peak in the cardiac cycle, can induce ventricular fibrillation (Maron and Estes 2005).

Although children and teenagers with thin chest walls are most vulnerable to commotio cordis (figure 8.6), deaths have been reported in adults. Sports such as baseball, ice hockey, lacrosse, and softball, which have hard projectiles that can strike the chest, have been associated with the greatest number of deaths. Commotio cordis also has occurred in sports such as soccer, football, rugby, and karate, in which the blow came from a soft projectile or a collision. It appears that the timing of the incident, rather than the degree of impact of the object, is the causative factor (Maron and Estes 2005). Commotio cordis is the only significant cause of traumatic sudden cardiac death in athletes.

Prevention

Because death can be the outcome, prevention has become the focus of attention for commotio cordis. Changes in practice have ranged from protective padding to softer balls that are used in Little League and softball. Because this may not completely resolve the problem, another solution is defibrillation in conjunction with cardiopulmonary resuscitation (CPR). Defibrillation interrupts the heart rhythm so the heart can "reboot" into a normal rhythm.

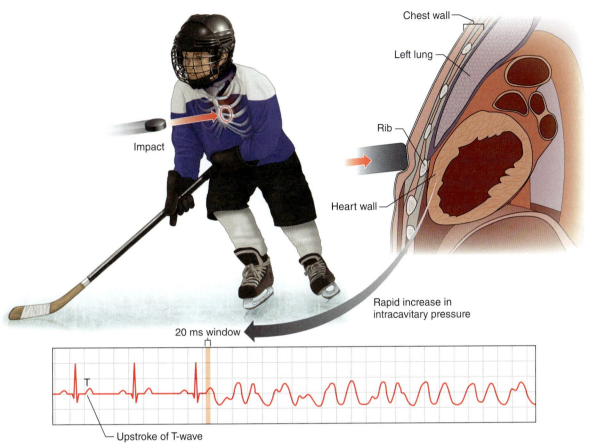

FIGURE 8.6   The type of injury associated with commotio cordis is a blow to the chest wall that interrupts the usual cardiac rhythm.

The American Heart Association estimates that communities with comprehensive CPR and automated external defibrillator (AED) training achieve 40% survival rates for cardiac arrest victims. If defibrillation is performed within 3 min, the likelihood of survival is high. For every minute of delay the chance of survival drops by as much as 10% (American Heart Association 2013).

The advent of the AED has provided greater public access to life-saving technology. These devices can be operated by trained laypeople and are increasingly affordable in all sectors. The AED is portable, rechargeable, simple to operate, and easy to maintain. The American Red Cross, American Heart Association, and National Safety Council offer AED certification courses in addition to CPR courses for the lay public. The NCAA Sports Medicine Guidelines require planned access to an AED and mandating CPR and first aid certifications for all who work with athlete practices, competition, and skill sessions. Athletic trainers are required to maintain certification in emergency cardiac care, including AED use. They need to have ready access to an AED in order to provide rapid cardiac assessment and care to those in fibrillation. Athletes who suffer a sudden collapse and have agonal or gasping breathing should be treated because they are suffering from a cardiac event (Casa et

CLINICAL TIPS

Emergency Planning

Every athletic site should have planned access to an AED, an emergency medical service (EMS), and an established emergency action plan (EAP), as well as medical personnel trained to respond to sudden collapse.

al. 2012; Solberg et al. 2015). An AED should be applied as soon as possible for heart rhythm analysis and possible defibrillation.

Hypertrophic Cardiomyopathy

Hypertrophic cardiomyopathy (HCM) is the leading cause of sudden cardiac death in athletes in the United States under the age of 35. The genetic disorder is characterized by an abnormally hypertrophied but nondilated left ventricle in the absence of physiological conditions such as physical training or pathological conditions like aortic stenosis or hypertension that would result in left ventricular hypertrophy (figure 8.7) (Maron, Ackerman, et al. 2005). More than 400 specific mutations within genes have been identified, and an autosomal dominant transmission of this disorder has been described. This is why familial history of sudden death at a young age is a critical history question in the PPE.

The prevalence of HCM is estimated at 1 in 500 in the general population and is more prevalent in males of African-American descent, at least in collegiate athletes (Maron, Ackerman, et al. 2005; Maron et al. 2014).

The walls of the left ventricle thicken in a variable pattern in HCM. As often as 28% of the time, physical obstruction of blood flow occurs during systole. Up to 80% of individuals with HCM have abnormally small coronary arteries that may cause myocardial ischemia (Maron, Ackerman, et al. 2005). Cellular abnormalities include myofibrillar disorganization and death with resultant fibrotic scarring.

Although outflow obstruction can occur, the presence of left ventricular diastolic dysfunction is more common. Either outflow obstruction or diastolic dysfunction can impair exercise performance even in the least symptomatic person (Maron, Ackerman, et al. 2005). Both decreased wall distensibility and incomplete myocardial relaxation contribute to altered left ventricular filling (Maron et al. 1987), which leads to left atrial dilation and potential development of emboli. Regional myocardial ischemia likely occurs because of the abnormally small coronary arteries and inadequate capillary density (Maron et al. 1987). Adding random fibrosis of the cardiac musculature produces a combination of ischemia, fibrosis, and impaired vasodilator reserve that can lead to arrhythmia and sudden death.

Signs and Symptoms

Symptoms of HCM are fatigue, dyspnea, exertional angina, and syncope or near syncope. These symptoms may not correlate with the degree of ventricular hypertrophy or be predictive for sudden death (Maron, Shirani, and Poliac 1996). Physical examination can provide valuable information, but the findings are not consistent. On palpation, an increased left ventricular impulse may be felt. Pulses may be **bifid** in character and exhibit a brisk upstroke. On cardiac auscultation, a classic, harsh precordial ejection murmur may be heard at the left lower sternal border toward the apex. The murmur increases with standing or Valsalva maneuver and diminishes with squatting; however, a murmur is not always present.

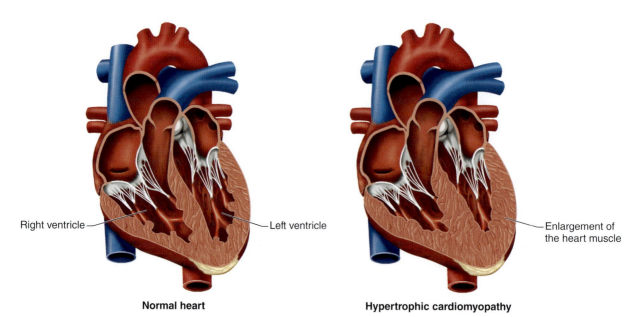

Right ventricle — — Left ventricle   — Enlargement of the heart muscle

Normal heart   **Hypertrophic cardiomyopathy**

FIGURE 8.7   Hypertrophic cardiomyopathy is characterized by an enlarged left ventricle and ventricular septum walls.

CONDITION HIGHLIGHT

Hypertrophic Cardiomyopathy (HCM)

Cardiovascular anomaly is the most common cause for sudden death in athletes. Most of these deaths are attributed to hypertrophic cardiomyopathy (HCM) (Maron et al. 2014; Drezner et al. 2007). HCM presents with a hypertrophic ventricle wall, typically the left, with the chamber size remaining normal (see figure 8.7). Since it is well documented that athletes, especially endurance athletes, benefit from an enlarged left ventricle due to training, their condition can also be confused with HCM. Signs and symptoms of HCM, such as shortness of breath and fatigue, can be dismissed by the athlete as deconditioning or fatigue. HCM is an inherited disorder, and it is unusual for an ECG to provide definitive evidence of the structural defect. Family history of a death at a young age, symptoms consistent with HMC, and an echocardiography demonstrating an enlarged ventricle with normal cavity all provide more definitive evidence that should be followed up with a cardiologist before allowing athletic participation. People with HMC are limited to low-intensity sports, but there is a suggestion that those with a family history of sudden death at a young age due to HCM are strong candidates for an implantable cardioverter defibrillator to allow for a more normal life (Maron 2015a).

It is important to consider differential diagnoses before determining clinical HCM. The clinical symptoms alone of exertional angina, syncope, and near syncope point to many conditions that could cause sudden death. They also can be related to benign conditions, such as dehydration or vasovagal syncope, or noncardiac conditions, such as asthma or gastroesophageal reflux disease. The potential for a serious, life-threatening condition, however, warrants an immediate referral.

Referral and Diagnostic Tests

Athletes with symptoms of exertional angina, syncope, or near syncope should be referred immediately to a physician who specializes in cardiology for evaluation. Fatigue and dyspnea uncharacteristic for a particular athlete warrant concern and certainly physician referral when accompanied by a heart murmur.

Standard laboratory tests, such as a resting 12-lead ECG or chest radiograph, have limited utility in screening for HCM. The most useful diagnostic test is echocardiography, or magnetic resonance imaging (MRI) with gadolinium contrast (Maron, Douglas, et al. 2005; Maron 2015b). Increased left ventricular wall thickness (>15 mm) is the most helpful diagnostic parameter. The majority of male athletes and all female athletes have a ventricular wall thickness of 12 mm or less (Pelliccia et al. 1991). Therefore, the range from 13 to 15 mm may pose a diagnostic dilemma because it is possible to have physiological hypertrophy in this wall thickness range; however, this hypertrophy has been reported only in male cyclists and rowers (Pelliccia et al. 1991). Another sign of HCM that can be seen on an echocardiogram is a ventricular septum or free wall thickness ratio greater than 1:3. Asymmetric wall thickening and decreased left ventricular diastolic cavity dimension (<45 mm) may also be present. In addition, the echo may reveal abnormal diastolic filling with decreased early filling and increased late filling and abnormal ultrasonic myocardial reflex activity in the athlete with HCM (Maron et al. 1993).

Discontinuing athletic activities for a few weeks to 1 mo for the athlete with these symptoms may help clinicians to determine whether the problem is HCM or simply athlete's heart (Maron et al. 1993). Hypertrophy of the ventricular wall will not resolve with detraining in a person with HCM.

As a diagnostic tool for HCM, echocardiography is the gold standard. Its value as a screening tool, however, is limited by its relative expense. If echocardiography were used as a preparticipation screening tool, the cost to prevent one death from HCM would exceed hundreds of millions of dollars. In the future, genetic markers may hold the greatest promise as effective screening tests, with 12 mutant genes and more than 400 specific mutations now implicated in the pathogenesis of clinically diagnosed HCM (Maron, Ackerman, et al. 2005).

Treatment and Return to Participation

In 2005, medical experts met to determine safe standards for athletic participation for athletes with cardiac conditions. The collection of these papers is referred to as the 36th Bethesda Conference. One of their many highlights was a classification of sports based on static (burst actions) and dynamic (aerobic) activities and their effect on the heart. These are summarized in table 8.1 and will be referred to often throughout this chapter. On the basis of the 36th Bethesda Conference recommendations, athletes with hypertrophic cardiomyopathy should be

TABLE 8.1 **Classification of Sports Based on Peak Static and Dynamic Components During Competition**

Classification	Low Dynamic (A)	Moderate Dynamic (B)	High Dynamic (C)
Low static (I)	Billiards Bowling Cricket Curling Golf	Baseball* Softball* Fencing Table tennis Volleyball	Badminton Cross-country skiing (classic technique) Tennis (singles) Field hockey* Orienteering Racquetball/squash* Race walking Distance running Soccer* Tennis
Moderate static (II)	Archery Auto racing*† Diving*† Equestrian*† Motorcycling*†	American football*† Field events (jumping) Figure skating* Rodeo*† Sprint running Surfing Synchronized swimming Rugby*	Basketball* Ice hockey* Cross-country skiing (skating technique) Lacrosse* Mid-distance running Swimming† Team handball
High static (III)	Bobsledding/luge*† Field events (throw) Gymnastics*† Karate/judo* Sailing Rock climbing Water skiing*† Weightlifting*† Wind surfing*†	Bodybuilding*† Downhill skiing*† Wrestling*	Boxing* Canoeing/kayaking Cycling*† Decathlon Rowing Speed skating*† Triathlon*†

* Danger of body collision. † Increased risk if syncope occurs.

Adapted from *Journal of the American College of Cardiology*, Vol 45(8), J.H. Mitchell et al., "Task Force 8: classification of sports," pg. 1366, copyright 2005, with permission from Elsevier.

restricted from participation in all competitive sports with the possible exception of low-intensity (class IA) sports such as golf, bowling, and billiards (Mitchell et al. 2005). Furthermore, the placement of an implantable cardioverter defibrillator (ICD) in a patient with HCM does not change the competitive sports recommendations for this disease.

Although the clinical significance and natural history of genotype positive–phenotype negative individuals remain unresolved, no compelling data are available at present with which to preclude these patients from competitive sports, particularly in the absence of cardiac symptoms or a family history of sudden death.

Prevention

Detection of HCM can be difficult, but the patient's medical history is invaluable. A comprehensive medical history can reveal an autosomal dominant transmission pattern, a family history of cardiac disease, or a record of other premature sudden death in family members. Unfortunately, medical histories have not been as useful as expected because of the variability of expression of the trait. Nonetheless, the athletic trainer and team physician should ask about a family history of cardiovascular disease in every athletic preparticipation examination, as discussed previously.

Obstacles in the United States to implementing additional screening tests (i.e., ECGs or echocardiograms) include the particularly large population of athletes to screen, major cost–benefit considerations, and the recognition that it is impossible to eliminate all risks associated with competitive sports. Although more and more large NCAA Division I programs use noninvasive cardiac testing, such as ECG or echocardiograms in the PPE, it is not yet commonplace (Asplund and Asif 2014).

Coronary Artery Abnormalities

Congenital coronary anomalies are a much less frequent cause of sudden death than HCM in athletes. They are characterized by either an aberrant (i.e., deviating or abnormal) coronary artery takeoff or the complete absence of a coronary artery (Vouhe 2015). Most reports rank coronary anomalies as the second leading cause of sudden death in athletes (Borjesson and Pelliccia 2009; Maron, Shirani, and Poliac 1996; Chappex et al. 2015), with most events happening during or just after strenuous exercise (Toukola et al. 2015).

Myocardial bridging refers to a coronary artery that is surrounded by myocardium for a portion of its course. This tunneling is seen in up to 25% of hearts at the time of autopsy after sudden death and usually involves the left anterior descending artery. Rarely does a congenital aberration result in clinical pathology, but the vascular compression from the ventricle during systole has been reported as an exercise-related cause of sudden death (Toukola et al. 2015).

Acquired coronary artery abnormalities that have been associated with exercise-related sudden death are atherosclerotic coronary artery disease, Kawasaki's disease, and coronary artery vasospasm.

Signs and Symptoms

Symptoms preceding death from coronary artery anomalies are infrequent but include anginal chest pain with exertion, exertional syncope, near syncope with exertion, or exertional dyspnea. If there is any symptom with myocardial bridging, it is usually angina because of myocardial ischemia (Betriu et al. 1980).

Referral and Diagnostic Tests

Any athlete presenting with unexplained exertional chest pain or an exertional syncopal episode must be referred immediately to a physician. An echocardiogram may demonstrate the anomalous takeoff. However, **cardioangiography** is usually required for a conclusive diagnosis (figure 8.8).

Treatment and Return to Participation

At present, no medical treatment exists that can permit continued athletic competition for athletes with congenital coronary anomalies, although the individual may benefit from β-adrenergic or calcium-blocking agents. In myocardial bridging, surgical resection may resolve the ischemia and allow a safe return to play.

It is recommended that the athlete with an anomalous coronary artery retire from competitive sports participa-

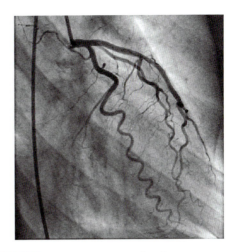

FIGURE 8.8 Cardioangiography showing a coronary stenosis caused by spasm.
© Katie Walsh Flanagan

tion (Graham et al. 2005). If possible, surgery to recreate the abnormal artery should be performed, and if after 3 to 6 mo the athlete is nonischemic during maximal exercise testing, then sport participation may be permitted (Graham et al. 2005).

If there is no evidence of myocardial ischemia after surgery in a patient with myocardial bridging, the patient may also participate in all sports (Graham et al. 2005; Thompson et al. 2005). Any evidence of ischemia, regardless of the cause, will restrict the athlete to low-intensity competitive sports (class IA) such as golf or bowling (Mitchell et al. 2005; Thompson et al. 2005).

Special Concerns in the Mature Athlete

Whereas atherosclerotic coronary disease resulting in myocardial infarction is the overwhelming cause of sudden death in athletes more than 35 years of age (Chappex et al. 2015), it is much less common in younger populations. The tragic death of Olympic skater Sergei Grinkov at 29 years of age, however, demonstrates that it can occur. Usually, major risk factors for coronary artery disease are present, such as family history, hypercholesterolemia, and hypertension.

Coronary artery vasospasm is a rare cause of exercise-related sudden death. Although most athletes who experience vasospasm are shown to have some evidence of atherosclerosis, there are reports of individuals with vasospasm and normal coronary arteries (Thompson et al. 2005). Although vasospasms can be treated with extended-release nitroglycerin and calcium channel blockers (Yasue et al. 2008), athletes with documented coronary artery vasospasm are limited to low-intensity competitive sports along with the other ischemic cardiac conditions (Thompson et al. 2005).

Diagnosis of a myocardial infarction (MI) is beyond the scope of this chapter but is mentioned here due to its relationship with coronary artery disease. When coronary arteries are ineffective in getting blood and oxygen to distal aspects of the myocardium, the tissue dies, resulting in a MI. Common symptoms of a MI are crushing substernal chest pain that can radiate into the left arm, neck, and jaw; diaphoresis; nausea; vomiting; and dyspnea. Sometimes the symptoms are quite nonspecific and easily mistaken for indigestion. Quite often a history of angina can be elicited from the patient.

While waiting for emergency transport, the patient may take an aspirin or prescribed nitroglycerin if available. Obviously, the patient is given nothing by mouth if unconscious or unable to swallow. Oxygen can also be given if available. The athletic trainer must be prepared to perform CPR and defibrillate.

In older athletes with coronary artery disease, several factors are considered when determining the risk for sudden death. They include resting ventricular function, exercise-induced ischemia, exercise-induced ventricular arrhythmia, and a degree of coronary artery stenosis (Marijon et al. 2015). Evidence of abnormalities places the athlete at significant risk and requires restriction to low-intensity competitive sports, such as golf or bowling (Thompson et al. 2005; Mitchell et al. 2005). Reevaluation is recommended every 6 mo. The athlete with minimal risk who has evidence of coronary artery disease may be advised to avoid intensely competitive activities, whereas other activity recommendations are evaluated yearly (Thompson et al. 2005).

Special Concerns in the Adolescent Athlete

Kawasaki's disease is a rare, inflammatory condition of unknown origin that usually occurs in young childhood. It is an acute, self-limited vasculitis that is the most common cause of pediatric acquired heart disease in the United States (Graham et al. 2005). Cardiac complications include coronary artery **aneurysm** in up to 20% of untreated patients (Graham et al. 2005).

Athletes with a history of Kawasaki's disease who have no evidence of cardiac involvement or have achieved complete resolution of cardiac involvement may participate in all sports (Graham et al. 2005; Maron, Douglas, et al. 2005). Minor residual abnormalities following resolution of coronary aneurysms may limit an athlete to participation in sports such as golf, bowling, baseball, volleyball, and doubles tennis (Graham et al. 2005; Mitchell et al. 2005). Unresolved aneurysms or stenoses place the athlete at significant risk for sudden death, and

only sports such as golf and bowling are recommended (Graham et al. 2005; Mitchell et al. 2005). Athletes with evidence of myocardial ischemia are restricted from all competitive sports (Thompson et al. 2005).

No guidelines are available for the young athlete with coronary artery disease. Any decision to permit athletic participation must be based on the extent of increased risk that a cardiac event will occur (Thompson et al. 2005). An athlete with these conditions needs to be under appropriate medical and surgical management.

Marfan Syndrome

Marfan syndrome is an autosomal dominant, heritable disorder of connective tissue, and it involves multiple organ systems (Maron, Ackerman, et al. 2005). Aortic dissection and rupture along with severe aortic regurgitation account for the majority of deaths in adolescents and adults with Marfan syndrome (Maron et al. 2014). Maron and other researchers (Maron, Shirani, and Poliac 1996; Borjesson and Pelliccia 2009) have reported that approximately 5% of sudden death events in young athletes are due to aortic rupture secondary to Marfan syndrome.

The prevalence of Marfan syndrome is estimated to be 1 in 5,000. There is no racial or ethnic predilection; males and females are equally affected. There is a 50% chance that a person with Marfan syndrome will pass along the trait, but at least 25% to 35% of cases occur sporadically without a family history (The Marfan Foundation 2015; Inna 2014).

Signs and Symptoms

Typically, people with Marfan syndrome have a tall stature, long, thin limbs, and an arm span-to-height ratio greater than 1.05 (figure 8.9). They have ligamentous laxity and are prone to scoliosis (Maron, Ackerman, et al. 2005; Inna 2014). It is critical to note that multiple variations can be seen in other organ systems affected by Marfan syndrome. It can be very difficult to make a definitive diagnosis, particularly if there is no family history. Table 8.2 contains the requirements for diagnosis. Conclusive diagnosis usually requires confirmation by several specialists under the direction of a primary care physician. Many common clinical manifestations worsen with growth, such as **pectus deformity** and scoliosis; diagnosis is sometimes delayed until adolescence or early adulthood when scoliosis becomes obvious. Rarely, a spontaneous, nontraumatic pneumothorax can be a diagnostic tip-off. Differential diagnoses for Marfan syndrome include any of the conditions listed in table 8.2 as well as endocrine disorders.

There is no single sign of Marfan syndrome; the diagnosis is based on determination of major signs over at

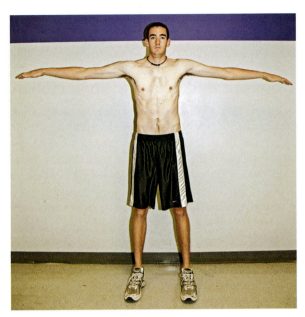

FIGURE 8.9 Marfan syndrome is characterized by an overly tall and thin physical stature with hypermobile joints, sternal deformity, and an arm span that exceeds the person's height.

© Katie Walsh Flanagan

least two different body systems, with minor involvement in an additional system and attributes in the family history (Inna 2014). The five systems that can be affected by Marfan syndrome are the skeletal, ocular, cardiovascular, pulmonary, and skin (integumentary) systems (see table 8.2). A diagnosis for a patient with a negative family history must contain the skeletal and one other system with at least one major involvement.

The major cardiovascular system criteria are dilation of the ascending aorta and dissection of the ascending aorta; minor criteria include mitral valve prolapse (Inna 2014). Any of these can predispose one to sudden death. Before the advent of echocardiography, such abnormalities were estimated to occur in 40% to 60% of patients (Pyeritz and McKusick 1976). It is now well established that more than 95% of patients with Marfan syndrome have cardiovascular abnormalities. Because it is impossible to determine whether a person has a potentially lethal cardiac abnormality without special studies, the athletic trainer and team physician need to promptly refer anyone suspected of having Marfan syndrome to appropriate specialists for further evaluation.

In an athlete with Marfan syndrome, the mitral valve can have multiple abnormalities that may lead to mitral

TABLE 8.2 Marfan Syndrome Diagnostic Criteria

System	Major involvement	Minor involvement

Skeletal	Pectus excavatum requiring surgery
	Arm span-to-height ratio greater than 1.05
	Positive wrist sign
	  (thumb and index finger overlap when
	  encircling the opposite wrist)
	Thoracolumbar scoliosis of more than 20°
	Spondylolisthesis
	Progressive collapse of hindfoot
		Moderate pectus excavatum
		Hypermobile joints
		Dental crowding due to high arched
		  palate

Cardiovascular	Dilated ascending aorta, involving sinuses
	  of Valsalva
	Dissection of ascending aorta
		MVP
		Dilatation of pulmonary artery
		Dilation or dissection of descending
		  thoracic or abdominal aorta
		  (if younger than 50)
		Calcification of mitral valve annulus
		  (if younger than 40)

Pulmonary	None listed	Spontaneous pneumothorax Apical blebs
Ocular	Lens dislocation	Myopia caused by hypoplastic iris or ciliary muscles Abnormally flat cornea

Skin and integument	Widening of the dura in the spinal cord in
	  the lumbosacral region
		Recurrent hernia
		Skin stretch marks (striae atrophicae)
		  not associated with pregnancy

MVP = mitral valve prolapse.

This table is not a complete list of attributes for diagnosis, but it contains the most common ones.

Based on Inna 2014; Maron, Ackerman, et al. 2005; Giese et al. 2007.

valve prolapse and to moderate or severe **mitral regurgitation** (figure 8.10). Regurgitation is evidenced on examination by **apical systolic murmurs**.

Aortic root and sinus dilation may be present at birth, whereas dilation of the ascending aorta usually does not begin until the child is older (el Habbal 1992). The rate of dilation is unpredictable, so it is wise to assess any enlargement beyond the time of long bone epiphyseal closure ascribed to pathological dilation (el Habbal 1992). The aortic root must dilate 50 to 55 mm in order to produce audible aortic regurgitation characterized by a diastolic murmur at the upper right sternal border. Prophylactic surgical repair of the aortic root is usually recommended when the root diameter reaches 55 mm (Gerry, Morris, and Pyeritz 1991).

The most dramatic cardiovascular manifestation is **aortic dissection**, which occurs in about two-thirds of cases (Marsalese et al. 1989). Once thought to be caused by cystic medial necrosis, it is believed to be the result of separation and fragmentation of elastic components of the aorta (Marsalese et al. 1989). The greater the degree of aortic dilation, the greater the risk of dissection.

With the many potential manifestations seen with Marfan syndrome, a multidisciplinary approach to management is usually optimal. Musculoskeletal manifestations may require surgical intervention if cardiopulmonary compromise or progressive spinal curvature beyond 45° occurs.

Ocular screening is conducted annually, but rarely is lens surgery necessary for the characteristic upwardly dislocated lens seen in 60% to 80% of patients (Maumenee 1981). An athlete should not be barred from participation because of dislocated lenses, but contact sports are restricted because of an increased risk for retinal detachment (Inna 2014; Maron, Ackerman, et al. 2005).

Prognosis and Return to Participation

Athletes with Marfan syndrome are restricted from participation in sports that risk body collision (Maron, Ackerman, et al. 2005). Athletes without a family history of sudden death and no personal evidence of mitral regurgitation or aortic root dilation may participate in class IA and IIA sports such as archery, diving, golf, bowling, and billiards (see table 8.1); otherwise, only low-intensity competitive sports (class IA) are permitted (Mitchell et al. 2005; Graham et al. 2005). Serial 6 mo echocardiographic evaluation is required for continued sport participation (Graham et al. 2005). These recommendations apply whether or not a β-blocker is used to help mitigate aortic root enlargement.

Prevention

An annual evaluation is the minimal requirement and includes a complete cardiac examination with echocardiography. Magnetic resonance imaging or transesophageal echocardiography is used to evaluate or monitor aortic dissection. More frequent examination is required when the aortic diameter increases. Quarterly monitoring of the aorta once the root has reached 50 mm is suggested because the risk for dissection significantly increases at this point (Gerry, Morris, and Pyeritz 1991; Inna 2014). Research suggests that prophylactic β-blocker therapy may slow the rate of aortic dilation (Inna 2014). Once

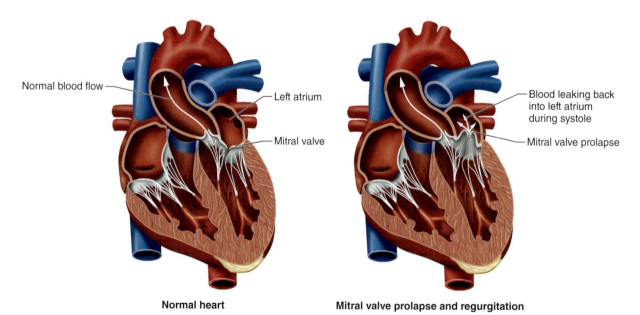

Normal heart

Normal blood flow

Left atrium

Mitral valve

Mitral valve prolapse and regurgitation

Blood leaking back into left atrium during systole

Mitral valve prolapse

FIGURE 8.10 Mitral valve prolapse and mitral valve regurgitation.

the aortic root diameter has reached 55 to 60 mm, surgical evaluation for aortoplasty, graft repair, or aortic valve replacement is advised (Gerry, Morris, and Pyeritz 1991). Anticoagulants may be required depending on the procedure performed.

Special Concerns in the Preadolescent and Adolescent Athlete

In children, mitral regurgitation may be a more significant problem than aortic root dilation. If mitral regurgitation is severe, mitral valve repair may be necessary, although the long-term results are not known. Mitral valve repair obviates the need for anticoagulation. This can allow the child to engage in mild to moderate physical activity. Competitive sports as well as activities with the danger of body collision need to be avoided (Maron, Ackerman, et al. 2005; Gerry, Morris, and Pyeritz 1991). Depending on the situation, the child may need to be excused from all physical education activities.

Myocarditis

Myocarditis is an inflammatory acute or chronic disease process of the cardiac myocytes, often resulting from enteroviral infections, most commonly coxsackievirus B. It can also occur in reaction to toxic agents or drugs such as cocaine (Maron, Ackerman, et al. 2005; Pugh, Bourke, and Kunadian 2012). It traditionally has been regarded as an important cause of unexplained sudden death in young people, and 5% to 22% of sudden cardiac deaths are attributed to it (Pugh, Bourke, and Kunadian 2012). Cardiac dysfunction arises from inflammation of the myocardium, with necrosis or degeneration of adjacent **myocytes**. Healed or active areas of such inflammation

---

🚩 **RED FLAGS FOR MYOCARDITIS**

- Body aches
- Fever
- Nausea
- Vomiting
- Diarrhea
- Mild fatigue
- Dyspnea
- Pitting edema
- Syncope
- Palpitations
- Exercise intolerance

---

may be a pathological substrate for cardiac arrhythmias, and physical activity may trigger a catastrophic event (Maron, Ackerman, et al. 2005).

Signs and Symptoms

Early in the course of the illness, the patient may experience what is thought to be a generalized viral illness with fever, body aches, nausea, vomiting, and diarrhea. However, the illness may be subclinical, and the patient can be asymptomatic aside from some mild fatigue. In a previously healthy person, symptoms of unexplained **congestive heart failure (CHF)** can herald myocarditis. These symptoms may include increased fatigue, chest pain, dyspnea, pitting edema, syncope, **palpitations**, and exercise intolerance. Sometimes the patient is asymptomatic, and sudden death may be the initial presentation (Maron, Ackerman, et al. 2005). Pericarditis is an inflammation of the pericardium surrounding the heart and may present with similar symptoms to myocarditis. Pericarditis is inflammation in the protective membrane surrounding the heart, not in the heart muscle. It is usually caused by a virus and can be seen in collagen vascular diseases.

The patient experiencing congestive heart failure gains weight, exhibits tachycardia, and hyperventilates. Auscultation often reveals a prominent S3 heart sound and rales in the lung bases.

Referral and Diagnostic Tests

An athlete who is having difficulty recovering from what appears to be a routine viral illness needs to be referred to a physician. Clinical tests such as a chest radiograph, ECG, and echocardiogram may demonstrate arrhythmias or acute CHF. Nuclear imaging can be used to pinpoint areas of acute inflammation. For cases in which the diagnosis is in question, endomyocardial biopsy is considered.

Treatment and Return to Participation

Treatment using diuretics and antiarrhythmic drugs is usually directed at preventing or treating CHF. Vasodilators and angiotensin-converting enzyme inhibitors are also used (Tang 2014). More than 30% of patients with myocarditis recover and return to full activity. One-third will experience residual problems, and the final third will need cardiac transplantation. Athletes suspected of having myocarditis need to refrain from all sports activity for 6 mo (a convalescent period) and then undergo an evaluation of cardiac status and ventricular function at rest and with exercise (Maron, Ackerman, et al. 2005). If cardiac function and dimensions have returned to normal and there are no clinically relevant arrhythmias, the athlete may return to competition (Maron, Ackerman, et al. 2005). Insufficient data are available to justify performance of an endomyocardial biopsy as a precondition for return to activity after the 6 mo recuperative period.

Prevention

Although the incidence of myocarditis is relatively small, the prognostic outcome for the majority of cases is poor. Health care providers should discourage ill athletes from participating in sport practice and events, particularly athletes with febrile illnesses. Such care not only will reduce the spread of infection but also may decrease the risk of contracting myocarditis.

Congenital Aortic Stenosis

Congenital aortic valve stenosis (AS) is most commonly related to a bicuspid valve malformation. The pathophysiology arises from impaired left ventricular outflow with compensatory hypertrophy of the interventricular septum and left ventricular (LV) free wall (figure 8.11). Of the recorded athletic deaths due to AS, the majority were Caucasian males, and death most often occurred during or immediately following exercise (Harris et al. 2015). Other causes of aortic stenosis are rheumatic heart disease and degenerative calcific changes (Bonow et al. 2005).

Signs and Symptoms

Patients may also develop significant myocardial ischemia and LV dysfunction from the increased pressure workload of the heart. This can result in hypotension and exertional syncope, which may be accompanied by lethal arrhythmias. Another cardiac and noncardiac condition to consider that may present in this fashion is hypertrophic cardiomyopathy. However, the characteristic murmur is definitive.

Referral and Diagnostic Tests

Patients with fatigue, dizziness, chest pain, syncope, or pallor on exertion require medical follow-up (Bonow et al. 2005). AS can be readily identified on clinical examination by its characteristic loud crescendo–decrescendo systolic murmur heard at the upper right sternal border (i.e., aortic area).

Treatment and Return to Participation

Untreated athletes with mild AS can participate in all sports if they have a normal ECG, exercise tolerance, and no history of exercise-associated chest pain, syncope, or arrhythmia with symptoms (Graham et al. 2005; Bonow et al. 2005). Athletes with moderate AS can participate in low static, low-to-moderate dynamic exercises and moderate static, low dynamic exercises (classes IA, IB, and IIA; see table 8.1) if they have mild or no LV hypertrophy by echocardiography, no LV strain on ECG, a normal exercise test, and absence of exercise-associated symptoms (Graham et al. 2005; Mitchell et al. 2005). However, athletes with severe AS or symptomatic patients with moderate AS are not candidates for competitive sport (Graham et al. 2005; Bonow et al. 2005).

Mitral Valve Prolapse

Mitral valve prolapse (MVP) is one of the most common cardiac abnormalities and is seen in approximately 2%

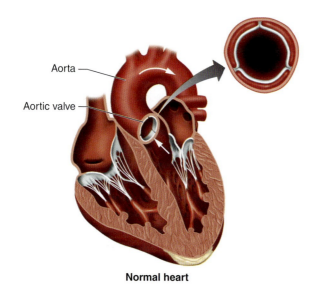

Normal heart

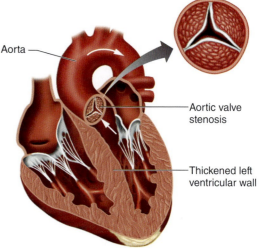

Heart with aortic valve stenosis

FIGURE 8.11 Aortic valve stenosis.

to 3% of individuals, usually women (Narayanan et al. 2015). Although MVP is often mentioned as a cause of exercise-induced sudden death, reports of sudden death are rare (Musante et al. 1987). The etiology of MVP is unknown.

Signs and Symptoms

Symptoms include chest pain, heart palpitations, and uncharacteristic shortness of breath. On occasion, patients complain of syncope or near syncope.

Referral and Diagnostic Tests

Any of the previously mentioned symptoms warrant referral to a physician. Diagnosis can often be made on the auscultative findings of a mid- to late-systolic apical click along with a systolic murmur. Patient positioning is important because both the click and the murmur vary with the patient's position. Squatting accentuates the click, and standing or Valsalva's maneuver increases the murmur (see figure 10.14). Echocardiography can confirm the diagnosis and record the presence of or degree of mitral regurgitation. Athletes who complain of palpitations or syncope require Holter monitoring. A Holter monitor is a portable device that records the ECG over a 24 h period. It has leads with electrodes that are attached to the patient's chest, and it feeds information to a cell phone-sized receiver (figure 8.12).

Treatment and Return to Participation

No treatment is needed in asymptomatic individuals, and athletic participation is unrestricted. Symptomatic individuals may need antiarrhythmic treatment. Arrhythmias are closely associated with MVP and are generally the cause of palpitations reported by patients. Although many arrhythmias have been associated with MVP, ventricular arrhythmias cause the most concern because, although rare, they have been assumed to cause sudden death (Maron, Ackerman, et al. 2005).

Participation in all competitive sports is allowed if the athlete with MVP does not show evidence of family history of sudden death due to MVP, moderate to severe mitral regurgitation, prior embolic event, or syncope caused by arrhythmia. If any of these conditions are detected, the athlete may participate only in class IA sports, such as golf and bowling (see table 8.1) (Maron, Ackerman, et al. 2005; Mitchell et al. 2005).

Arrhythmias

The electrical pathway that synchronizes and controls the contraction of the atria and the ventricles can malfunc-

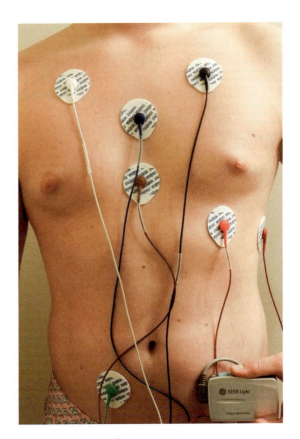

FIGURE 8.12 A Holter monitor.

Photo courtesy of Kathleen Knott / Johns Hopkins University

tion without warning. Most of these malfunctions are innocent, but some are pathological. Arrhythmias can recur frequently or disappear for years, and they vary with activity. Most benign arrhythmias in the athlete are due to increased vagal tone and disappear with exercise. Pathological arrhythmias can compromise blood flow and blood pressure. Some can result in sudden death. It is now well understood that a subset of arrhythmias and heart blocks is inherently safe in athletic participation if certain criteria are met.

As discussed earlier, the electrical activity of the heart is generated via the SA node that the ECG depicts as two events, depolarization (contraction) and repolarization (relaxation).

Arrhythmias are divided into two groups depending on the structures they affect: supraventricular and ventricular. Wolff-Parkinson-White syndrome and long QT syndrome are associated with sudden death and are discussed later. Other abnormal arrhythmic conditions are beyond the scope of this chapter.

A patient with a suspected rhythm or conduction disturbance needs to undergo a 12-lead ECG (see figure 3.9), echocardiography, stress test, and prolonged ambulatory ECG recordings (using a Holter monitor) as warranted. If this evaluation reveals no evidence of structural heart disease and the patient has no symptoms, the 36th Bethesda Conference deems a number of conditions acceptable for full participation in sports (Zipes et al. 2005).

Wolff-Parkinson-White Syndrome

Wolff-Parkinson-White (WPW) syndrome manifestations include ventricular preexcitation and tachycardia resulting from electrical conduction over accessory pathways. Occurring in 0.1% to 3% of the population, WPW syndrome is characterized by a short PR interval (<0.12 s) and a prolonged QRS complex (>0.12 s) with a distinctive early depolarization, the delta wave.

It is fortunate that the incidence of WPW in athletes is very low, for it is rarely provoked by exercise testing. Sudden death as the initial manifestation of WPW is rare but well documented, and it appears to be confined to those patients with accessory pathways that have short refractory periods. In some patients, the occurrence of secondary ventricular fibrillation after paroxysmal WPW tachycardia has been occasionally reported (Zipes et al. 2005).

Referral and Diagnostic Tests

Those athletes with symptoms of palpitations, near syncope, syncope, or periods of impaired consciousness must have an assessment of functional capabilities and electrophysiological properties of the accessory pathway, in addition to a standard cardiac evaluation (Zipes et al. 2005).

Treatment and Return to Participation

Surgical treatment for symptomatic WPW is common. If a short refractory period is found, **radiofrequency catheter ablation** is often considered. This technique, carried out with a catheter inserted through the lower extremity veins, simply destroys the accessory pathway of the ventricle, thereby allowing the heart to resume its normal electrophysiological characteristics (Zipes et al. 2005).

Asymptomatic athletes over age 20 who are without structural disease are unrestricted for athletic participation; younger patients may require more in-depth evaluation before they play in moderate- to high-intensity competitive sports (Zipes et al. 2005). Athletes with atrial fibrillation or flutter with a resting rate less than 240 beats/min without syncope or near syncope are at low risk for sudden death and can participate fully. Those patients with higher rates or symptoms are limited to class IA activities and should consider ablation (Zipes et al. 2005; Mitchell et al. 2005). After ablation, asymptomatic athletes with no inducible arrhythmia, normal AV conduction, and no spontaneous recurrence of tachycardia for several days are cleared for full participation (Zipes et al. 2005).

Long QT Syndrome

A ventricular repolarization abnormality (i.e., QT prolongation) that can be idiopathic or acquired characterizes **long QT syndrome (LQTS)** (figure 8.13). It affects 1 in 2000 people and has a low rate of death in athletes (Johnson and Ackerman 2013; Zipes et al. 2005). Affected individuals may be at high risk for syncope and ventricular arrhythmias. The idiopathic form is inherited (congenital) in both an autosomal dominant manner and an autosomal recessive manner. There are actually five genes responsible for inherited varieties of LQTS. Seventy-five percent of those who have LQTS have one of these varieties and, surprisingly, they have different triggers. One gene is triggered by physical exertion, another by rest and inactivity, and still another by auditory or emotional triggers (Zipes et al. 2005). Acquired forms of the disorder are usually the result of drug or electrolyte abnormalities. Regardless of how one has developed LQTS, all affected patients share similar signs and symptoms.

Long QT syndrome is rare in the general population and almost unknown in athletes (Johnson and Ackerman 2013). Most patients are identified when a family member experiences syncope or sudden death (Moss and Robin-

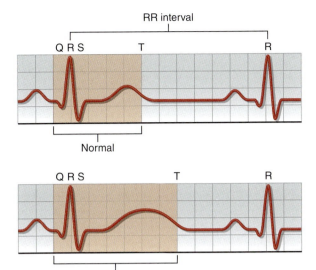

FIGURE 8.13 An ECG of the long QT syndrome (LQTS).

son 1992). Evaluation for long QT syndrome, particularly in a child, is prompted by unexplained seizures or syncope (Singh et al. 1993).

Signs and Symptoms

Patients experience a varied clinical course from no symptoms to syncope with sudden death. Syncope is almost always due to a transient malignant arrhythmia, usually a **torsades de pointes** type of polymorphic ventricular tachycardia.

Referral and Diagnostic Tests

Any athlete with exertional syncope or near syncope needs a prompt physical evaluation. The diagnosis of long QT syndrome can be based on an electrocardiogram, but many asymptomatic people have normal ECGs. The corrected QT interval (QTc) must meet specific criteria to be considered prolonged but is affected by gender, age, and heart rate (Zipes et al. 2005). Borderline prolongation must be interpreted carefully, looking for reproducibility and other evidence of abnormal repolarization, such as prominent U waves and alterations in the T wave (Johnson and Ackerman 2013). In 10% to 15% of athletes, the QT interval is prolonged, particularly in endurance athletes, but no relationship between QT prolongation and ventricular arrhythmias in athletes has been observed. Tests such as Holter monitoring, echocardiography, and exercise stress testing may be useful for confirming the diagnosis in equivocal cases (Moss and Robinson 1992). Genetic testing for the five cardiac ion-channel genes responsible for 75% of long QT syndrome is now available commercially.

Treatment and Return to Participation

β-blockers are the most effective antiarrhythmic agents for long QT syndrome. In acquired long QT syndrome, identifying and correcting the agent or abnormality may be all that is necessary for resolution. According to the 36th Bethesda Conference guidelines for competitive sport participation for athletes with prolonged QT syndrome, those who either have (1) an out-of-hospital cardiac arrest, or (2) a suspected long QT syndrome–precipitated syncopal episode should be restricted from all competitive sports (except those in the class IA category) regardless of genotype (Zipes et al. 2005; Mitchell et al. 2005). Asymptomatic patients with baseline QT prolongation should be restricted to class IA sports. The restriction limiting participation to class IA activities may be liberalized for the asymptomatic patient with genetically proven type 3 long QT syndrome. Patients with genotype-positive or phenotype-negative long QT syndrome may be allowed to participate in competitive sports. Although the risk of sudden cardiac death is not zero in such individuals, there is no compelling data available to justify excluding them from competitive activities. Because of the strong association between swimming and type 1 long QT syndrome, these athletes should refrain from competitive swimming. Patients with long QT syndrome and an ICD or pacemaker should not engage in sports with a danger of bodily collision because such trauma may damage the pacemaker system. The presence of an ICD should restrict patients to class IA activities (Mitchell et al. 2005; Ponamgi, DeSimone, and Ackerman 2015). There is, however, a study with over 353 participants with long QT syndrome, 130 of whom were athletes. None had a sport-related event, which suggests that the 36th Bethesda Conference guidelines for athletes with this disorder may be too restrictive (Johnson and Ackerman 2013).

Syncope

Syncope, or fainting, can be a challenging and frustrating condition for the practitioner as well as the patient to encounter. The many causes of syncope range from benign conditions, such as vasovagal reaction, to life-threatening conditions, such as hypertrophic cardiomyopathy. In many cases, no definitive cause can be established.

Signs and Symptoms

The most frequent cause of syncope in young people is neurocardiogenic (i.e., vasovagal) in response to a trigger. For this chapter, the focus is on underlying cardiac pathology syncope, but triggers can range from changing positions (e.g., prolonged sitting to standing);

stress during or immediately following office medical procedures (e.g., biopsy, sutures); pain; severe emotions; lack of sleep, hydration, or food; extreme temperatures; and the use of certain drugs, among other things. Symptoms are a prodrome of nausea, dizziness, blurred vision, and diaphoresis. The mechanism of neurocardiogenic syncope is believed to be the result of activated cardiac mechanoreceptors set off by forceful systolic contraction, causing increased vagal stimulation with resultant bradycardia and hypotension. Decreased venous return from abrupt postural changes in susceptible individuals as well as intense catecholamine release, as seen in anxious, fearful, or panic situations, can result in neurocardiogenic syncope. Athletic trainers may see a vasovagal response in the athlete who reacts to pain, observes an injection, or receives minor surgery. These are all anxiety-producing situations, and the athlete (or coach) can be apparently healthy one minute and suddenly collapsed on the floor the next. These causes are different from syncope caused by an organic or physiological abnormality. Nevertheless, the immediate treatment is similar.

Referral and Diagnostic Tests

Any case of exertional syncope or near syncope, including postexercise events, requires evaluation by a physician. A thorough history and physical examination are essential in the athlete with syncope. The history of the syncopal event may dictate what laboratory tests are indicated to confirm the diagnosis. Standard laboratory tests include orthostatic vital signs, hemoglobin and hematocrit, blood glucose, electrolytes, and a resting ECG. Situations that call for a more extensive cardiac assessment are exercise-induced syncope without definitive etiology, a family history of premature sudden cardiac death, or physical examination findings of a significant heart murmur or Marfan syndrome. An athlete with a history suggestive of neurological syncope or an abnormal neurological examination receives an extensive neurological assessment as well.

Most cases of neurocardiogenic syncope do not require an extensive workup if the athlete is young and the history is consistent with vasovagal reaction. However, Vettor states that those who suffer exercise-induced syncope must be evaluated for underlying cardiac pathology (Vettor et al. 2015).

Treatment and Return to Participation

Immediate treatment for an athlete who has sustained syncope is to evaluate airway, breathing, and circulation (i.e., ABC) status. If the athlete is pale and sweating and has good airway, breathing, and circulation, the immediate treatment is to raise the feet, thereby assisting the venous return to the vital organs, particularly the heart and brain. Further assessment continues as the athlete regains consciousness and can assist with the medical history, including drug or supplement ingestion. Besides the aforementioned cardiac anomalies, the athlete may simply have skipped a meal, been dehydrated, or been exhausted.

Secondary treatment for syncope depends on its etiology. If the syncope is cardiac in origin (e.g., long QT syndrome), β-blocker medication and disqualification from sport are in order. In other cardiac conditions, such as WPW syndrome, ablation of the accessory pathway cures the problem, and the athlete can return to full athletic participation. If the syncope is neurological in origin (e.g., epilepsy), medical treatment may permit full to modified athletic participation. If the cause of the syncope is asthma-related, medical treatment may permit full to modified athletic participation. If the syncope is vasovagal, correcting the problem can be as easy as improving nutrition or hydration or adding some salt to the diet to maintain electrolyte balance in sweating athletes.

In the athlete, syncope is a serious condition that requires a thorough evaluation. Straightforward episodes of vasovagal or **orthostatic syncope** dictate a cost-effective assessment. Questionable cases and those with syncope predicated by exercise must be examined for cardiac or neurological etiologies. Return to participation is dictated by the etiology of the syncope and how well the underlying problem can be controlled or eliminated. Vasovagal syncope is not cause for any athletic restriction.

Prevention

Prevention depends on what is causing the syncope. Maintaining proper nutrition, sleeping habits, and hydration can usually prevent vasovagal syncope. When exercising in the heat, the athlete who does not usually salt food might benefit from some additional salt in the diet because electrolytes lost in sweat could be the culprit causing the syncope.

Pathological Conditions of the Vascular System

Hypertension

Systemic hypertension is the most common cardiovascular disorder among athletes. Most of the time there is no identifiable cause. The elevated blood pressure (>140/90 mmHg in adults) results from increases in total peripheral resistance mediated by changes in plasma epinephrine and norepinephrine along with the **renin–angiotensin system** (MacKnight 2003).

Untreated hypertension can lead to serious consequences, such as heart disease, atherosclerosis, renal disease, visual changes, and neurological impairment. It is also a major independent factor for coronary artery disease for all people regardless of sex, race, or age (Rosendorff et al. 2015). Therefore hypertension should be identified as soon as possible and treated appropriately.

Signs and Symptoms

Although most cases are asymptomatic, hypertension is more likely to occur in people with a family history of the disease. It is also more common in those who are obese and in African-Americans. Symptoms on presentation can include headaches, malaise, visual problems, and exercise intolerance.

Referral and Diagnostic Tests

Annual blood pressure screening is an essential part of early diagnosis. Usually, three separate measurements that demonstrate elevated blood pressure—seated, standing, and supine—are needed to confirm the diagnosis (see chapter 2). Updated and more stringent diagnostic guidelines were issued by the American Heart Association in 2015 (table 8.3). Proper conditions, positioning, and equipment minimize false-positive measurements. Clinical findings that may be detected in those with hypertension include cardiac hypertrophy, tachycardia, decreased pulses, bruits, retinal changes, thyroid abnormalities, and tremors.

When evaluating a patient with suspected hypertension, the examiner obtains a thorough history of diet, exercise, weight, and drug use (MacKnight 2003). High sodium intake can contribute to hypertension. It is important to consider exercise history as well because even an athlete can overtrain, resulting in blood pressure changes or deconditioning between seasons. Both situations cause susceptibility if there is a familial tendency toward hypertension. Body weight is often elevated, which is commonly seen in specific sports (linemen in football, throwers in track and field) and can contribute to the problem. Many drugs can contribute to or exacerbate hypertension. Common offenders include caffeine, nasal decongestants, nicotine, appetite suppressants, and nonsteroidal anti-inflammatory drugs. In addition, many drugs banned for those participating in athletic competition, such as ephedrine, cocaine, steroids, erythropoietin, and amphetamines, elevate blood pressure (MacKnight 2003).

Assessment includes an ECG to evaluate for cardiac hypertrophy. The physician orders urine tests for blood and protein and blood work that specifically checks lipid levels, electrolytes, and liver and kidney function. Thyroid function is assessed as needed. If there are cardiac concerns, an exercise stress test may be indicated in addition to the ECG.

Treatment and Return to Participation

Treatment can be nonpharmacological and/or pharmacological and generally is based on a step approach. Strategies such as smoking cessation, diet and weight control, alcohol moderation, and exercise all have a role in the management of hypertension (MacKnight 2003). For most people, medications are needed to effectively lower and maintain blood pressure. This may be especially true in athletes, as they are already exercising, rarely smoke, and typically have their weight under control. With this in mind, lifestyle changes are encouraged and may limit the number of medications required for blood pressure control.

The several classes of hypertension drugs act in different ways. For the active athlete, **angiotensin-converting enzyme (ACE) inhibitors** are the drugs of choice because they have fewer side effects with exercise. Commonly prescribed diuretics increase the chance for dehydration and heat illness. β-blockers restrict exercise capacity, exacerbate asthma, and are banned in certain competitive sports.

Patients with mild to moderate hypertension (systolic, 140–160 mmHg; diastolic, 90–99 mmHg) can participate in all sports if there is no evidence of end-organ damage or heart disease. Activities are focused on dynamic exercise, but static activities are not prohibited. Blood pressure needs to be under control or in the mild range (<140/90 to 159/99 mmHg) before an athlete engages in highly competitive sports or highly strenuous physical training. Blood pressure for a hypertensive athlete should

TABLE 8.3 Blood Pressure Levels Recommended by the American Heart Association

Blood Pressure	Systolic (mmHg)	Diastolic (mmHg)
Normal	<120	<80
Prehypertension	120–139	80–89
High blood pressure (hypertension)		
Stage 1 (hypertension)	140–159	90–99
Stage 2 (hypertension)	≥160	≥100
Hypertensive crisis	>180	>110

A physician should evaluate low or high readings.

Modified from American Heart Association, 2016, *Understanding blood pressure readings.* Available: www.heart.org/HEARTORG/Conditions/HighBloodPressure/AboutHighBloodPressure/Understanding-Blood-Pressure-Readings_UCM_301764_Article.jsp#.VjZCJ-lX_dk.

be checked every 2 to 4 mo (American Heart Association 2014a).

Patients with severe hypertension (>180/110 mmHg) are restricted from strenuous exercise until their blood pressure can be controlled. Dynamic physical activities, however, are encouraged because few data suggest that strenuous dynamic exercise in persons with severe hypertension will lead to progression of the hypertension or exercise-induced sudden death.

Prevention

Prevention of hypertension includes careful monitoring to make sure it remains consistently within safe participation guidelines. The NCAA mandates annual blood pressure assessment as a critical aspect of the PPE (Parsons 2014). Early recognition of consistent elevated blood pressure can be addressed with nutrition, exercise, and, if need be, pharmacological interventions discussed earlier.

Deep Vein Thrombosis

Deep vein thrombosis (DVT) is a condition in which a blood clot becomes lodged in a large vein. This results in venous blockage with stasis distal to the clot. Most of these clots occur in the lower legs (figure 8.14). However, a DVT can occur in any limb. For instance, subclavian

vein thrombosis, although rare, has been reported in baseball pitchers (Hurley et al. 2006).

Many factors contribute to the formation of a DVT. In an active population, a DVT is usually caused by trauma to the extremity from injury or surgery. Other less common causes include prolonged sitting on a plane, in a bus, or in a car; hypercoagulability disorders such as **factor V Leiden anticoagulant gene mutation**; pregnancy; and **polycythemia**. Women who use oral contraceptives, particularly women who smoke, also have an increased risk of blood clots (National Institutes of Health 2011).

It is possible to confuse a DVT with a more superficial **thrombophlebitis**, **postphlebitic syndrome**, ruptured Baker's cyst, or even cellulitis, as they all have similar presentations with a swollen extremity. Even the common problem of calf muscle strain may be confused with a DVT. Usually the mechanism of injury can help differentiate a strain from a DVT. If the patient has had recent surgery, traveled long distances while sitting down, or been subject to a known trauma, a DVT is highly possible.

Signs and Symptoms

The symptoms of DVT are often nonspecific; some DVTs are actually asymptomatic. The key symptoms are limb pain and swelling. In the leg, these symptoms are worsened by standing and walking. On examination, there is usually distal edema of the affected extremity. This can be confirmed by comparison with the contralateral extremity. In the lower leg, the examiner squeezes a passively dorsiflexed calf, as a test for Homans' sign, realizing the test is not specific for a DVT nor is it commonly present with DVT (Delis et al. 2001). Measuring the patient's temperature can be important because fever may be the clue to a DVT proximal to the knee, which is closely associated with the often-fatal **pulmonary embolus**. The Wells' Clinical Prediction Rule for DVTs (Wells et al. 1997), which provides a score for predisposing factors, signs, and symptoms of a DVT, has been validated as being useful for patients at low risk of a blood clot (Tamariz et al. 2014). Pitting edema, calf swelling greater than 3 cm, and tenderness along distribution of the affected veins and collateral superficial veins are all score-worthy signs of a DVT (Wells et al. 1997). The thrombus is generally confirmed through Doppler ultrasound testing but may require invasive **contrast venography**.

Treatment and Return to Participation

Treatment requires anticoagulation, which can be started on an outpatient basis but may require hospitalization. After adequate anticoagulation is reached with heparin, the patient usually must keep taking other anticoagulants such as warfarin (Coumadin) for 3 mo or more (Schreiber

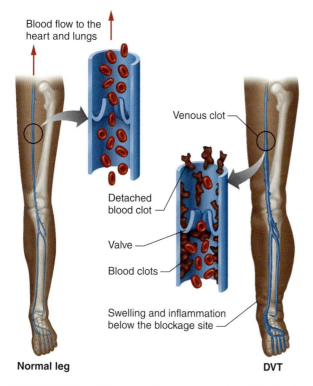

Blood flow to the heart and lungs

Venous clot

Detached blood clot

Valve

Blood clots

Swelling and inflammation below the blockage site

Normal leg   **DVT**

FIGURE 8.14 A foot swollen as a result of blocked venous return caused by a deep vein thrombosis (DVT).

RED FLAGS FOR DEEP VEIN THROMBOSIS AND PULMONARY EMBOLISM

Suspicion of DVT or PE rests with athletes who have recently had surgery, been bedridden, or had sustained sitting (such as in bus or air travel). Athletes with unexplained pain, limb swelling (either upper or lower), edema, or shortness of breath should be evaluated for possible DVT or PE. Shortness of breath, chest pain, and hemoptysis are more indicative of a PE.

2015). Anticoagulation medications must be monitored and adjusted following blood tests every week or so until the medication level is stabilized. Another, more expensive, injectable drug, enoxaparin (Lovenox), is also available and requires less monitoring than other anticoagulants. Note that mixing alcoholic beverages with anticoagulant medications is dangerous; alcohol can increase the blood-thinning properties of the drugs. Serious, if not deadly, ramifications can be caused by such combinations, and they need to be fully explained to the patient. Patients also need to be aware that anti-inflammatory medications alter the blood-clotting process and may exacerbate bleeding time. While patients are taking anticoagulants, collision or contact sports are not advised. In addition to medications, the patient's diet needs to include adequate but not excessive vitamin K.

Athletes undergoing continued anticoagulation therapy should not participate in collision or contact sports. Once anticoagulation is completed, and if hypercoagulable evaluation is negative, a gradual return to play may be granted with careful monitoring for recurrence.

Prevention

Simple prevention is difficult, with the exception that everyone should avoid prolonged sitting, such as when traveling by plane or automobile. Also, as women age they may need to consider an alternative form of contraception to birth control pills. Postsurgical and hypercoagulability situations require subspecialty care. Prompt recognition of symptoms by the athletic trainer is essential to initiate proper care of DVTs and to prevent catastrophic results.

Pulmonary Embolus

A pulmonary embolus (PE) can be a catastrophic complication of a DVT. PE occurs when a blood clot becomes lodged in one of the pulmonary blood vessels. If the vessel is large enough, gas exchange can be interrupted

long enough for death to occur before the clot can be dissolved (figure 8.15). Injury and trauma can also elicit a hypercoagulability response in otherwise healthy athletes (Coleman et al. 2015).

Signs and Symptoms

Symptoms are not specific and can lead to a delay in diagnosis. Common symptoms include acute dyspnea and chest pain. Coughing, or coughing up blood, are also signs of a PE (National Institutes of Health 2011). If the embolism is large, the patient may experience a sense of impending doom. Fatigue and exercise intolerance may occur. Common clinical findings include tachycardia and tachypnea. Low-grade fever may develop, and hemoptysis may occur. There may be signs of a DVT, although many instances of PE occur without warning.

Because the symptoms of a PE are nonspecific, many serious conditions need to be considered in the differential diagnosis. Cardiovascular conditions range from angina and pericarditis to aortic aneurysm and myocardial infarction. Pulmonary conditions include pneumonia, pneumothorax, and pleuritis. Gastrointestinal conditions, such as ulcers, gastritis, and esophageal rupture, can produce atypical chest pain and warrant consideration.

Referral and Diagnostic Tests

When a PE is suspected because of acute dyspnea or chest pain, the patient needs emergent medical attention. A high index of suspicion is often needed to diagnose a PE because standard tests are going to be of limited

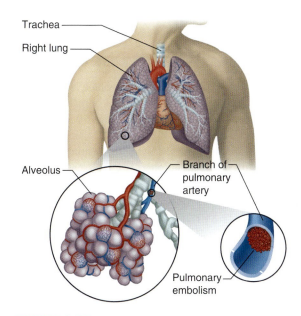

FIGURE 8.15 Pulmonary embolisms cause life-threatening emergencies when they occlude pulmonary vessels.

value. Special hospital studies, such as ultrasound, computed tomography scan, **ventilation–perfusion scan**, or pulmonary arteriography, are performed to confirm the diagnosis.

Treatment and Return to Participation

As for a DVT, anticoagulation treatment is the mainstay of medical therapy, and hospitalization may be required in the early stages of treatment. Ninety percent of those treated with anticoagulants recovered with no ascertainable sequelae of DVT (Schreiber 2015). At least 3 mo of anticoagulation therapy is needed. Continuation of therapy depends on the risk factors for recurrence. Athletic participation is limited in the same manner as for a DVT.

Prevention

In most cases, the cause of the PE is not determined. For those with a defined cause such as hypercoagulability, long-term anticoagulation may be necessary (Schreiber 2015). A person who is at risk for PE but cannot take anticoagulation therapy may need to have a filtering device inserted into the vena cava, where it will catch clots, to keep a life-threatening clot from reaching the lungs. In both instances, athletic participation is significantly restricted depending on the activity and the level of participation. A study providing early prophylactic anticoagulation medication to those hospitalized following trauma, including those with long bone fractures of the lower extremity and severe head or chest trauma, did not demonstrate that the early intervention prevented early PE (Coleman et al. 2015).

Peripheral Arterial Disease

Peripheral arterial disease (PAD), which is also called peripheral vascular disease, is caused primarily by atherosclerosis. It usually presents after age 50 and is more common in older adults. Risk factors include smoking, hypertension, diabetes, and **hyperlipidemia** (Vaidya et al. 2014). In the heart, coronary artery disease is a subclassification of PAD.

Signs and Symptoms

The hallmark of PAD is intermittent **claudication**, which leads to cramping, weakness, pain, or numbness in the affected muscles (American Heart Association 2014b). Most commonly, this is in the lower leg and is provoked by exercise of a given intensity and duration. In the beginning, the symptoms are relieved by rest. However, as PAD progresses, pain can also occur at rest. The key signs are diminished or absent pulses, arterial bruits, dry skin, and ulcerations on the heels and toes that are slow to heal.

PAD could be mistaken for many common problems, such as shin splints, muscle cramps, or arthritis. Lumbar spinal stenosis causes pseudoclaudication, symptoms of which occur with walking or prolonged standing and are relieved by sitting and flexing the spine. Individuals with these conditions do not have any pulse abnormalities or skin changes from arterial insufficiency. Claudication can also occur as the result of vein damage; this causes venous stasis, edema, and pain while resting. Other arterial diseases, such as arteritis and **Raynaud's disease** (see chapter 14), can mimic PAD. Neurological causes of peripheral pain, such as lumbar disc disease or diabetic peripheral neuropathy, may be confused with PAD. Another condition to rule out is compartment syndrome of the lower leg, which has both acute and exertional onset.

Referral and Diagnostic Tests

Clinical suspicion of PAD warrants referral to a physician for assessment. The athletic trainer becomes suspicious when an athlete complains of cramping or weakness in the lower extremities that worsens with exercise. One way to test for PAD is to measure the ankle–brachial index (ABI) (Vaidya et al. 2014). This test determines the ratio of ankle to brachial systolic blood pressures. The gold standard test is invasive angiography.

Treatment and Return to Participation

Treatment focuses on correcting the contributing factors such as smoking, hypertension, and hyperlipidemia. To decrease the risk of stroke or heart attack, a daily aspirin is recommended (Vaidya et al. 2014). Regular exercise with breaks when the symptoms occur may be more beneficial than any medication. Initiating a walking program and gradually adding other physical activities such as biking or swimming are excellent exercise programs for the patient with PAD. For patients with PAD, surgical referral for arterial bypass is an important consideration. Treating or resolving the risk factors can decrease the potential for deterioration. Return to participation depends on the type and level of activity. Risk factor modification is the best preventive strategy for patients with a propensity for PAD.

Anemia

Anemia refers to a decreased number of red blood cells or a decreased hemoglobin concentration in the blood. It is a common medical condition, and it can be a sign of a chronic disease such as cancer. The size of the red blood cell differentiates anemias into three general categories: microcytic, normocytic, and macrocytic.

Microcytic anemias include iron deficiency, **thalassemia**, lead poisoning, **sideroblastic anemia**, and anemias of chronic disease. Normocytic anemias include blood loss, hemolysis, chronic disease, dilutional pseudoanemia, and sickle cell disease. Macrocytic anemias include nutritional anemias related to deficiency of vitamins B_{12} and folate, drug-induced aplastic and **hemolytic anemias**, malignancy, and other hemolytic anemias, such as enzyme deficiencies or red blood cell membrane defects.

In the athlete, decreased hemoglobin is usually the result of iron deficiency, exertional hemolysis, or dilutional pseudoanemia. These disorders are more common in endurance athletes, particularly females (Eichner 2010). Because many other conditions can result in anemia, and the treatments can vary, it is important to be certain of the diagnosis.

Iron deficiency anemia is the most common true anemia seen in athletes. It is rare in male athletes unless they experience a gastrointestinal bleed, whereas as many as 5% of female athletes have iron deficiency anemia, and up to 16% of female athletes are iron deficient (Eichner 2010). This is due to menstrual blood loss combined with inadequate dietary iron intake.

Dilutional pseudoanemia has been labeled sports anemia. It is not a true anemia. The volume of red blood cells is actually normal, but the increased plasma that comes about from endurance training appears to dilute the hemoglobin levels (Eichner 2011).

Signs and Symptoms

Anemia can produce symptoms of weakness, fatigue, dizziness, and headache. Athletes are often asymptomatic if the anemia developed slowly. Decreased performance typically brings the anemia to the athlete's attention. Clinical findings include tachycardia, **orthostatic hypotension**, dyspnea, tachypnea, and pallor. Mouth and tongue abnormalities suggest nutritional deficiencies. Less common clinical findings, such as jaundice and **hepatosplenomegaly**, indicate serious pathology and require urgent medical referral (Harper 2014).

Craving ice or constantly eating crunchy, raw vegetables may suggest iron deficiency anemia (Eichner 2010). Nonsteroidal anti-inflammatory drugs (NSAIDs) can cause gastrointestinal irritation with resultant blood loss, and continual alcohol use can cause similar findings.

Antibiotic use (e.g., penicillin, sulfa, cephalosporin) can trigger hemolytic anemia as well as acute illnesses such as infectious mononucleosis or mycoplasma pneumonia (see chapter 5).

Dilutional pseudoanemia can be indistinguishable from very mild iron deficiency anemia (Eichner 2010). Because lead poisoning and sideroblastic anemia are extremely rare in the athlete, a microcytic anemia is usually a choice between iron deficiency and thalassemia. Other conditions to consider are exertional hemolysis and systemic illnesses such as infectious mononucleosis. The symptoms of hypothyroidism or depression also can mimic those of anemia.

Referral and Diagnostic Tests

An athlete who presents with symptoms of fatigue and loss of energy and who bruises easily should be referred to a physician for a complete blood count (CBC) as well as other tests. Initial tests also include a peripheral blood smear. The CBC measures hemoglobin concentration. The typical cutoff criterion for anemia is below 14 g/dl for men and below 12 g/dl for women (see table 3.3) (Eichner 2011; Harper 2014).

As previously mentioned, the size of the red blood cell classifies the anemia into one of three general categories: microcytic, normocytic, and macrocytic. The mean corpuscular volume (MCV), which is one of the tests contained in the CBC, allows for this classification. Microcytic anemia is defined by an MCV of less than 75 femtoliters (fl). An MCV of 75 to 95 fl defines normocytic anemia; and an MCV of greater than 98 fl defines a macrocytic anemia. The degree of abnormality in the MCV can provide a clue to the diagnosis. Although both iron deficiency and thalassemia conditions have a low MCV, an MCV of less than 60 fl is more suggestive of thalassemia than iron deficiency anemia. Table 3.3 gives normal values for the CBC.

Looking at the size, shape, and color of the red blood cells provides valuable information to determine the type of anemia. Using the previous example of iron deficiency and thalassemia, the peripheral blood smear for both conditions will show microcytic cells. The cells in iron deficiency are hypochromic compared with the normochromic cells seen in thalassemia.

Many tests can be ordered to determine the presence of anemia:

- *Stool blood:* Can be done in the physician's office, or the patient can collect stool on special cards at home; can determine microscopic blood in the stool, which indicates a gastrointestinal source

- *Serum ferritin:* A measure of tissue iron stores, which are low (<12 ng/dl) in iron deficiency anemia and normal to elevated in other microcytic anemias; serum ferritin can be low and the individual not be anemic; although some authorities think that decreased ferritin is associated with decreased exercise performance, scientific evidence does not support this claim

- *Serum iron:* Decreased in iron deficiency anemia and in anemia of chronic disease; elevated in thalassemia and sideroblastic anemia

- *Total iron-binding capacity (TIBC):* Increased in iron deficiency anemia and may be normal or increased in thalassemia; decreased in anemia of chronic disease and can be decreased in sideroblastic anemia
- *Reticulocyte count:* A marker of red blood cell production; should be elevated in anemia, but it is inappropriately low in iron deficiency anemia
- *Hemoglobin electrophoresis:* Can be ordered to identify genetic hemoglobinopathies, such as thalassemia or sickle cell disease
- *Vitamin B₁₂ or folate:* May be decreased in the malnourished athlete (e.g., an eating disorder) with macrocytic anemia
- *Bone marrow biopsy:* Invasive test reserved to determine very serious anemias, such as **aplastic anemia** that can be caused by drugs such as nonsteroidal anti-inflammatory drugs (NSAIDs) or antibiotics

Treatment and Return to Participation

Iron deficiency anemia is not difficult to treat; however, before treatment one must identify and correct any source of abnormal blood loss. The patient takes 325 mg of ferrous sulfate three times per day for optimal treatment of iron deficiency anemia. When a patient cannot tolerate that dosage because of gastrointestinal irritation (constipation), taking one dose with dinner is acceptable. A response is expected within 2 wk, showing a weekly increase in hemoglobin. When the hemoglobin is back to normal (typically 3 to 6 wk), daily iron therapy is continued for another 3 to 6 mo to reestablish iron stores (Harper 2014).

When it is difficult to decide between dilutional pseudoanemia and iron deficiency anemia, an empirical trial of iron therapy is tried. If after 1 to 2 mo of therapy the hemoglobin has increased, then the patient has iron deficiency anemia. In thalassemia minor, no treatment is required. In fact, iron therapy can be harmful.

Dilutional pseudoanemia does no harm, and competition is not restricted. Because iron deficiency anemia can impair athletic performance, training and competition are limited to what the athlete can tolerate. Full training and competition are dictated by the athlete's degree of anemia and the demands of the sport.

Prevention

Prevention of iron deficiency anemia focuses on consuming adequate amounts of iron in the diet. Here are foods that are rich in iron:

- Organ meat (e.g., liver, heart, kidney)
- Lean red meat
- Dark poultry
- Shellfish (e.g., oysters, clams, shrimps)
- Eggs
- Legumes (e.g., beans, dried peas, lentils)
- Leafy green vegetables
- Iron-fortified cereals

The best source of iron is lean red meat. Although some vegetables, such as spinach and beans, contain iron, these sources are not as bioavailable. Also, some foods, such as breads, pastas, and cereals, are iron fortified. To enhance absorption, advise the athlete to avoid coffee or tea and to drink orange juice or other drinks with vitamin C. In addition, cooking in cast iron cookware can provide some iron leaching into the food.

Hemolysis

Exertional hemolysis is defined as the intravascular breakdown of red blood cells as a result of the rigors of physical activity. Initially reported in runners, it was called *foot strike hemolysis* because it was believed to occur from the physical pounding of the soles of the feet. However, the process has been seen in a variety of sports from weightlifting to swimming.

The hemolysis may result in anemia and decreased iron stores. The hemoglobin released in the plasma binds to haptoglobin, which carries it to the liver for salvage. When hemoglobin stores are saturated, it may be secreted into the urine with iron. It would be rare for hemolysis to present with signs and symptoms because it is typically displayed as asymptomatic microscopic hematuria.

Signs and Symptoms

In an athlete with substantial hemolysis, symptoms of mild anemia, such as fatigue and weakness, may be present. It is more likely that the athlete will be asymptomatic. In anemia, dark-colored urine suggests **hemoglobinuria**. In **hemolysis**, it is more likely that the urine will have a combination of myoglobin from muscle breakdown and some hemoglobin, particularly if the inciting activity is intense or prolonged (Eichner 2011). Because clinically significant exertional hemolysis is extremely rare, its diagnosis is one of exclusion. Pathological causes of hemolytic anemia, including red cell trauma from other sources such as cardiac valvular disease, enzyme defects, toxin and metabolic disorders, and paroxysmal nocturnal hemoglobinuria, are differential diagnoses and need to be excluded.

Referral and Diagnostic Tests

A physician orders the following diagnostic tests to confirm hemolysis: A CBC usually shows normal to mildly decreased hemoglobin and red cell concentrations, MCV is elevated but rarely exceeds 108 fl, blood smear is normal, reticulocyte count is elevated, and the serum haptoglobin concentration is low (Eichner 2011). Examination of the urine may detect the presence of hemoglobin.

Treatment and Return to Participation

In most cases of exertional hemolysis, there is no anemia. Therefore no treatment is needed as long as the person has adequate iron stores. Excellent prognosis and full return to participation are the norm for athletes who have exertional hemolysis. Prevention is important in the rare case of a problem.

Prevention

Prevention of hemolysis depends on the mechanism of injury. If excessive impact is to blame, then steps need to be taken to reduce the impact. Examples include better-cushioned shoes, softer running surfaces, and varying the activity with cross-training.

Sickle Cell Trait or Anemia

Sickle cell trait or anemia is caused by a genetic defect in the hemoglobin of the affected person. The altered hemoglobin, called hemoglobin S, causes a chronic hemolytic anemia because the abnormally sickle-shaped defective red blood cells logjam, producing ischemia in distal areas. This is characterized by decreased red blood cell survival, microvascular occlusions from sickling in which the cells stick together, and increased susceptibility to certain infections (figure 8.16). These complications result in significant morbidity and a decreased life expectancy (Anderson and Eichner 2007).

People with sickle cell trait (SCT) have the abnormal gene from one parent, whereas those with **sickle cell anemia**, also termed sickle cell disease, have abnormal genes from both parents. Most people with sickle cell anemia in the United States are of African-American descent. In the athlete with sickle cell anemia, the average hemoglobin concentration is 50% to 66% of normal counts, which is prohibitive for binding oxygen to the red blood cells. Only in very rare instances would a person with sickle cell anemia be able to participate in sports and that would be restricted to the least physically demanding.

On the other hand, people with sickle cell trait are not prohibited from athletic participation. Those with the trait

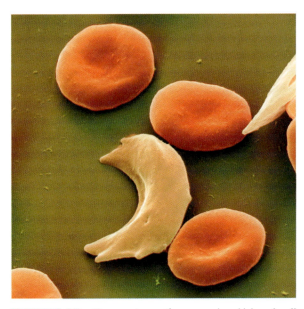

FIGURE 8.16 Comparison of a normal red blood cell and a sickle cell.
Eye of Science / Science Source

are not anemic, and they have a normal life expectancy. Approximately 1 in 12 African-Americans has sickle cell trait. In contrast, only 1 in 10,000 Caucasians carries the trait.

Unfortunately, there have been some rare deaths in athletes with sickle cell trait associated with extreme environmental conditions, such as altitude or hot, humid conditions, in combination with high-intensity workouts. The causes of death have been unclear, although sickling has been postulated as a potential culprit. Ischemia resulting from sickling may cause **rhabdomyolysis**, **lactic acidosis**, and shock (Parsons 2014). People with sickle cell trait are prone to heat illness because they have an inability to concentrate their urine, which makes them prone to dehydration. It is not known if this has been a factor in these rare deaths. All 50 states test for SCT at birth, and confirmation of this status is mandated by the NCAA prior to participation in athletics (Anderson and Eichner 2007; Parsons 2014). The presence of SCT is not prohibitive in athletics, but knowledge of it can preemptively allow education and awareness that could prevent a sickling collapse.

Signs and Symptoms

The signs and symptoms of sickle cell anemia or trait often present in specific environments. Early, preseason practice in a hot, humid environment or events at high altitude tend to lead to attacks in a previously undiagnosed athlete. In addition, intensive exercise such as sprinting and intervals can be the trigger, and sickling can begin as

RED FLAGS FOR SICKLE CELL TRAIT OR ANEMIA

- Heat intolerance
- Severe muscular cramping
- Affected muscles feel normal, not hard or contracted
- Hyperventilation
- Tachycardia
- Hypotension
- Symptomatic indicators in high-altitude environments
- Symptomatic indicators after intense exercise
- Sudden onset, early in the practice or training session

soon as 2 to 3 min into intense, all-out exertion (Parsons 2014; Anderson and Eichner 2007). Often the athlete develops an ischemic-like pain from working muscles robbed of blood supply, similar to the pain of intermittent claudication when leg arteries are narrowed by atherosclerosis. With sickling, the athlete's legs become weak and wobbly (without a prodrome of muscle twinges) and can no longer hold up the patient. On examination, the muscles look and feel normal as opposed to heat cramping, which presents with more excruciating pain and large, rock-hard muscles in full contraction (Anderson and Eichner 2007). This is an emergency situation. The collapse of an athlete from sickle cell anemia or trait, if not witnessed, can be confused with heat cramps, heatstroke, malignant hyperthermia, syncope, or cardiac arrest.

Referral and Diagnostic Tests

Athletes suffering from heatstroke usually do not collapse within the first 30 min of practice, and those suffering from cardiac collapse are typically unable to communicate. Collapse due to sickling is sudden; it occurs early in an intense activity, and the victim can verbally articulate. Sickle cell trait collapse requires emergency transport to a hospital equipped to handle such an emergency. If prompt diagnosis and management are not undertaken, the athlete may go into shock, experience multisystem organ failure, and die. Diagnosis of sickle cell trait can be made with a Sickledex test, with confirmation by **hemoglobin electrophoresis**.

Treatment and Return to Participation

Recognition, emergent first aid (ABCs, oxygen), administration of high-flow oxygen (15 lpm) with a nonrebreather mask, and transport to the hospital emergency department for appropriate care are necessary and may decrease the likelihood of the patient going into acute renal failure or multisystem organ failure.

If the athlete survives an episode of complete sickle cell anemia or trait collapse, restriction from similar exercise settings or environmental conditions is warranted. This may mean that the athlete is disqualified from that competitive sport.

Prevention

The following are some guidelines for working with athletes with sickle cell trait:

- Athletes should build up slowly in training with paced progressions, allowing longer periods of rest and recovery between repetitions.
- Encourage participation in preseason strength and conditioning programs to enhance the preparedness of athletes for performance testing, which should be sport specific. Exclude participation in performance tests such as timed/repeat sprints.
- Athletes should cease activity with the onset of symptoms.
- Allow athletes with sickle cell trait to set their own pace.
- Encourage the athlete to participate in a year-round strength and conditioning program that is consistent with the individual's needs, goals, abilities, and sport-specific demands. Extended recovery between repetitions of sprints and/or interval training should be allowed.
- Carefully monitor athletes with SCT who are new to altitude.
- Ambient heat stress, dehydration, asthma, illness, and altitude predispose the athlete with sickle cell anemia to the onset of crisis with physical exertion.

The medical staff must adjust work/rest cycles for environmental heat stress, emphasize hydration, control asthma, withhold participation when the athlete is ill, and watch closely at high altitudes (Pelliccia, Zipes, and Maron 2008; Anderson and Eichner 2007). Since 2009, the NCAA has mandated that all athletes be confirmed for status of sickle cell trait (Parsons 2014). Those involved with the athlete, including peers, parents, and coaches, need to understand the warning signs of collapse and the consequences of inaction. Health care professionals need to consider screening other physically active patients for sickle cell trait, which is relatively inexpensive.

Summary

Conditions that affect the cardiovascular system can have catastrophic sequelae in athletes. Appreciating the anatomy and physiology of the cardiovascular system is one way to understand the demands placed on this system. Another is to understand the various cardiac arrhythmias and abnormalities, their effect on the human body, and the implications of both on strenuous activity. This chapter highlights some cardiovascular abnormalities that can create problems for athletic participation, how to recognize them, and when to refer an athlete who exhibits them to a physician.

The preparticipation examination is critical to the identification of cardiovascular problems. The initial examination offers the best opportunity to seek additional medical evaluation. Having access to AEDs and trained personnel is crucial, as is knowledge of the venue-specific emergency plan. Many athletes with cardiovascular conditions have long and productive careers within safe parameters because of early discovery and proper treatment of their conditions.

 Apply It! The case study for this chapter looks at a female collegiate athlete complaining of chest tightness. Read the scenario and answer the questions at www.HumanKinetics.com/MedicalConditionsInTheAthlete.

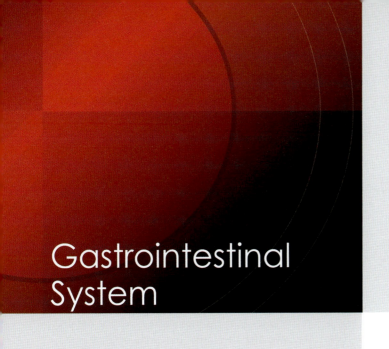

Gastrointestinal System

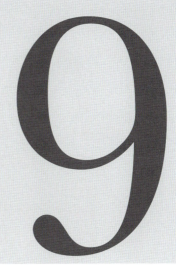

OBJECTIVES

At the completion of this chapter the reader should be able to do the following:

- Describe the basic anatomy of the abdomen and gastrointestinal system.
- Perform a basic examination of the gastrointestinal system, including history, inspection, auscultation, percussion, and palpation.
- Recognize conditions of the gastrointestinal system that require referral.
- Describe appropriate initial management of common disorders of the gastrointestinal tract.
- Recognize conditions of the gastrointestinal system that may preclude the athlete from participation, and recognize which symptoms are self-limiting.

Health care providers hear complaints about abdominal pain or discomfort every day. Nausea, diarrhea, and constipation account for some of these complaints; heartburn and gastroesophageal reflux account for others. For the physically active, the stress of hectic schedules and travel for those involved in competition and the consumption of greasy or spicy foods are certainly among the causes. Often gastrointestinal disorders are transient, and although they may affect performance or the ability to compete, they are not serious conditions. Fortunately, because they work closely with the athletes, the athletic trainer can identify more serious gastrointestinal conditions that require further medical evaluation and treatment.

This chapter reviews the anatomy and physiology of the gastrointestinal system and procedures for evaluating the abdominal area, including auscultation, palpation, and percussion. This chapter also presents common disorders of the gastrointestinal system, including the signs and symptoms, diagnostic tests, and differential diagnoses. Treatment of selected conditions and implications for athletic participation are also discussed.

Overview of Anatomy and Physiology

The gastrointestinal system is composed primarily of a long tube between the mouth and the anus that serves to process food and fluids (figure 9.1). From the ingestion of solids and liquids to the absorption and balancing of electrolytes and finally waste production and excretion, the alimentary tract performs several vital functions. For athletes, it is unlikely that sport will cause significant gastrointestinal problems, but gastrointestinal problems are common, and they can affect athletic performance.

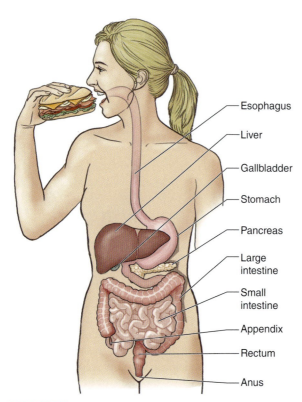

- Esophagus
- Liver
- Gallbladder
- Stomach
- Pancreas
- Large intestine
- Small intestine
- Appendix
- Rectum
- Anus

FIGURE 9.1   The gastrointestinal system is composed of a long tube between the mouth and the anus that serves to process food and fluids.

The major organs of the gastrointestinal tract start with the esophagus, which connects the mouth to the stomach via a muscular band called the gastroesophageal junction or lower esophageal sphincter. The mouth and teeth, although part of the gastrointestinal tract, are discussed in chapter 13. Within the pouch of the stomach, hydrochloric acid and enzymes, such as pepsin and gastric lipase, serve to break down food for later absorption in the intestines. The stomach empties through another muscular ring, the pyloric sphincter, into the duodenum, the first portion of the small intestine.

The small intestine is about 21 ft long; it comprises the duodenum, jejunum, and ileum; and it completes the digestive breakdown of food with enzymes produced by the pancreas and liver. Nutrients are absorbed throughout the length of the small intestine as it coils back and forth and joins the large intestine in the lower right portion of the abdomen. This connection also has the ileocecal valve, which is designed to prevent fecal material in the large intestine from backing up into the small intestine. There is a small blind pouch called the *cecum* at this end of the large intestine, and the small wormlike (vermiform) appendix originates from the base of the pouch. The large intestine or colon serves to absorb water and produce neutralizing mucus as it ascends up the right side of the

abdomen (the ascending colon), traverses across the upper abdomen (the transverse colon), and then descends down the left side (the descending colon). The colon also hosts numerous bacteria that further decompose food residue. As the descending colon comes to an end at the lower right side of the abdomen, it produces an S-shaped curve called the sigmoid colon. This in turn empties into the rectum, and together they serve as the primary storage location for solid or semisolid waste. Finally, the rectum ends with the sophisticated musculature of the anal canal and then the anus.

Among the many important organs in the abdomen, the gastrointestinal tract includes the liver, gallbladder, pancreas, and spleen as well as the kidneys and related structures (figure 9.2). Each of these essential organs helps digestive and absorptive functions of the gastrointestinal system.

The liver is a large organ located under the right diaphragm that has several crucial functions in metabolism: storing vitamins and iron, filtering toxins from the blood, and producing critical blood proteins. Bile is produced in the liver and stored in the saclike gallbladder, where it is periodically released into the duodenum to help in the absorption of fats. The pancreas sits below the stomach and assists digestion by producing several enzymes that are also released into the duodenum. In addition, the pancreas produces the essential hormones insulin and glucagon that are released into the bloodstream to maintain blood sugar (i.e., glucose) levels.

Most abdominal organs and the inner lining of the abdominal cavity are covered with a protective membrane called the peritoneum. When this becomes inflamed or irritated by blood or infection, the entire abdomen can become very tender, and the muscles of the abdominal wall may become rigid. Individual sensory nerves do not innervate each organ within the peritoneum, which is why abdominal pain is not necessarily specific to the origin (location) of pathology.

The rectus abdominis muscle and the internal and external oblique muscles serve to protect the organs of the abdominal cavity (figure 9.3). Just like muscles elsewhere in the body, they can be injured by overuse, acute strain, or contusions. For an athlete with abdominal pain, distinguishing whether the pain is from the internal organs or the overlying muscles is important. Sometimes this distinction can be difficult, or there may be problems with both.

When referring to the abdomen, clinicians will typically divide it into quadrants. The midline extends from the center of the sternum through the pubic bone, and the horizontal line extends through the umbilicus. This creates right and left upper and lower quadrants, commonly referred to as RUQ, LUQ, RLQ, and LLQ. Here are structures that are within these quadrants:

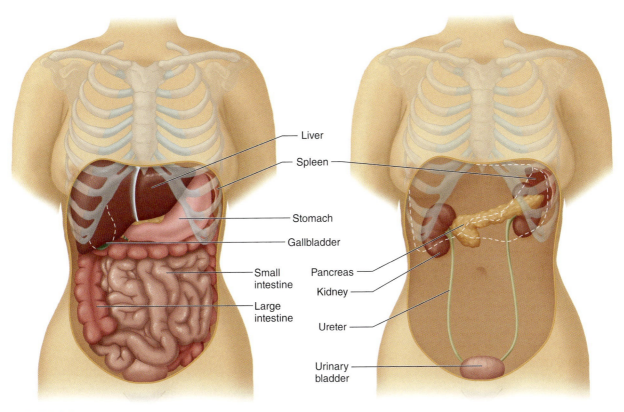

FIGURE 9.2   Structures of the abdominal cavity.

Right upper quadrant
    Liver
    Gallbladder
    Duodenum
    Head of pancreas
    Right adrenal gland
    Portion of right kidney
    Portions of ascending and transverse colon

Left upper quadrant
    Left lobe of liver
    Spleen
    Stomach
    Body of pancreas
    Left adrenal gland
    Portion of left kidney
    Portions of ascending and transverse colon

Right lower quadrant
    Lower pole of right kidney
    Cecum and appendix
    Portion of ascending colon
    Bladder
    Ovary
    Uterus (if enlarged)
    Right spermatic cord
    Right ureter

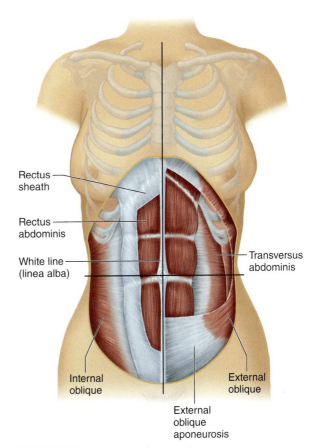

FIGURE 9.3   Abdominal musculature.

Left lower quadrant
Lower pole of left kidney
Sigmoid colon
Portion of descending colon
Bladder
Ovary
Uterus (if enlarged)
Left spermatic cord
Left ureter

This distinction becomes important and helpful in diagnosing many conditions (Ball et al. 2014). Appendicitis, for example, will typically cause RLQ pain, whereas constipation can cause LLQ pain. Here are common causes of abdominal pain in different anatomical locations:

Right upper quadrant
Cholecystitis
Duodenal ulcer
Hepatitis
Pneumonia

Left upper quadrant
Abdominal aortic aneurysm
Gastric ulcer
Pneumonia
Splenic laceration or rupture

Periumbilical
Abdominal aortic aneurysm
Diverticulitis
Early appendicitis
Intestinal obstruction

Right lower quadrant
Appendicitis
Ectopic pregnancy
Hernia
Ovarian cysts
Pelvic infection
Renal stone

Left lower quadrant
Constipation
Diverticulitis
Ectopic pregnancy
Hernia
Ovarian cysts
Pelvic infection

Other clinicians may use the nine-region classification, which uses two imaginary horizontal lines and vertical lines to divide the abdomen into regions (figure 9.4). Anatomical correlates of the nine regions of the abdomen are listed here:

Epigastric region
Pyloric end of stomach
Duodenum
Pancreas
Portion of liver

Umbilical region
Omentum
Mesentery
Lower part of duodenum
Jejunum and ileum

Hypogastric region
Ileum
Bladder
Uterus (in pregnancy)

Right hypochondriac region
Right lobe of liver
Gallbladder
Portion of duodenum
Hepatic flexure of colon
Portion of right kidney
Suprarenal gland

Left hypochondriac region
Stomach
Spleen
Tail of pancreas
Splenic flexure of colon
Upper pole of left kidney
Suprarenal gland

Right lumbar region
Ascending colon
Lower half of right kidney
Portion of duodenum and jejunum

Left lumbar region
Descending colon
Lower half of left kidney
Portion of jejunum and ileum

Right iliac region
Cecum
Appendix
Lower end of ileum
Right ureter
Right spermatic cord
Right ovary

Left iliac region
Sigmoid colon
Left ureter
Left spermatic cord
Left ovary

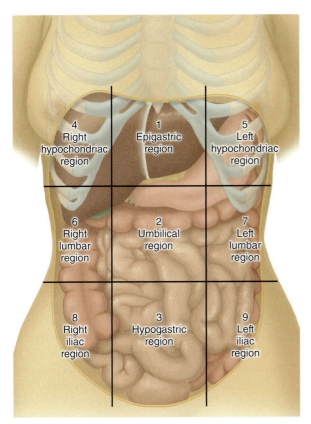

FIGURE 9.4 The nine regions of the abdomen.

Evaluation of Abdominal Pain

The patient with abdominal pain may not have a problem with the gastrointestinal tract at all. Many possible conditions, including diseases of the heart, lungs, kidneys, and musculoskeletal system, can present as "abdominal pain." Some differential diagnoses for abdominal pain include the following:

- Muscle contusions
- Gastroenteritis
- Appendicitis
- Peptic ulcer disease
- Cholecystitis
- Splenic rupture
- Diverticulitis
- Pelvic inflammatory disease
- Pancreatitis
- Other conditions: myocardial infarction, pneumonia, pericarditis, pneumothorax, kidney disease, reproductive system problems

Key questions to ask to evaluate abdominal pain are as follows:

- Onset of pain: Sudden or gradual?
- Duration of pain: Present for hours? Days? Weeks?
- Temporal factors: Constant pain or intermittent?
- Relationship to meals: Better with food or worse?
- Quality of pain: Burning, cramping, stabbing?
- Radiation of pain: Does it seem to spread up or down?
- Severity of pain: Determine by use of pain scale
- Aggravating or alleviating factors: Better lying down or sitting up? Have over-the-counter medicines, such as antacids or others, been tried?
- Associated symptoms: Nausea, vomiting, diarrhea, constipation, fever?
- Last bowel movement?
- Medications or supplements that may cause symptoms?

CONDITION HIGHLIGHT

Stitch in the Side

A condition that has frustrated athletes and health care providers is exercise-related transient abdominal pain (ETAP), commonly called a *side stitch*. It is characterized as a sharp, acute, cramping sensation in the abdomen that occurs during exercise. When an athlete reduces her level of exertion, the pain will often spontaneously resolve. ter Steege et al. reported significantly more frequent episodes in women (8.2% vs. 1.8%) than in their male counterparts (2012). Complaints were also more common in 10k runners when compared to longer distance runners. Theories for the cause of the pain include ischemia of the diaphragm, stress on subdiaphragmatic ligaments, and irritation of the parietal peritoneum (Waterman and Kapur 2012).

All proposed treatments to date are anecdotal, and prevention tips are inconsistent. Better conditioned athletes report fewer instances of ETAP, so one can rationalize that if the athlete can continue to increase his or her fitness, the incidence of ETAP should decrease.

For female patients, it is important to obtain an appropriate menstrual cycle history. Pain that is perceived as being abdominal may be from the reproductive system, such as ovarian cysts, menstrual cramps, pelvic infections, or complications of pregnancy.

As with other conditions, the examiner must determine whether there was any trauma involved and the details of that injury. A past medical history or family history of gastrointestinal problems can also help in the diagnosis, as can social history factors, such as alcohol intake (Bickley 2012). Taking a thorough history, including training regimen or use of training logs, may be helpful in diagnosing the endurance athlete with GI complaints (deOliveria, Burini, and Jeukendrup 2014; Viola 2010, Morton and Callister 2015). Signs or symptoms that may indicate a severe or life-threatening condition constitute red flags with abdominal pain (see the sidebar "Red Flags for Abdominal Pain"). Beyond the obvious issues, such as unstable vital signs or altered mental status that are always red flags, these findings are serious enough that a physician should be contacted immediately, or the patient should be taken to an emergency department.

Physical examination of the abdomen involves the skills of inspection, auscultation, palpation, and percussion. Inspection consists of carefully examining the abdomen when the athlete is lying comfortably supine. Initially, the examiner notes the presence of scars that may indicate prior surgery—thus reducing concern about acute appendicitis or gallstones—and looks for obvious bruising or contusions as well as swelling or distention. A yellowish tint can indicate jaundice from liver disease, or a faint bluish discoloration around the umbilicus may indicate intraabdominal bleeding. The examiner watches the movement of the abdomen as the patient breathes in and out for asymmetry that can indicate intraabdominal masses or hernia.

In distinguishing abdominal muscle pain from problems of the abdominal organs, it is helpful to have the patient tense the muscles by doing a partial sit-up. As the patient's head is raised from the table, the muscles are held taut and muscle pain is aggravated, so this can help pinpoint a problem that is muscular.

Auscultation is always performed before palpation in the examination of the abdomen. In the examination of the heart and lungs, palpation is done before auscultation; however, palpation of the abdomen may create abdominal sounds that were not there before palpation. Auscultation should reveal the normal clicks and gurgling of bowel sounds that may be heard anywhere from a few times to dozens of times every minute. Chapter 2 covers use of the stethoscope and basic auscultation techniques. The examiner needs to be alert to abnormal sounds, such as high-pitched tinkling sounds or rushing water sounds, as well as the potentially absent sounds that can indicate intraabdominal pathology. Some patients may have quieter abdomens; bowel sounds are not considered absent until the examiner has listened continuously for 5 min with no sound heard.

Percussion is a skill that requires considerable practice; it is not covered in detail in this text. It may be used to assess the size and density of abdominal organs or to detect the presence of air or fluid in the abdominal cavity. In general, the examination follows a standard sequence for abdominal percussion (figure 9.5) or percussion to determine the size of the liver (figure 9.6). As indicated in chapter 2, percussion may be direct or indirect.

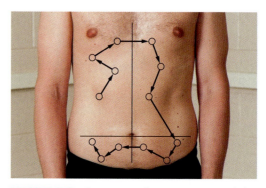

FIGURE 9.5 Sequence for percussion of the abdomen.

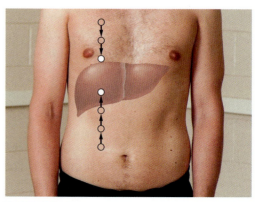

FIGURE 9.6 Percussion sequence to determine liver size.

RED FLAGS FOR ABDOMINAL PAIN

- Vomiting bright red blood or black material that looks like coffee grounds
- Fever of 38.3 °C (101 °F) or more, accompanied by severe abdominal pain
- Persistent vomiting, such that the person cannot keep any fluids down for more than 24 to 36 h (in younger athletes the time window is shorter)

The examiner should practice percussing normal tympanic and dull sounds of the four quadrants exhibited by various positions of percussion. Tympany is the predominant sound throughout the abdomen and hollow organs because of the air contained in the stomach and intestines (table 9.1). A dull sound is present over solid masses adjacent to hollow organs.

Examiners use indirect percussion to tell when they are directly over solid organs or hollow organs of the abdomen. A change in sound from tympanic to dull is easier to detect, so examiners usually start over an area known to be normally tympanic. Percussion is most commonly performed to determine the size of the liver and spleen. Examiners must understand the surface anatomy of the liver (figure 9.7) in order to assess the liver through indirect percussion.

The patient lies supine during palpation. If the patient has difficulty relaxing the abdominal muscles to allow the examiner to adequately palpate deeply, the knees may be bent slightly to encourage relaxation of the abdominal muscles. Palpation is used to assess masses or areas of tenderness at both the superficial and deep levels (Ball et al. 2014).

At first, the abdomen is palpated lightly (pressing only about 1 cm deep) in all quadrants to assess for muscular tenderness or rigidity as well as any superficial masses. The palmar aspect of the fingers is used in a steady, even fashion, avoiding any sharp or sudden jabbing motions. Pain or resistance to even this light palpation generally indicates either injury or inflammation of the abdominal musculature or peritoneal lining.

If significant tenderness is not present with light palpation, the examiner presses more firmly and deeply and continues to press as deeply as the patient will comfortably allow, generally to a depth of at least 3 or 4 cm (figure 9.8). In this manner, the examiner may be able to feel the edges of the liver in the RUQ (figure 9.9) or an enlarged spleen in the LUQ. Tenderness in the RLQ with deep palpation may indicate appendicitis, pelvic, or ovarian problems in a female athlete.

To more adequately palpate the liver, the athletic trainer stands on the right side of the patient with the left hand placed under the patient. The left hand presses

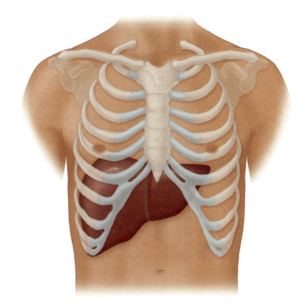

FIGURE 9.7 Surface anatomy of the liver.

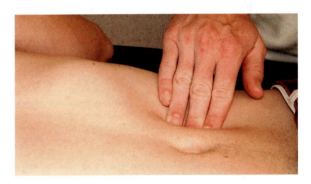

FIGURE 9.8 Deep palpation of the abdomen. If the patient tolerates light palpation of the abdomen, the examiner can press firmly and deeply to patient's tolerance (3 to 4 cm) and try to feel the edges of the abdominal organs.

© Micki Cuppett

up at the 11th or 12th rib, causing the liver to be lifted toward the anterior abdominal wall. The right hand simultaneously palpates the liver. The clinician asks the

TABLE 9.1 **Percussion Notes of the Abdomen**

Sound	Description	Location
Tympanic	Drumlike high-pitched, hollow sound	Over air-filled structures
Hyperresonant	Low-pitched, hollow quality between that of tympany and resonance	Distended bowel, hyperinflated lung, emphysema, or pneumothorax
Resonance	Sustained note of moderate pitch	Over normal lung tissue
Dullness	Short, soft, high-pitched sound with little resonance	Over solid organs such as the liver

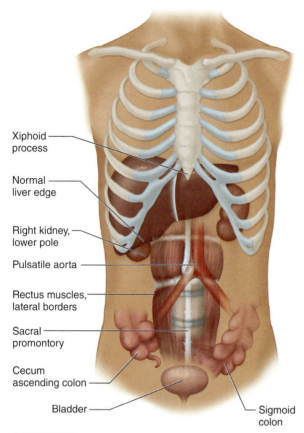

Xiphoid process

Normal liver edge

Right kidney, lower pole

Pulsatile aorta

Rectus muscles, lateral borders

Sacral promontory

Cecum ascending colon

Bladder

Sigmoid colon

FIGURE 9.9   Structures felt by deep palpation of the abdomen.

patient to breathe regularly and then tries to feel the edge of the liver with the right hand as the patient breathes (figure 9.10). The edge of the liver should be smooth and firm. Palpation of the liver does not normally cause pain, so the athletic trainer should be suspicious if direct palpation of the liver is painful for the athlete. Often the

liver is not palpable except in a very thin person or if it is enlarged.

The examiner pays special attention to the spleen while palpating the LUQ. The same basic technique may be used as when palpating the liver, namely, to reach across the patient with the right hand, placing it beneath the costovertebral angle (figure 9.11). The fingers of one hand are placed just below the patient's left costal margin to lift the spleen anteriorly. The patient takes a deep breath while the examiner moves the fingers of the other hand up and under the ribs toward the spleen. The inspiring breath will push an enlarged spleen down to meet the fingers of the other hand; the examiner may be able to feel the spleen just below the left costal margin. A normal-sized spleen is typically not palpable. Pain with palpation of the spleen indicates the patient should be referred to a physician.

Evaluation of the Athlete With Acute, Traumatic Abdominal Pain

As with any traumatic injury, an assessment of the mechanism of injury is important. A sharp blow with the end of a hockey stick is obviously more likely to cause damage than a blow with an elbow. Fortunately, the abdominal organs are generally well protected, and most trauma results only in contusions to the muscles. After confirming that there is no damage to the underlying organs, these injuries can be treated just like any other muscle contusion.

The spleen is the most commonly injured solid abdominal organ (Gannon and Howard 2010). The spleen that is not enlarged is generally well protected by the lower ribs on the left. When trauma results in rib fracture, however, the ribs can lacerate the spleen. The spleen can become

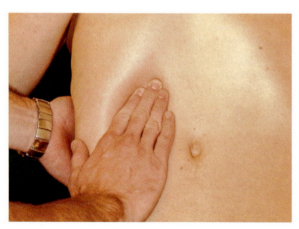

FIGURE 9.10   Palpation of the liver.
© Micki Cuppett

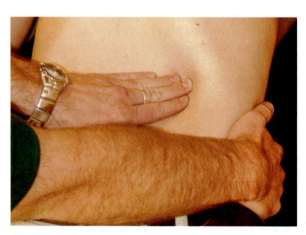

FIGURE 9.11   Palpation of the spleen.
© Micki Cuppett

enlarged (i.e., splenomegaly) from various causes; most commonly the enlargement resulting from **infectious mononucleosis** is temporary and lasts a few weeks. This enlargement will cause the spleen to extend downward beyond the protection of the ribs and make it vulnerable to direct trauma that can cause splenic contusion or laceration. (See chapter 15 for more information about mononucleosis.)

Less commonly, the liver can also be lacerated or contused by direct trauma. The pancreas is deep enough in the abdomen that contusion is rare, but it should be suspected if there is persistent abdominal pain with radiation through to the back. Injury to the hollow organs (i.e., stomach, intestines) is rare and generally occurs only

CLINICAL TIPS

Abdominal Examination

History
- Pain: onset, duration, quality, severity, radiation
- Associated symptoms: nausea, vomiting, diarrhea, constipation, fever, fatigue, painful urination
- Aggravating or alleviating factors
- Medications
- Appetite and food intolerance
- Bowel habits

Observation
- Shape and symmetry
- Assessment of skin and scars

Auscultation
Note: Do before percussion and palpation of the abdomen!
- Bowel sounds
- Vascular sounds

Percussion
- The four quadrants
- Liver span and spleen

Palpation
- Light palpation to assess tenderness in all four quadrants
- Deeper palpation for masses in all four quadrants
- Palpation of spleen, liver, kidneys, and McBurney's point

when there is enough force to cause crushing damage against the spine.

When an athlete sustains an injury to the abdomen, the health care provider initially assesses the overall status and vital signs. Unfortunately, sideline evaluations can be normal or reveal only vague, nonspecific findings even in athletes with significant injuries. If there is diffuse abdominal tenderness or rigidity, pain in the back without trauma to the back, low blood pressure, or rapid heart rate, or if the mechanism of injury suggests injury to the liver or spleen, then the athlete must be seen by a physician before resuming play.

Nausea, Vomiting, and Diarrhea

Nausea, vomiting, and diarrhea can be the result of any one of many conditions, including self-limited viral illness, food poisoning, side effects of medications, dietary indiscretions, or stress. They may also be signs of more serious conditions, such as appendicitis, pancreatitis, or pelvic inflammatory disease. In most cases, however, nausea, vomiting, and diarrhea are self-limiting conditions that can be managed with over-the-counter medicines and common sense.

An important consideration is the severity and duration of symptoms of nausea, vomiting, or diarrhea in terms of the athlete's hydration status. With mild or intermittent symptoms, most people will still take in enough oral fluids that they can go for several days without significant concerns about dehydration. However, when symptoms are more severe, then intravenous fluids may be needed to treat dehydration that could develop over 24 to 36 h. When these symptoms have been present for more than 24 to 36 h or are accompanied by significant pain or fever, referral is made to a physician.

The character of the vomited material must be determined. Undigested food or minimal amounts of yellow to green stomach acid or bile are common and not worrisome. If the athlete has been persistently vomiting bilious material or has noted any blood, dark coffee-ground material, or foul-smelling stool-like material, then urgent referral is needed.

Similarly, for the athlete with diarrhea, it is important to obtain a description of the character of the stool. Loose or watery brown stools are most common and reflect a more benign process. If the diarrhea is bloody or maroon in color or seems to be more like mucus than water, then referral is needed.

Treatment

The athlete who feels nauseated or queasy but has not been vomiting and has little or no pain or fever can safely and effectively take over-the-counter **antiemetic agents** containing a high-concentration carbohydrate and phosphoric acid solution, such as Nausetrol or Emetrol. When used as directed on the label, these agents can safely treat the symptoms and will not mask a more serious condition. If they fail, numerous prescription medicines can be used, including promethazine (Phenergan) and prochlorperazine (Compazine).

Once the patient has started to vomit, the stomach must be given enough time to settle down between vomiting spells. A common scenario is the person who vomits, then feels better, and decides to drink some water or other fluids in order to both quench thirst and avoid dehydration. If this happens too soon after the last vomiting spell, the hypersensitive stomach will start the vomiting again. This behavior of drinking too quickly is very common in the person who "just can't stop vomiting." After any spell of vomiting, the person should not drink anything at all, not even a sip of water, for about 1 h (sometimes 2 h). Once the stomach has remained quiet for that time, then one of the over-the-counter or prescription antinausea (or antiemetic) medicines listed previously can be used. The athlete who can tolerate these medicines can slowly advance to sips of water or electrolyte solutions (e.g., Gatorade, Powerade, Pedialyte). Finally, the patient can add more carbohydrates to the diet in the form of grains and fruits as tolerated. The BRAT (i.e., bananas, rice, applesauce, toast) diet has long been used in children with nausea, vomiting, and diarrhea. These foods are tolerated well by both children and adults and may be helpful in quieting the gastrointestinal tract while recovering from nausea, vomiting, and diarrhea. Acidic, spicy, or greasy foods should be avoided for 1 or 2 d to be certain the athlete can tolerate them and to prevent a recurrence of vomiting.

For the treatment of diarrhea, loperamide (Imodium) obtained over the counter can be very effective in the control of diarrheic episodes, but it may have side effects of drowsiness and dizziness that may impair performance. Loperamide can decrease stool frequency and volume to allow the patient to continue a somewhat normal routine. Use of antidiarrheals when invasive pathogens are suspected is controversial because they can delay the clearance of pathogens from the bowel, thereby prolonging the disease. However, in the afebrile athlete with a nonbloody stool, they can be a very effective and safe method of treatment (Barr and Smith 2015). The athlete must hydrate as discussed previously with electrolyte solution and water and adhere to a bland diet until symptoms subside.

Return to Participation

The decision on when to return to participation depends on the sport in question and the severity and duration of symptoms. It is unlikely that mild illnesses that cause nausea, vomiting, or diarrhea in the absence of fever will be significantly aggravated by athletic activity; rather, athletic performance may be significantly impaired by the illness. A mild case of nausea, vomiting, or diarrhea may have little impact on most sports. For sports in which stamina plays a greater role, such as cross country running, the athlete may see a significant impairment of performance with mild to moderate symptoms; the same symptoms may have little to no effect on the athlete for whom performance time is relatively short, such as in weightlifting or gymnastics. A good rule of thumb for most athletes with afebrile illnesses is to avoid activities when there are symptoms below the neck (e.g., chest congestion, vomiting, diarrhea) and play as tolerated when symptoms remain above the neck (e.g., headache, sore throat, earache).

Viral Gastroenteritis

Viral **gastroenteritis**, or acute gastroenteritis, is a very common condition caused by any one of several viruses including adenovirus, astrovirus, echovirus, and Norwalk agent (Barr and Smith 2015.) These viruses cause a self-limited inflammation of the stomach and intestines that is usually completely resolved within 2 to 3 d. The infections are contagious and can spread through a family or college dormitory or by the actions of food handlers.

Signs and Symptoms

Signs and symptoms of viral gastroenteritis include watery diarrhea, nausea with or without vomiting, and fever. The affected athlete may also have diffuse aches, pains, and chills. Management includes general supportive measures and attention to hydration as noted previously.

Treatment and Return to Participation

Over-the-counter loperamide (Imodium) is very effective for diarrhea but may have side effects of drowsiness

---

CLINICAL TIPS

Vomiting

The patient who is vomiting should not drink anything at all for about an hour to allow the stomach time to quiet down. If the stomach remains quiet for an hour or so, only then should the patient progress to sips of liquid.

and dizziness that can significantly affect performance. Referral is considered if there is no response to over-the-counter medicines, if symptoms persist for more than 48 h, or if the athlete has an accompanying high fever. The athlete can return to participation whenever symptoms are resolved and hydration is adequate. With usual good hygiene, the risk of spread to fellow athletes is extremely low.

Food Poisoning or Bacterial Diarrhea

The term *food poisoning* is often overused. People who experience the sudden onset of gastrointestinal symptoms often will attribute it to something they ate or drank. Food poisoning generally should be suspected when multiple people who ate the same food become ill at about the same time. Sampling and culturing the person's stool can confirm the diagnosis. Food poisoning typically occurs when food is improperly handled, cooked, stored, or refrigerated. In some cases, the problem is the bacterium itself, and in other cases, it may be from the toxin or toxins produced by the bacterium. The most common causes are *Campylobacter, Salmonella,* and *Staphylococcus* species, but several other bacteria can also cause problems, including *Shigella* species, *Bacillus cereus, Yersinia,* and *Escherichia coli* (Ferri 2016).

Signs and Symptoms

Bacterial diarrhea is typically more severe and lasts longer than viral gastroenteritis. It may cause higher fevers or severe abdominal cramps and is more likely to result in weight loss and dehydration. Depending on the bacterium, the onset may occur 4 to 6 h after eating the contaminated food (e.g., *Staphylococcus*) or 3 to 10 d later (e.g., *Salmonella*). This variable duration obviously makes it difficult to pinpoint a specific food.

Treatment and Return to Participation

Initial management of the diarrhea can include over-the-counter medicines as for viral gastroenteritis. If the athlete is significantly ill or there is blood in the stool, then referral is needed for thorough evaluation and treatment. This may include stool specimens and antibiotics. If several athletes become ill at the same time, then it may be important to trace back to a shared meal as the source. If the problem was simply poor refrigeration of a single food, then the problem may resolve on its own. However, the problem may be an infected food worker who may continue to spread the infection until treated. The athlete may return to participation when symptoms have been completely resolved and strength and hydration are back to normal.

Parasitic Infection

Parasitic infections of the gastrointestinal tract are less common than bacterial or viral infections but may still cause significant problems. The most common parasites are single-celled organisms called protozoa. *Giardia* is a common waterborne protozoan that is found worldwide, especially in people who drink from more remote streams when hiking or camping. *Entamoeba* species are parasitic protozoa that are also found worldwide but are much more common in tropical regions (Domino et al. 2016). In addition, tapeworms, roundworms, and flukes can be parasitic in humans. These infestations are uncommon, and discussion is beyond the scope of this text.

Giardia-induced diarrhea is characterized by the significant gas that typically results. The diarrhea may be acute or chronic and intermittent. The diarrhea is often explosive in nature, with patients complaining of dull abdominal cramping and bloating with gas and flatulence. *Entamoeba* may cause a variety of symptoms from chronic intermittent diarrhea, abdominal pain, and weight loss to profound bloody diarrhea and fever (Ferri 2016).

Parasitic infections must be recognized by the athletic trainer as different from self-limited viral and bacterial diarrhea and promptly referred for the appropriate antibiotic treatments. The treating physician is the one to make decisions about return to participation.

Stress-Induced Gastrointestinal Symptoms

It is well known that stress can cause a wide variety of gastrointestinal symptoms from diffuse abdominal pains and cramps to heartburn, nausea, vomiting, diarrhea, constipation, and anorexia (deOliveria, Burini, and Jeukendrup 2014; ter Steege et al. 2012; Leggit 2011). The diagnosis of stress-induced or functional gastrointestinal

CLINICAL TIPS

Evaluating Abdominal Pain

When evaluating abdominal pain, keep the differential diagnoses list practical. Sure, the athlete could have parasitic infection, pancreatitis, diverticulitis, or other condition, but the chances are that the athlete will have something much more common.

problems is a diagnosis of exclusion. The patient is thoroughly evaluated for other causes of the symptoms, and only when these have been excluded can the problem be considered stress induced. Even highly stressed athletes can develop other, easily treatable conditions, and therefore the health care provider must not be too quick to attribute symptoms to stress.

Treatment and Return to Participation

If the athlete has been thoroughly evaluated and other causes have been ruled out, the athletic trainer can play an important role in the management of stress-induced gastrointestinal symptoms. It is very important to understand and to remind the athlete that the symptoms are not imaginary. Recent medical research has increasingly helped in understanding the vital connection between the mind and the body: Biochemicals of the brain can become imbalanced, causing major depression or symptoms of anxiety. These conditions can affect the rest of the body and impair healing or worsen other chronic illnesses. Stress does cause very real symptoms of stomach pain, nausea, or even vomiting or diarrhea. The athletic trainer can assist in management through close communication with the team physician and allowing the athlete to have time off as needed or playing through the symptoms as needed in each case.

Constipation

Constipation is commonly misunderstood as a simple decrease in the frequency of bowel movements, with many people feeling that they must have a bowel movement every day or there is something wrong. A better definition is a subjective discomfort from a difficulty in passing stool or a change in the consistency such that stools are excessively hard or small. People have a wide range of tolerance, but constipation can cause significant abdominal pain, cramps, and general discomfort.

CLINICAL TIPS

Dehydration and Constipation

Dehydration is a common cause of abdominal pain and constipation in athletes. Certainly hydration is important for all athletes, but the athlete who experiences frequent bouts of constipation or abdominal pain should monitor hydration levels and increase fluid intake as tolerated.

An initial evaluation to determine the cause of the constipation is helpful. Hundreds of medications, such as narcotic or nonsteroidal anti-inflammatory pain relievers and antidepressant medicines, can cause temporary or persistent constipation (Kuster et al. 2013).

Referral and Diagnostic Tests

Referral to a physician is indicated if the athlete fails to respond to over-the-counter agents or if the problem persists over a period of weeks and the athlete cannot participate without restriction.

Treatment and Return to Participation

Treatment is best directed at increasing fluid and fiber intake. Fiber intake may be dietary by means of whole grains and vegetables or over-the-counter fiber supplements, such as Metamucil or Citrucel. These fiber supplements can be taken indefinitely as needed. The stronger over-the-counter agents, such as milk of magnesia (magnesium hydroxide) or magnesium citrate, are effective but may be too strong for some people and lead to temporary diarrhea (Ferri 2016). These medications are for short-term use because long-term use can lead to a form of dependence.

Heartburn and Gastroesophageal Reflux Disease

The terms heartburn and esophageal reflux, or **gastroesophageal reflux disease (GERD)**, are generally interchangeable and refer to a very common condition in which stomach acid travels up through the lower esophageal sphincter (LES) into the esophagus or even into the back of the throat. Although more common after age 60, it can affect athletes of any age and is estimated to cause frequent symptoms in 14% of adults. More than 60 million persons in the United States report symptoms of GERD at least weekly (Anderson, Strayer, and Mull 2015). There are many things that will decrease the pressure of the LES, including foods such as chocolate and high-fat meals and common medications such as calcium channel blockers (used for hypertension) and nitrates (used for heart disease). Other causes include family history, obesity, and tight-fitting clothing. Behavioral factors include overeating in general and especially exercising or lying down with a full stomach. Certain foods are also well-known triggers for some people, including citric acid-based or tomato-based foods, mints, alcohol, carbonated beverages, and caffeine-containing foods.

Signs and Symptoms

In addition to the heartburn sensation, signs and symptoms of GERD include chest pain (potentially severe), belching, regurgitation of food and acid, chronic cough, and laryngitis. It is essential to remember that not all people will feel a heartburn sensation with this condition. Some people experience only a chronic cough or frequent asthmatic attacks from acid that goes up the esophagus and then into the airways. GERD should be considered in any patient with a chronic cough, chronic laryngitis, or atypical asthma. GERD is not simply an annoying condition. In some cases, after persisting for years, heartburn and GERD can cause significant damage to the lining of the esophagus (esophagitis), which can increase the risk for esophageal cancer. These complications are rare in people under age 40 but are more common in those who also smoke cigarettes and drink alcohol (Domino et al. 2016).

Referral and Diagnostic Tests

Any athlete who does not respond to over-the-counter medicines or who needs these medicines on a daily basis for weeks should be referred for further evaluation. There are various types of diagnostic tests that can be done, including a barium esophagogram or *upper GI series* that involves swallowing some barium and having a series of X-rays taken. More commonly, this would include the use of an endoscope to directly visualize the lining of the esophagus. This is called esophagogastroduodenoscopy (EGD) and is done as a simple outpatient procedure.

Treatment and Return to Participation

Management of GERD is initially directed toward appropriate lifestyle management. The athlete may need to do some self-assessment to determine how much of which foods and behaviors will cause symptoms and adjust accordingly. Although over-the-counter medicines can be very effective, it is rather foolish to take a pill when simple avoidance of the offending agent will handle the problem. The over-the-counter medications work by decreasing the acidity of the stomach and thus diminishing the symptoms and not by stopping the reflux itself. Several effective agents include antacids (e.g., Maalox, Mylanta, Rolaids, Tums) and H_2 blockers (e.g., cimetidine [Tagamet HB], famotidine [Pepcid AC], ranitidine [Zantac]) (Domino et al. 2016). The most effective, yet also the most expensive, over-the-counter agents are the proton pump inhibitors omeprazole (Prilosec), lansoprazole (Prevacid), and esomeprazole (Nexium). If taken before known triggering behaviors or foods, these agents can prevent symptoms, or they can be taken as needed

after symptoms start (Anderson, Strayer, and Mull 2015; Leggit 2011). Some patients need stronger prescription medications and higher doses. A failure to respond to over-the-counter medications does not mean the patient does not have GERD.

Heartburn and GERD are rarely severe enough to interfere with athletic activity. Athletes should be reminded not to eat for 2 to 3 h before activity to avoid triggering symptoms during their sport (Leggit 2011; Waterman and Kapur 2012).

Gastritis and Peptic Ulcer Disease

Gastritis is a diffuse or patchy inflammation of the lining of the stomach. **Peptic ulcer disease (PUD)** is a more serious condition in which there is a deeper ulcer in the stomach (i.e., gastric ulcer) or, much more commonly, in the duodenum (i.e., duodenal ulcer). Although gastritis can have several causes, in otherwise healthy and younger athletes it is usually from (1) processes of erosion and then an ulcer caused by nonsteroidal anti-inflammatory drugs (NSAIDs) or alcohol and/or (2) infectious processes caused by the bacterium *Helicobacter pylori*. PUD may also be caused by *Helicobacter pylori* (Anderson, Strayer, and Mull 2015; Domino et al. 2016). These conditions are more common in people over age 40 but may be seen in children as well. Other factors can contribute to the development of gastritis, including smoking, severe stress, and steroids.

Signs and Symptoms

Symptoms of gastritis include generally mild to moderate persistent mid-abdominal pain, loss of appetite, and nausea. Eating often aggravates the pain. The patient with PUD will have similar symptoms but will often have more severe pain that is worse a couple of hours after eating but gets better with food. Pain can wake the patient from sleep. Both these conditions can lead to gastrointestinal bleeding. Gastritis is less likely to bleed, but PUD can sometimes cause severe and dangerous bleeding. If the blood passes through the digestive tract, it may present as very dark or black stools with a very sticky, tarlike consistency. Blood in the stomach is also an irritant and may cause the patient to vomit, in which case the condition may present as red blood- or coffee grounds-appearing material in the vomit (partially digested blood takes on the appearance of dark coffee grounds). On occasion, a patient may have bleeding gastritis or PUD with no apparent gastrointestinal distress, and thus any black, tarry stools or blood or coffee-ground vomit are causes for concern and prompt referral.

Treatment and Return to Participation

The over-the-counter antacids, H_2 blockers, and proton pump inhibitors discussed previously can all provide substantial relief from symptoms of gastritis or PUD. Nonetheless, any patient with gastritis or PUD should see a physician regularly because of the potential for severe complications. Testing for and treating potential *Helicobacter pylori* infection can bring about a cure and thus avoid the long-term need for acid suppression.

Symptoms can be quite variable. In most cases, they will not interfere with athletic activity, and the athlete can fully participate in sports. However, the athlete should not participate if there is unexplained blood or coffee ground-like material in the vomit or black and tarry stools.

Irritable Bowel Syndrome

Irritable bowel syndrome (IBS) is defined as abdominal discomfort or pain associated with altered bowel habits for at least 3 d/mo in the previous 3 mo, with the absence of organic disease (Wilkins et al. 2012). The peak prevalence of IBS is from ages 20 to 39, and it is estimated to affect 5% to 10% of the population. It is 1 ½ times more common in women than in men, tends to be familial, and is often triggered by stress (Brandt et al. 2009). There are various theories as to its underlying cause, with some experts believing it is due to an overly sensitive gastrointestinal (GI) tract, others reporting an overgrowth of intestinal bacteria, and others believing it to be an underlying neurological disorder that disrupts normal GI motility. There are no definitive diagnostic tests for this, and our treatments have limited effectiveness; thus patients can often be very frustrated by this disorder.

Signs and Symptoms

IBS has several different symptoms and some people have just one or two, whereas others have several symptoms together or different symptoms at various times. Some people have diarrhea predominantly, some have the constipation-predominant type, and some have diarrhea alternating with constipation. Some people have neither significant constipation nor diarrhea but instead have persistent upper abdominal bloating and generalized discomfort. Some have diffuse abdominal pain, with or without fecal urgency (a sudden sensation of an urgent need for a bowel movement). Some types of abnormalities associated with bowel movements are most common with IBS, and abdominal pain is often relieved by a

Diagnostic Tests for Gastrointestinal Disorders

- Radiological studies
- Radiograph of abdomen
- Upper gastrointestinal (GI) series (barium swallow)
- Ultrasound
- Computerized tomography (CT) scan
- Endoscopy
- Upper endoscopy (esophagogastroduodenoscopy [EGD])
- Lower endoscopy (colonoscopy or flexible sigmoidoscopy)
- Laboratory testing
- Complete blood count (CBC)
- Chemistry panel (sodium, potassium, blood urea nitrogen [BUN], creatinine)
- Serology for *Helicobacter pylori*
- Liver enzymes (alanine transaminase [ALT], aspartate transaminase [AST], γ-glutamyltransferase [GGT], bilirubin)
- Pancreatic enzymes (amylase, lipase)
- Stool studies
- Evaluation for red or white blood cells
- Stool cultures
- Microscopic evaluation for parasites

bowel movement, although some will have a sense of incomplete bowel evacuation. Patients may also complain of occasional mucus mixed with stool or abdominal distention and nausea. IBS is also associated with many other chronic pain and mental health disorders ranging from migraines to fibromyalgia and from depression to anxiety. Differential diagnoses of IBS include inflammatory bowel syndrome, celiac disease, colorectal cancer, diverticular disease, gastrointestinal infection, lactose intolerance, or ischemic colitis.

Referral and Diagnostic Tests

No specific test exists for IBS, and thus any athlete with these symptoms is referred for evaluation for other causes of symptoms, including inflammatory bowel diseases (see subsequent sections), celiac disease, tumors, or infections. After a thorough history and physical, the testing is then designed to assess for other causes of chronic abdominal distress. Routine testing for celiac disease in patients with diarrhea-predominant or mixed presentation IBS should be considered (Brandt et al. 2009). Laboratory work such as complete blood count, thyroid function studies, and stool studies for parasites are low-yield tests and not recommended in routine diagnostic evaluation of IBS (Wilkins et al. 2012). Red flag features such as anemia, rectal bleeding, nocturnal symptoms, or weight loss may suggest the use of colonoscopy to assess for colon cancer, inflammatory bowel disease, celiac disease, or other abdominal diseases (Carter, Lang, and Eliakim 2013).

Treatment and Return to Participation

Management of IBS consists of ongoing reassurance to the patient and supportive encouragement, as there are no agents shown to control all symptoms. The best responses seem to come from constant vigilance toward a high-fiber diet and stress management. Then the most distressing symptom is treated on an as-needed basis. Diarrhea and constipation can each be managed with over-the-counter

medicine, but athletes must avoid inadvertently cycling back and forth between the two. Prescription antispasmodic medicines (dicyclomine) can sometimes be used to control cramping and pain. Behavioral modification can be very helpful as an adjunct to medical treatment (Brandt et al. 2009).

The athlete with IBS can fully participate in sports depending on the severity of symptoms. Although some athletes may cope with symptoms during critical games or performances, others may become incapacitated at these times. Professional assessment and management of stress, including techniques such as biofeedback, can be very helpful for these athletes.

Celiac Disease

Celiac disease is an autoimmune disorder that affects the gastrointestinal tract and is thought to be triggered by dietary gluten in affected individuals. The disease is characterized by chronic inflammation of the small intestinal mucosa, which leads to atrophy of the small intestinal villi and subsequent malabsorption (Pelkowski and Viera 2014). Celiac disease affects approximately 1% of the U.S. population and typically occurs in persons of European ancestry as well as persons of Middle Eastern, Indian, South American, and North African descent. It is two to three times more common in women. Celiac disease is *not* a food allergy.

Signs and Symptoms

Typical presentation includes chronic diarrhea with cramping and gas pains. Patients often have weight loss, or in the adolescent, delayed onset of growth or puberty. A history of nervousness and/or depression is often present, as is a family history of autoimmune disease. Other complaints may include bone or joint pain, migraines, weakness, fatigue, and anemia (Volta et al. 2015; Vivas et al. 2015; Byrne and Feighery 2015; Mancini, Trojian, and Mancini 2011). Physical examination is often normal, but the patient may present with abdominal distension or dermatitis herpetiformis.

Referral and Diagnostic Tests

Lab tests are performed for differentiating celiac disease and to rule out more common diseases. These include a basic metabolic panel, CBC (iron deficiency), TSH (thyroid disease), vitamin D level, and allergy testing. If celiac disease is suspected from history and physical exam, the initial serologic test is a tissue transglutaminase (tTG) antibody level. This antibody is found in every tissue in the body and acts to join proteins together. In people with celiac disease, tTG activates specific immune cells and triggers the inflammatory response

CLINICAL TIPS

IBD vs. IBS

Many people confuse inflammatory bowel disease (IBD) with irritable bowel syndrome (IBS), but they are very different and should be easily differentiated through history. People with IBS complain of abdominal cramps with diarrhea or constipation that is relieved with a bowel movement. Those with IBD often report with diarrhea, blood in the stool, and weight loss.

that leads to atrophy of the villi in the small intestine (Mancini, Trojian, and Mancini 2011). The diagnosis is often confirmed with repeat blood tests after 4 wk on a gluten-free diet. Endoscopy with biopsies of the duodenal mucosa may be necessary to confirm the diagnosis. Celiac disease should be differentiated from GERD, pancreatic insufficiency, Crohn's disease, or other inflammatory bowel diseases.

Treatment and Return to Participation

The general treatment is to remove gluten from the diet. The patient can substitute rice, corn, and soybean flour for products that contain gluten. Periodic blood tests are performed to measure the levels of the antibodies. The levels will normalize with gluten abstinence. Abstinence will be required for life because the immune response to gluten will recur if gluten is consumed again. Usually no medications are prescribed for celiac disease, but athletes may benefit from iron, vitamin, and calcium supplements. The most difficult aspect for the athlete with celiac disease is the dietary restrictions while traveling with the team or with set team meals. The athletic trainer may need to check on the gluten-free status of many of the standard gluten-containing products provided by the athletic department, such as energy drinks or meal replacement bars (Mancini, Trojian, and Mancini 2011).

Inflammatory Bowel Diseases

Crohn's disease and ulcerative colitis are severe inflammatory diseases of the small intestine and colon and together are referred to as **inflammatory bowel dis-**

eases (IBD). Although these conditions can occur in families, the underlying cause is unknown. Each condition has certain specific characteristics; for example, Crohn's disease more commonly affects the small intestine, and ulcerative colitis is more likely to have symptoms beyond the gastrointestinal tract (Juckett and Tirivedi 2011). This text discusses both conditions together.

Signs and Symptoms

Crohn's disease and ulcerative colitis typically present with chronic abdominal pain, cramping, and weight loss. The diarrhea is often bloody and can lead to anemia. Some patients also develop other symptoms beyond the gastrointestinal tract, including arthritis and eye and skin conditions.

Referral and Diagnostic Tests

Any athlete with bloody diarrhea or persistent gastrointestinal symptoms needs to be referred to a physician. Evaluation will routinely include direct visualization of the colon by means of colonoscopy and often a biopsy of a small piece of the bowel wall to make the diagnosis. Laboratory testing can also reveal anemia and other evidence of inflammation that accompany these conditions (Trivedi and Keefer 2015).

Treatment and Return to Participation

Ulcerative colitis and Crohn's disease require regular and close management by a physician. Although several prescription medications can help to control symptoms, the medicines have significant side effects (Cars et al. 2016;

CONDITION HIGHLIGHT

Gluten Sensitivity and Intolerance

Over the past 10 yr, the number of people choosing a gluten-free diet (GFD) is much higher than the projected number of celiac disease patients (Lis et al. 2015). This has fueled a global market of gluten-free products and highlights several conditions related to the ingestion of gluten. There are three main forms of gluten reactions: allergic, autoimmune (celiac disease), and immune-mediated conditions (gluten sensitivity) (Sapone et al. 2012). Wheat allergy is an adverse reaction to wheat proteins with onset in minutes to hours after gluten ingestion. It may affect the skin, GI tract, or respiratory tract. Celiac disease or other autoimmune gluten disorders generally present months to years after gluten exposure. There is a third condition where some people experience distress from eating gluten-containing products and show improvement with a GFD. It is distinct from celiac disease and wheat allergies (Vivas et al. 2015). Gluten sensitivity cannot be distinguished clinically; **serology** tests need to be conducted. Patients with GI discomfort or distress following gluten ingestion should be referred for a follow-up blood test and immune-allergy tests.

Ha and Khalil 2015). In addition, even when symptoms seem controlled, the athlete needs to be monitored for potential complications, including an increased risk for colon cancer (Ferri 2016).

Athletic performance will vary depending on the severity of disease and the degree of control with medications. The disease state may or may not interfere with participation, depending on whether it is currently flaring up or well controlled. In addition, the medications used to treat the disease can cause problems and side effects, such as severe headaches, depression, or fatigue. Athletes must closely monitor their own symptoms and stay in contact with the treating physician.

Appendicitis

Appendicitis is the most common cause for urgent abdominal surgery in the United States, with about 7% of the population requiring an appendectomy at some point in their lives. It is caused by an acute obstruction and inflammation of the appendix (DeFilippis and Callahan 2013).

Signs and Symptoms

Many signs and symptoms point toward appendicitis, and the diagnosis is usually suspected on the basis of several symptoms and then confirmed at surgery. The pain of appendicitis generally starts as a nonspecific discomfort located around the umbilicus or in the midline epigastric region. As it progresses, the pain will usually begin to localize to the RLQ and be improved when the patient flexes the right hip (DeFilippis and Callahan 2013). A patient typically progresses from anorexia, with the complete loss of appetite, to abdominal pain to nausea and mild vomiting. Patients may have a slight fever and either constipation or diarrhea. As the pain progresses, the athlete will often lie motionless with the right thigh drawn up, and attempts to straighten the thigh will increase the pain. The athlete's abdomen may be very tender to even light touch around McBurney's point in the RLQ, halfway between the right anterior superior iliac spine (ASIS) and the umbilicus, and it may be very rigid (figure 9.12).

Other conditions can mimic appendicitis; some of these are fairly benign but others can also be serious, such as acute pelvic inflammatory disease.

Referral and Diagnostic Tests

Appendicitis is a surgical emergency because of the risks for rupture of the appendix and severe intraabdominal infection that can result. Any athlete with sudden and severe RLQ pain and tenderness associated with anorexia, nausea, or vomiting should be sent to the emergency

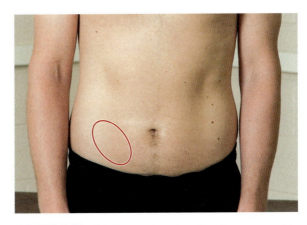

FIGURE 9.12 McBurney's point: Tenderness at this point, halfway between the umbilicus and the right anterior superior iliac spine (ASIS), generally indicates appendicitis when accompanied by fever and nausea.

department of the closest hospital. Although some cases may progress over a few days, it is more typical to see progression over several hours (DeFilippis and Callahan 2013). Athletes at away games who are more than a couple hours from home may need to be seen in the emergency department at an away hospital and should not wait until they get home.

Treatment and Return to Participation

Even with advanced diagnostics, such as computerized tomography (CT) scans, it is not always possible to diagnose appendicitis until surgery, and it is expected and understood that some cases of suspected appendicitis will have a normal appendix surgically removed. The timing of the return to participation is best deferred to the surgeon. It depends on the sport in question, the type of surgical procedure (open versus **laparoscopic**), and the extent of potential surgical complications.

 RED FLAGS FOR APPENDICITIS

- Diffuse epigastric or periumbilical pain early
- Pain localization to right lower quadrant (RLQ) within 12 to 18 h
- Point of maximal tenderness at McBurney's point
- Low-grade fever
- Nausea or vomiting

Cholecystitis and Cholelithiasis

Inflammation of the gallbladder is called **cholecystitis** and is most commonly caused by gallstones, or **cholelithiasis**. Gallstones are common, occurring in about 8% to 10% of the U.S. population. They are more common over the age of 30 years, in women, and in American Indians and Hispanics (Domino et al. 2016).

Signs and Symptoms

Gallstones often cause no symptoms at all, but they are the underlying cause of more than 90% of the cases of cholecystitis. Symptoms are generally caused by a stone blocking the bile duct that drains the gallbladder. The patient may have intermittent RUQ pain, nausea, vomiting, or simply indigestion. Symptoms are often worse after a high-fat meal. They may be mild and minimally distressful or sudden and very severe. If the duct is blocked for a prolonged time, the athlete may develop jaundice or severe pain and fever. On examination of the abdomen, the patient typically has tenderness in the RUQ and may exhibit a sudden stopping or arrest of inspiration when the examiner deeply palpates the liver while the patient takes a deep breath. This is called **Murphy's sign**.

Referral and Diagnostic Tests

Any patient with significant RUQ pain and tenderness needs to be seen by a physician. Typical evaluation will include an ultrasound of the gallbladder, which is highly accurate at diagnosing gallstones and can also indicate thickening of the wall of the gallbladder with cholecystitis.

Treatment and Return to Participation

Gallstones and cholecystitis are treated surgically by removal of the gallbladder (i.e., cholecystectomy). This procedure can usually be done by laparoscopic surgery with a short overnight hospital stay and a return to most activities within a few days. Sometimes open surgery is needed, and then the patient may be hospitalized for several days and may recover slowly over weeks.

Overall, prognosis is excellent for cholecystitis and cholelithiasis. Return to play after surgery depends on the type of surgery, and the decision is best left to the surgeon. For many patients, however, the symptoms of gallstones may be fairly mild and intermittent, and the patient can simply remain on a very low-fat diet to get through the season and have elective surgery after the season.

Colorectal Cancer

Colon cancer is a common neoplasm arising from the lining of the large intestine. In the United States, colon cancer is currently the second leading cause of all cancer deaths behind lung cancer. According to the American Cancer Society's 2014 statistics, 136,830 people are predicted to be diagnosed with colorectal cancer in the United States, and about 50,130 are predicted to die of the disease (American Cancer Society 2014). Colon cancer incidence increases with age, with a peak incidence in the seventh decade of life (Moghadamyeghaneh et al. 2015).

Many risk factors are known to increase the incidence of colorectal cancer. The lifetime risk of colorectal cancer is about 1 in 50 in the general population, but the risk increases two to three times for those with a first-degree relative with colon cancer (Jensen et al. 2015). Younger patients with colorectal cancer tend to have a more aggressive form of the disease compared with older adult patients. Several other risk factors increase one's likelihood of developing colon cancer, including hereditary polyposis syndromes, obesity, and dietary factors such as heavy consumption of processed and red meat (American Cancer Society 2014).

Signs and Symptoms

The signs and symptoms of colon cancer vary widely. Patients may present with vague abdominal pain, weight loss, red blood or maroon-colored stool, anemia, or a change in bowel habits from diarrhea to constipation to changes in the caliber of the stool.

Referral and Diagnostic Tests

If colon cancer is suspected, referral should be made to a physician capable of performing a colonoscopy to make a definitive diagnosis. After the diagnosis of colon cancer is made, referral should be made to a colorectal surgeon if resection of the colon needs to be performed. Referral may also be made to an oncologist depending on the stage of the disease.

Treatment and Return to Participation

The treatment for colorectal cancer depends entirely on the stage at diagnosis. Early cancers that have not spread can be treated by surgical removal of the cancerous growth or of that portion of the colon. More advanced cancers that have spread to local lymph nodes or distant organs involve surgical resection as well as adjunctive radiation, chemotherapy, or both.

The importance of early diagnosis cannot be over-emphasized in colon cancer. When diagnosed early, more than 90% of patients can be "cured" (or have a 5 yr survival rate of >90%) (Moghadamyeghaneh et al. 2015). Unfortunately, many cases are not found until they are advanced and are spreading through the body. The decision of return to participation depends on the type of treatment. For simple removal of a cancerous polyp, the athlete may return to full activity right away. If part of the colon is removed, the surgeon needs to make the decision on the basis of the extent of the patient's cancer, the surgery involved, and the patient's recovery rate.

Summary

Athletic trainers must remember that not all abdominal distress is caused by gastrointestinal disease; they must be alert to possible cardiac, pulmonary, and reproductive system causes of symptoms in the abdomen. Other than appendicitis, most gastrointestinal problems in athletes are not true emergencies. The athletic trainer can initially manage symptoms safely with over-the-counter medications, and eventually with referral to the physician only if the over-the-counter medications do not elicit an adequate response. Severe gastrointestinal symptoms with accompanying high fever, however, need to be assessed by a physician.

Gastrointestinal problems may or may not interfere with performance, and return to participation is generally based on the severity of the symptoms. In addition, many gastrointestinal disorders are chronic and intermittent in nature. The athletic trainer can help the athlete in managing these symptoms as needed.

 Apply It!   The case study for this chapter looks at a minor league baseball player who has intermittent epigastric pain. Read the scenario and answer the questions at www.HumanKinetics.com/MedicalConditionsInTheAthlete.

10

Genitourinary and Gynecological Systems

OBJECTIVES

At the completion of this chapter the reader should be able to do the following:

- Explain the anatomy of the genitourinary and gynecological systems.
- Explain the physiology of ovulation and menstruation.
- Describe common genitourinary and gynecological disorders that athletic personnel encounter in the care of the athlete.
- Differentiate conditions of the genitourinary and gynecological systems that warrant referral.
- Summarize preventive strategies for genitourinary and gynecological disorders and for sexually transmitted infections (STIs).
- Refer patients with signs or symptoms of an STI to a physician.
- Describe the physiological changes that occur in pregnancy.
- Recommend limitations for pregnant athletes.

Whereas injury to the genitourinary and gynecological systems is rare in athletics, disorders of these systems are common in the athletic population. This chapter focuses on these systems and discusses how an athletic trainer might recognize and refer conditions to these systems to a physician. Although athletic trainers do not perform most of the evaluations in this chapter, they do have a relationship with their athletes whereby they may be able to gather enough symptomatic data to warrant referral to the team physician. In addition, knowledge of the types of diagnostic tests will better enable the athletic trainer to explain them to the affected athlete.

Overview of Anatomy and Physiology

The genitourinary system is common to both males and females, with few exceptions. Here we discuss the basic anatomy and physiology of the system before diverging into the anatomical differences between males and females. Following the anatomy discussion is an overview of the physiology of ovulation, menstruation, and pregnancy.

Anatomy of the Kidneys, Ureters, and Urinary Bladder

The kidneys act to remove excess water, salts, and products of metabolism from the blood in order to maintain proper acid–base status. The body's waste products are then conveyed in the urine to the urinary bladder by the ureters. Normally, a person has two kidneys, two ureters, and a single urinary bladder (see figure 9.2). The kidneys lie posterior to the peritoneum in the retroperitoneal space on the posterior abdominal wall, alongside the spine and against the psoas major muscles. The kidneys are bean-shaped organs whose upper poles are protected by the lower bony thorax, and each has an associated adrenal gland superior to it. Because of the large size of the right lobe of the liver, the right kidney lies at a slightly lower level than the left. In muscular individuals and those with well-developed abdominal musculature, the kidneys are generally not palpable on examination.

The anatomy surrounding the two kidneys differs from an anterior perspective. The right kidney is associated with the liver and is separated from it by the hepatorenal recess. The left kidney is associated with the left adrenal gland, stomach, spleen, pancreas, a portion of the small bowel, and the descending colon. In the posterior, both kidneys lie well protected by the costovertebral angle between the 12th rib and the vertebral spine (figure 10.1). They are also attached superiorly to the diaphragm and move slightly on respiration.

The kidneys are enclosed in a strong fibrous capsule that is surrounded by a layer of fat called **perirenal fat**. The unique characteristics of the density of the kidney itself and the perirenal fat allow for the kidneys to be visualized on abdominal radiographs. The kidney is a solid organ with a thick cortex under the fibrous capsule (figure 10.2). Filtration begins at the medulla, continues on the interior in the calix structures, and ends in the collection area before the ureter.

The ureters are muscular ducts, or tubes, that carry urine from the kidneys to the urinary bladder. Urine passes from the kidneys through the ureters by peristaltic waves of muscular contraction. The ureters are approximately 25 cm long and are retroperitoneal. Each descends almost vertically along the psoas major muscle just anterior to the tips of the transverse processes of the lumbar vertebrae (L2–L5). In the female, the ureters and uterine arteries are closely associated. The uterine artery crosses

the ureter at the side of the cervix; therefore, during a surgical procedure to remove the uterus and cervix, the ureter may be inadvertently damaged.

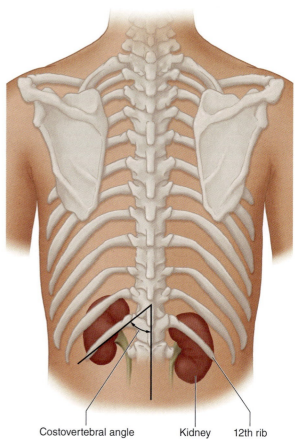

Costovertebral angle   Kidney   12th rib

FIGURE 10.1   Posterior view of the kidneys protected within the costovertebral angle between the 12th rib and the spine.

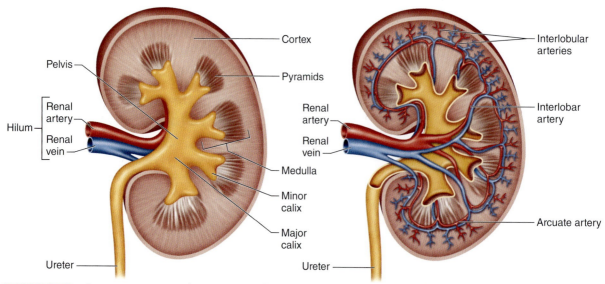

FIGURE 10.2   Cross section reveals two views of the internal structure of the kidney.

The urinary bladder is a muscular sac or vesicle that functions to store urine (figure 10.3). Its shape, size, position, and relation to other structures vary with the amount of urine it contains. It is composed chiefly of smooth muscle. In the adult, the empty urinary bladder lies posterior to the symphysis pubis within the pelvis. As it fills, it ascends into the lower abdomen. A full bladder may reach as high as the level of the umbilicus. The ureters enter at the superolateral aspect of each side of the bladder. The bladder is then drained by a single urethra that empties from the central inferior aspect.

The blood supply to the kidneys is provided by the right and left renal arteries, respectively. These branch off from the descending aorta at nearly right angles. Venous drainage is provided by the right and left renal veins that empty into the inferior vena cava. Blood supply to the ureters is more complex, but it is principally supplied by arterial branches from the renal, aortic, common iliac, vesicular, or uterine arteries. The main arteries supplying the urinary bladder are branches of the internal iliac arteries. In the female, however, branches of the uterine and vaginal arteries also supply a portion of the blood supply to the bladder. Venous drainage occurs via the vesicular venous plexus that drains to the internal iliac vein.

The urinary bladder is supplied by parasympathetic motor fibers to the detrusor muscle of the bladder and sensory fibers. The sensory fibers are stimulated by stretching of the bladder, causing a sensation of fullness and activating the micturition, or urination, reflex. Micturition is preceded by contraction of the diaphragm and abdominal wall. The neck of the bladder descends, the detrusor muscle contracts by reflex, and urine is voluntarily expelled from the bladder.

Anatomy of the Urethra

The urethra is a fibromuscular tube that conducts urine from the bladder (and semen from the ductus deferens in the male) to the exterior. The urethra originates at the central lower portion of the urinary bladder, traverses the pelvis, and terminates at the external urethral orifice.

The female urethra is approximately 4 cm long. It is closely associated, often fused, with the anterior vaginal wall. The urethral orifice is located between the clitoris (anteriorly) and the vagina (posteriorly).

The male urethra is considerably longer, averaging 20 cm in length. The male urethra consists of three parts: prostatic, membranous, and spongy. The proximal prostatic portion descends through the prostate gland. The membranous portion of the urethra descends from the lower portion of the prostate to the bulb of the penis. This portion of the urethra is surrounded by a sphincter (i.e., muscle). The lowermost portion of the membranous urethra is most susceptible to rupture or penetration by a catheter. The spongy portion of the urethra lies in the corpus spongiosum and traverses the bulb, shaft, and glans of the penis, terminating at the external urethral orifice or meatus.

Male Genital Anatomy

The male genital organs comprise the penis, ejaculatory duct, prostate gland, bulbourethral gland (Cowper's gland), and paired testes, each with an epididymis, ductus or vas deferens, and seminal vesicle (figure 10.4). Spermatozoa, formed in the testes and stored in the epididymides, are contained in the semen, which is secreted by the testes and epididymides, seminal vesicles,

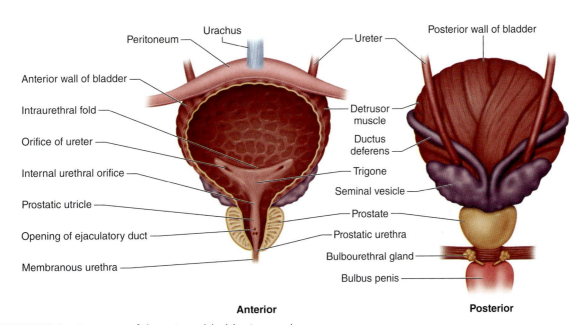

FIGURE 10.3 Anatomy of the urinary bladder in a male.

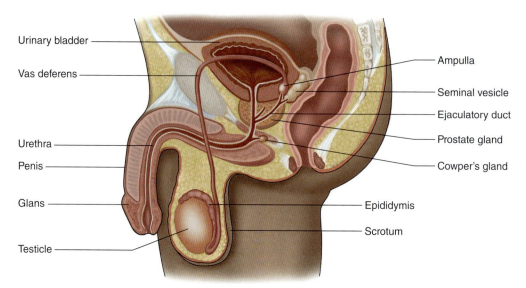

FIGURE 10.4 Anatomy of the male genitourinary system.

prostate, and bulbourethral glands. The sperm, on leaving the epididymides, pass through the ductus deferens and ejaculatory ducts to reach the urethra and pass through the external urethral orifice.

The testes are paired ovoid glands located in the scrotum and responsible for the production of spermatozoa and steroid hormones. They reside away from the core of the body to maintain a slightly lower temperature of approximately −17.2 °C (1 °F) to −16.7 °C (2 °F) below that of the body proper. The left testicle often lies slightly lower than the right testicle in the scrotum. The epididymis is associated with the posterior portion of each testicle. The testes and epididymides are covered by a dual-layered tunica vaginalis testis, which is derived prenatally from the processus vaginalis of the peritoneum (figure 10.5). The potential cavity between these two layers or some part of the processus vaginalis may become distended with fluid, forming a hydrocele.

The testes and epididymides receive their blood supply from the testicular artery, and venous drainage occurs via the pampiniform plexus, which forms the bulk of the spermatic cord. The veins of the pampiniform plexus can become varicose, leading to the formation of a varicocele. Lymphatic drainage from the testes empties into the lower aortic lymph nodes.

The scrotum is a cutaneous pouch that houses the testicles and epididymides. A median raphe indicates the subdivision of the scrotum by a septum into right and left compartments. Smooth muscle, known as the dartos muscle, is firmly attached to the overlying skin. The dartos muscle contracts in response to cold, exercise, and sexual stimulation. Loose connective tissue underlying the dartos allows free movement and is the site for the accumulation of edema.

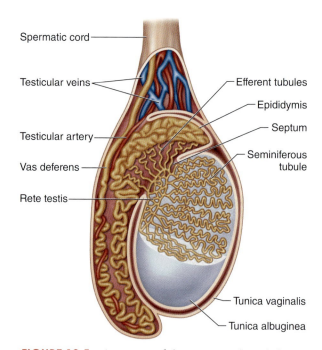

FIGURE 10.5 Anatomy of the testis and epididymis. Turner's syndrome results because of the absence of one X chromosome.

The prostate gland is a fibromuscular pelvic organ surrounding the male urethra and containing glands that contribute to the semen. It is located behind the symphysis pubis and directly in front of the rectum, which is where it can be palpated by a digital rectal examination. Venous drainage and lymphatic drainage of the prostate are important because these contribute to the distinct areas for the spread of prostate cancer. Venous drainage occurs via the prostatic venous plexus that drains into the internal iliac vein and communicates with the vertebral plexus, thereby allowing **metastatic** spread of prostate cancer to the vertebrae. Lymphatic drainage terminates in the internal and external iliac lymph nodes.

Female Genital Anatomy

The female genital organs comprise the ovaries, fallopian tubes, uterus, vagina, and external genitalia, specifically the mons pubis, labia majora and minora, vestibule of the vagina, bulb of the vestibule, vestibular glands, and clitoris (figure 10.6).

The ovaries are paired organs that produce oocytes (eggs) and secrete steroid hormones. The ovaries are situated on the lateral wall of the pelvis, where they can be palpated bimanually. The paired fallopian tubes allow the passage of oocytes from the ovaries as well as spermatozoa from male ejaculation, and a fallopian tube is the usual site of fertilization. From there, it conveys the early embryo to the uterus. Fallopian tubes are also where tubal pregnancies occur, and they are susceptible to scarring associated with ascending infections (e.g., pelvic inflammatory disease [PID]), which can ultimately render the tube unable to transmit either oocytes or spermatozoa, resulting in infertility.

The uterus is a muscular organ that lies within the pelvis (figure 10.7). The uterus accepts the fertilized egg

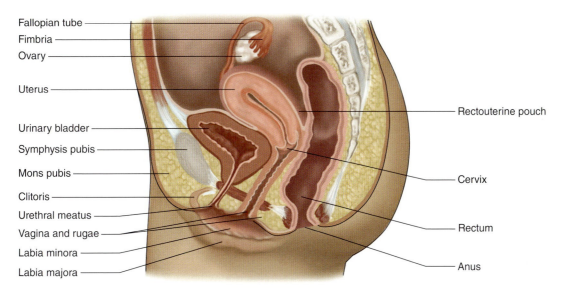

FIGURE 10.6   Anatomy of the female genitourinary system, lateral view.

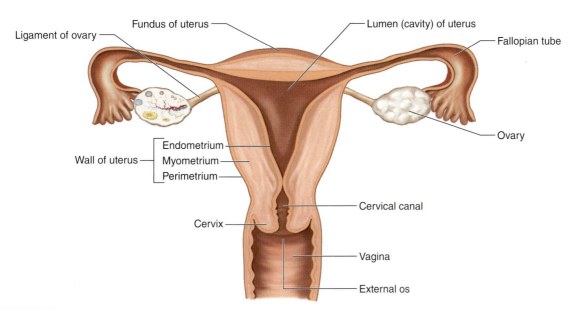

FIGURE 10.7   Anatomy of the uterus, anterior view.

and is the site for implantation and development of the fetus. The upper uterine segment receives the fallopian tubes. The lower uterine segment terminates in the cervix, which opens to the vagina. The uterus has three distinct layers: a mucosa or endometrium, a muscular coat or myometrium, and a serosa or perimetrium.

The vagina lies posterior to the urinary bladder and anterior to the rectum. It serves as a receptacle for the penis, as the lower end of the birth canal, and as the excretory duct for the products of menstruation. The anterior and posterior walls of the vagina are approximately 7.5 and 9 cm long, respectively. The opening of the vagina into the vestibule may be partially closed by a membrane called the hymen. The opening is located posterior to the urethral orifice and anterior to the anus. The vagina and cervix can be inspected through a speculum placed in the vagina. A Papanicolaou (Pap) smear is taken from the cervix to aid in the detection of cervical cancer.

Blood supply to the ovaries (that is, to the ovarian arteries arising from the lower abdominal aorta), fallopian tubes (via the ovarian and uterine arteries), and uterus (via the uterine artery) forms a complex **anastomosis**. The vagina and cervix are supplied by branches from the internal iliac arteries. Venous drainage for the ovaries is distinct for each side. The right ovarian vein drains to the inferior vena cava, whereas the left ovarian vein empties into the left renal vein. The veins of the fallopian tubes drain into the ovarian and uterine veins. The uterine veins form a uterine venous plexus on each side of the cervix and drain to the internal iliac veins. The uterine venous plexus connects with the superior rectal vein, forming a portal–systemic anastomosis. The vaginal veins form the vaginal venous plexuses and lie along the sides of the vagina, draining into the internal iliac veins. Lymphatic drainage, again, is related to the metastatic spread of cancer. The ovaries drain to the lumbar lymph nodes. The fallopian tubes have their lymphatic drainage directed to the lower lumbar lymph nodes with the ovaries and uterus. The uterus drains to the lower aortic and external iliac

lymph nodes. The superior and middle portions of the vagina drain into the external and iliac lymph nodes, and the lower portion of the vagina drains into the superficial inguinal lymph nodes. The cervix drains to the external and internal iliac nodes and sacral lymph nodes.

Physiology of Ovulation and Menstruation

Normal menstrual cycles depend on an intact hypothalamic–pituitary axis, functioning ovaries, and a normal outflow tract. The menstrual cycle, which averages 28 d, requires a well-coordinated series of events (figure 10.8). The normal menstrual cycle is divided into two parts: a proliferative, or follicular, phase and a secretory, or luteal, phase. During the follicular phase, estrogen and luteinizing hormone (LH) levels increase as follicle-stimulating hormone (FSH) levels decrease. The endometrium thickens during this phase. Before ovulation, estrogen sharply declines, followed by a surge in LH and a steady rise in progesterone. It is shortly after this that ovulation occurs, followed by a slight increase in core body temperature. The remnant of the follicle (i.e., corpus luteum) supplies the progesterone for the second half of the cycle. During this time, the endometrium prepares itself for implantation. If fertilization and implantation do not occur, the corpus luteum involutes and progesterone levels decline, prompting menses, which is the discharge of the endometrium from the uterus through the vagina.

Physiological Changes of Pregnancy

Noteworthy physiological changes occur in pregnancy. Cardiac output (CO), defined as stroke volume (SV) × heart rate (HR), increases during pregnancy as a result of increases in both SV and HR. Plasma volume also increases with pregnancy (Perales et al. 2015; May et al. 2015). The high flow of blood exiting the heart can often create a benign heart murmur. Blood pressure, defined as CO × systemic vascular resistance (SVR), actually decreases because of a decrease in SVR. Healthy women who exercised during pregnancy experienced reduced resting HR and increased endothelial cells in umbilical cord blood (Perales et al. 2015; Onoyama et al. 2016).

Respiratory changes also occur in pregnancy and result in increased tidal volume, which translates into increased minute ventilation at rest despite a normal respiratory rate. Of note, the forced expiratory volume in 1 s (FEV_1) does not change, which is important for asthmatic athletes because peak flow meter values would not need to be altered. Overall airway resistance is also decreased in pregnancy.

Physiological responses to exercise are somewhat different in pregnancy than in the nonpregnant female. Respiratory rates increase with mild exercise in preg-

---

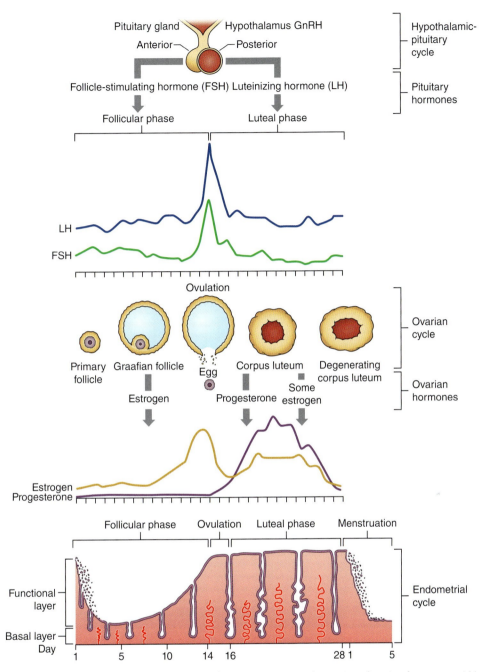

FIGURE 10.8   Diagram of the female menstrual cycle. GnRH = gonadotropin-releasing hormone; LH = luteinizing hormone; FSH = follicle-stimulating hormone.

nancy compared with nonpregnant women, whereas maximal oxygen consumption ($\dot{V}O_2$max) is less in pregnant women than in nonpregnant women. The respiratory quotient ($\dot{V}CO_2/\dot{V}O_2$) is also increased in exercising pregnant women, suggesting that there may be a greater dependence on carbohydrates as the preferred fuel source. This may also explain the fact that hypoglycemia can develop more rapidly during prolonged strenuous exercise in pregnant women. In addition, the core temperature of

a pregnant woman is higher than that of a nonpregnant woman, which requires caution in the expectant mother who exercises, especially in hotter climates.

Anatomical considerations because of the enlarging uterus result in common changes in pregnancy. Urinary frequency increases during pregnancy as a result of pressure of the uterus on the urinary bladder. Low back pain is another common complaint and is again the result of the enlarging uterus. In this scenario, however, changes in biomechanics lead to increased lumbar lordosis that is more commonly the cause of the low back discomfort. Lower extremity edema may also develop and is more common later in pregnancy.

Evaluation of the Genitourinary and Gynecological Systems

Evaluation of the genitourinary and gynecological systems by the athletic trainer begins with a thorough and complete history. Maintaining a clear and professional demeanor with the patient is key, as is using correct medical terminology and anatomical terms. It is strongly advisable to have a person of the athlete's gender present when taking the history to increase the patient's comfort, and it is a good professional practice. Ask pertinent history questions, and ask about signs, symptoms, onset, and other details that can assist in a diagnosis. The goal is to collect enough information to refer the patient to the correct provider. Visual inspection and palpation of the genitourinary and gynecological systems is best left to the medical professionals who have expertise and specialties in these areas. These providers may order distinctive tests based on their findings, and they only need the history, not any other evaluative information, to assist them.

Pathological Conditions of the Genitourinary System

Kidney Stones

Kidney stones, also known as renal or urinary calculi, arise in the kidney when urine becomes supersaturated with a salt that is capable of forming solid crystals. Although they are commonly referred to as "kidney stones," they may be found in the ureters, urinary bladder, or urethra as well. Renal calculi are commonly composed of calcium oxalate (50%), calcium phosphate (10%–20%), struvite (7%), and cystine (3%) (Ferri 2016). In the United States, the lifetime prevalence for kidney stones is 13% in males and 7% in females. There is a reported 5 yr recurrence rate of 35%–50% following an initial kidney stone (Qaseem et al. 2014). Caucasian males are affected more commonly than African-American males, although African-American males have a higher incidence of associated infection with renal calculi. Females of all races have been noted to have a higher incidence of infected **hydronephrosis**. The age of onset of symptomatic renal calculi is generally in the third or fourth decade.

Most stones pass spontaneously, but some patients require hospitalization for unremitting pain, dehydration, associated urinary tract infection, or inability to pass the stone.

Signs and Symptoms

Most kidney stones originate within the kidney and proceed distally, creating various degrees of urinary obstruction as they become lodged in the narrow canal areas. Acute passage of a kidney stone from the kidney through the ureter gives rise to pain so excruciating that it has been likened to that of childbirth. The location and quality of pain are related to the position of the stone within the urinary tract. The severity of pain is related to the degree of obstruction, the presence of ureteral spasm, and the presence of any associated infection. The pain typically begins suddenly at night or in the early morning, but it can follow heavy exercise and may present with a more gradual onset (Favus 2015). The pain is

Types of Kidney Stones

Each of the following five commonly identified types of kidney stones has its own causes:

1. *Calcium stones* are composed of calcium oxide, calcium phosphate, calcium oxalate, and uric acid. Common causes of calcium stones include hyperparathyroidism, increased gut absorption of calcium, a renal phosphate leak, hyperuricosuria, hyperoxaluria, hypocitraturia, and hypomagnesemia.

2. *Struvite stones* are composed of magnesium ammonium phosphate. These stones are associated with chronic urinary tract infections secondary to gram-negative rods.

3. *Uric acid stones* are associated with high purine intake (diet rich in organ meats, legumes, fish, meat extracts, or gravies), gout, and malignancy.

4. *Cystine stones* are caused by an intrinsic metabolic defect resulting in failure of renal tubular reabsorption of cystine, ornithine, lysine, and arginine.

5. *Indinavir stones* typically appear in patients with human immunodeficiency virus (HIV) infection who are treated with the protease inhibitor indinavir (Crixivan). These stones are composed entirely of the protease inhibitor.

typically described as unilateral flank pain that radiates to the groin (Ferri 2016). The person is often writhing in pain, moving about and unable to lie still. Nausea and vomiting are common. Examination demonstrates flank tenderness, costovertebral angle tenderness, and occasionally testicular pain, notably in the absence of any testicular tenderness. The abdominal examination is often normal, although bowel sounds may be hypoactive because of a mild ileus. The presence of a fever raises the possibility of an infectious complication and warrants immediate referral.

Once a kidney stone passes to the urinary bladder it is often asymptomatic and can be passed during urination. During passage of the stone the athlete will usually note burning and some blood-tinged urine depending on the size of the stone.

The differential diagnoses for kidney stones is long and often depends on what side of the body is involved, as well as on the sex and age of the individual. The list includes urinary tract infection, **pyelonephritis**, urinary obstruction, renal vein thrombosis, testicular torsion, pelvic inflammatory disease, ectopic pregnancy, bowel obstruction, appendicitis, cholecystitis, **biliary colic**, and constipation (Favus 2015; Ferri 2016). Among those older than 60 years of age, an **abdominal aortic aneurysm (AAA)** may also be included as a differential diagnosis (Borrero and Queral 1988).

In a series of 134 patients with symptomatic AAA presenting to the emergency department, 18% had an initial misdiagnosis of a kidney stone (Borrero and Queral 1988).

Referral and Diagnostic Tests

An athlete with symptoms suggestive of a kidney stone should be referred immediately to the team physician if this is the first episode. Any athlete with new or recurrent presentation and an associated fever needs to be referred immediately for physician evaluation and a urology consultation. Also, an athlete with recurrent symptoms who cannot tolerate oral fluids and has unrelenting pain with a history of renal failure or a single kidney should be referred for immediate physician evaluation and possible observation or hospitalization.

The mainstay of diagnostic testing for kidney stones is a urinalysis. Blood is often visible in the urine and may be detectable in more than 90% of symptomatic individuals using both a urine dipstick and microscopy. Urine pH can also be helpful because a urine pH greater than 7 suggests the presence of urea-splitting organisms and struvite stones. Alternatively, a urine pH less than 5 suggests the presence of uric acid stones. The presence of pyuria (>5 white blood cells per high-power field) in a centrifuged urine specimen should prompt a careful search for an associated infection (Ferri 2016). (Normal urine values are listed in table 3.2.) In these cases, a complete blood count (CBC) and differential, serum creatinine, and urine culture are in order.

Imaging studies may also be performed and are often done to confirm the initial diagnosis. The imaging study most often used is the infused or noninfused helical computerized tomography (CT) scan (Favus 2015). This is a rapid test with sensitivity in the range of 95% to 100%. Ultrasonography is also widely used and has sensitivity similar to that of the CT exam, but the CT exam is less operator dependent. It should be noted that in ultrasonography there is no exposure to radiation, and therefore this is an ideal imaging tool for pregnant women. Radiographs may also be obtained and may demonstrate a radiopaque stone. Radiographs are occasionally used to monitor the passage of a stone under certain circumstances. An **intravenous pyelogram (IVP)** may be used in the diagnosis of kidney stones but has essentially been replaced by CT.

Treatment and Return to Participation

The crux of treatment for the uncomplicated passage of a kidney stone is pain management and maintenance of adequate hydration. Pain management is often obtained with nonsteroidal anti-inflammatory agents or narcotic analgesics, such as morphine sulfate or meperidine (Demerol) (Favus 2015). An antiemetic medication also may be added when nausea is present and deters the use of oral analgesics or hydration. The forcing of oral or intravenous fluids has not been shown to alter outcomes or to improve the passage of a stone; therefore the focus should remain on maintenance of hydration. A strainer is useful to filter the urine during the passage of the stone in order to collect the stone for analysis. Antibiotics are necessary in the presence of an associated infection.

The overall prognosis for kidney stones is very good. Fifty percent of stones pass uneventfully within 48 h (Ferri 2016). Recurrence rates escalate with time, but on the basis of the type of stone present, treatment options to reduce the risk of recurrence are available. Return to sport can follow passage of the kidney stone and adequate rehydration. However, even after the diagnosis of a kidney stone, any athlete who develops fever, increasing pain, or emesis should be referred for immediate physician evaluation.

Prevention

Individuals who have had a kidney stone may benefit from maintaining adequate hydration and avoiding dehydration (Fink et al. 2013; Cheungpasitporn et al. 2015; Qaseem et al. 2014). This may decrease the chance of urinary saturation with stone-forming salts. Contributors to recurring kidney stones have been reported to be obesity, diabetes, hyperparathyroidism, intestinal malabsorption, and anatomical abnormalities (Fink et al. 2013). Daily consumption of coffee, tea, beer, or wine may decrease the risk of stone formation, whereas daily apple or grapefruit juice may increase the risk of stone formation. Sodium intake should be restricted to help prevent recurrence. Increasing the amount of dietary bran may decrease bowel time and limit the formation of urinary calculi (Ferri 2016). It should be noted that, although nearly 60% of kidney stones are calcium derivatives, dietary intake of calcium should not be eliminated or reduced below a reasonable level (Qaseem et al. 2014).

Sports Hematuria

Sports hematuria is the benign, self-limiting presence of three or more red blood cells per high-power field in a centrifuged urine specimen and is directly associated with exercise or activity. Sports hematuria is asymptomatic and has been documented to occur in both contact and noncontact sports. The degree of hematuria is believed to be related to the intensity and duration of the exercise. In most circumstances, the hematuria will resolve within 72 h of onset in athletes without any coexisting urinary tract pathology (Varma, Sengupta, and Nair 2014). Active people under age 30 had higher incidences of postexertional hematuria than did older participants (Varma, Sengupta, and Nair 2014; Bernard 2009).

The incidence of sports hematuria is estimated to be as high as 80% in swimming, lacrosse, and track and field; 55% in football and rowing; and 20% in marathon runners. These incidence levels have led to the development of several possible causes of sports hematuria (e.g., increased permeability of the glomerulus, direct or indirect trauma to the kidneys, renal ischemia, dehydration, release of a hemolyzing factor), all of which appear to be related to exercise duration and exercise intensity (Varma, Sengupta, and Nair 2014; Shephard 2015).

Signs and Symptoms

By definition, sports hematuria is asymptomatic. The finding of hematuria may occur during a routine urinalysis, such as those that may be performed during a physical examination or preparticipation examination. On occasion, athletes will present with gross hematuria (i.e., visible presence of blood in the urine) after a prolonged and strenuous workout. However, microscopic hematuria is not visibly apparent but is noted during a dipstick or urine analysis. Regardless of how hematuria is determined, the general rule is that sports hematuria will resolve within 72 h without any further intervention than rest. One study with 500 runners noted that postexertional hematuria continued to 7 d in some (12%) and beyond 7

d in 7% of participants. It was determined that the three who had persistent (beyond 14 d) hematuria had other kidney pathologies (Varma, Sengupta, and Nair 2014).

The differential diagnosis includes distinguishing true hematuria from false-positive urine blood dipsticks. True hematuria may result from a urinary tract infection, urethritis, interstitial nephritis, renal papillary necrosis, nephrolithiasis (kidney stone), polycystic kidney disease, kidney laceration, a neoplasm arising from any structure in the urinary tract, urinary bladder cancer, and prostatitis in males (Ferri 2016). Causes of a false-positive urine dipstick examination for blood include those related to drug intake (i.e., phenazopyridine, rifampin, nitrofurantoin, phenytoin), food dyes, menses, and myoglobin in the urine. Also, menstruating females may present with "hematuria," but it is actually menstrual blood. It is appropriate to question the female athlete presenting with hematuria whether or not she is currently menstruating. However, the health care provider should not dismiss signs or symptoms that could indicate a concurrent condition.

Referral and Diagnostic Tests

The finding of asymptomatic hematuria in an athlete during some form of routine testing needs to be reviewed by the team physician. As a general rule, these athletes are retested at 24 to 72 h to document resolution. Any athlete with symptomatic hematuria or systemic symptoms is referred to a physician for immediate evaluation.

Although sports hematuria is a benign condition, not all hematuria is benign, and therefore the evaluation must include some basic tests. A urinalysis or dipstick test will demonstrate the presence of blood in the urine. Because drugs, dyes, and myoglobin can mimic hematuria by causing a false-positive result on the urine dipstick, microscopic examination of a spun urine specimen will confirm the presence of red blood cells. If symptoms of dysuria (i.e., painful urination) are present, a urine culture may be performed. If hypertension, renal disease, repeated urinary tract infections, or pyelonephritis is found in the athlete's history, an initial serum creatinine may be performed. As a general rule, if hematuria persists beyond 72 h, further evaluation is warranted. Additional tests include a renal ultrasound, CT, and possible **cystoscopy**.

Treatment and Return to Participation

The treatment of sports hematuria is simply rest for 24 to 72 h. Resolution is the rule, and it should be documented with a repeat urinalysis after rest. The prognosis is excellent because sports hematuria is a benign and self-limiting condition (Varma, Sengupta, and Nair 2014; Shephard 2015).

Urinary Tract Infection

Urinary tract infection (UTI) is the most common bacterial infection seen in ambulatory care settings in the United States, and it occurs in either the upper or lower urinary tract (Ferri 2016). These infections most commonly involve the urinary bladder, but they can also involve the urethra, ureters, and kidneys (i.e., pyelonephritis). UTIs are a leading cause of morbidity and health care expenditures in persons of all ages.

Anyone can develop a UTI; however, sexually active young women are at the highest risk. Several factors have been attributed to this higher risk: a short urethra; sexual activity; delays in micturition, particularly after intercourse; and the use of diaphragms and spermicides (Fiore and Cox 2015). Fortunately, the risk of a complicated UTI in this population is very low, yet up to 20% of young women with a UTI will develop recurrent UTIs (Mohsin and Siddiqui 2010).

UTIs in men are less common than in women but can occur. Catheter-associated UTIs are also known to occur.

Signs and Symptoms

In most people, a UTI is signaled by a constellation of symptoms, including dysuria, increased frequency of urination, and voiding small amounts of urine relative to their normal pattern. On occasion, lower pelvic discomfort or cramping may also be present. The presence of gross hematuria, abnormal vaginal bleeding, or fever warrants prompt physician attention.

Differential diagnoses for UTIs include urethritis, noninfectious cystitis, pyelonephritis, vulvovaginitis, sexually transmitted infections (STIs), dehydration, mittelschmerz, endometriosis, and **balanitis**.

Referral and Diagnostic Tests

Because of the relative discomfort associated with a UTI and the possibility of developing an ascending infection, symptomatic athletes need to be referred to a physician for evaluation and treatment.

The diagnosis of an uncomplicated UTI is often made on the basis of the history, physical examination, and examination of a urine specimen. A urine dipstick test is the most reliable examination for determining a UTI. The presence of nitrates or leukocytes confirms the diagnosis. A urine specimen can also be examined specifically for the presence of leukocyte esterase, nitrite (a surrogate marker for bacteria), and the finding of leukocytes on microscopic examination. A urine Gram stain can also aid in the identification of bacteria. The finding of a single bacterial organism, under high-power oil immersion, on an unspun urine specimen correlates with a count of more than 100,000 colony-forming units of bacteria per millili-

ter on urine culture (Medina-Bombado and Jover-Palmer 2011). Because of its limited added value in determining treatment for most uncomplicated UTIs, a urine culture may not be performed in the initial evaluation. The evaluation of a recurrent, complicated, or catheter-associated UTI often necessitates obtaining a urine culture (Ferri 2016; Fiore and Cox 2015).

Urine culture results must be viewed in light of certain threshold values that have been shown to correlate with significant **bacteriuria**. In young women, a urine culture producing more than 100,000 colony-forming units of bacteria per milliliter of urine is considered a positive culture because of its high specificity for the diagnosis of a true infection. In men, a urine culture yielding more than 1000 colony-forming units of bacteria per milliliter is considered a positive culture, and in catheterized patients, this value falls to more than 100 colony-forming units of bacteria per milliliter.

The use of additional urological testing for anatomical abnormalities is generally unrewarding. However, a urological evaluation should still be performed in prepubescent children, in adolescent males with a first UTI, and in men with pyelonephritis or recurrent UTI (Fiore and Cox 2015).

Treatment and Return to Participation

UTIs are treated with antibiotics. An uncomplicated UTI can be treated with antibiotics such as trimethoprim-sulfamethoxazole, ciprofloxacin, or ofloxacin for a 3 d course (see chapter 5). Recurrent UTIs in women or men should be treated with a 7 to 10 d course of antibiotics with antibiotic choice based on the results of the urine culture. If a woman experiences more than three UTIs in a year, prophylactic antibiotics may be used to prevent recurrence. Studies demonstrated the effectiveness of prophylactic antibiotic use after coitus, when given continually at a lower dose than treatment dose, for recurrent UTIs (Fiore and Cox 2015). Complicated UTIs require a longer course of treatment and should be treated for 10 to 14 d.

The prognosis for an uncomplicated UTI is excellent and generally will not preclude participation in athletics.

CLINICAL TIPS

Significance of Dipsticks

Ready access to and knowledge of how to correctly use urinary dipsticks is critical in the early diagnosis of a urinary system condition. Properly used, these can quickly determine if there is hematuria, infection, or dehydration.

For the few athletes who develop a complicated UTI, return-to-play decisions need to be based on the athlete's unique complication. Athletes with fever or poor fluid intake as a result of nausea or vomiting should be observed and should return to play only after symptoms resolve with treatment.

Prevention

Common sense will help prevent recurrent UTIs. Modification of risk factors for UTIs includes avoiding delays in urination and limiting the use of either diaphragms or spermicides. Wearing breathable (cotton) underwear also reduces the chances of contracting a UTI. Although there are some data supporting the effectiveness of cranberry supplements, other urban myths such as postcoital voiding, increased fluid consumption, and avoiding bubble baths have shown no reproducible evidence in preventing UTIs (Fiore and Cox 2015).

Urethritis and Cystitis

Urethritis is an inflammation of the urethra, whereas cystitis is an inflammation of the urinary bladder and ureters. Both conditions are actually subcategories of UTIs. Both present with similar signs and symptoms and are caused by irritation of the urinary system (bladder, ureters, and/or urethra). Urethritis is sometimes used to describe a syndrome of sexually transmitted infections (STIs), but it can have both infectious and noninfectious causes. The two most common categories of infections linked to the urethritis are gonococcal urethritis (GU) and nongonococcal urethritis (NGU). STIs will be discussed later in the chapter. Infectious causes of urethritis are typically sexually transmitted and include *Neisseria gonorrhoeae* (GU) and nongonococcal organisms such as *Chlamydia trachomatis, Ureaplasma urealyticum, Mycoplasma hominis,* and *Trichomonas vaginalis* (NGU) (Workowski 2015). Less common infectious causes of urethritis include herpes genitalis and syphilis, and they may also be associated with communicable conditions such as epididymitis, **orchitis**, prostatitis, or UTIs. The incidence of GU is in decline. Conversely, the incidence of NGU is rising and is notably higher during the summer months. Urethritis affects males and females equally, although up to 50% of females may be asymptomatic, and homosexual males are more commonly infected than heterosexuals or homosexual females. Infectious urethritis may occur in any sexually active person, but the incidence is highest among people 20 to 24 years of age (Workowski 2015; Ferri 2016).

Signs and Symptoms

Signs and symptoms of urethritis are similar to those of a UTI. Symptom onset typically occurs between 4 and 14 d after contact with an infected partner. Urethral discharge may be present and may be yellow, green, brown, or blood tinged. Dysuria is usually localized to the urethral orifice and is worst with a first-morning void. Urethral itching or hematuria may be present, but up to 25% of those with urethritis have no signs or symptoms (Ferri 2016). Males may report heaviness or aching in the testicles, although associated tenderness should suggest orchitis or epididymitis. Females may report a worsening of symptoms with their menses. The presence of fever, chills, sweats, or nausea suggests a more systemic infection and warrants immediate referral to a physician (Porter and Kaplan 2011).

The differential diagnosis for urethritis is best considered by gender. Differential diagnoses to be considered in both men and women include recent passage of a kidney stone as well as STIs such as chlamydia, gonorrhea, herpes, mycoplasma, syphilis, and trichomoniasis. Other etiology without gender considerations that need to be ruled out include dermatological diseases involving the urethral orifice (e.g., contact dermatitis secondary to spermicides), **molluscum contagiosum**, urethral stricture, urethral trauma, urethral warts, urethral diverticulum, and urethral cancer. Differential diagnoses affecting females include rigorous sexual intercourse (termed *honeymoon cystitis*), **oophoritis**, pelvic inflammatory disease, salpingitis, vaginitis, and vulvovaginitis. Differential diagnoses exclusive to males are epididymitis and chronic bacterial prostatitis (Porter and Kaplan 2011).

Referral and Diagnostic Tests

Athletes suspected of having urethritis or cystitis are referred to a physician for diagnosis and treatment. In the interim, the athlete should be counseled to refrain from sexual intercourse until seeing the physician so as to avoid further irritation or possible infection of other people, if an STI.

The diagnosis of urethritis is most often based on history and examination. A urinalysis is not particularly helpful in establishing the diagnosis, but it may be helpful in the exclusion of cystitis or pyelonephritis. Microscopic examination of the specimen will reveal pyuria (>8 WBCs/μL) and possible microscopic hematuria. A dipstick test is specific for WBCs (>10 WBCs/μL) (Porter and Kaplan 2011). Further testing should be done if an STI is suspected.

More than 30% of individuals with NGU do not have leukocytes in their urine. A urethral culture may be performed to examine for the presence of gonococcus or chlamydia. In cases of confirmed GU or NGU, testing for syphilis, hepatitis B, and human immunodeficiency virus (HIV) is encouraged (Workowski 2015). Women of childbearing age who have experienced unprotected intercourse need a pregnancy test before treatment.

Treatment

Antibiotics are the mainstay of treatment for urethritis. Symptoms will resolve in all patients with urethritis over time regardless of treatment. The use of antibiotics in the treatment of infectious urethritis is to prevent morbidity and to reduce transmission to others. The antibiotic choices are based on the likelihood of whether it is GU or NGU. Current recommendations are to treat for both GU and NGU. Azithromycin in a single 2 g dose treats both GU and NGU, is the treatment of choice for urethritis, and is well tolerated. Ceftriaxone (intramuscularly), cefixime (oral), ciprofloxacin (oral), or ofloxacin (oral) can be used in single doses to treat GU only. Doxycycline can be taken for 7 d to treat NGU only. In the case of recurrent NGU, a prolonged course of erythromycin for 14 to 28 d is recommended (Ferri 2016). Antibiotic treatment is recommended for sexual partners of those with culture-positive urethritis, including *Trichomonas*. Men infected with NGU must have all sex partners within the 60 d preceding diagnosis referred for evaluation and treatment. Prevention of reinfection includes abstinence from sexual activity until the patient and partner(s) have been effectively treated (Workowski 2015).

Treatment and Return to Participation

The overall prognosis for urethritis is excellent. The use of antibiotics helps to decrease any associated morbidity and prevent further transmission. Anyone with urethritis is counseled to abstain from sexual intercourse until all partners have been treated and is further encouraged to use barrier devices (condoms) when engaging in sexual intercourse with multiple partners. Uncomplicated urethritis should not interfere with an athlete's ability to train or compete.

Prevention

Prevention of urethritis equates to education. Sexually active athletes are encouraged to use barrier methods during intercourse. Education about STI risk factors can be beneficial. Risk factors include intercourse at a young age, unprotected intercourse, multiple sexual partners, intercourse with partners known to have infections, and drug abuse. The early diagnosis and treatment of athletes with urethritis help to limit the transmission, as do the identification and treatment of all partners.

Sexually Transmitted Infections

Sexually transmitted diseases (STDs) and infections (STIs) are really sexually transmittable infections as they pass via sexual contact but some may occur in the absence of sexual activity. The name STD is now typically referred to as STI. STI covers a broader range as it includes persons who are infected and may infect others but who may not have signs of a disease (table 10.1). STIs are unique in that they tend to affect males and females differently, and their presentations are different depending on sex. Males tend to come forth more regularly with signs and symptoms of an STI, whereas women do not, chiefly because their anatomy may preclude obvious

TABLE 10.1 Sexually Transmitted Diseases and Infections

Disease	Incubation	Transmission	Signs and symptoms	Treatment	Long term
HIV	1–6 mo	Sexually transmitted	Malaise, fever	ZDU for maintenance	AIDS
HPV	1–6 mo	Sexually transmitted	Genital warts	Symptomatic	Chronic carrier
Syphilis	1–13 wk	Sexual contact	Chancre, dermatological signs, constitutional symptoms	Penicillin	Incapacitating cardiovascular disease, often with neurological signs
Gonorrhea	Men: 2–14 d Women: 7–21 d	Sexually transmitted	Dysuria, discharge, frequency of voiding	Ceftriaxone, doxycycline	Hydrocele and abscesses in men; salpingitis in women
Chlamydia	7–28 d	Sexually transmitted	Dysuria, meatal itching, asymptomatic	Tetracycline or doxycycline	Pelvic inflammatory disease if left untreated
Herpes 2	4–7 d	Sexual contact	Lesions	Acyclovir	Chronic carrier

AIDS = acquired immunodeficiency syndrome; HIV = human immunodeficiency virus; HPV = human papillomavirus; ZDU = zidovudine.

symptoms. Many women may forgo medical evaluation and self-treat if they think they have a urinary tract infection. General signs and symptoms of STIs are similar in both sexes: dysuria (i.e., painful urination); urge to void but production of small volume; and urethral discharge, itching, and burning.

Catch-all terms associated with STIs are **nongono-coccal** or **nonspecific urethritis** (**NGU** or **NSU**). Both occur in men and women and are caused by organisms that are not necessarily sexually transmitted. The signs and symptoms of these are similar to other STIs in that patients present with dysuria, a frequent need to void, and discharge. These symptoms can be less intense than those of other STIs and can occur up to 6 wk after exposure, unlike the 2 to 8 d incubation period for gonorrhea. A large number of causative agents include *Escherichia coli*, herpes simplex, trauma, chemical contact, or chlamydia. NGU is not a true sexually transmitted infection. Undetected, this infection can spread to the testes, epididymis, prostate, and seminal vesicles in males. In females, the inflammation can spread to the labia, ovaries, uterus, and fallopian tubes, producing pelvic inflammatory disease (PID) (Workowski 2015).

Prevention

Most STIs can be prevented by using barrier protection such as a condom during sexual intercourse, knowing the medical history of the sex partner, and avoiding risky behaviors that include multiple sex partners, unsafe sexual practices, and excessive drinking of alcohol, which may lead to risky behaviors. Some STIs, such as herpes, can be contagious even if there is a barrier because the barrier must completely cover the lesion to deter the infection.

Athletes must understand that having an STI does not provide immunity from another infection in the manner seen with childhood diseases discussed in chapter 15. The only certain way to avoid STIs is to abstain from sexual relations or to maintain mutually monogamous sexual intimacy with a partner who has proven to be uninfected. An infected person needs to abstain from sexual contact until the course of treatment has been completed and all lesions have completely healed (Porter and Kaplan 2011).

Concerns With Adolescents and Public Health Implications

Athletes under the age of 18 who are sexually active and report their anxiety about a possible STI to the athletic trainer are of special concern. In addition to state statutory rape laws, each state has specific laws regarding the reporting of this type of medical information to another person, parent, or guardian. The athletic trainer should consult the school counselor or nurse about applicable laws. The health of the athlete is of utmost importance. The treating physician has the obligation to report infectious diseases to the appropriate agency, but athletic trainers need to be aware of the ramifications for children with STIs.

Human Immunodeficiency Virus and Acquired Immunodeficiency Syndrome

Human immunodeficiency virus (HIV) is a blood-borne virus, usually transmitted by sexual intercourse, shared intravenous materials, transplantation of infected organs, or mother-to-child transmission during birth or breast-

---

CONDITION HIGHLIGHT

Herpes Simplex Virus

Herpes simplex virus (HSV) has two forms: HSV-1 (oral herpes, often called fever blisters or cold sores) and HSV-2 (genital herpes). The Centers for Disease Control and Prevention call HSV among the most prevalent STIs. In the United States, by the age of 30, 50% of people of higher socioeconomic status and 80% of those of lower socioeconomic status are seropositive; but this does not indicate these people are symptomatic (Salvaggio 2015). Transmission of HSV-1 usually occurs through oral secretions or sores, and it is spread via kissing or sharing cups or utensils, toothbrushes, and so on. HSV-1 can cause genital herpes; but most cases of HSV-2 are caused by infection from HSV-1. Both types of herpes can be transmitted even if sores are not present. HSV-2 can be passed to infants via childbirth. Although many have no overt signs of HSV, the typical presentation is lesion with vesicles (blisters). Other signs and symptoms include fever (102 °F–104 °F), lymphadenopathy, and listlessness. Once one is infected, many things can trigger an outbreak of herpes, including illness, stress, fatigue, sunlight, menstruation, and physical trauma to the area affected. There is no cure for herpes, but drugs such Famvir, Zovirax, and Valtrex are used to treat the symptoms of herpes.

feeding (Bennett 2015). It is the precursor to acquired immunodeficiency syndrome (AIDS), the late-stage result of HIV infection, for which there is no known cure. HIV may lay dormant for years after infection; however, it is estimated that 90% of those infected with HIV will eventually develop AIDS if left untreated (Ferri 2016).

Transmission via saliva, urine, tears, insects (including mosquitoes), or bronchial secretions has not been recorded, but the virus has been found in these fluids (Ferri 2016). Transmission of HIV through sexual contact is much rarer than is transmission of hepatitis B virus (HBV) because HIV is not as hardy but that should not preclude caution. The presence of a concurrent STI increases the likelihood of acquiring HIV (Bennett 2015).

The incubation period for HIV can last several months or years before the onset of symptoms, but most infected individuals will test positive for the virus within 6 mo. Some patients develop a self-limiting mononucleosis-like illness weeks to months after exposure to HIV, but the acute illness lasts only a few weeks and is often dismissed.

In 2010–2014, the Centers for Disease Control and Prevention reported a rise in HIV infection in the United States for persons ages 25 to 29. The rates of infection for American Indians, Alaska natives, and Asians also increased; Hispanics/Latinos and whites remained stable; and African-Americans and persons of multiple races decreased. In 2014, males accounted for 81% of all diagnoses of HIV infection among adults and adolescents (Centers for Disease Control and Prevention 2015d).

Generally, the public is not in danger of contracting HIV unless they are a population at risk (e.g., sexual behaviors, needle sharing). The U.S. Preventive Services Task Force strongly recommends HIV testing for all adolescents and adults at increased risk for HIV infection, including pregnant women. Health care workers infected with HIV may be required to notify their employers of their status and be restricted in the types of procedures they can perform (Bennett 2015). Of particular concern are pregnant women infected with the HIV virus. In a joint statement, the American Congress of Obstetricians and Gynecologists and the American Academy of Pediatrics put forth a policy in 2011 strongly supporting universal HIV testing as a component of prenatal care, and it has been jointly reaffirmed annually since then (American Congress of Obstetricians and Gynecologists 2015a). Studies have shown that HIV-infected pregnant women have a 90% chance of bearing a noninfected child if they follow the guidelines for prevention of perinatal transmission (American Congress of Obstetricians and Gynecologists 2015b).

Signs and Symptoms

After infection, a broad variety of clinical issues may occur. AIDS-related complex (ARC) is the term used for HIV-positive patients who have not yet developed opportunistic infections that are associated with AIDS. General signs and symptoms of ARC include malaise, intermittent fever, diarrhea, anemia, weight loss, lymphadenopathy, **hairy leukoplakia**, and **thrush**. Some life-threatening cancers, including **Kaposi's sarcoma**, non-Hodgkin's lymphoma, and lymphoma of the brain, may be acquired through AIDS-related infection in patients who never manifested ARC symptoms (Porter and Kaplan 2011; Ferri 2016).

The AIDS virus itself is considered an opportunistic infection, settling on whole body systems or organs. Signs and symptoms are presented chiefly via other known pathologies but are in fact caused by AIDS. Associated illnesses include encephalitis, meningitis, tuberculosis, central nervous system (CNS) infections, vascular and digestive complications, peripheral neuropathies, and renal pathologies (Bennett 2015).

Because HIV/AIDS can manifest as a multi-organ system problem, the differential diagnoses for these diseases are lengthy, ranging from malaise and simple gastrointestinal disturbances to pneumonia, cancer, or complex regional pain syndrome.

Referral and Diagnostic Tests

Athletes who present with unexplainable fatigue or slow-healing wounds are referred to a physician for further evaluation. If an athlete has reason to warrant HIV testing, a blood test is necessary to confirm the disease. A high-sensitivity enzyme-linked immunoabsorbent assay (ELISA) is used for screening (Bennett 2015). False-positive test results are known to occur, so reactive tests are supplemented by additional studies, such as the **Western blot** or the indirect fluorescent antibody (IFA) test. There are commercially available at-home or so-called rapid tests for HIV but not all are FDA-approved diagnostic tests for HIV. Consumers must understand that both false-positive and false-negative results are possible (Centers for Disease Control and Prevention 2015d).

Treatment and Return to Participation

Since there is no vaccine to prevent HIV, and there is no cure, treatment of HIV and AIDS is actually management of the symptoms. HIV and AIDS weaken the immune system, and management entails maintaining overall health, allowing opportunistic infections to invade. Highly active antiretroviral therapy (HAART) is the principal method of preventing immune deterioration (Bennett 2015). Long-term HAART yields a gradual improvement of immune responses and, coupled with other prophylactic medications, can retard or stabilize the HIV infection.

An HIV-positive athlete is not banned from sport, and as long as health care providers practice approved blood-borne pathogen policies, the chance of transmission via sport is negligible. The illnesses associated with AIDS may preclude athletic endeavors but that is up to the individual athlete and the physician. Because HIV attacks the immune system, infected athletes would be wise to keep their distance from sick teammates.

The National Collegiate Athletic Association (NCAA) does not require that HIV-positive college athletes report or acknowledge infection to the organization or on health screenings. HIV is, however, reportable to the local health authority, and it is mandatory to report AIDS in the United States and most countries (Parsons 2014).

Genital Warts

Genital warts are caused by human papillomavirus (HPV) and are typically acquired via sexual contact. They are also called venereal warts or condylomata acuminata and result in a fibrous overgrowth of the dermis. There are more than 60 identified strains of HPV, any of which can cause genital warts. These warts tend to grow rapidly in areas of the skin and mucous membranes that experience heavy perspiration or poor hygiene, and they often accompany other sexually transmitted infections (Gearhart 2015). In the past decade, the prevalence of HPV has increased to twice the rate of genital herpes in the United States, and young adults (ages 15 to 25) account for nearly one-half of all infections each year. The association with genital herpes is disconcerting because HPV has an association with cancer that herpes does not share. Several types of HPV are the viruses that cause cervical cancer (see "Ovarian and Cervical Cancer" later in this chapter). The incubation period for HPV is 1 to 6 mo.

Women who have a history of specific types of genital warts need to be monitored over time because these warts can develop into an invasive cervical carcinoma. In addition, some types have developed into bladder cancer. Genital warts are not common before puberty or after menopause (Gearhart 2015). HPV also causes nongenital warts, such as the common and plantar warts (see chapter 16).

Signs and Symptoms

Genital warts look like common warts, that is, typically painless, minute, pink or red, soft, moist outgrowths that can appear in clusters. They can resemble cauliflower and are found in warm, moist areas of the body. In women, they are found on the vulva, vaginal walls, cervix, and perineum. Males with HPV may present with warts in the urethra or penile shaft and in the perianal area or rectum in homosexual men. Genital warts do not resemble acne or express any discharge.

Differential diagnoses for genital warts include secondary syphilis, cervical cancer, and skin tags.

Referral and Diagnostic Tests

Athletes with wart-like genital growths are referred to a physician for assessment. Genital warts are diagnosed on the basis of their appearance; however, lingering or unusual warts must be differentiated from secondary syphilis by biopsy. Women with cervical warts must obtain a clear Pap smear before undergoing any further diagnostic tests on warts.

Treatment and Return to Participation

Although genital warts are typically removed by electro-cauterization, cryotherapy, laser, or, if necessary, surgical excision, these remedies are not infallible. There is no single curative treatment, and only visible warts are usually treated. Urethral warts are removed via resectoscope with the patient under general anesthesia and circumcision in males to prevent recurrence (Gearhart 2015). Urethral lesions also need to be monitored for the rare occasion of urethral obstruction. Direct injection of interferon-α may remove genital warts that have returned after previous removal but will not reduce the rate of return. HPV and genital warts do not prohibit sport participation.

In 2006, the Food and Drug Administration approved a vaccine for four types of the HPV virus that cause cervical cancer. It is approved for both young men and women (see "Ovarian and Cervical Cancer" later in this chapter).

Syphilis

Syphilis, a sexually acquired disease caused by the organism *Treponema pallidum,* has systemic ramifications. The disease has been called the "great imitator" because so many of its symptoms reflect other diseases (Ferri 2016). Although syphilis is a preventable and curable affliction, new cases are seen in the United States each year. The most recent report shows a trend upward with 63,450 new cases in 2014 (up from 36,000 reported cases in 2010), including nearly 20,000 primary and secondary cases in 2014 (up from 10,000 in 2006) (Centers for Disease Control and Prevention 2015f). Although no particular group is without representation, homosexual men are the fastest growing population with 83% of the new diagnoses.

Syphilis presents with a series of clinical manifestations interrupted by years of latency. No body system is protected from the disease, and it can be transmitted to the fetus from an infected mother. Acquired, not congenital, syphilis is discussed here. Unlike HBV, *T. pallidum* is an unstable organism that cannot live long outside its human host. Transmission occurs from person to person via direct contact with a syphilis sore (Ferri 2016). Syphilis has an incubation period of 1 to 13 wk, but it is more typical to develop signs and symptoms between weeks 3 and 4 postinfection. Within hours of exposure, *T. pallidum* infiltrates the lymphatic system and subsequently moves throughout the entire body. The CNS is affected during the secondary stage of the disease.

Signs and Symptoms

There are four distinct stages of syphilis (see the sidebar "Stages of Acquired Syphilis"); signs and symptoms depend on the stage of the disease. Primary syphilis begins with a chancre or sore at the point of contact with the infected person. This occurs most often on the external genitalia and mouth (Centers for Disease Control and Prevention 2015f). The chancre may be a single firm, round, painless sore or multiple sores. This sore forms a painless ulcer and exudes a clear serum. More often than not, the person with the disease is unaware of it because the sores heal on their own untreated, and many patients are asymptomatic for years. Untreated, however, the syphilis infection progresses to the secondary stage.

Signs of secondary syphilis include skin rash and mucous membrane lesions that can appear 4 to 12 wk after infection. Although most rashes are **antipyretic**, they are rough and red with reddish brown spots. Sixty to eighty percent of infected people present with secondary rashes on the palms or soles (figure 10.9), but they can develop anywhere on the body and may be so subtle that they are overlooked (Ferri 2016; Centers for Disease Control and

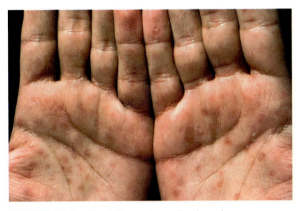

FIGURE 10.9   Syphilis rash on the hands.
Martin M. Rotker / Science Source

Stages of Acquired Syphilis

Primary Stage
Usually within 3 wk of exposure

- Chancre
- Contagious

Secondary Stage
Usually 4–12 wk after exposure

- Dermatological presentations, including rash and mucous membrane erosion
- Cerebrospinal fluid (CSF) abnormalities
- Lymphadenopathy
- Contagious

Early Latent Stage

- Less than or equal to 1yr
- Usually asymptomatic
- May never progress to later stage

Late Latent Stage (or Tertiary)

- More than 1 yr since exposure
- Symptomatic but not contagious
- Cardiovascular syphilis marked by aortic insufficiency, coronary stenosis, aortic aneurysm
- Neurosyphilis marked by personality changes, hyperactive reflexes, decreased memory, slurred speech, optic atrophy, seizures, hemiparesis

Prevention 2015f). These rashes often heal spontaneously, only to reappear. Other signs and symptoms associated with the secondary stage include fever, lymphomegaly, pharyngitis, myalgia, malaise, headache, weight loss, and patchy hair loss (Centers for Disease Control and Prevention 2015f). Again, if left untreated, secondary syphilis progresses to latent-stage syphilis.

The early latent period of the disease is usually a time without symptoms; it may last the remainder of the patient's life or may spontaneously relapse. This period begins approximately 1 yr after infection and may be treated by penicillin given for another reason other than the syphilis.

Late latent (or tertiary) stage syphilis is the final stage of this devastating disease. When other body systems are affected by the syphilis infection, profound sequelae, including cardiovascular, neurological, musculoskeletal, and visual system deterioration occur. Untreated syphilis can cause death (Porter and Kaplan 2011). In addition, there is a fivefold increased risk of acquiring the HIV infection in patients who have syphilis (Centers for Disease Control and Prevention 2015d).

The differential diagnoses for primary syphilis include genital herpes, scabies, ulceration, and trauma. Alternative diagnoses for secondary syphilis, which presents primarily as a dermatological reaction, include dermatitis, drug reaction rash, rubella, mononucleosis, ringworm, warts, and fungal infection. Latent stages of syphilis are more troublesome because they can manifest in any body organ or system and go undetected until serological tests for *T. pallidum* have been performed (Chandrasekar 2015).

Referral and Diagnostic Tests

Primary syphilis is diagnosed from exudates removed from the chancre followed by serological workup if the results are unremarkable.

The serological test for syphilis (STS) is the most common screening tool used for diagnosis. This test is often used by allied health workers to determine whether subsequent evaluation is warranted. Two other tests, the Venereal Disease Research Laboratory (VDRL) test and the rapid plasma reagin (RPR) test, are also common screening tools for syphilis. Because the CSF shows abnormal findings in less than 30% of patients, it is seldom used as an indicator of the disease (Porter and Kaplan 2011; Chandrasekar 2015).

Treatment and Return to Participation

Treatment for primary and secondary syphilis includes the physician taking a full sexual history from the patient, including all sexual partners during the past 3 mo in the case of primary syphilis and during the past 12 mo for secondary infections.

Penicillin is the appropriate medication for all forms of syphilis, and a single intramuscular injection of penicillin will cure a patient who has had syphilis less than 1 yr (Chandrasekar 2015; Centers for Disease Control and Prevention 2015f). If the patient is allergic to penicillin, erythromycin or tetracycline can be administered at a dosage of 500 mg every 6 h for 15 d (see chapter 5).

Syphilis is a reportable disease, and sexual partners of the infected person must be notified by the reporting agency, tested, and given treatment.

Gonorrhea

Gonorrhea is a sexually transmitted disease caused by a gram-negative organism, *Neisseria gonorrhoeae*, and it is a major cause of PID in women. It can affect the epithelium of the urethra, cervix, rectum, pharynx, and conjunctiva. Incidence rates have been rising since 2009, and the CDC reported over 350,000 new cases in 2014 (Centers for Disease Control and Prevention 2015c). The greatest incidence occurs in people age 20 and older, primarily in men. The rate among African American men was 10.6 times greater than the infection rate of Caucasian men (Centers for Disease Control and Prevention 2015c). The infection has a relatively short incubation period of 2 to 21 d. Transmission almost always is via direct sexual contact, with the rare exceptions of infants during vaginal birth and health care personnel through broken skin.

If gonorrhea is left untreated, serious, sex-related complications may include male postgonococcal urethritis, epididymitis, and prostatitis; women can develop PID or **salpingitis**, an inflammation of the fallopian tube, and both of these can lead to acute pain, infection, possible tubal scarring and adhesions, and resultant infertility (figure 10.10).

Both men and women may develop systemic or disseminated gonococcal infection (DGI), which presents with malaise, mild febrile illness, pustular lesions, and arthritis. Systemic disease is associated with bacteremia that may manifest as ocular infections, septic arthritis, skin lesions, and tenosynovitis.

Signs and Symptoms

Men and women have differing presentations and complications with this disease. Women may not seek treatment as soon as men because their symptoms are mild and may be more easily dismissed. In men, the symptoms begin as a discomfort in the urethra, moving quickly to dysuria and a purulent, yellow-green urethral discharge. Women's symptoms include dysuria, frequency of voiding, painful intercourse, mid- and lower abdominal pain, and vaginal discharge (Ferri 2016; Wong 2015).

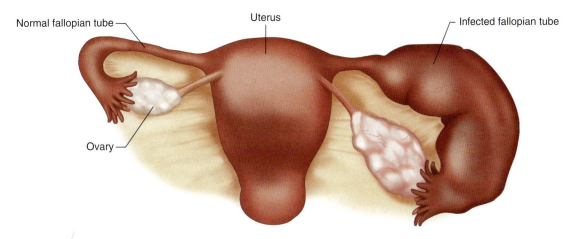

Normal fallopian tube

Uterus

Infected fallopian tube

Ovary

FIGURE 10.10 Salpingitis is an inflamed or infected fallopian tube that can result from unresolved gonorrhea.

Differential diagnoses for gonorrhea include syphilis, chlamydia, urinary tract infection, injury, or infection related to a lost or forgotten tampon in women.

Referral and Diagnostic Tests

Athletes manifesting symptoms consistent with gonorrhea are immediately referred to a physician. A patient suspected of having gonorrhea is also tested for syphilis (STS) before initiating treatment. Gonorrhea may occur concurrently with other STIs; it is important to treat them all. Specific tests for gonorrhea include a urethral swab of the discharge, which confirms the disease in 90% of infected men but only 60% of infected women (Porter and Kaplan 2011; Centers for Disease Control and Prevention 2015c). Culture with exudates from the urethra, cervix, rectum, and pharynx can confirm diagnosis.

Treatment and Return to Participation

Because strains of drug-resistant gonorrhea have emerged, the use of penicillin has been challenged. The current drug of choice is ceftriaxone (125 mg intramuscularly), but because this STI often occurs in conjunction with chlamydia, the latter also must be treated (Wong 2015). The referring physician will typically use a combination of medications, keeping in mind the complexity of treating two STIs and the challenge of drug resistance.

As with syphilis, all of the patient's sexual contacts must be located, cultured, and treated.

Chlamydia

Chlamydia includes all members of the genus *Chlamydia,* gram-negative bacteria with a unique developmental cycle within host cells. Almost every species of bird and mammal is infected with chlamydia and because of its parasitic reproductive process is capable of producing

a broad spectrum of diseases. It causes many different diseases in humans, largely in the eye, respiratory system, and genital tract. The strain of chlamydia most commonly associated with a sexually transmitted infection is *Chlamydia trachomatis,* and it is the most frequently reported STI in the United States (Torrone, Papp, and Weinstock 2014). Chlamydial infection is the most common reportable disease in the United States, with 1.4 million new infections in 2014, and it tends to be linked with other STIs such as gonorrhea, NGU, and syphilis (Centers for Disease Control and Prevention 2015b). Approximately one-half of NGU cases are caused by *C. trachomatis,* which has an incubation period of 2 to 3 wk. The infection is on the rise, as a nearly 10% increase has been reported over each of the last several years (Centers for Disease Control and Prevention 2015b).

The primary danger from chlamydia is the possible repercussions from untreated disease. Female sequelae include risk of infertility, ectopic pregnancy, and chronic pelvic pain (Centers for Disease Control and Prevention 2015b). Males risk urethral infection, epididymitis, infertility, and Reiter's syndrome (Ferri 2016).

Signs and Symptoms

The signs and symptoms of chlamydia are consistent with those of other STIs, but those with the disease may remain asymptomatic (Centers for Disease Control and Prevention 2015b). It presents with urethral discharge, dysuria, fever, and meatal itching.

Other STIs, such as gonorrhea and NGU, need to be ruled out when chlamydia is suspected. In addition, differential diagnoses include urinary tract infection, yeast infection, and dermatitis.

Referral and Diagnostic Tests

Diagnosis of chlamydia is based on cultured secretions obtained from the infected area by swab. Physicians have found little benefit from serology for this diagnosis (Qureshi 2015).

Treatment and Return to Participation

Because chlamydia is often concurrent with gonorrhea and tends to persist after gonorrhea is successfully treated, physicians should evaluate and provide remedies for both diseases. Untreated, the disease can lead to infertility, PID, ectopic pregnancy, and chronic pelvic pain (Qureshi 2015). Chlamydia is resistant to penicillin and cephalosporins and must be treated with azithromycin, tetracycline, erythromycin, or doxycycline to be eradicated. The U.S. Preventive Services Task Force recommends routine screening of young women for chlamydia in an effort to prevent the sequelae that can follow the disease. Chlamydia is also a disease that must be reported to the local health authority in most states (Centers for Disease Control and Prevention 2015b).

Pathological Conditions Related to the Male Genitourinary System

Testicular Torsion

The testicle is covered by the tunica vaginalis, which attaches to the posterolateral surface of the testicle and allows for limited mobility. In the event that the testicle is able to twist or freely rotate (i.e., torsion; see figure 10.11), venous occlusion can occur, which subsequently leads to arterial ischemia, causing infarction of the testicle.

The incidence of testicular torsion in males younger than 25 is approximately 1 per 4,000. The highest incidence is among males aged 12 to 18, with a peak incidence at age 21 (Lu et al. 2015). Torsion predominantly affects the left testicle. Recall that typically, the left testicle lies slightly lower than the right. A subgroup of individuals has a higher frequency of testicular torsion because of an extremely narrow attachment of the epididymis to the tunica vaginalis (**bell clapper deformity**). This attachment allows the testicle to rotate freely on the spermatic cord within the scrotal sac. This congenital abnormality is found in as many as 12% of males. Testicular torsion can also occur after exercise, sexual activity, or trauma, or it may develop at rest. There are some studies (56 and 64 patients, respectively) that demonstrate that incidences of testicular torsion are higher in warmer temperatures, which suggests that colder weather has an effect on reducing the frequency of these types of injuries (Karakan et al. 2015; Gomes et al. 2015). Other than early identification of the bell clapper deformity, no preventive measures can prevent a testicular torsion. Wearing an athletic supporter or tighter fitting undergarments may lower the risk of torsion.

Signs and Symptoms

The history of testicular torsion includes the sudden onset of severe unilateral scrotal pain. The most common symptoms include scrotal swelling, abdominal pain, nausea, and vomiting. Younger patients may be reluctant to disclose scrotal pain, and they may present with lower abdominal pain (Rupp 2015). Less frequently a fever or urinary frequency may be documented. Examination of the scrotum reveals a tender and painful testicle that is

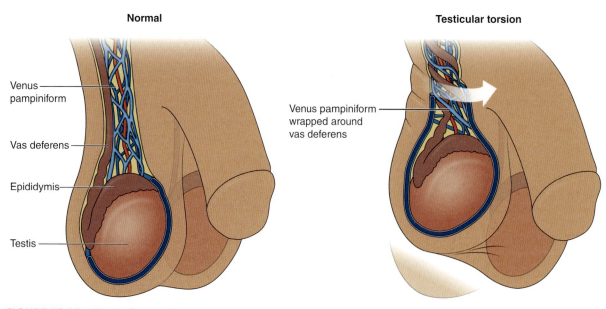

FIGURE 10.11   Testicular torsion.

Testicular Torsion in Youth

Adolescent and younger athletes often report vague thigh or knee pain when referring to testicular pain. Whether this is due to an inability or unwillingness to focus on their testicle issue, athletic trainers need to keep an index of suspicion for testicular torsion if athletes have a mechanism consistent with this trauma. This is especially true in the absence of clinical findings of thigh or knee pathology.

often elevated in relationship to the contralateral testicle. The involved testicle often is in a horizontal position rather than its usual vertical orientation. The testicle may be enlarged with scrotal swelling and erythema. In general, elevation of the involved testicle provides no relief of pain as compared with epididymitis, in which pain relief is notable with elevation of the involved testicle.

Referral and Diagnostic Tests

Testicular torsion is a urological emergency. Patient history and physical examination may not confirm testicular torsion, and imaging studies (including ultrasonography and nuclear scans) may be helpful in confirming the diagnosis (Rupp 2015).

The possibility of testicular torsion requires immediate and emergent evaluation by the team physician or immediate referral to an emergency department. Diagnosis and treatment within 6 h of the onset of pain result in an 80% to 100% salvage rate for the affected testicle. Beyond this time frame, the salvage rate steadily decreases and approaches 0% at 12 h (Tajchner, Larkin, and Bourke 2009).

RED FLAGS FOR TESTICULAR TORSION

Testicular torsion is a urological emergency requiring emergent medical attention. It presents as follows:

- Scrotal swelling
- Abdominal pain
- Nausea and vomiting
- Tender testicle
- Elevated testicle compared with uninvolved one
- Possible horizontal rather than vertical orientation

Imaging studies can provide useful information, but because testicular torsion is a clinical diagnosis, treatment should not be delayed for imaging if the diagnosis is clear. For those cases in which the diagnosis is less clear, color Doppler ultrasonography can be performed (Baldisserotto 2009; Yusuf and Sidhu 2013; Barkin, Rosenberg, and Miner 2014; Liang et al. 2013). A color Doppler is used to assess arterial blood flow to the testicle. A radionuclide scan can also be performed to assess arterial blood flow, with decreased uptake indicating a lack of blood flow to the testicle.

Because testicular torsion is a urological emergency, there is little room for error in diagnosis. The differential diagnoses, however, should include epididymitis, orchitis, hydrocele, varicocele, a hernia, and acute appendicitis. Traumatic hematoma and testicular carcinoma should also be considered differential diagnoses for testicular torsion (Liang et al. 2013; Lu et al. 2015).

Treatment and Return to Participation

Early diagnosis and referral are the keys to successful treatment. Once testicular torsion is diagnosed, a manual reduction can be attempted by the physician. Because most testicular torsion involves a "turning in" toward the midline, the process of detorsion involves rotating the affected testicle 180° from medial to lateral. The physician may need to repeat the rotation two or three times for a complete detorsion. Success is determined by a marked decrease in pain. Detorsion can be accomplished manually in 25% to 80% of affected individuals (Rupp 2015; Liang et al. 2013). If manual detorsion is not successful, surgery is indicated for definitive treatment and involves detorsion and orchiopexy, which is surgical fixation of the testicle.

The prognosis for testicular torsion depends on rapid referral and diagnosis. If detorsion is obtained within 6 h of the onset of symptoms, nearly 100% of torsive testicles can be salvaged. A delay in treatment up to 12 h results in decreasing rates of salvage. Return to participation is based on the result of the torsion and physician clearance.

Hydrocele

Hydroceles are fluid collections within the tunica vaginalis of the scrotum or along the spermatic cord (figure 10.12). Most hydroceles are developmental in origin because of persistence of a patent processus vaginalis. However, for unknown reasons, hydroceles can also develop as a result of an imbalance between scrotal fluid production and absorption. It is estimated that approximately 6% of adult males have a clinically apparent hydrocele.

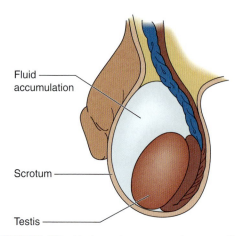

FIGURE 10.12   Hydrocele is a painless swelling in the scrotum.

Signs and Symptoms

Hydroceles are usually asymptomatic. Increased fluid collections, however, can cause a scrotal aching. A hydrocele typically manifests itself as a nontender fullness in the hemiscrotum and is palpable just anterior to the testicle. They can be congenital, and they may also resolve spontaneously (Porter and Kaplan 2011). Inability to clearly delineate or palpate the testicular structures or the presence of tenderness raises the possibility of an alternative diagnosis.

Both hydroceles and varicoceles are differential diagnoses for each other. In addition, the differential diagnoses include the following:

- Epididymitis
- Orchitis
- Testicular tumor
- Testicular torsion

For hydrocele, another differential diagnosis is an inguinal hernia. For varicocele, another differential diagnosis is spermatic vein compression.

Referral and Diagnostic Tests

Athletic trainers should immediately refer any male with painful scrotal swelling to a physician. Although a hydrocele is not an emergency, nontender scrotal swelling that is consistent with a hydrocele needs to be examined by a physician to document its presence. An experienced physician can confirm the diagnosis of a hydrocele. An ultrasound may be performed to confirm the diagnosis in some cases (Barkin, Rosenberg, and Miner 2014).

Treatment and Return to Participation

Asymptomatic adults with an isolated hydrocele can be observed indefinitely or until they become symptomatic.

Surgical intervention is warranted for the following indications: inability to distinguish hydrocele from an inguinal hernia, failure to resolve spontaneously after an appropriate interval of observation, inability to clearly examine the testes, or association of hydroceles with suggestive pathology, such as testicular torsion or tumor (Barkin, Rosenberg, and Miner 2014). Return to sport may take 2 to 6 wk after a simple hydrocele repair.

The presence of a hydrocele does not preclude participation in athletics. If the hydrocele is symptomatic or has been surgically repaired, the treating physician will need to make a decision regarding return to play.

Varicocele

A varicocele is a dilation of the pampiniform venous plexus and the internal spermatic vein within the scrotum (figure 10.13). The etiology of a varicocele is unclear. Varicoceles occur in approximately 20% of the adult male population; however, about 40% of infertile men may have a varicocele (White 2015).

Signs and Symptoms

Approximately 80% to 90% of varicoceles occur on the left side of the scrotum because of anatomical vascular differences (White 2015). Men are generally asymptomatic but will occasionally report an aching pain or heaviness in the scrotum. Physical examination demonstrates a soft thickening just above the testicle and has been described as feeling like a "bag of worms." Radiological testing discovered bilateral varicoceles in 35% to 40% of men with a unilateral palpable varicocele (White 2015). Varicoceles are staged according to size:

- *Large:* Those easily identified by inspection alone
- *Moderate:* Those identified by palpation without Valsalva maneuver
- *Small:* Those identified by palpation, using Valsalva maneuver to increase intraabdominal

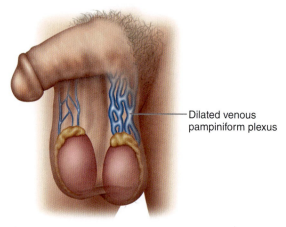

FIGURE 10.13   Varicocele in the spermatic cord.

pressure, which will impede venous drainage and increase varicocele size

Referral and Diagnostic Tests

The development of a new varicocele or sudden onset of testicular swelling or pain requires immediate physician evaluation. Any male athlete with a known varicocele who develops increasing testicular pain also warrants physician evaluation. Referral to a urologist for a surgical opinion is indicated when there is significant testicular pain, impairment of testicular function as evidenced by decreased semen quality, or testicular atrophy (volume <20 ml or length <4 cm) (Roque and Esteves 2016).

The diagnosis of a varicocele is typically clear by physical examination; Valsalva maneuver may aid diagnosis (figure 10.14). If the physical examination is equivocal, a Doppler ultrasonogram may be performed to demonstrate the varicocele. Athletes who have a new or sudden-onset varicocele or a nonreducible varicocele in the recumbent position may warrant abdominal CT to evaluate for renal or vascular pathology as a cause of spermatic vein compression (Roque and Esteves 2016).

Treatment and Return to Participation

There is no medical treatment per se for an asymptomatic varicocele. Surgical treatment via laparoscopy, if warranted, involves the ligation of the involved veins in order to prevent continued abnormal blood flow.

The presence of a varicocele poses no known risks to the athlete involved in individual or team sports. After surgical correction of a varicocele, return to play is generally within 2 to 6 wk but will depend on the circumstances for the athlete and the recommendations of the surgeon. The use of a protective cup is recommended for involvement in contact or collision sports if early return is allowed (White 2015).

Testicular Cancer

Testicular cancer is an abnormal growth of cells in the testicles. It accounts for 1% to 2% of all cancers in men and typically affects a single testicle. Because of the high cure rate if diagnosed early, most men with this cancer are cured. Although the number of new cases of testicular cancer has risen steadily since 1975, so too has the survival rate, which is now 95% (National Cancer Institute 2015).

Testicular cancer typically affects men between the ages of 16 and 44. According to the National Cancer Institute, statistics indicated that in 2015, about 8,430 men were diagnosed with testicular cancer but only 380 would die of the disease (National Cancer Institute 2015). Caucasian men experienced the largest increase in incidence. Asian and African-American populations have a low incidence of testicular cancer. The average age at diagnosis is 33 (National Cancer Institute 2015). There is increasing evidence that there may be a slight genetic component to this cancer (Greene, Kratz, and Mai 2010). Conditions that are associated with an increased risk of testicular cancer include cryptorchidism (i.e., failure of one or both testicles to descend into the scrotum during development), family history of testicular cancer, maternal exposure to diethylstilbestrol (DES) while pregnant, testicular atrophy, and some possible environmental and drug exposures (Greene, Kratz, and Mai 2010; National Cancer Institute 2015).

Signs and Symptoms

Any new or unexpected change in the testicles should prompt an evaluation by a physician. The most common findings noted by the athlete or during the testicular self-examination include a painless swelling (58%), a growth (27%), or pain in the testicle (33%). Less commonly, a sense of heaviness or prolonged aching in the testicles may be noted. Rarely, breast tenderness (3%)

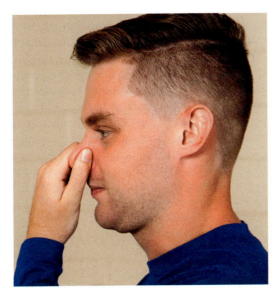

FIGURE 10.14 In Valsalva maneuver the athlete is asked to exhale against a closed epiglottis (bearing down).

> ⚑ **RED FLAGS FOR TESTICULAR CANCER**
>
> - Painless testicular swelling
> - Testicular growth
> - Painful testicle

may occur as the initial sign and is the result of hormonal changes caused by the cancer.

Referral and Diagnostic Tests

Any male with an abnormal testicular examination, a new painless testicular growth, swelling, or testicular pain should be referred to the team physician for further evaluation. Physical examination of the testicles by the athlete or a physician can determine whether a palpable mass or swelling is present. An ultrasound of the scrotum and testicles is then performed to document the presence or absence of an abnormality. Confirmatory testing is by tissue diagnosis that is most commonly obtained by radical orchiectomy (i.e., surgical removal of the testicle and spermatic cord). In the presence of testicular cancer, a chest radiograph and CT of the abdomen and pelvis are performed to evaluate for metastatic spread of the disease.

The differential diagnoses for testicular cancer include orchitis, epididymitis, hydrocele, and varicocele.

Treatment and Return to Participation

The initial treatment for testicular cancer is a radical orchiectomy involving the testicle and spermatic cord. Therapy is then based on tumor type (i.e., **seminoma**, nonseminoma, or other), microscopic appearance, location and extension of the tumor, and both physician and patient preference. Treatment options include chemotherapy, radiation therapy, and surgical resection of lymph node (Greene, Kratz, and Mai 2010; Travis et al. 2014). Men undergoing orchiectomy are often counseled to consider sperm banking because radiotherapy or chemotherapy can have long-term effects on testicular function. Overall treatment success is high for testicular cancer. Follow-up care is essential, is based on tumor type, and involves periodic chest radiographs, CT scans, and blood tests for tumor markers.

Cure rates for testicular cancer are high, ranging from greater than 80% for more disseminated cancers to nearly 100% for cancers localized to the testicle. During treatment, individual participation in athletics may be limited because of pain or discomfort from the treatment. Specific decisions about the degree of involvement in athletics will need to be made by the treating physician in conjunction with the athlete. After complete recovery, patients can obtain a testicular prosthesis via surgical implantation. After successful treatment of testicular cancer, there are no contraindications to participation in athletics, although the use of a support cup is recommended in contact or collision sports to protect the remaining testicle.

Prevention

There is no known way to prevent testicular cancer. Recommendations are for men (particularly those ages

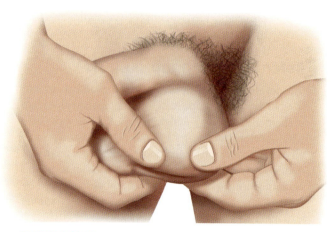

FIGURE 10.15 Testicular self-examination.

16 to 44) to perform monthly testicular self-examinations (TSE). These consist of examining and palpating the scrotum for lumps or swelling and bringing any abnormality to a physician's attention. Here is how to complete a TSE:

- Stand in front of a mirror and look for scrotal swelling.
- Examine each testicle individually with both hands, fingers under the testicle, while rolling the testicle gently with the thumbs, palpating for lumps or swelling (figure 10.15).
- Palpate the epididymis superior and posterior to each testicle.
- Perform once each month, preferably after a shower; the heat of the shower will enable the scrotal skin to relax and be more pliable.

A monthly testicular self-examination can help in the early recognition and diagnosis of testicular cancer, thereby improving overall survival (Travis et al. 2014). In a large international systematic review, researchers discovered that few men were informed about the danger of testicular cancer and fewer performed regular TSEs (Saab, Landers, and Hegarty 2016). Specifically, they reported that African-Americans were the least knowledgeable about testicular cancer and TSEs. In their report, they cite education as paramount to prevention, and they note that organizations can assist with education. The Testicular Cancer Awareness Foundation used 89% of its funding to educate young men to perform routine self-exams (Saab, Landers, and Hegarty 2016).

Prostate Cancer

As discussed at the beginning of this chapter, the prostate gland is responsible for contributing to the seminal fluid and is located directly anterior to the rectum (see figure 10.4). Prostate cancer is an abnormal growth of cells within the prostate gland. It is the second leading cause of cancer deaths for men in the United States, and African-American men have a higher death rate from this cancer than those in all other racial groups (Centers for Disease Control and Prevention 2016). The incidence of prostate cancer increases with age, with an estimate that 1 in 10 men will develop prostate cancer in his lifetime. Risk factors for the development of prostate cancer include advancing age, a family history of prostate cancer, and race (Centers for Disease Control and Prevention 2016; Heidenreich et al. 2014). Since 2002, the incidence of prostate cancer and its death rate have steadily and significantly decreased (Centers for Disease Control and Prevention 2016).

Prostate cancer prevention involves risk factor modification and regular prostate screening. Men at risk for the development of prostate cancer should consider diets low in animal fats and chromium, regular exercise, and digital rectal examinations every year starting at age 40.

Signs and Symptoms

No reliable signs or symptoms suggest the early presence of prostate cancer. Advanced or metastatic prostate cancer may result in fatigue associated with anemia, weight loss, hematuria, urinary retention (caused by obstruction), urinary incontinence, back pain, pathological fractures, or spinal cord compression.

Conditions that involve the prostate gland and should be excluded when determining if the patient has prostate cancer include benign prostatic hypertrophy, both acute and chronic prostatitis, **prostatic calculi**, prostate cysts, and **prostatic tuberculosis**. Other cancers that can mimic prostate cancer include lymphomas.

Referral and Diagnostic Tests

Any male athlete suspected of having prostate cancer should be referred to his physician, and any male athlete over age 40 is encouraged to obtain a yearly digital rectal examination.

The early diagnosis of prostate cancer is based on a medical history, physical examination that includes a digital rectal examination (DRE) in order to palpate the prostate, and, if enlarged, a serum **prostate-specific antigen (PSA)** test. It is worth mentioning that the upper limit of normal for PSA is related to age, and elevated PSA levels may not always be present in relatively higher-grade prostate cancers. It should be noted that the PSA test has a 75% sensitivity but only a 40% specificity for detecting prostate cancer (Barkin, Rosenberg, and Miner 2014). Both malignant and benign cells are produced by PSA, and there is growing evidence that PSA alone

is not a strong indicator of prostate cancer; if it is used, it must be confirmed by other diagnostic tests specific for prostate cancer (Barkin, Rosenberg, and Miner 2014; Heidenreich et al. 2014; Adami 2010; Denham, Bender, and Paradics 2010). In itself, elevated PSA could indicate prostatitis, UTI, recent sexual activity, or a recent, vigorous DRE (Barkin, Rosenberg, and Miner 2014).

When cancer is suspected, an ultrasound examination with a transrectal needle biopsy can often provide a definitive tissue diagnosis. Once prostate cancer is diagnosed, further testing and imaging for staging of the cancer are performed. These tests generally include complete blood count, serum chemistries, liver function tests, PSA, free PSA to total PSA ratio, alkaline phosphatase, and urinalysis. Imaging studies can include chest radiographs, CT or magnetic resonance imaging (MRI) of the abdomen and pelvis, ProstaScint scan (i.e., immunoscintigraphy used to detect extraprostatic spread), and bone scan.

Treatment and Return to Participation

The treatment strategies for prostate cancer are changing with new advances. Treatment options include surgical removal (prostatectomy), radiation, radiation via external or internal radioactive seeds implanted into the prostate gland, and hormone therapy. At present, general recommendations favor early versus delayed treatment and radiation or hormone therapy for locally advanced prostate cancer, depending on the stage of the cancer. In lower stages, the treatment may be *active surveillance*, whereby the patient is monitored and only treated if his cancer causes symptoms or grows (Centers for Disease Control and Prevention 2016). The management of metastatic prostate cancer involves the addition of palliative radiation therapy to sites of painful metastases. Specific treatment regimens will be outlined for the athlete by his physician.

Mortality rates from prostate cancer are declining in the United States. Early diagnosis can lead to the detection of prostate cancer confined to the prostate gland and subsequently improve survival (Centers for Disease Control and Prevention 2016). The overall prognosis in terms of survival is related to tumor size, lymph node involvement, and the presence or absence of metastases. For small cancers, localized within the prostate gland itself, overall survival is excellent, and a cure may be expected. In contrast, the 10 yr survival rate for men with aggressive cancers that have metastasized is 25% (Centers for Disease Control and Prevention 2016).

Athletes may return to play during treatment for prostate cancer if they feel well and experience no significant side effects from their treatment regimen.

Pathological Conditions of the Gynecological System

Vaginitis

Vaginitis is an inflammation, usually derived from infection, of the vagina. Vaginitis can also be due to a fungal condition or caused by an estrogen deficiency (Ferri 2016). In the sexually active athlete, bacterial vaginosis (BV), trichomoniasis, and candidiasis are three common conditions that may account for 90% of all cases of vaginitis (Ferri 2016).

The normal vaginal environment is relatively stable. The high estrogen levels in women of childbearing age help protect the vagina by increasing vaginal thickness. Bacteria are an important component of this environment and help to maintain an acidic pH (Porter and Kaplan 2011). An abnormality or disruption in this system can create an environment that allows for the growth of pathogens and subsequent infection. Examples may include frequent douching, antibiotics or certain other medications, intercourse, foreign objects in the vagina, STIs, and pregnancy. Chemicals or foreign objects can also cause inflammation of the vagina. In addition, wearing certain undergarments (i.e., thongs) can transport bacteria from the anus, thereby introducing foreign bacteria to the vagina.

Bacterial vaginosis occurs when the normal balance of bacteria in the vagina is disrupted. A shift in the dominance or overgrowth of certain bacteria causes symptoms. This is not an STI, but it may be more common in sexually experienced persons, and it may occur secondary to sexual intercourse, which can change the vaginal environment.

Candidiasis also is not an STI, but it is more common than BV in the sexually naive person. Candidiasis is often called a yeast infection; women with diabetes or who are immunocompromised are at greater risk. Other risk factors may include pregnancy, obesity, and wearing nonbreathable or close-fitting underwear.

For **trichomoniasis**, an STI, prevention consists of abstinence from sexual intercourse or protection with a condom. The prevention of vaginitis caused by BV or *Candida* is aided by the promotion of a normal vaginal environment, which is facilitated by avoidance of douching, wearing breathable cotton underwear, and the use of condoms during intercourse.

Signs and Symptoms

Vaginal discharge is a common symptom in vaginitis. However, the description of the discharge differs depending on the cause. BV discharge is typically thin, white, or gray in color, and malodorous. The athlete may also experience vaginal itching.

An athlete with a *Trichomonas* infection may not have any symptoms, but a discharge described as thick, frothy, and green or yellow is not uncommon. The athlete may experience vaginal itching or discomfort with voiding, although this does not occur in most cases.

Last, athletes with candidiasis or fungal vaginitis may experience a thick white discharge resembling cottage cheese that is associated with itching or burning. This may also involve the vulva and surrounding skin and is thus termed vulvovaginitis (Ferri 2016).

The differential diagnosis for an athlete with vaginal discharge includes STIs. Other causes of vaginal inflammation include contact dermatitis, in which the skin reacts to some chemical or object that has come in contact with it; a retained foreign object, such as toilet tissue, tampon, or condom; chemical irritants; and much less commonly a neoplasm, such as cervical or vaginal cancer.

Referral and Diagnostic Tests

Any athlete with vaginitis benefits from referral to a physician because diagnosis requires a pelvic examination, and treatment typically involves prescription medication.

Initially, a sexually active athlete with vaginal discharge is evaluated for STIs in general. The diagnosis of the common causes for vaginitis involves sampling the discharge or vaginal fluid, measuring the pH of the secretions, and performing microscopic examination of the vaginal fluid. Trichomonads can be seen microscopically and are described as "swimming" on the slide. Microscopic findings for BV include "clue cells," which are vacuolated epithelial cells. Demonstration of pseudohyphae and budding yeast on a potassium hydroxide (KOH) preparation suggests candidiasis.

Another diagnostic tool, in which KOH is added to the sample, is called the whiff test. If the discharge is due to BV, a particular fishy odor may be noted. Measurement of the vaginal pH is also helpful with diagnosis. BV and trichomoniasis tend to occur when the pH is less acidic (>4.5). Other, more sophisticated tests are available but not necessarily needed for the diagnosis.

Treatment and Return to Participation

Metronidazole is used to treat both BV and trichomoniasis. The athlete must abstain from alcohol while taking the medication because the combination can cause nausea and vomiting. Treatment for vulvovaginal candidiasis includes the use of antifungal agents, either oral or topical, many of which are available over the counter (Ferri 2016) (see chapter 5). On occasion, vaginitis of fungal origin is resistant to initial therapy, and further evaluation and treatment are required. Including yogurt with active cultures in the diet can help with certain cases of vaginitis, such as those related to an athlete taking antibiotics, because yogurt helps promote stabilization of the normal bacterial flora. Partners of those found to have a *Trichomonas* infection also need to receive treatment to prevent further spread.

The prognosis is good for common causes of vaginitis, and interference with athletic activity is not typical; therefore return to play is not usually delayed. Problems related to BV and trichomoniasis, however, can occur during pregnancy and may include the risk of premature labor and premature rupture of membranes. In addition, athletes with frequently recurring vulvovaginitis may have an underlying disorder, such as diabetes or a compromised immune system, although other systemic symptoms or complaints would likely be present in these cases.

Special Concerns

None of these causes of vaginitis are reportable to a public agency; however, a partner of an athlete with trichomoniasis must be treated for the disease in order to prevent its spread or recurrence.

It is especially important to treat vaginitis caused by BV or trichomoniasis in the pregnant female because it may place her at risk for complications such as premature labor. Complications can be prevented by prompt diagnosis and treatment. The health care provider must encourage any athlete with recurrent or chronic vaginitis that resists treatment to be carefully evaluated for underlying causes to ensure that she is receiving the proper treatment.

Pelvic Inflammatory Disease

In generally accepted terms, primary pelvic inflammatory disease (PID) is defined as a bacterial infection of the upper genital tract that originates in and ascends from the lower genital tract (figure 10.16). It includes a host of inflammatory disorders such as endometritis, salpingitis, and many sexually transmitted infections (Centers for Disease Control and Prevention 2015e). Sites of inflammation or infection include the endometrium, perimetrium, fallopian tubes, ovaries, and pelvic peritoneum. These infections usually are a result of sexually transmitted organisms, such as *Chlamydia trachomatis* and *Neisseria gonorrhoeae*.

Signs and Symptoms

The signs and symptoms of PID vary over a large spectrum, from mild or relatively few symptoms to severe symptoms. Diagnosing even the mildest cases is important, however, because sequelae from this disease can be problematic. Typically, symptoms begin within the first couple of weeks after menses, and subtle findings can include abnormal vaginal bleeding or **dyspareunia** (i.e., painful intercourse). Because no examination finding or laboratory test is optimal in diagnosing PID, the Centers for Disease Control and Prevention (CDC) list the following minimal criteria: lower abdominal tenderness, **adnexal** tenderness, and cervix motion tenderness without evidence of a different, obvious source (Centers for Disease Control and Prevention 2015e).

To further clarify diagnosis, the CDC also includes the following: fever above 38.3 °C (101 °F); elevated

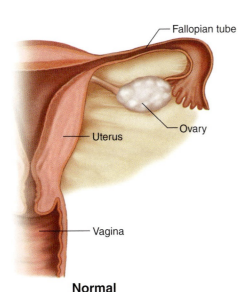

Normal

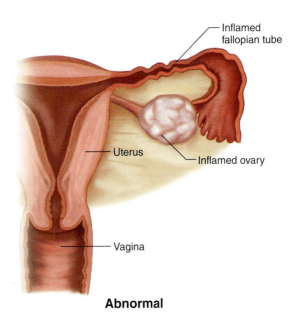

Abnormal

FIGURE 10.16 Pelvic inflammatory disease.

erythrocyte sedimentation rate (ESR); elevated C-reactive protein (CRP); the presence of leukocytes on a saline preparation of vaginal secretions; abnormal cervical or vaginal discharge, particularly mucopurulent discharge; and documented cervical infection with *Neisseria gonorrhoeae* or *Chlamydia trachomatis*. More definitive answers may require surgical sampling of tissue, which is not without its own risks and can lead to false-negative results.

The differential diagnosis of a female athlete thought to have PID may include inflammation or infection that has occurred in close proximity to the upper genital tract. Appendicitis, classically described as periumbilical pain that radiates to the right lower quadrant, is another process that is typically diagnosed clinically and may be entertained as a possible cause of symptoms. This, however, would have no particular relationship to menses, and such a diagnosis would be more likely for someone with anorexia, nausea, and vomiting without symptoms of PID. Other possibilities include, but are not limited to, tubal pregnancy, corpus luteal cyst, endometriosis, mittelschmerz (typically described as a dull pain of short duration at mid-cycle), gastroenteritis, and lymphadenitis of the intestinal lymph nodes. A careful history of symptoms, including fever, genitourinary complaints, and onset of pain, especially in relation to the menstrual cycle, and an evaluation for risk factors can provide useful information in the diagnosis of PID.

Referral and Diagnostic Tests

Symptoms or a health history that raises suspicion for PID warrants urgent referral to a physician. If appendicitis or other emergent surgical problems are suspected, immediate referral to a physician or emergency department is necessary.

Every female athlete of reproductive age presenting with pelvic complaints or symptoms requires a pregnancy test to evaluate the possibility of pregnancy. Because of the varying presence of signs and symptoms, it is prudent to obtain a urinalysis to evaluate for urinary tract problems. Other specific tests include a cervical or vaginal

smear to be evaluated for the presence of leukocytes, overwhelming bacterial load, or trichomonads and possibly a Gram stain to identify specific organisms. A cervical culture for gonorrhea and chlamydia is performed. Blood tests with a CBC and differential, ESR, and CRP also are performed. If the diagnosis is unclear, a pelvic ultrasound may be performed to evaluate for other abnormalities (Centers for Disease Control and Prevention 2015e).

Treatment and Return to Participation

Treatment of PID must be initiated as soon as the diagnosis is made to prevent long-term sequelae. Assigning the most appropriate antibiotics for the specific condition is critical, but health care providers must also take into account patient compliance and accessibility and affordability of the chosen medication (Centers for Disease Control and Prevention 2015e). Inpatient versus outpatient setting is controversial; however, it is generally accepted that certain patients need to be treated in a hospital setting:

- Patients who require surgical intervention for an ectopic pregnancy or abscess that requires drainage
- Pregnant patients
- Patients not responding to outpatient therapy
- Patients noncompliant with therapy or follow-up within 48 to 72 h
- Patients who are immunocompromised

Medical treatment for PID includes antibacterials (Duarte, Fuhrich, and Ross 2015). Chapter 5 lists outpatient and inpatient medications geared toward treating the most common bacterial organisms.

The prompt diagnosis and treatment of PID are crucial because of the sequelae, which include infertility, increased risk of ectopic pregnancy, recurrent infections, and chronic pelvic pain. The risk of infertility is relatively high, increases with subsequent infections, and depends on the severity of the infection and therefore the time between infection and initiation of treatment.

Before return-to-sport participation by the affected athlete, adequate antibiotic therapy is instituted, fever is resolved, nausea and vomiting are rectified to ensure adequate hydration status, and pelvic or abdominal pain is minimized. If a surgical procedure was performed, the surgeon will determine when return to activity will be allowed.

Prevention

Early diagnosis is important but is not nearly as crucial as prevention. Athletes, both male and female, should understand the problems associated with PID

🚩 **RED FLAGS FOR PELVIC INFLAMMATORY DISEASE**

Female athletes with any of the following signs or symptoms should be referred to a physician:

- Abnormal vaginal bleeding
- Lower abdominal tenderness
- Fever
- Abnormal vaginal discharge
- Amenorrhea (3 mo or more)

and the importance of preventing the transmission of STIs, especially in light of the fact that many who have *Neisseria gonorrhoeae* or *Chlamydia trachomatis* may be asymptomatic. The only proven method to prevent the transmission of many STIs, besides abstinence, is a correctly used condom. It should also be noted that intrauterine devices and douching may actually increase a woman's risk for disease.

Special Concerns

An athlete who is diagnosed with PID should be tested for other STIs, notably HIV and syphilis, and advised to receive hepatitis B vaccinations if she has not been previously immunized. A Pap smear also is performed to look for pathological changes caused by human papillomavirus (HPV). In addition, the athlete's sexual partner(s) need to be evaluated for gonorrhea and chlamydia infection and treated if there was sexual contact within 60 d of the patient's symptoms. The athlete should abstain from sexual activity until fully treated. Follow-up testing in 4 to 6 wk for gonorrhea and chlamydia may be warranted and recommended by the physician (Ferri 2016; Centers for Disease Control and Prevention 2015e). Last, information about STIs and their prevention needs to be made available to all athletes, and adherence to safe sex practices is encouraged.

Dysmenorrhea

Dysmenorrhea is described as severe cramps and pain associated with menstruation or painful menstruation and is categorized as either primary or secondary. Primary dysmenorrhea is not associated with gross pathology but rather involves a type of prostaglandin that acts to constrict blood vessels in the uterus, causing ischemia and subsequently painful uterine contractions during menstruation. It is a common gynecological condition, found in 45% to 95% of menstruating women (Iacovides, Avidon, and Baker 2015).

Secondary dysmenorrhea, by contrast, is caused by a gross pathological process involving the uterus. This can include endometriosis—in which endometrial tissue is found outside the uterus—PID, uterine fibroids or polyps, pelvic tumors, ectopic pregnancy, and spontaneous abortion. In these cases, the painful uterine contractions are a result of the associated condition.

Signs and Symptoms

Primary dysmenorrhea may be more common in the first few years after menarche and in those whose gravity and parity status is low. The athlete may also have a significant family history for this condition. In addition, smoking, early menarche, and a history of heavy flow and long menstrual periods may be risk factors associated with more severe dysmenorrhea. Symptoms may include not only cramping of the lower abdomen or back, with occasional radiating pain to the thighs, but also nausea, vomiting, diarrhea, headaches, and other systemic problems. The pain and associated symptoms typically begin just before or at the onset of menses and last through the first day or two of menstruation. Physical examination yields no obvious pathology. Dysmenorrhea was highly correlated with absenteeism in school for adolescent girls, and missing class or practice on a reasonably monthly schedule could indicate a suspicion for this condition (Zannoli et al. 2014). In a critical review of the literature, authors found that, compared with women without dysmenorrhea, women with primary dysmenorrhea had a diminished capacity for pain and were at risk for other chronic pain conditions later in life (Iacovides, Avidon, and Baker 2015; Grandi et al. 2013).

Secondary dysmenorrhea may not be as closely tied to the onset of menses, and symptoms last for a longer time but may still have some relation to the menstrual cycle. Physical examination may or may not provide an etiology, and symptoms may vary depending on the underlying pathology. If an athlete has been diagnosed with primary dysmenorrhea and treatment, such as nonsteroidal anti-inflammatory agents or oral contraceptives, has failed, then a pathological cause must be considered, and the athlete should be reevaluated. It is important to listen to the athlete and get a good history of the frequency and quality of pain. In a study of 144 women with chronic pelvic pain who reported severe dysmenorrhea, 96 (66.7%) were found to have endometriosis (Apostolopoulos et al. 2015).

Differential diagnoses for dysmenorrhea include endometriosis, PID, uterine fibroids or polyps, pelvic tumors, ectopic pregnancy, or spontaneous abortion.

Referral and Diagnostic Tests

Athletes who experience severe menstrual pain, who have pertinent systemic complaints as mentioned previously, or who have abnormal menstruation need to be routinely referred to a physician for evaluation.

As always, a thorough history and physical examination are warranted with a presentation of dysmenorrhea. A careful health history of the patient's menstruation includes age of onset, length, frequency, flow, and regularity of cycling; sexual activity history; family history; and type and severity of associated symptoms. Any female being evaluated for dysmenorrhea warrants a pregnancy test, regardless of sexual history. Depending on the history and the physical examination, other diagnostic tests may be necessary. Options include pelvic ultrasound; laparoscopy, which is a direct visualization of the pelvic organs via a surgical procedure; hysteroscopy, which views the inside of the cervix and uterus with an endoscope; and radiological procedures. In some cases, tissue sampling or endometrial biopsy may be required for review by a pathologist.

Treatment and Return to Participation

The management of dysmenorrhea varies according to its etiology. For primary dysmenorrhea, nonsteroidal anti-inflammatory drugs (NSAIDs) as well as oral contraceptives have been the mainstay of treatment (Marjoribanks et al. 2015). NSAIDs should be taken just before the onset of menses and continued through the first few days of the menses. They function to decrease levels of the inciting prostaglandins. Oral contraceptives alone or in combination with NSAIDs can be beneficial. Patients should be cautioned about the long-term adverse effects of NSAIDs, as many athletes take them often for myriad ailments, not just during their menses. Adverse effects of oral contraceptives can include anorexia, thrombosis, nausea, depression, dizziness, weight change, nervousness, varicose veins, breakthrough bleeding, gallbladder disease, and cerebral hemorrhage, among other serious conditions. Risks of oral contraception increase with smoking, and oral contraceptives are contraindicated for patients with a history or family history of breast cancer, vascular diseases, or jaundice; these women should use alternative methods of birth control. Studies on the effects of oral hormones on young women's breast and cervical cancer risk are controversial (Samra-Latif 2015).

Treatment for secondary dysmenorrhea depends on the pathological etiology as previously discussed. Secondary dysmenorrhea should be considered in someone with primary dysmenorrhea who does not respond well to treatment. Older female athletes with dysmenorrhea are more likely to have a secondary or pathological cause for their discomfort and warrant close evaluation.

Dysmenorrhea can certainly be disabling to those affected; however, several treatment options exist for the varying etiologies, and prognosis generally is good. Sport participation may be limited only by the athlete's symptoms, unless the athlete is being treated for a certain pathological condition that may, as directed by the physician, exclude her from strenuous physical activity.

Prevention

There is no primary prevention for primary dysmenorrhea. Secondary prevention for primary dysmenorrhea stems from its treatment. Starting NSAIDs before menses, when pain would typically develop, or taking oral contraceptives lends itself to this secondary prevention. For secondary dysmenorrhea, only certain causes, such as PID and STIs, are preventable by employing safe-sex practices.

Amenorrhea

Amenorrhea is typically categorized as primary or secondary. Primary amenorrhea is classically defined as the absence of menarche (i.e., onset of menses) by age 16. Secondary amenorrhea is less well defined but alludes to the fact that a female's menstruation has stopped after having previously been normal. Depending on the source, secondary amenorrhea may be defined as either (1) the absence of menses for 3, 4, 6, or 12 mo in a previously menstruating female or (2) fewer than three menstrual cycles per year (Ferri 2016). To add further confusion, oligomenorrhea is used to describe menstrual cycles with intervals greater than 36 d but less than 90 d. Because the cause of oligomenorrhea is often the same as for amenorrhea, this section focuses mainly on amenorrhea with the knowledge that the discussion may apply to many cases of missed menstrual periods in general.

The cause of amenorrhea, both primary and secondary, is highly variable. To understand the various etiologies, a basic review of ovulation is necessary. The ovulatory pathway consists of the hypothalamic–pituitary axis, the ovaries, a feedback loop, the uterus, and a subsequent outflow tract. The hypothalamus secretes gonadotropin-releasing hormone (GnRH), which stimulates the pituitary gland to secrete follicle-stimulating hormone (FSH) and luteinizing hormone (LH). These hormones then stimulate the ovaries to produce estrogen and progesterone, which each directly affect the menstrual process (see figure 10.8). Low circulating levels of these hormones, in turn, directly feed back to the hypothalamus, causing it to produce more GnRH. One can therefore imagine both hormonal and anatomical problems that can interfere with normal ovulation.

The source of amenorrhea depends on the cause. In general terms, anatomical defects can occur that are congenital, genetic, or acquired. Ovarian failure can occur prematurely. Chronic anovulation or the absence of ovulation in the presence of estrogen, such as in **polycystic ovarian disease** or certain tumors, can occur. Chronic anovulation also can occur in the absence of estrogen or in **hypogonadism**, such as occurs with **athletic amenorrhea**, stress, anorexia nervosa, and pituitary tumors. Research has demonstrated that high-intensity training may delay the onset of menses and contribute to the cessation of menarche if the athlete has already begun menstruation (Rauh, Nichols, and Barrack 2010; Bonci et al. 2008; Mountjoy et al. 2014). Female athletes who display the combination of amenorrhea, disordered eating, and low bone density have a condition that used to be termed the *female triad*. The International Olympic Committee recently renamed this condition *relative energy deficiency in sport* (RED-S) because, except for amenorrhea, males suffer from the same energy-deficient condition that creates many medical issues for the athlete (Mountjoy et al. 2014).

Signs and Symptoms

Signs and symptoms of amenorrhea vary greatly and depend on the etiology of the amenorrhea. For primary amenorrhea, genetic disorders and anatomical abnormalities of the reproductive system must be considered. A classic example is a genetic defect called **Turner's syndrome**; patients with Turner's syndrome may present, in addition to primary amenorrhea, physical findings such as short stature, webbed neck, shield chest, increased carrying angle of the elbows, and other possible findings.

Problems with the outflow tract can also cause amenorrhea. If there is no exit path for the sloughed endometrial lining, then the athlete perceives there is no menses, but she may have severe cramping and pain from retained tissue and blood with each menstrual period. Obstruction can be congenital, such as an imperforate hymen or **labial agglutination**, or it can occur secondarily, such as with **uterine synechiae** or as seen in **Asherman's syndrome** scarring after a surgical procedure.

Proceeding further up the ovulatory chain, ovarian failure from various causes can lead to amenorrhea. It can be related to genetic defects, autoimmune disorders, or prior chemotherapy and can be associated with various symptoms. Not uncommonly, an athlete may have symptoms similar to those of menopausal women, such as hot flashes, vaginal dryness, and mood changes. The athlete may also have systemic symptoms common to particular autoimmune or endocrine disorders. For example, an athlete with hypothyroidism may exhibit fatigue, weight gain, constipation, or cold intolerance.

Problems with the hypothalamic–pituitary axis are varied as well. Deficient, absent, or inappropriate secretion of GnRH from the hypothalamus is common in female athletes, which in turn results in amenorrhea. Not all female athletes are affected, and some are at greater risk than others. The athlete's diet, her particular sport and level of activity, and her genetic composition may all contribute to athletic amenorrhea (Mountjoy et al. 2014; Bonci et al. 2008). Diagnosis of athletic amenorrhea is important because a hypoestrogenemic state, such as with athletic amenorrhea and ovarian failure, can adversely affect bone mineral density, leading to fractures. The athletic trainer needs to look for signs or symptoms of disordered eating in the evaluation of the athlete because this remains a common and well-described entity (see chapter 17) (Rauh, Nichols, and Barrack 2010; Bonci et al. 2008; Mountjoy et al. 2014).

Another potential cause for amenorrhea that involves the hypothalamic–pituitary axis is inhibition of GnRH by increased prolactin levels, which can occur as a result of a pituitary tumor that could have neurological manifestations, such as headaches and visual disturbances, as well as a complaint of galactorrhea. Polycystic ovary syndrome is a common condition that is manifested by findings such as **hyperandrogenism** (with associated acne and **hirsutism**), obesity, and hyperinsulinemia (Ferri 2016).

Referral and Diagnostic Tests

Athletes with primary amenorrhea are referred to a physician for a complete evaluation. An athlete who has had normal menstrual cycles but who misses three consecutive periods or who is oligomenorrheic needs to be evaluated by a physician. However, missing just one or two menses is not always benign, and one must not allow the number of missed menses to define the line between passiveness and concern.

The workup for amenorrhea involves assessment of the neuroendocrine system, genetics, anatomy of the athlete, and a pregnancy test. A complete medical history, including exercise, nutrition, and menstrual history, and a physical examination should be performed. Laboratory evaluation may include a urine pregnancy test and blood tests for thyroid-stimulating hormone (TSH), FSH, estradiol, and prolactin. Testing for levels of LH, dehydroepiandrosterone (DHEA), and testosterone may be indicated depending on the history and physical examination. In addition, the physician may elect to perform a progestin challenge to see if the endometrium has been primed by estrogen and if there is a patent outflow tract. With proper estrogen priming of the endometrium, its lining should slough after withdrawal of progesterone, as it would with normal menstruation.

Other laboratory evaluations may include karyotyping to check for any chromosomal abnormalities. This will also provide evidence of the presence or absence of a Y chromosome. Depending on the history, laboratory, and examination findings, neuroimaging may be helpful to look for an intracranial mass, specifically involving the pituitary. Other imaging may include evaluation of the reproductive tract and the gonads.

A bone density assessment should be considered in all female athletes with a prolonged history of oligomenorrhea or more than 6 mo of amenorrhea, particularly in those with a history of disordered eating (Mountjoy et al. 2014; Gamboa et al. 2008; Bonci et al. 2008).

Treatment and Return to Participation

The treatment of amenorrhea depends on its etiology and the sequelae one is trying to eliminate or prevent. One such problem is low bone mineral density or other effects of a hypoestrogenemic state. Treatment may consist of dietary changes to improve overall energy balance, hormone replacement therapy, and a decrease in the athlete's activity level (Bonci et al. 2008). In some causes of amenorrhea, surgery could be required, such as for an athlete with a pituitary tumor or an outflow tract abnormality. Treatment for polycystic ovarian disease may include oral birth control pills and medications to control the **hyperinsulinemia**. Knowing the underlying cause of the amenorrhea is the key in determining treatment (Hilibrand et al. 2015; Bonci et al. 2008).

In the case of athletic amenorrhea, treatment involves both pharmacological and nonpharmacological measures. Oral contraceptives are the mainstay of pharmacological treatment for athletic amenorrhea and should be strongly considered if nonpharmacological measures fail. In the presence of either osteopenia or osteoporosis, nasal calcitonin should be considered. Neither bisphosphonates nor selective estrogen receptor modulators (SERMs) have been well studied in young premenopausal women. Nonpharmacological measures include dietary changes and adjustments in physical activity in order to promote an overall positive energy balance, daily calcium and vitamin D supplements, nutrition counseling, and screening or treatment for disordered eating (Mountjoy et al. 2014; Gamboa et al. 2008; Rauh, Nichols, and Barrack 2010).

As with treatment, prognosis relies on the etiology of amenorrhea. The concern for female athletes with amenorrhea caused by low gonadotropin stimulation is the increased risk for low bone mineral density and its sequelae, such as stress fractures. Correcting the underlying conditions, or providing hormone replacement when the cause of the hypoestrogenemia cannot be corrected, is important in trying to prevent adverse outcomes for the athlete.

Because the etiology of amenorrhea is broad, return-to-play recommendations for each type are not presented here. Rather, for female athletes with athletic amenorrhea, although there may be multiple contributing factors, an intense exercise routine can play a major role. Simply reducing the athlete's level of activity and ensuring an adequate and well-balanced diet may help the athlete to return to a regular menstrual pattern. Therefore, returning to play is not prohibited, but it may be limited, at least initially. Such decisions and treatment plans require the involvement and communication of the athlete, athletic trainer, physician, registered dietitian, coach, and perhaps a mental health provider (Bonci et al. 2008; Mountjoy et al. 2014).

Special Considerations

As discussed previously, special care must be taken when evaluating an athlete for amenorrhea because of its possible complications. In addition to medical intervention, changes in exercise routine may be required. Nutritional evaluation is also important, especially with athletic amenorrhea or in the presence of an eating disorder. The relevance of age in the return-to-play decision depends on the cause of the amenorrhea and required treatment.

Mittelschmerz

Mittelschmerz is pain secondary to ovulation and hence tends to occur at mid-cycle, also referred to as *intermenstrual pain* (O'Toole 2013). The pain associated with ovulation is thought to be due to fluid that is released from the ovary, along with the ovum, during ovulation. This fluid can be irritating to intraabdominal tissue and can cause pain for the female athlete.

Signs and Symptoms

Pain can vary from one person to another, and it can be sudden, severe, and sharp. The pain tends to be located in the lower abdomen, usually occurs on one side, and can be accompanied by light vaginal spotting (Porter and Kaplan 2011). This is probably secondary to the unilateral release of the ovum. The affected side may change from one month to the next. Typically, the pain will last minutes to hours and, occasionally, a day or two. Because mittelschmerz is related to ovulation, there will be a history of pain that occurs between menstrual periods.

Lower abdominal pain in a female athlete can pose a diagnostic dilemma because the differential diagnoses can be varied. However, as previously mentioned, a good history can be extremely useful. Certain signs or symptoms are considered serious; periumbilical or right lower quadrant pain associated with nausea, vomiting, or fever should always raise concern for appendicitis. A history (including sexual and menstrual data) along with a physical examination and possibly imaging and laboratory studies can help in diagnosing PID (see "Pelvic Inflammatory Disease"). Ectopic pregnancy may also be associated with lower abdominal pain and needs to be included in the differential diagnosis, especially if there is a history of PID or prior ectopic pregnancies. Endometriosis, UTI, kidney stones, constipation, and gastroenteritis should also be considered depending on history, onset, and symptoms.

Ovulation must be occurring for a diagnosis of mittelschmerz; therefore, it is not a diagnosis in an athlete who is no longer menstruating.

Referral and Diagnostic Tests

A female athlete who presents with new-onset lower abdominal pain or pelvic pain needs to be referred to a physician for evaluation. If the athlete's pain is associated with nausea, vomiting, or fever, she should be immediately referred to a physician. She should also be referred if the pain is prolonged (lasts more than 2 d), if the pain is severe or unrelieved by over-the-counter medications, or if there is a suspicion of pregnancy or an STI.

There is no diagnostic test for mittelschmerz; rather, it is a diagnosis of exclusion. A good health history, including menstrual history, is very helpful. Depending on the history and type of pain, a pelvic examination may be warranted to exclude other etiologies. On occasion imaging, such as ultrasound, can be helpful in looking at anatomy and ruling out certain structural causes. In addition, one should always have a low threshold for ordering a urine pregnancy test.

Treatment and Return to Participation

The standard treatment for mittelschmerz includes over-the-counter pain medications, such as NSAIDs and acetaminophen (Tylenol). Heating packs can alleviate some of the discomfort. Oral contraceptives prevent pain by preventing ovulation.

The prognosis for mittelschmerz is generally good, and athletic activity is not contraindicated. Although the pain is generally tolerable, it can be significant for some. The use of oral contraceptives has proven useful in relieving the pain of mittelschmerz (Kaunitz 1999). Again, pain unrelieved by standard medications may warrant referral to a physician.

Ovarian and Cervical Cancer

Ovarian cancer is a malignant cell growth originating from an ovary; it is the leading cause of death from a gynecological malignancy. Cervical cancer is a malignancy originating from the cervix and has significant morbidity and mortality as well. It is one of the most common cancers in females, and it has a high cure rate if detected early (American Cancer Society 2016).

Ovarian cancer is typically seen in older women, with symptoms usually presenting late in its course. Risk appears to be proportional to the number of times a woman ovulates. For example, women who have never had children are at increased risk. Oral contraceptives that prevent ovulation may decrease a woman's risk. Age is another factor and is related to the greater number of ovulatory cycles experienced. Other risks include family history, personal history of breast or colon cancer, and history of prolonged hormone replacement. The Mayo Clinic also identifies multiple sex partners, early sexual activity, STIs, cigarette smoking, and a weak immune system as possible risk factors for cervical cancer (Mayo Clinic 2016). Genetic predisposition is an important risk factor, especially with the *BRCA1* or *BRCA2* gene mutation.

Human papillomavirus (HPV) plays a significant role in the development of cervical cancer (Arends, Wyllie, and Bird 1990). Several HPV genotypes exist, but only a few are associated with cervical cancer. This may be why sexual activity plays an important role in the development of this malignancy. Risk factors include sexual activity beginning at a young age, a higher number of sexual partners, a history of other STIs, and smoking.

Signs and Symptoms

Signs and symptoms are not usually present with either ovarian or cervical cancer in the early stages because symptoms may occur only after the tumor has grown large enough to have some mass effect. Unfortunately, by this time, the tumor has likely metastasized to other sites. Symptoms may vary, depending on the size and location of the tumor and sites of metastasis. Gastrointestinal disturbances, such as constipation or diarrhea, may occur with either malignancy. A woman may also experience early satiety or unexplained weight changes. Vaginal bleeding and discomfort may occur with cervical cancer, as may urinary complaints. Extension of cervical cancer may obstruct lymphatic and venous drainage, causing lower extremity edema, perhaps unilaterally (Mayo Clinic 2016). Symptoms involving other organs depend on metastatic spread. Symptoms for either cancer can be nonspecific and of little diagnostic value.

Because the symptoms of ovarian or cervical cancer can be vague or nonspecific, the differential diagnoses can be broad. For both ovarian and cervical cancer, a definitive diagnosis is based on tissue biopsy. For ovarian cancer, a benign ovarian mass or complex cystic ovarian disease is considered in the differential diagnosis, as is localized spread of cancer from surrounding tissues. The differential diagnoses for cervical cancer include severe cervical dysplasia, vaginal dysplasia or cancer, and uterine cancer with localized spread to the cervix.

Referral and Diagnostic Tests

Any suspicion of malignancy requires referral to a physician for evaluation. An athlete with a past history of or family history of malignancy and with unexplained symptoms as previously described needs to be referred. In addition, a female athlete should be encouraged to have routine pelvic examinations and Papanicolaou (Pap) smears as outlined by her physician.

Diagnosing ovarian cancer may prove somewhat difficult. Finding an adnexal or pelvic mass on examination is of concern, especially in an older woman or one with other risk factors for ovarian cancer. Unfortunately, no good screening test is available. Serum tumor markers are used in the initial evaluation of ovarian cancer, but they are not appropriate for use as screening tests at this time. Pelvic ultrasound may demonstrate an ovarian mass if suspected or symptoms warrant this examination. Laparoscopy plays an important role in diagnosis and staging of ovarian cancer because no one laboratory test or imaging technique is sufficient.

The incidence of cervical cancer has decreased in recent years, largely because of screening examinations with the use of the Pap smear test. Cells from the cervix are taken and evaluated for atypical or abnormal appearance, with further evaluation and treatment depending on the results. The U.S. Preventive Services Task Force currently recommends that every woman be screened by Pap smear at least every 3 yr (barring any previous abnormal results) beginning no longer than 3 yr after first sexual activity or by age 21, whichever comes first. Some people may not need routine screening, such as women over age 65 who have had normal screenings in the past, or women who have had total hysterectomies but without a history of malignancy or a questionable malignancy. These cases, however, must be individualized and the decision made by the woman in consultation with her physician (Carter 2015).

Treatment and Return to Participation

The treatment of ovarian cancer largely depends on the stage of disease, which is determined by surgical exploration. There are four stages (I, II, III, IV), with stage IV being the least favorable. The degree of tumor extension plays a large role with regard to staging. Therapies include surgical removal of involved tissue and chemotherapy. Invasive cervical cancer therapies include surgery, radiation therapy, and chemotherapy. Here again, the choice depends on the stage of malignancy (Carter 2015).

Several treatments are available for cervical dysplasia (i.e., precancerous lesions) discovered by Pap smear. Treatment may be as simple as frequent follow-up and repeat Pap smears, or it may include colposcopy with biopsy or removal of the abnormal tissue.

Morbidity and mortality due to ovarian and cervical cancer are high because of the nature of the disease process and its lack of symptoms early in its course. Screening for cervical cancer by Pap smear has allowed for great progress in the prevention of invasive disease. Much progress has also been made in the fight to prevent cervical cancer with the advent of Gardasil and Cervarix, which are three-series vaccines designed to help prevent infection by HPV.

Athletic participation for women undergoing treatment for ovarian or cervical cancer is limited by the toll of treatment, which can include nausea, vomiting, fatigue, and diarrhea. Treatment requires a multidisciplinary approach, and good communication among all involved is important for the athlete's well-being.

Prevention

Many risk factors for ovarian cancer are difficult to avoid. Probably the best form of prevention is routine medical examinations with special attention placed on those persons with risk factors, such as family history and prior medical history of gynecological malignancy.

Cervical cancer has risk factors associated with sexual activity. Therefore, changes in sexual behavior or practices as previously described may decrease an athlete's risk. Routine examinations, including screening for cervical lesions, cannot be overemphasized. Gardasil has added much in the way of cervical cancer prevention. Current CDC age recommendations for administration to females are 11 to 12 yr, although it can be given as early as age nine. It is also recommended for girls and women between the ages of 13 and 26 who have not received the series and who, of course, have no contraindications. Gardasil is also approved for males to prevent HPV, and it is recommended they begin the vaccination between the ages of 9 and 15. In a study of U.S. southwestern university women, researchers found that 55% reported having received the vaccination against HPV. Native American, Hispanic, and African American women had vaccination rates of 71%, 68%, and 58%. The ethnic group with the lowest vaccination rate was Caucasian women, who had a 31% rate (Nuno et al. 2016). These results are very different from those of a study in a southeastern U.S. university performed six years earlier, where white women had a 77% rate of vaccination against HPV (Daley et al. 2010). There should be a greater effort to educate all on the importance of HPV vaccination in the prevention of cervical cancer.

Breast Cancer

The breast consists of glands, blood and lymph tissue, fat, and fibrous or connective tissue (figure 10.17). Underlying the breast is muscle. The lymph tissue drains to nodes in the axillae. To facilitate milk delivery, the breast has numerous milk glands, which open to lobules. Several lobules make up a lobe, and these lobes empty into ducts that deliver the milk to the nipple. The lymphatic system is also an important aspect of the breast (figure 10.18), and it can act as a conduit for cancer to metastasize to other areas.

A neoplasm arising from the breast tissue is a breast cancer in both males and females. Approximately 10% to 15% originate in the ducts of the breast, with another significant portion originating within the lobules. These cells can escape the breast or metastasize and affect other areas of the body. With the exception of skin cancer, breast cancer is the most commonly diagnosed cancer among American women. According to the Centers for Disease Control and Prevention, in 2015, an estimated 40,150 women and 405 men would die from breast cancer, with 224,150 newly diagnosed cases in women and 2,125 in men (Centers for Disease Control and Prevention 2015a).

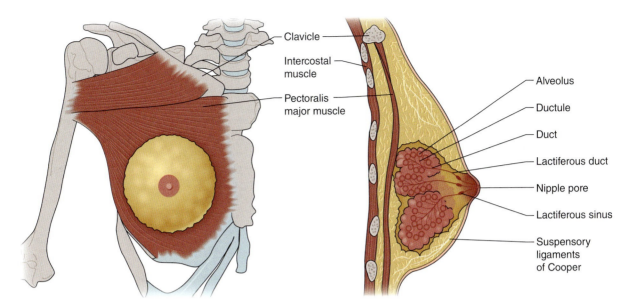

FIGURE 10.17   Anatomy of the female breast.

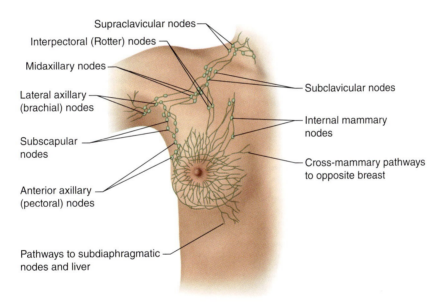

FIGURE 10.18   Lymphatic system surrounding the breast.

Risk factors associated with breast cancer include a person's sex, age, prior history of breast cancer, family history of breast cancer, and genetics. One's overall exposure to estrogen, either physiological or by replacement, may increase the risk for breast cancer. Therefore, women who have taken hormone replacement for several years, women who began menstruation at an early age, women who experienced menopause at a late age, and women who never had children or began childbearing at a later age may all be at increased risk.

The three major types of breast cancer are described on the basis of their location of origin and histology: infiltrating ductal carcinoma or ductal carcinoma *in situ*

if localized, infiltrating lobular carcinoma or lobular carcinoma *in situ* if localized, and inflammatory breast carcinoma.

Signs and Symptoms

Early stages of breast cancer usually are silent. The initial tumor is typically painless, and the first sign may be a breast or axillary lump or mass not previously evaluated, skin puckering, or abnormality noted on a mammogram. Many of these lumps are benign and associated with fibrocystic change, which may be manifested by breast tenderness just before menstruation. The lump in this case

RED FLAGS FOR BREAST CANCER

- Nipple discharge, especially when unilateral
- Change in size or shape of the breast
- Change in appearance of the skin overlying the breast, especially pitting, in which the skin begins to resemble an orange peel
- Inversion of the nipple, especially when recent in onset and unilateral

is a fluid-filled cyst rather than a solid, fixed nodule. Other warning signs include nipple discharge, change in size or shape of the breast, change in appearance of the skin overlying the breast, and recent inversion of the nipple (American Cancer Society 2015; Centers for Disease Control and Prevention 2015a).

Although breast cancer in men is rare, it does occur. Concerns about breast cancer expressed by the male athlete should not be taken lightly.

The finding of a breast mass can be frightening. Not all masses are cancerous, and in fact, most are probably benign. In the very young athlete (i.e., before puberty), a lump may appear around the nipple that is followed by a similar occurrence on the other side, with both remaining unchanged until some time during puberty. A fibroadenoma, which is a firm but painless mass, is typically a benign lesion that tends to occur in the young athlete during the late teens to early 30s. It is typically well circumscribed and mobile on examination. These lumps tend to persist and sometimes calcify. Fibrocystic change is a common benign breast lesion that consists of fluid-filled cysts within the breast tissue. These cysts or lumps are typically tender, especially just before menses, and may be fluctuant on examination.

Referral and Diagnostic Tests

Although many breast lumps are benign and can have characteristic findings, the importance of a medical evaluation of a lump cannot be underestimated. Any athlete with any signs or symptoms of a breast or axilla mass or breast changes needs to be referred to a physician.

The diagnosis of breast cancer starts with a thorough medical history and physical examination, including breast palpation by a trained medical provider. In the presence of a suspicious palpable breast mass, imaging of the breasts by mammography, MRI, or ultrasound may help further clarify the malignant potential of the mass. A potential difficulty in younger female athletes involves their relatively dense breast tissue, which may make clear imaging of a mass more difficult.

Other diagnostic tools are more invasive and involve sampling or removing tissue for pathological examination. These tools include fine needle aspiration, in which a needle is introduced into the lump and cells are aspirated for cytological examination; core needle biopsy, which introduces a large needle to obtain tissue for pathological review; and surgical biopsy, which involves surgical removal of a portion of the mass or the entire lump and surrounding tissue. These tissue samples are used to make a definitive diagnosis.

Treatment and Return to Participation

Treatment for breast cancer largely depends on its progression, which is measured on the basis of a staging system. This system assigns stages based on the tumor's size, lymph node involvement, and location of any metastatic spread. For instance, stage 0 is noninvasive cancer such as ductal carcinoma *in situ* or lobular carcinoma *in situ*. This type of cancer is localized but has the potential for spreading. Stage IV represents the other end of the spectrum: The cancer has metastasized beyond the breast and its lymph nodes. In addition to staging, other factors are extremely important when treating breast cancer. These include the patient's age, general state of health, previous medical history, sex, pregnancy status, and menopausal status, as well as the specifics of the tumor itself, such as the presence of certain receptors on the tumor cells.

Multiple therapies exist, including surgery, chemotherapy, radiation therapy, hormone therapy, and biological therapy. Surgery ranges from the common removal of the mass and surrounding tissue, including a sampling of the axillary lymph nodes, to the uncommon removal of the entire breast and its lymph nodes. Often some other form of therapy is used in addition to surgery, especially if only a portion of the breast is removed. This may include radiation, chemotherapy, or hormone therapy, which are also used before surgery for certain larger cancers that may require shrinkage preoperatively (Centers for Disease Control and Prevention 2015a; American Cancer Society 2015).

The prognosis varies from person to person, but overall it is related to the stage of the cancer. Stage IV obviously offers the worst prognosis for 5 yr survival. Other factors include those used for determining particular treatments, such as the patient's overall health, age, and tumor receptor status. The time to return to sport can range from days to weeks or months and is determined by the overall tumor burden, including metastases, side effects from the treatment, and the athlete's overall condition.

Prevention

Because many risk factors associated with breast cancer are not controllable, screening is very important. Screening includes monthly breast examinations performed by the patient and examinations performed by a medical professional every 2 to 3 yr between the ages of 20 and 40 and yearly thereafter. Women should become familiar with the usual appearance of their breasts so they can detect any changes that might be warning signs for breast cancer. A monthly breast self-examination is performed by first palpating for lumps or abnormalities. Here is how to perform a breast self-examination:

- Perform the examination 7 to 10 d after the first day of the menstrual cycle.
- Stand before a mirror and visually inspect the breast in three positions:
  1. Standing with arms at side
  2. Holding arms behind head and pressing forward
  3. Hands on hips, rolling shoulders and elbows forward
- Raise one arm, and using at least three or four fingers, palpate the other breast using these motions (figure 10.19):
  1. Palpate the breast in a circular motion, covering the whole breast, moving in toward the nipple
  2. Palpate the breast in toward the nipple
  3. Palpate the breast in an up-and-down motion
- Palpate the axillary area because it is rich with lymph nodes and should not contain unusual lumps or masses.
- Squeeze the nipple and look for any discharge.
- Repeat the preceding steps for the other breast.
- Complete this examination both in the shower and while lying supine.

Mammography is another screening tool, and the American Cancer Society recommends that it be done yearly after age 40. Recommendations for breast examinations and mammography may need to be altered if the athlete has a past medical history or family history of breast cancer. In patients without breast symptoms, mammograms can be offered annually between the ages of 40 and 54. At age 55, women without breast symptoms can choose to have mammograms every 2 yr, or they can decide to continue with annual evaluations. Screening should continue as long as the patient is in good health and expected to live 10 more years or longer (American Cancer Society 2015). It is important for older athletes to seek the advice of their physicians regarding screening.

Preemptive breast removal, that is, breast removal for someone without cancer or a lump, may seem extreme but is not uncommon. For example, a person with a strong family history of breast cancer or who is known to carry a gene associated with breast cancer (*BRCA1* or *BRCA2*) may elect to have breast removal to preempt the cancer.

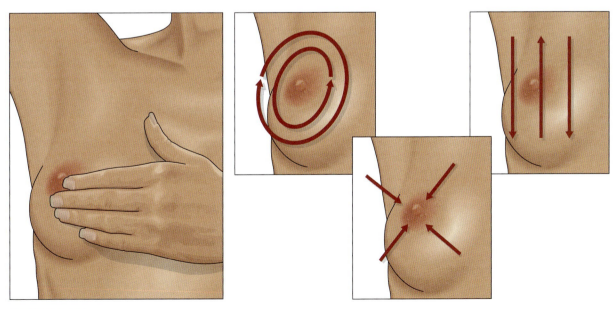

FIGURE 10.19 Breast self-examination.

Pregnancy

Normal pregnancy consists of a series of remarkable changes that occur within the female body. Multiple organ systems are affected in order to support a growing fetus while maintaining the health of the mother. A few of these important normal changes are highlighted here and a single pathological condition, ectopic pregnancy, is discussed.

Before becoming pregnant, a woman should maintain proper nutrition, start the use of prenatal vitamins, and discontinue using or avoid potentially harmful substances such as tobacco, alcohol, and illicit drugs. Folic acid is present in most prenatal vitamins and is important in helping to prevent neural tube defects in the fetus. It should be taken by all pregnant women.

The initial signs and symptoms of pregnancy include a missed menstrual period and breast swelling or tenderness. Nausea and vomiting, known as morning sickness, may also be present early in the pregnancy and if severe, may compromise hydration, nutrition, and weight gain. Severe cases of nausea and vomiting, termed *hyperemesis gravidarum,* can lead to hospitalization for fluid replacement, electrolyte correction, and control of emesis. In general, however, symptoms are not this severe, and they typically subside. In fact, the pregnant woman's fluid status increases during pregnancy. Blood volume increases, as does intracellular and extracellular fluid. Fluid tends to accumulate more during the day, and swelling to distal extremities is very common (Perales et al. 2015).

Physiological changes also occur in pregnancy. Plasma volume and cardiac output increase as a result of increases in stroke volume and heart rate. In addition, blood pressure decreases in the normal pregnancy because of an overall decrease in systemic vascular resistance. Respiratory changes include an increased tidal volume, increased minute ventilation, and decreased overall airway resistance. Despite these changes, the woman's FEV_1 and respiratory rate usually remain unchanged at rest (May et al. 2015; Perales et al. 2015).

Gastroesophageal reflux is another common symptom occurring among pregnant women and is due to both anatomical and physiological changes. An athlete may note that certain foods aggravate reflux, and avoidance of these foods is prudent. If avoidance of the offending foods does not help, pharmacological therapy may be necessary. This therapy can consist of calcium-containing antacids, histamine (H_2) antagonists, or proton pump inhibitors as prescribed.

Low back pain is a common complaint as well and is largely due to the woman's altered center of gravity secondary to the enlarging fetus, uterus, and breast tissue. Low back pain is generally more of a problem during the latter stages of pregnancy. Interestingly, although the woman's bones may adjust to the various stresses placed on them, they appear to suffer no ill effects from the high calcium demands of the fetus.

Throughout the course of pregnancy, a woman's breasts enlarge and may become tender. It is also possible for a pregnant woman to notice that she is expressing fluid from her breasts before the birth of her child. The fluid expressed is known as colostrum and is a normal change associated with pregnancy.

Exercise and physical activity for healthy women should be encouraged in pregnancy. Women who exercise regularly in pregnancy have the benefits of improved cardiac function, limited weight gain, improved mental health, and decreased time in labor (Perales et al. 2015; May et al. 2014). Few scientific data address the participation in vigorous and competitive sport by the pregnant athlete, but some recommendations are noteworthy. Pregnant athletes should avoid exercise in the supine position as much as possible, particularly after the first trimester. Scuba diving, downhill skiing, contact sports, and the use of hot tubs, steam baths, and saunas place the fetus at potential risk and are discouraged during pregnancy (American Congress of Obstetricians and Gynecologists 2011b). In addition, pregnant athletes are generally discouraged from participation in contact or collision sports after the 14th week of pregnancy, although this is based on indirect evidence. Further, a pregnant athlete who participates in competitive endurance sports should consider participation at the noncompetitive level for the duration of the pregnancy.

Whereas exercise during pregnancy is safe in most cases, in some situations, exercise needs to be discontinued pending a complete evaluation by a physician (Parsons 2014; American Congress of Obstetricians and Gynecologists 2011b). The American College of Obstetrics and Gynecologists lists contraindications to exercise in pregnancy, including vaginal bleeding, pregnancy-induced hypertension, an incompetent cervix, preterm labor, premature rupture of membranes, and intrauterine growth restriction. Warning signs that suggest the immediate cessation of exercise include back, pubic, or abdominal pain; dizziness; nausea; uterine contractions; excessive fatigue; and decreased fetal movements (American Congress of Obstetricians and Gynecologists 2011b). When in doubt, the athlete should discuss these issues with her physician. According to the NCAA recommendations (Parsons 2014), the pregnant athlete should do the following:

- Avoid supine exercise after the first trimester.
- Be discouraged from heavy weightlifting.
- Be discouraged from activities that require the Valsalva maneuver.

RED FLAGS FOR TERMINATING EXERCISE WHILE PREGNANT

Signs to terminate exercise while pregnant and follow-up with your obstetrician:

- Vaginal bleeding
- Shortness of breath before exercise
- Dizziness
- Headache
- Chest pain
- Calf pain or swelling
- Preterm labor
- Decreased fetal movement
- Amniotic fluid leakage
- Muscle weakness

- Avoid activities associated with a high risk of falling (gymnastics, horseback riding, or downhill skiing).
- Consider noncompetitive activity for those athletes involved in endurance sports.
- Avoid contact sports after the 14th week of pregnancy, even though there are no data regarding contact sports and pregnancy.
- Avoid any physical activity pending evaluation by an obstetrician when the mother has a previously diagnosed medical condition that may affect normal pregnancy, such as uncontrolled diabetes, hypertension, or cervical defects.
- Remain well hydrated.
- Avoid overheating.

Ectopic Pregnancy

An infrequent yet important complication of pregnancy is an ectopic pregnancy. Ectopic pregnancy occurs when the fertilized egg implants outside the normal endometrial lining of the uterus (figure 10.20). This is lethal for the fetus and can be for the mother as well. Appropriate diagnosis is therefore extremely important. The implantation can occur in many places, but most occur in the ampulla of the fallopian tube, which is the long length of tube leading to the uterus.

Common causes of ectopic pregnancy include anatomical abnormalities, such as scarring or obstruction of a portion of the egg's path that hinders the normal migration of the fertilized egg to its proper implantation site in the uterus. Some risk factors include a prior ectopic pregnancy, a history of PID, use of an intrauterine device, a history of tubal ligation, an abnormally formed uterus, and cigarette smoking. Diagnosis of an ectopic pregnancy involves serial measurement of serum β-HCG (human chorionic gonadotropin) levels and pelvic or abdominal imaging with ultrasound (American Congress of Obstetricians and Gynecologists 2011a).

Signs and Symptoms

Signs and symptoms of ectopic pregnancy include abnormal vaginal bleeding, bleeding outside of the usual menstrual cycle, sudden or sharp abdominal or pelvic pain, dizziness, and possible referred pain to the shoulder (American Congress of Obstetricians and Gynecologists 2011a). Symptoms may include amenorrhea, vaginal bleeding, and pain. An athlete may have hemodynamic compromise in severe cases when rupture of the fallopian tube and hemorrhage have occurred.

Some women may be unaware that they are pregnant, and any signs or symptoms associated with ectopic

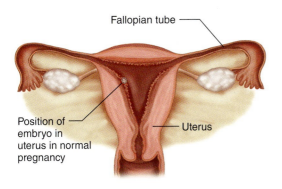

Normal pregnancy

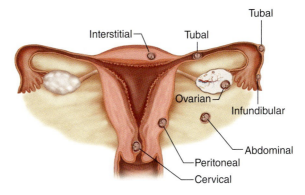

Possible sites of embryo in ectopic pregnancy

FIGURE 10.20 Ectopic pregnancy.

pregnancy should be followed up with a history of the last menstrual period. The placenta produces a hormone, human chorionic gonadotropin (HCG), which can be detected in pregnant women's blood or urine. The presence of HCG confirms pregnancy. A pelvic exam and ultrasonography are performed to further confirm the pregnancy and assess the fetal tissue.

Treatment and Return to Participation

Treatment most commonly involves aborting the fetus through the use of either methotrexate or surgical intervention. Methotrexate can be considered, under favorable circumstances, in order to avoid the risks and trauma of surgery. Methotrexate stops fetal growth and allows the body to absorb it over time. It is not, however, recommended if the growth of pregnancy is large or the fallopian tube is ruptured (American Congress of Obstetricians and Gynecologists 2011a). Each method of treatment carries its own risks, however, and is generally prescribed by the obstetrician in conjunction with the woman's personal wishes.

The prognosis for recovery from an ectopic pregnancy is generally very good as long as the pregnancy is identified early in its course. In the event of either a delayed diagnosis or rupture of the fallopian tube, the prognosis is considered guarded. Ectopic pregnancy can easily become fatal for the mother. If diagnosis is delayed and rupture occurs, it can result in hemorrhage and hemodynamic collapse. The successful treatment of an ectopic pregnancy may be followed by infertility. Several weeks of follow-up with a physician are required for both medication and surgical interventions, and the athlete must be fully recovered before beginning to return to full activity.

Summary

Athletes are unique individuals by nature of their high-intensity exercise and the physical demands placed on their bodies, but like everyone else, they can develop any number of genitourinary or gynecological problems. Some of these conditions are unique to athletes, such as sports hematuria and amenorrhea in the athlete, and others are common to athletes and nonathletes alike.

The team of professionals caring for athletes must all be aware of the common medical problems that can occur in this group so they can receive prompt attention and diagnosis. Because of the sensitive nature of these systems and the unique relationship of the athletic trainer to the athlete, familiarity with the signs and symptoms is especially critical to proper assessment and the subsequent early return of the athlete to sport.

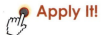 **Apply It!** The case study for this chapter looks at a collegiate volleyball player who complains of painful urination. Read the scenario and answer the questions at www.HumanKinetics.com/MedicalConditionsInTheAthlete.

Neurological System

OBJECTIVES

At the completion of this chapter the reader should be able to do the following:

- Describe the anatomy and function of the nervous system.
- Recognize and assess an athlete with a suspected sport-related concussion.
- Describe a return-to-play progression for an athlete after sport-related concussion.
- Recognize and refer an athlete with signs or symptoms of a life-threatening neurological condition.
- Identify conditions that make an athlete susceptible to migraines and stroke.
- Recognize the symptoms of complex regional pain syndrome.
- Describe chronic neurological conditions and their effect on athletic participation.
- Differentiate when to make a referral to a physician for further neurological evaluation.

Neurological disorders in athletes are generally divided into two categories: immediately life-threatening conditions such as encephalitis, meningitis, or stroke; and those with chronic implications, which may include Guillain-Barré syndrome, multiple sclerosis, migraines, amyotrophic lateral sclerosis (ALS), complex regional pain syndrome (CRPS), or epilepsy. In addition, there has been increased emphasis on sport-related concussion because of the incidence of and possible short- and long-term consequences of concussive injuries. All of the conditions discussed in this chapter have one basic tenet: Early recognition of the symptoms and rapid referral can lead to better outcomes. Infectious neurological conditions (encephalitis and meningitis) are discussed in chapter 15.

Although chronic neurological conditions are less common, they produce symptoms that can interfere with normal daily function and prevent vigorous activity for periods of time. Most have no clear or distinguishable signs, and only the patient's symptoms can guide the clinician to a correct diagnosis. These conditions can also cause emergent situations that require immediate medical referral.

Many symptoms associated with neurological conditions are vague and fleeting and are sometimes passed off as a result of overtraining or fatigue, both of which are common to the athlete. This chapter reviews the pertinent neurological anatomy and highlights signs and symptoms associated with specific neurological conditions. A strong knowledge base, coupled with an inclusive medical history, will enable the athletic trainer to recognize important symptoms and properly refer the athlete to a physician.

Overview of Anatomy and Physiology

The neurological system consists of the brain, spinal cord, and nerves that arise from it. Understanding the anatomy and physiology of this system is critical to evaluating conditions specific to it. Depending on the location of the neurological tissue, it may or may not regenerate if damaged. Signs and symptoms of injury or insult to this system typically present some distance from the actual damage and increase the challenge in determining the cause of an injury. Appreciating the anatomy and physiology will enable the practitioner to make a better decision about the cause of the condition and therefore assist with a diagnosis and treatment.

Skull

The human skull is made up of two main components: the cerebral cranium, which protects the brain and brainstem, and the anterior facial bony structure. The cerebral cranium consists of these bones: frontal, temporal, parietal, occipital, sphenoid, and ethmoid. The facial skeleton is made up of these bones: mandible, zygomatic, maxillary, and nasal (figure 11.1).

Meninges

The meninges lie just under the skull and provide three protective layers: the outermost dura mater, the arachnoid mater, and the pia mater (figure 11.2). The dura mater is a thick, tough, fibrous membrane functionally composed of two layers, with the periosteum against the skull and the inner dura supporting structures of the brain. The real and potential spaces formed between these membranes allow for arteriovenous connections that can be disrupted by hematomas (i.e., accumulations of blood between the spaces) caused by trauma.

Blood supply to the meninges comes from vessels that follow grooves in the skull. Although the periosteum adheres directly to the skull bones, a potential epidural space exists and ruptured vessels or infection can cause an actual space to form as seen when a hemorrhage causes an epidural hematoma. In the spine, a true epidural space, separating the dura from the periosteum of the vertebral bones, contains fat and epidural veins.

The inner lining of the dura mater forms folds in the cerebral hemispheres. The membranous plate known as the falx cerebri divides the hemispheres into right and left halves. Another plate formed by the dura, the tentorium cerebelli, separates the cerebral hemispheres from the cerebellum and brainstem.

Large sinuses or cavities that lie within the dura mater allow for the venous return from cerebral veins located between the two layers. The walls of these sinuses are made up primarily of dura. The function of the superior sagittal sinus is to collect venous blood, as well as excess cerebrospinal fluid (CSF), which drains through its arachnoid villi. The blood flows into the transverse sinuses, which also receive blood from other veins of the brain. Together with the sigmoid sinuses, these major venous pathways leaving the brain become the internal jugular vein.

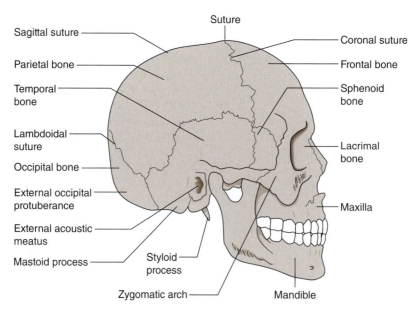

FIGURE 11.1 Bony structures of the head and face.

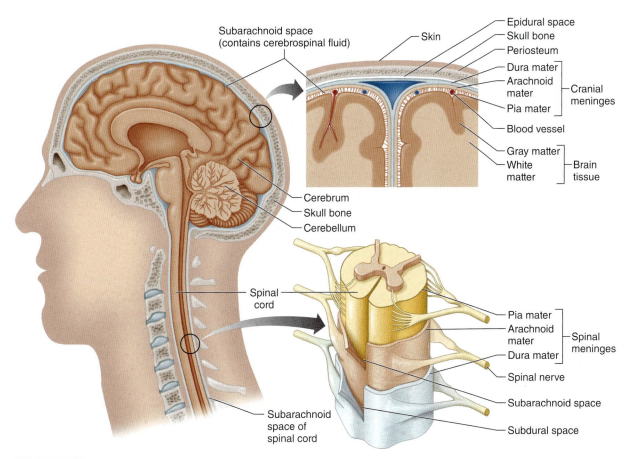

FIGURE 11.2 Sagittal view of the head, showing the skull, meninges, and spaces surrounding the brain.

The cavernous sinuses are smaller and receive venous blood from the hypothalamus. They are of clinical importance because the internal carotid artery and several nerves pass through them after entering the cranium at the base of the skull.

The arachnoid mater is named for its delicate, spiderweb-like consistency. The arachnoid mater and dura mater are separated by the subdural space, which is a potential space that contains only a small amount of CSF and numerous small veins. If the membrane is disrupted, it can become distended with blood, pus, or other fluids under pathological conditions. The subarachnoid space separates the arachnoid from the pia mater and is filled with fibrous connecting trabeculae, the major arteries, and CSF.

The pia mater is the innermost layer of the meninges and is very thin, adhering directly to the surface of the brain and spinal cord. It follows every fold and enters every crevice, making it difficult to distinguish this membrane from the surface to which it adheres. No potential or actual spaces exist between the pia mater and neural tissue.

Meninges also provide a protective covering to the brainstem and spinal cord, which is why infections affecting the meninges can be detected via a lumbar tap that draws CSF from the membranes covering the spinal cord.

Cerebrum

The two cerebral hemispheres are composed of neural tissue. These hemispheres are divided into four principal lobes: frontal, temporal, parietal, and occipital (figure 11.3). The lobes have been extensively researched in attempts to isolate the locations of specific physiological functions and pathological processes. The most commonly used classification is Brodmann's classification system, which identifies functional cortices of each lobe by numbers (see figure 11.4).

The frontal lobe contains the primary motor area (area 4), the premotor area (area 6), the frontal eye field (area 8), Broca's speech area (areas 44 and 45), and the frontal association area (areas 9, 10, and 11). The primary motor cortex is highly organized in a somatotopic fashion with the lips, tongue, face, and hands on the lowest part, moving upward to trunk, arms, and hips, and ultimately to the feet, lower legs, and genitalia that hang over the edge into the interhemispheric fissure. This cortical area

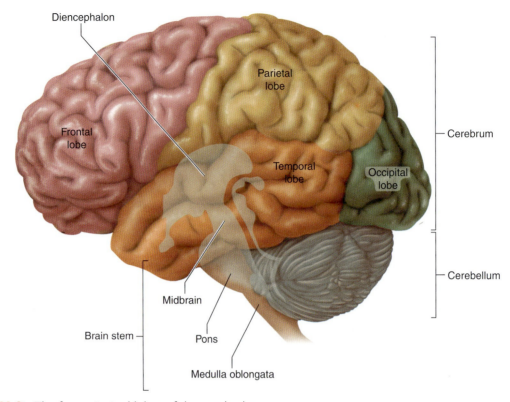

FIGURE 11.3 The four principal lobes of the cerebral cortex.

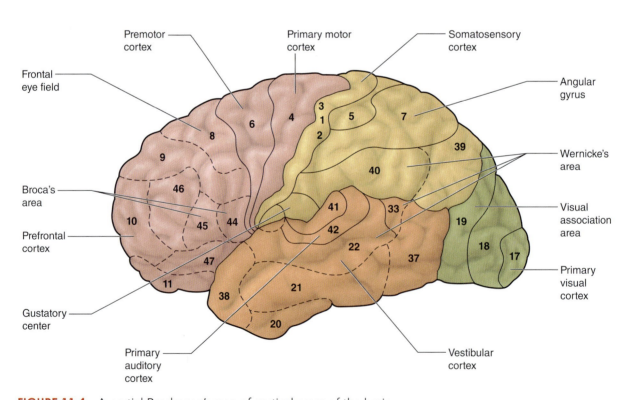

FIGURE 11.4 A partial Brodmann's map of cortical areas of the brain.

is responsible for voluntary movement of skeletal muscle of the contralateral side of the body. The frontal eye fields coordinate contralateral deviation of the head and eyes.

Clinically, seizure activity within this cortex results in convulsions of the parts of the body represented in the area of electrical disruption. Damage to this cortex can lead to contralateral flaccid paresis or paralysis, and spasticity is usually present if there is concomitant injury to the premotor area. The left hemisphere usually influences and correlates with right hand dominance. Broca's area is located in the dominant hemisphere only, and when this area is damaged, Broca's aphasia is the resulting disorder. Also known as *expressive aphasia,* Broca's aphasia presents with intact comprehension and impaired expression of speech.

The parietal lobe contains the primary sensory cortex (areas 1, 2, and 3), the sensory association areas (areas 5 and 7), and the cortical taste area embedded in the facial sensory area (areas 1, 2, and 3). The primary sensory cortex, like the motor cortex, is also organized in a somatotopic way. This cortex receives sensory information from the skin and mucosa of the body and face. The types of sensory information processed here include pain, temperature, touch, and proprioception. Pathological injuries to this cortex, such as those that occur with cerebrovascular accidents (CVAs), also known as strokes, lead to paresthesias, impaired sensation, and, rarely, complete anesthesia of the representative body areas on the contralateral side of the body.

The occipital lobe contains the primary visual cortex (area 17) and the visual association areas (areas 18 and 19). The visual cortex receives information from the ipsilateral half of each retina. Therefore, the right visual cortex receives information from the right half of each retina, which correlates clinically with the left visual field. Irritative lesions to this area, such as seizures or migraines, can lead to visual hallucinations; cortical damage, such as that caused by CVAs, results in contralateral homonymous visual field defects. Pathology of the visual association areas can lead to impairments of spatial orientation and visual disorganization in the same visual field.

The temporal lobe contains the primary auditory cortex (area 41), auditory association area (area 42), temporal association area (represented here by anterior area 22), and Wernicke's speech comprehension area (posterior area 22). The primary auditory cortex receives auditory input from the cochlea of both ears. Irritation of this area can cause buzzing or roaring sounds, and damage can cause hearing deficits ranging from mild, caused by a unilateral lesion, to severe loss or deafness, caused by bilateral lesions. Wernicke's area, like Broca's area, is located in the dominant hemisphere only and is involved in higher auditory processing and in speech comprehension. Injury to this area can lead to word deafness, or **Wernicke's aphasia**.

Although specific areas of the brain may be critical to certain functions, other brain areas can also be involved, and these areas can play a more dominant role when the brain must adapt to neural loss resulting from trauma or disease.

Brainstem

The brainstem acts as the main conduit for information between the brain and the spinal cord by way of three large bundles of fibers called the cerebellar peduncles. These bundles contain the ascending and descending tracts carrying motor and sensory information, descending tracts of the autonomic nervous system, and pathways of the monoaminergic system. In addition, the brainstem contains almost all of the cranial nerve nuclei and houses the center that controls respiration, cardiovascular system functions, level of consciousness, sleep, and alertness.

The brainstem comprises the medulla oblongata, the pons, and the midbrain. Each of these areas is associated with neural fibers related to specific body functions. The medulla oblongata contains the ascending and descending tracts, the nuclei of cranial nerves (CN) IX, X, and XII, and the inferior cerebellar peduncles. The pons consists of longitudinal neural tracts; the raphe nucleus, which is important in pain modulation and in controlling the level of arousal during the sleep–wake cycle; the nuclei of CN V, VI, and VII; auditory pathways; and the middle cerebellar peduncles. The midbrain contains ascending and descending longitudinal neural tracts; the nuclei of CN III and IV; the substantia nigra, which connects with the basal nuclei; the superior and inferior colliculi, which are involved in the visual and auditory pathways; pathways of the monoaminergic system, which interact with the raphe nucleus and its functions; periaqueductal gray matter, which contains autonomic pathways and endorphin-producing cells that modulate pain; and the superior cerebellar peduncles.

Autonomic Nervous System

The autonomic nervous system innervates glands, smooth muscle, and cardiac muscle. It is divided into the parasympathetic and sympathetic nervous systems. The parasympathetic nervous system is also referred to as *craniosacral* because of its origins in the brainstem and the sacral levels of the spinal cord. The cranial division consists of parasympathetic fibers in four of the cranial nerves (III, VII, IX, and X) that innervate the head and the thoracic and abdominal viscera. The sacral division comprises parasympathetic fibers from segments S2 to S4 and innervates the bladder, genitalia, descending colon, and rectum. The sympathetic nervous system is also referred to as *thoracolumbar* because it arises from the thoracic and lumbar areas of the spinal cord. These sympathetic fibers usually travel with the peripheral nerves or along the wall of a blood vessel to their target vessels in skeletal muscle.

The major functions of the parasympathetic and sympathetic nervous systems, which are generally antagonistic, are as follows:

Parasympathetic Nervous System

- Constricts the pupils
- Decreases the heart rate
- Increases gastrointestinal peristalsis and secretion
- Expels wastes

Sympathetic Nervous System

- Increases heart rate and breathing
- Dilates blood vessels in skeletal and cardiac muscles and constricts them in the gastrointestinal tract
- Dilates the bronchial passages
- Dilates the pupils
- Erects the hairs for protection and display
- Increases sweat secretion
- Mobilizes glucose

The sympathetic nervous system is responsible for the fight-or-flight response and is catabolic, expending energy as it prepares the body for danger. The parasympathetic nervous system dominates during times of rest.

Disruption of the sympathetic system can lead to several clinical conditions. **Horner's syndrome** is a neurological condition manifested by facial flushing of the affected side, **ipsilateral miosis**, and moderate **ptosis** of an eye. It is caused by a lesion or tumor at the level of the carotid plexus, cervical sympathetic chain, upper thoracic cord, or brainstem. Sympathetic pathway disruption at the level of the peripheral vascular system can lead to the severe vasoconstrictive episodes characteristic of Raynaud's disease (see chapter 14). Reflex sympathetic dystrophy and causalgia also involve abnormalities at the level of the peripheral blood vessels leading to sympathetic overactivity.

Cerebellum

The cerebellum is located dorsal to the pons and medulla oblongata and consists of two hemispheres connected by the vermis. The cerebellar peduncles connect the cerebellum to the brainstem and contain communicating neural pathways. The cerebellum controls function in the higher-level coordination of voluntary movements and in the maintenance of balance, equilibrium, and muscle tone. Injuries to this structure generally result in the loss of muscle tone (hypotonia) and the loss of muscle coordination (**ataxia**). Other clinical signs of cerebellar disease include nystagmus, **dysmetria**, intention tremor, and **dysdiadochokinesia** (Baugh et al. 2014).

Spinal Cord

The spinal cord is the body's communication system, transmitting nerve impulses to the brain from the spinal nerves that innervate sensory organs and muscles. The cord is divided into white and gray matter. The gray matter consists of neurons or nerve cells. The anterior, or ventral, gray matter contains nerve cells for axons in the ventral roots that carry motor output. The intermediolateral gray matter contains nerve cells that carry autonomic nerve fibers. The posterior, or dorsal, gray matter contains sensory fibers that convey pain, temperature, proprioception, and touch input. These nerve cells are further mapped out into laminae on the basis of the types of information being carried. The white matter surrounds the gray matter and consists of the ventral, lateral, and dorsal columns, which contain myelinated and unmyelinated nerve fibers.

The dorsal columns comprise the ascending sensory tracts called the fasciculus gracilis and the fasciculus cuneatus. Together they relay information about touch, proprioception, and two-point discrimination. The lateral columns contain the spinothalamic tracts, dorsal and ventral spinocerebellar tracts, and the spinoreticular pathway. The crossing over, or decussation, that occurs between the axons of the dorsal columns and the spinothalamic

---

CLINICAL TIPS

Upper and Lower Motor Neurons

- *Upper motor neurons* pertain to the brain or spinal cord. Damage to these structures presents as weakness, paralysis, increased muscle tone, spasticity, hyperactive deep tendon reflexes, and the presence of Babinski's reflex. Typically, damaged or destroyed upper motor neurons do not regenerate.

- *Lower motor neurons* pertain to nerve cell bodies or axons or both, and they are located in the anterior horn of the spinal cord and peripheral nerves. Damage to these nerves causes decreased muscle tone, flaccidity, diminished or absent deep tendon reflexes, muscular twitching, and progressive atrophy of the affected muscles. Most lower motor neurons are able to regenerate if they are located outside of the spinal cord.

tracts in the spinal cord is clinically important. Brain injuries involving these areas lead to contralateral deficits, whereas injuries within the spinal cord result in ipsilateral touch and proprioception deficits and contralateral pain perception deficits.

Injuries to the motor tracts result in two different clinical conditions based on the level of injury. Injuries at or peripheral to the anterior horn cells in the spinal cord gray matter present as lower motor neuron syndromes; injuries in the lateral white column or above are associated with upper motor neuron syndromes.

Spinal Nerves

The 31 paired spinal nerves in the body arise from the spinal cord as ventral or dorsal roots. The dorsal roots contain sensory fibers carrying pain and temperature information from the muscles; they also contain axons from muscle spindles and skin and joint mechanoreceptors. The ventral roots are composed primarily of motor neuron fibers from skeletal muscle, as well as muscle spindle fibers, autonomic axons, and axons carrying thoracic and abdominal visceral sensory information.

The spinal nerves combine to form the cervical, brachial, lumbar, and sacral plexuses and then innervate the limbs via peripheral nerves (figure 11.5a). Therefore, peripheral nerves generally contain fibers from several different spinal nerves. Dermatomes represent areas of skin supplied by specific spinal nerves. They are clinically significant in diagnosing the sensory area of nerve injury (see the sidebar "Dermatomes"). Nerve injury must be distinguished from the cutaneous innervation of the peripheral nerves. A myotome is a muscle or group of muscles supplied by one ventral (motor) nerve. Motor deficits may be attributed to damage in specific myotomes.

Myelination is a process in which a nerve is enveloped in a myelin sheath. In the peripheral nervous system, this is accomplished by the encircling of a nerve axon by Schwann cells. Gaps between the Schwann cells are called the nodes of Ranvier (figure 11.7), and they expose unmyelinated axons. The significance of this is that nerve conduction in these myelinated nerves is saltatory, jumping from node to node, which increases the conduction velocity. This type of myelination ceases just before the

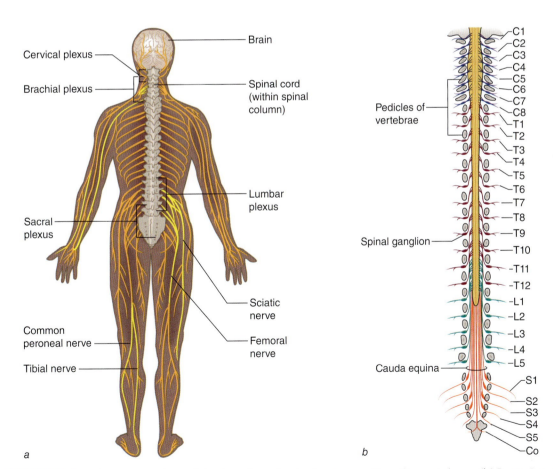

a   *b*

FIGURE 11.5 *(a)* Posterior view of the location of spinal nerves exiting the vertebrae. *(b)* Posterior view of the spine and spinal cord.

Dermatomes

Nerves exit the spinal cord in an orderly manner similar to a ladder. A dermatome is an area of skin supplied mainly by one spinal cord segment through a particular spinal nerve (figure 11.6). Fortunately, dermatomes overlap, so if one nerve is severed, sensations can be transmitted by the nerve above or below it. By following this generalized map of the spinal cord and spinal nerves and their related dermatomes, you can find useful landmarks that aid in assessment.

- The thumb, middle finger, and fifth finger are each in the dermatomes of C6, C7, and C8.
- The head and neck are at the level of C2 and C3.
- The chest is at the levels of C5 through T7.
- The groin is in the region of L1.

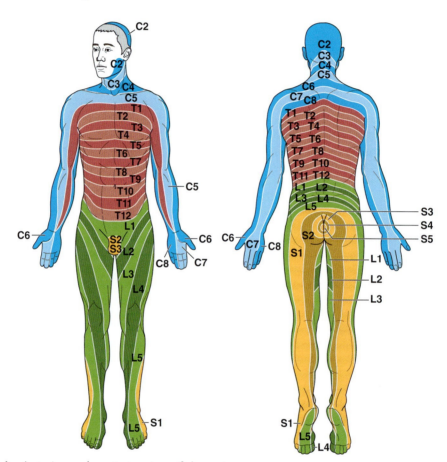

FIGURE 11.6   Anterior and posterior view of dermatomes.

interface of the dorsal or ventral nerve root with the spinal cord. At this juncture, between the peripheral nervous system (PNS) and the central nervous system (CNS), known as the Obersteiner-Redlich zone, astrocytes and oligodendrocytes form the myelin covering.

Demyelinating conditions such as multiple sclerosis, which affects the CNS, and Guillain-Barré syndrome, which affects both the PNS and CNS, can lead to varying degrees of sensory and motor loss. Remyelination often takes place in the PNS; however, it occurs sluggishly, if at all, in the CNS.

Evaluation of the Neurological System

Unlike most other body systems, evaluation of the neurological system depends largely on symptoms, and practitioners would be wise to be attuned to patient

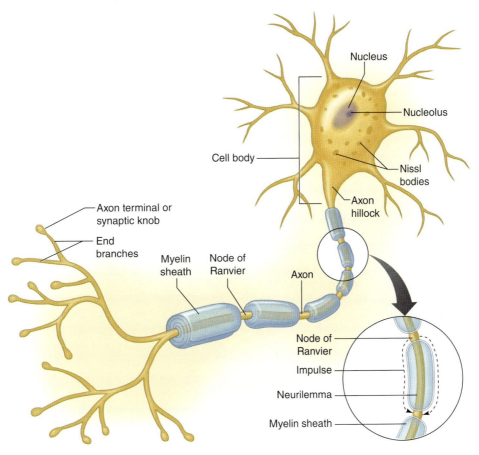

FIGURE 11.7   A neuron. Note the unmyelinated areas in the nodes of Ranvier.

complaints and comments. Although there can be signs (physical evidence of something) of a neurological deficit, they are not as common as symptoms. In a thorough evaluation of neurological conditions, clinicians should know the warning signs and listen to patients' descriptions of symptoms.

Warning Signs of Neurological Diseases

Assessment of the neurological system begins with the athlete's clinical history, coupled with listening carefully to the complaints and terms the athlete uses to describe the condition. In general, neurological diseases can present with either positive or negative manifestations.

Positive manifestations represent inappropriate excitation of the nervous system. These include hypersensitivity; seizures; movement disorders that include tremors, spasms, and tics; and upper motor neuron signs, such as spasticity, hypertonicity, and hyperreflexia. Athletes' descriptions of such positive symptoms may include heaviness, weakness, cramps, slow reaction, tiredness, tremors, visual disturbances, incoordination, a deadened

feeling, numbness, tingling, or pins and needles. Negative manifestations represent a loss of function. These include paresis, paralysis, hyposensitivity, dementia, aphasia (whether receptive-sensory, expressive-motor, or anomic), **syncope**, neck stiffness, gait dysfunction, movement disorders, incoordination, sensory ataxia or proprioception loss, and lower motor neuron signs such as hypotonicity–flaccidity, hyporeflexia, and atrophy. In the case of sport-related concussion (SRC), the history component of the evaluation is crucial in identifying signs and symptoms, determining the presence or absence of amnesia and loss of consciousness, and evaluating the athlete's mental status.

The physical examination begins with a visual inspection of the spinal column, assessing for deviations, muscular imbalance, or surgical scars. The athlete's musculature, although typically stronger on the dominant side, should not be unilaterally hypertrophic. The health care provider assesses bilaterally for tremors, atrophy, and muscular tone. The dermatomes are bilaterally assessed for sensation as described in chapter 2, followed by bilateral comparison of the reflexes. Evaluation of the cranial nerves (described in the next section) and muscular strength tests follow. Muscular strength tests include both range of motion and break tests for the brachial plexus, as well as heel and toe walking for the lower extremities. The practitioner notes any weakness or differences and refers the athlete to a physician when a discrepancy occurs in either. Functional knowledge of the myotomes and dermatomes is instrumental in assessing any neurological issue. The physical examination for SRC should include the assessment of cognition and coordination (balance) along with the aforementioned evaluation of strength, myotomes, and dermatomes.

Clinical neurological signs can help in differentiating muscle weakness. The pattern of muscle weakness varies depending on the area of injury within the motor unit: upper motor neuron, lower motor neuron, neuromuscular junction, muscle itself, or manifestation as functional weakness. Upper and lower motor neurons have already been discussed. Neuromuscular junction disorders are characterized by signs of injury that include fatigable weakness, normal or decreased muscle tone, and normal deep tendon reflexes. Decreased or absent reflexes present with injury at the muscle level (myopathy). Functional weakness, in contrast to actual weakness, is associated with decreased power in the presence of normal tone, reflexes, and muscle girth.

Understanding the basic anatomy and physiology of the neurological system also helps in identifying injuries to higher neurological systems. Cerebral injuries may present with aphasias, apraxias, paresis, paralysis, sensory deficits, and visual and auditory dysfunction. Cerebellar damage leads to varying degrees of ataxia and incoordination, as well as dysmetria and tremors. Neurological injury to the brainstem may manifest with cranial nerve palsies (CN III to CN XII). In addition to these symptoms, many other common signs associated with neurological disease have special terminology.

Neurological presentations can range from emergent to urgent to routine in severity and in their need for medical evaluation and management. "Red Flags for Urgent Intervention" provides a framework of warning signs and symptoms that warrant immediate referral to a physician or an emergency department. Indications for referral of specific disorders are addressed in the section "Pathological Conditions."

Cranial Nerves and Cranial Nerve Testing

The cranial nerves emerge from the cranium, as opposed to spinal nerves, which emerge from the spinal cord (figure 11.8). The cranial nerves provide sensory and motor innervation to the head and neck, including sensation and voluntary and involuntary muscle function. Testing these nerves is essential to ascertaining their integrity as well as noting discrepancies that may indicate a medical condition.

The olfactory nerve (CN I) can be tested by placing different-smelling substances underneath a single nostril with the other nostril occluded. Both nares are tested because injuries to this nerve are usually unilateral. The clinical spectrum of pathology can range from normal function to anosmia, in which the patient can discern only ammonia, to organic dysfunction, in which the patient cannot recognize any smells. Use caution when evaluating an athlete who appears to be disorientated. Do not use a noxious odor to provoke a response to CN I in athletes suspected of a concussion or cervical spine injury.

The optic nerve (CN II) carries visual information within the complex visual system. The fibers of the optic nerve carrying information from the right half of the retina cross over and join with those same fibers of the contralateral optic nerve. Together, these fibers form the optic tract. The optic tract then forms optic radiations that eventually synapse on the primary visual cortex. Different clinical visual defects will occur depending on the area of lesion within the optic pathway. Complete assessment of the optic nerve requires testing the visual fields, acuity, and pupillary light reflex.

To test the visual fields, the health care provider faces the athlete, who is looking straight ahead. The athletic trainer moves the fingers of one hand within the athlete's peripheral vision and monitors the athlete's response about which finger is moving. Next, the practitioner focuses on individual eye deficits by repeating this test while the athlete closes one eye. The Snellen eye chart, which is described in chapter 12, is used to test visual

---

🚩 RED FLAGS FOR URGENT INTERVENTION

- Any alteration in the level of consciousness
- Fixed or abnormal pupil reactions, abnormal eye movements, or acute visual impairments
- Any focal neurological symptoms occurring after head trauma
- Paralysis or progressive (either unilateral or bilateral) muscle weakness
- Bowel or bladder incontinence
- Acute severe headache, especially associated with nausea and vomiting or focal neurological deficits
- Prolonged or recurrent generalized seizure

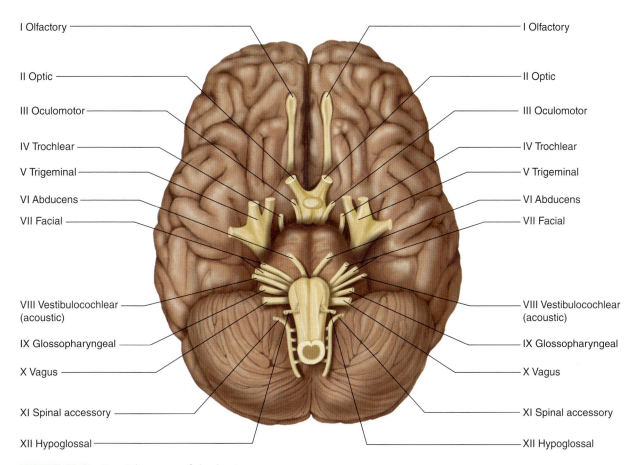

I Olfactory

II Optic

III Oculomotor

IV Trochlear

V Trigeminal

VI Abducens

VII Facial

VIII Vestibulocochlear
(acoustic)

IX Glossopharyngeal

X Vagus

XI Spinal accessory

XII Hypoglossal

I Olfactory

II Optic

III Oculomotor

IV Trochlear

V Trigeminal

VI Abducens

VII Facial

VIII Vestibulocochlear
(acoustic)

IX Glossopharyngeal

X Vagus

XI Spinal accessory

XII Hypoglossal

FIGURE 11.8   Cranial nerves of the brain.

acuity. Alternatively, the athlete may be asked to read something.

The oculomotor nerve (CN III) controls the pupillary light reflex. When a light is shone in an athlete's eye, the pupil normally constricts (direct response); the pupil of the other, unstimulated eye should constrict as well (consensual response). Any deviation from this is abnormal. This nerve is also responsible for eye adduction (toward the midline) and downward movement.

The trochlear (CN IV) and abducens (CN VI) nerves can also be tested by monitoring the movements of the extraocular muscles. The athlete is asked to visually follow a finger, while maintaining a static neck position, as it is slowly moved within the visual field. Then the athletic trainer passes the finger across the midline space toward the athlete's nose, watching for movement of both eyes in toward the midline and testing for convergence. Saccadic eye movements are tested by having the athlete look in each direction and watching the coordination and quality of movement. The trochlear nerve (CN IV) is responsible for upward eye movement, and the abducens nerve (CN VI) coordinates eye movement laterally away from the nose (figure 11.9).

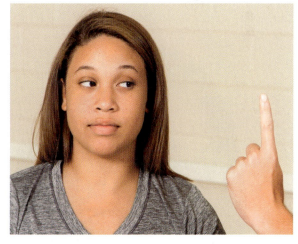

FIGURE 11.9   A test for the abducens nerve (CN VI) is to have the athlete move the eyes laterally, following the finger of the examiner.

The health care provider tests the response of the trigeminal nerve (CN V) and the facial nerve (CN VII) by observing for symmetry when the athlete bares teeth and clenches eyes closed (figure 11.10). Sensory testing of the trigeminal nerve is performed with a light touch and pinprick in the divisions of the trigeminal nerve on both sides. If any abnormalities are found, further tests are warranted. When testing the motor function of the trigeminal nerve, the athletic trainer has the athlete clench teeth and then place a hand under the athlete's chin to resist jaw opening. Any noticeable muscle atrophy or elicited muscle weakness indicates an abnormal test. Sensory testing of CN VII and CN IX (glossopharyngeal) appraises the athlete's ability to distinguish taste. For example, the athlete might be asked to tell the difference between sweet and sour.

Testing of the vestibulocochlear nerve (CN VIII) involves auditory testing of hearing and equilibrium. Auditory testing is performed using the Rinne test and the Weber test (see chapter 13). In both tests, a vibrating tuning fork is placed at various points on the patient's head, and the patient is asked to identify which placement is louder. Conductive deafness occurs when conduction of sound is impaired, as opposed to sensorineural deafness, in which there is neurological disruption. Auditory testing may also be conducted by creating a sound—such as snapping fingers—behind each of the athlete's ears and looking for a response.

Tests of the glossopharyngeal (CN IX), vagus (CN X), and hypoglossal (CN XII) nerves involve observing the athlete's tongue and mouth anatomy and watching for deviations in tongue movement when the mouth is opened and the tongue stuck out. The athlete is asked to push tongue against cheek or a depressor to demonstrate strength. The athletic trainer watches the uvula for deviation from midline as the patient says "aah." The vagus nerve (CN X) controls the gag reflex, which is assessed by touching each side of the pharyngeal wall behind the tonsils and observing movement of the uvula. The vagus nerve is also responsible for movement of the larynx and pharynx, which can be tested together by observing the quality and coordination of movement while the athlete swallows water.

The athletic trainer tests the spinal accessory nerve (CN XI) by focused examination of the sternocleidomastoid and trapezius muscles on both sides of the body. The strength of the trapezius muscle is assessed through a resisted shoulder shrug (figure 11.11), and the sternocleidomastoid muscle is assessed by resisting both turning and lifting of the chin. The presence of atrophy or weakness during resisted muscle movement suggests nerve injury.

Pathological Conditions

Pathological conditions discussed in this chapter are divided into sections as follows: brain and spinal cord disorders (sport-related concussion, stroke, Guillain-Barré syndrome); paroxysmal disorders (headaches, seizures); neuromuscular disorders (multiple sclerosis [MS], amyotrophic lateral sclerosis [ALS]); and pain disorders (complex regional pain syndrome).

The presentation and diagnosis of many neurological conditions are based on a process of exclusion. The phy-

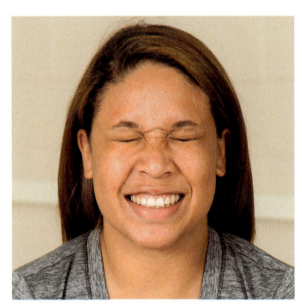

FIGURE 11.10 The trigeminal (CN V) and facial (CN VII) nerves are tested by clenching the teeth and making facial expressions, respectively.

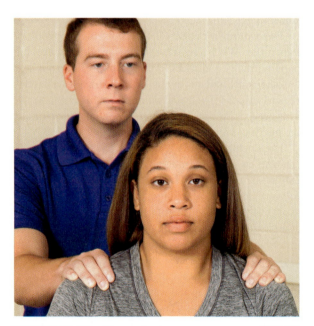

FIGURE 11.11 The spinal accessory nerve (CN XI) is tested by a resisted shrug, which determines the bilateral integrity of the trapezius muscle.

sician must exclude all other possible explanations for the symptoms in order to arrive at the correct diagnosis. Conditions such as Guillain-Barré syndrome, MS, ALS, and complex regional pain syndrome all have a rather insidious onset, and no single diagnostic test confirms the presence of the affliction. A thorough history is paramount in helping the clinician to arrive at the correct diagnosis. Patients often dismiss symptoms and attribute them to fatigue (vision problems, balance issues, headaches), and a complete medical history should illuminate the symptoms specific to the neurological condition.

Brain and Spinal Cord Disorders

Sport-Related Concussion

This section on sport-related concussions contributed by Tamara C. Valovich McLeod.

Sport-related concussion (SRC) is a common injury in recreational activities and sports that may have possible short- and long-term sequelae. Reports have estimated that approximately 1.6 to 3.8 million SRCs occur annually (Langlois 2006). It is also speculated that these numbers may be higher because of SRCs that are not recognized by the athlete and thus not reported (Guskiewicz et al. 2013; Baugh et al. 2014). Data from two national injury surveillance systems found that concussions represented 8.9% of all high school and 5.8% of all collegiate athletic injuries (Gessel et al. 2007).

An evidence-based definition was published after the Third International Conference on Concussion in Sport, held in 2008 (Benson et al. 2009), and again after the fourth conference in 2012 (Guskiewicz et al. 2013). This definition, provided in the sidebar "Definition of a Sport-Related Concussion," is more comprehensive and identifies clinical, pathological, and biomechanical features of concussion that are important in identifying these injuries (Benson et al. 2009). Immediate referral to the nearest emergency department is indicated for any athlete demonstrating any of the following signs and symptoms:

- Deterioration of neurological function
- Decreasing level of consciousness
- Decreasing or irregular respirations or pulse
- Unequal, unreactive, or dilated pupils
- Signs or symptoms of associated injuries
- Skull fracture (including cerebrospinal fluid from the nose or ears) or bleeding
- Decreasing mental status and seizures

Signs and Symptoms

The health care provider should be able to identify signs and symptoms associated with SRC. These signs and symptoms are often categorized as somatic (physical), emotional, cognitive, or sleep-related (Kontos et al. 2012). Symptoms that warrant referral to a medical facility are listed in the physician referral guidelines. Each athlete may present differently with respect to the severity and duration of symptoms. In an NCAA concussion study (McCrea et al. 2003), there was an increase in reported symptoms immediately after concussion, followed by a

---

CONDITION HIGHLIGHT

Definition of a Sport-Related Concussion

Concussion is defined as a complex pathophysiological process affecting the brain, induced by traumatic biomechanical forces. Several common features that incorporate clinical, pathological, and biomechanical injury constructs that may be used in defining the nature of concussive head injury include the following:

- Concussion may be caused by a direct blow to the head, face, or neck or by a blow elsewhere on the body with an "impulsive" force transmitted to the head.
- Concussion typically results in the rapid onset of short-lived impairment of neurological function that resolves spontaneously.
- Concussion may result in neuropathological changes, but the acute clinical symptoms largely reflect a functional disturbance rather than structural injury.
- Concussion results in a graded set of clinical syndromes that may or may not involve loss of consciousness. Resolution of the clinical and cognitive symptoms typically follows a sequential course; however, in a small percentage of cases, postconcussive symptoms may be prolonged.
- No abnormality on standard structural studies is seen in concussion.

gradual decrease in symptom complaints throughout the first week, with 91% of athletes returning to their baseline symptom levels by day 7 postinjury. Headache is the most common symptom reported and tends to last the longest.

Differential Diagnosis and Referral

As part of the initial assessment of SRC, the health care provider should try to rule out more severe head injuries such as skull fracture, cerebral contusion, and epidural hematomas (Guskiewicz et al. 2013; Broglio et al. 2014; Harmon et al. 2013). Assessment of these injuries may reveal acute localized swelling, deformity, prolonged loss of consciousness (LOC), intractable vomiting, and often multiple positive neurological examination findings such as cranial nerve abnormalities and motor or sensory weakness. Positive findings during an initial examination for loss of consciousness on the field, amnesia lasting longer than 15 min, deterioration of neurological function or consciousness, unequal or unreactive pupils, or other systemic declines should warrant immediate transfer to an emergency department capable of managing a neurosurgical emergency (Broglio et al. 2014). The clinician should continue to monitor the athlete for any signs of changing or deteriorating condition in the acute injury phase and throughout the first week postinjury that would increase suspicion of a subdural hematoma. Patients should be given a home instruction form that lists the warnings for immediate referral and other information about home care of the SRC (figure 11.12).

Physician referral is also indicated for athletes who are not experiencing a typical recovery, for those who may still be symptomatic in the weeks after their initial injury, and for those who demonstrate an increase in symptoms in the postacute phase. At this time, referral to a specific specialty may be necessary. For example, an athlete with sleep disturbances may benefit from a referral to a neurologist, whereas an athlete with cognitive difficulties may be best referred to a neuropsychologist (Broglio et al. 2014).

Diagnostic Tests

Because SRC is a functional injury and does not normally include structural injury to the brain, most diagnostic tests will result in negative imaging findings, thus making neuroimaging of little value for most SRCs (Guskiewicz et al. 2013; Broglio et al. 2014; Harmon et al. 2013; Giza et al. 2013). Suspicion of an intracranial hemorrhage or hematoma should result in immediate referral for a computed tomography (CT) scan, functional magnetic resonance imaging (MRI), or other imaging study. Moreover, the sudden presence or deterioration of symptoms that had previously resolved or had remained stable necessitates

Concussion Legislation and Policy

Health care providers need to be aware of the laws and policies regarding SRC. In 2009, the first law was passed in the state of Washington, and since that time, all 50 states and the District of Columbia have passed concussion laws. All 51 of the laws apply to high school student-athletes, with 50 laws also applying to middle school students, and 42 applicable to youth athletes (Baugh et al. 2014). The language in most laws differs, but most include three common components: (1) concussion education and informed consent, (2) removal from play, and (3) return-to-play guidelines (Harvey 2013). The laws differ in the areas of required coach or health care provider training, liability waivers, designation of qualified medical providers, and the delivery mode for concussion education. A few studies have begun to evaluate the impact of these laws and have found an increase in coach knowledge (Chrisman et al. 2014; Shenouda et al. 2012) and health care utilization (Bompadre et al. 2014; Gibson et al. 2015; Mackenzie et al. 2015) after implementation of the law. Health care providers should understand the concussion laws in the states in which they practice to be sure they comply with all aspects of the laws.

In addition to state laws, many sport organizations, school districts, and schools have their own concussion policies. Most states have an interscholastic athletic association that oversees all sports and activities in its state, and most of these associations have concussion policies, which may be similar to or more conservative than the state law. Other organizations, such as Pop Warner Football (Pop Warner 2015) and USA Soccer, have developed concussion policies as well.

Patient Instructions for Sport-Related Concussions

I believe that _____ sustained a concussion on _____. To make sure he or she recovers, please follow the following important recommendations:

1. _____ must report to the athletic training facility on _____ at _____ for a follow-up evaluation.

2. If any of the problems below develop before the follow-up visit, please call _____ at _____ or contact the local emergency medical system or your family physician.

   ○ Decreasing level of consciousness
   ○ Increasing confusion
   ○ Increasing irritability
   ○ Loss of or fluctuating level of consciousness
   ○ Numbness in the arms or legs
   ○ Pupils becoming unequal in size
   ○ Repeated vomiting
   ○ Seizures
   ○ Slurred speech or inability to speak
   ○ Inability to recognize people or places
   ○ Worsening headache

   Otherwise, you can follow the instructions outlined below.

It is OK to

- Use acetaminophen (Tylenol) for headaches
- Use ice pack on head and neck as needed for comfort
- Eat a carbohydrate-rich diet
- Go to sleep
- Rest (no strenuous activity or sports)

There is NO need to

- Check eyes with flashlight
- Wake up frequently (unless otherwise instructed)
- Test reflexes
- Stay in bed

Do NOT

- Drink alcohol
- Drive a car or operate machinery
- Engage in physical activity (e.g., exercise, weightlifting, physical education, sport participation) that makes symptoms worse
- Engage in mental activity (e.g., school, job, homework, computer games) that makes symptoms worse

Other recommendations:

Recommendations provided to _____

Please feel free to contact me if you have any questions. I can be reached at _____.

Please follow up in the athletic training facility on _____ (date).

FIGURE 11.12 Take-home instructions for patients with sport-related concussions.

Reprinted from S.P. Broglio et al., 2014, "National Athletic Trainers' Association Position Statement: Management of sport concussion," *Journal of Athletic Training* 49(2): 245-265.

neuroimaging for a subdural hematoma, which may not be noted on a CT scan or MRI for 1 to 2 wk after the initial concussion (Broglio et al. 2014). However, a negative imaging finding does not rule out an SRC, and it should not be used to prematurely return a patient to activity.

Assessment

The assessment of SRC should begin off-season or during preseason in conjunction with the preparticipation physical examination (PPE) to obtain an adequate concussion history and to assess baseline measures of symptom reports, postural stability, and neurocognition. The PPE should include a thorough neurological injury history, including a history of sport-related concussion and other concussive injuries (e.g., motor vehicle accidents, falls) (Preparticipation Physical Evaluation Working Group 2010). The PPE should contain an adequate series of questions regarding concussion history, including queries about perceived previous concussions and those focusing on earlier concussion-related symptoms sustained during both sport and non-sport activity. Knowledge of an athlete's concussion history is important as research has demonstrated a relationship between previous concussions and increased risk for later injury (Harmon et al. 2013; Scopaz and Hatzenbuehler 2013; Broglio et al. 2014). In addition, baseline measures of symptoms, neurocognitive function, and postural stability should be obtained from the athlete when he or she is healthy for future comparison with postconcussion scores.

After a concussion, the athlete should be assessed immediately for symptom reports, mental status, and postural stability. Serial assessments using tools, such as the graded symptom checklist (GSC) or scale should take place at planned intervals (postgame, 24, 48 and 72 h postinjury) to assess the athlete's recovery. The GSC asks patients to relay symptoms, such as blurred vision, dizziness, "in a fog" feeling, headache, nausea, irritability, and so on, and the athletic trainer notes changes in the number of symptoms reported or if new symptoms arise. Once the athlete reports the disappearance of symptoms, the more complex neurocognitive assessments should be administered to determine whether cognitive recovery has occurred as well. Scores on all assessment tools should meet or improve on baseline scores before a return-to-play progression is begun.

Self-Report Symptoms

Athletic trainers typically use instruments to identify postconcussion signs and symptoms (PCSS). There are several variations of PCSS tools, including both symptom checklists and graded symptom scales (GSSs), that differ in the number of symptoms they list and whether symptoms are grouped into the factors mentioned pre-

viously (Gioia et al. 2009; Broglio et al. 2014). A PCSS checklist is composed of a list of commonly noted concussion symptoms to which the athlete responds simply yes or no as to whether he or she is experiencing each symptom. A GSS is a more objective measure that provides detailed information about concussion severity or duration. Using a Likert scale, the athlete notes the extent to which he or she is experiencing each symptom. The summative score can then be calculated. The first score is the sum of Likert scale responses and represents a "total symptom score." The second score is the total number of symptoms for which the athlete indicated a severity or duration score greater than zero (Broglio et al. 2014). In addition to these stand-alone PCSS tools, some of the computerized neurocognitive tests and the Sport Concussion Assessment Tool-3 (SCAT-3) (Casa et al. 2013) have a GSS built into the tool.

A meta-analysis investigating the degree to which concussion affected self-report symptoms, neurocognitive ability, and postural stability found a significant increase in self-report symptoms in the immediate postinjury phase and during follow-up examinations within the first 14 d postinjury. This further highlights the need for clinicians to use some tool to assess PCSS in all athletes with a suspected concussion (Broglio and Puetz 2008). Clinicians should ensure that the checklist or scale chosen is appropriate for their patients, as children and adolescents must be assessed with appropriate symptom inventories (Gioia et al. 2009; Broglio et al. 2014).

Mental Status Testing

Mental status tests are often used on the sideline or in the acute postinjury phase to determine the presence of cognitive deficits in an athlete with a suspected concussion. These tests differ from the computerized neurocognitive tests in that they are simple cognitive screening tests and are most sensitive to deficits in cognition within the first 48 h postinjury (Barr and McCrea 2001). These tests may be more informal and can include questions of orientation and memory (Maddock's questions [Maddocks, Dicker, and Saling 1995]), repeating digits backward or forward, serial subtraction of 3's or 7's (Young et al. 1997), or repeating days of the week or months of the year in reverse order. In addition, several more formal mental status tests have been used in the evaluation of SRC, including the Standardized Assessment of Concussion (SAC) (Barr and McCrea 2001) and SCAT-3 (Casa et al. 2013).

The SAC has adequate reliability, validity, and sensitivity to change subsequent to SRC (Barr and McCrea 2001; McCrea 2001; McCrea, Kelly, and Randolph 2000; McCrea et al. 2002) and has been evaluated as an assessment tool in collegiate (McCrea et al. 2003; McCrea et al. 2005), high school (McCrea 2001; McCrea, Kelly, and Randolph 2000), and youth sports athletes (Valovich McLeod 2006; Valovich McLeod et al. 2004). The SAC was found to indicate the largest negative effect (decrease in cognition) of all cognitive tests studied, including pencil-and-paper and computerized batteries, during the immediate postinjury assessment (Broglio and Puetz 2008). This finding supports single studies that evaluated the SAC and found it to be the most sensitive in detecting cognitive deficits in the first 48 h after concussion (McCrea et al. 2005).

Neurocognitive Testing

Although mental status testing is important on the sideline and in the immediate postinjury phase, those tests are not sensitive enough to determine the extent of more complex cognitive deficits. Nor are they useful in making return-to-play decisions during the later stages of recovery. Pencil-and-paper neurocognitive batteries or, more commonly, computerized neurocognitive concussion programs are used once an athlete is asymptomatic to determine whether cognitive deficits still exist. Clinicians using neurocognitive assessments should be aware of factors that might affect test performance and the interpretation of the scores, including demographic variables (age, ethnicity, native tongue, education level), medical conditions (learning disabilities, attention deficit disorder, anxiety, sleep disorders, concussion history), preinjury cognitive function, and previous exposure to neurocognitive testing (learning effects) (Grindel, Lovell, and Collins 2001).

Pencil-and-paper batteries are typically put together by neuropsychologists trained to administer and interpret these types of assessments. A baseline battery may last up to 30 min, with postinjury assessments being slightly shorter, and is composed of several different neurocognitive tests that assess domains sensitive to impairment after SRC. These include attention, concentration, processing speed, learning, memory, and executive functioning (Barr 2001). Some of the more common computerized neurocognitive examinations available on the market today, along with their assessment domains, are listed here.

- ANAM (Automated Neuropsychological Assessment Metrics Sports Medicine): Attention, concentration, reaction time, memory, processing speed, decision making
- Axon Sports CCAT: Attention, processing speed, learning, working memory speed, working memory accuracy
- Concussion Resolution Index: Simple reaction time, complex reaction time, processing speed
- ImPACT (Immediate Post-Concussive Assessment and Cognitive Testing): Verbal memory, visual memory, processing speed, reaction time, impulse control
- CVS (Concussion Vital Signs): Concentration, attention, memory, reaction time, processing speed

Significant deficits in neurocognitive function have been noted during both initial assessment and subsequent follow-up evaluations, with the effect of concussion on neurocognition resulting in a smaller but still significant negative effect during the first 14 d postinjury (Broglio and Puetz 2008). The largest negative effect on cognition reported at the follow-up assessment was found with pencil-and-paper batteries, indicating they were more sensitive to detecting cognitive deficits. Mild to moderate negative effects in cognitive function immediately after concussion and little effect, indicating full neurocognitive recovery, by 7 to 10 d postinjury were also reported in a prior meta-analysis of concussion and neurocognitive function (Belanger and Vanderploeg 2005). Although both of these meta-analyses found a lesser effect with computerized neurocognitive programs, these programs may be more cost- and time-effective as well as clinician-friendly in the assessment of SRC.

Postural Stability Testing

The assessment of postural control or postural stability has become another central component of concussion evaluation plans. Computerized force plate systems (Guskiewicz 2001), such as the NeuroCom Sensory Organization Test, and clinical balance measures (Riemann and Guskiewicz 2000), such as the Balance Error Scoring System (BESS), have been advocated as means to assess postural stability, and these have been shown to be sensitive to deficits in postural stability until about 5 d postinjury (Guskiewicz 2001). In addition, large negative effects were found in postural control measures both immediately after SRC and during follow-up assessments (Broglio and Puetz 2008).

The BESS has several clinical advantages compared with force plate measures of postural stability, including cost-effectiveness (requiring only a stopwatch and a foam pad), efficiency (taking only 5 min to administer), and portability (foam pad is transported easily). The BESS consists of six separate 20 s balance tests completed in three different stances on both firm and foam surfaces (figure 11.13): *(a)* double leg stance, *(b)* tandem leg stance (nondominant leg placed behind dominant leg), *(c)* single leg stance (standing on nondominant leg), *(d)* double leg stance on foam, *(e)* tandem leg stance on foam, and *(f)* single leg stance on foam (Riemann and Guskiewicz 2000). During each of the test conditions, error scores are recorded when the athlete compensates to aid balance. Errors include each instance of opening eyes; lifting hands off hips; stepping, falling, or lifting foot or heel; remaining out of position more than 5 s; or hip in more than 30° of abduction or flexion. Recent advancements in mobile technology have also led to the development of several applications for balance assessment using smartphones and tablets.

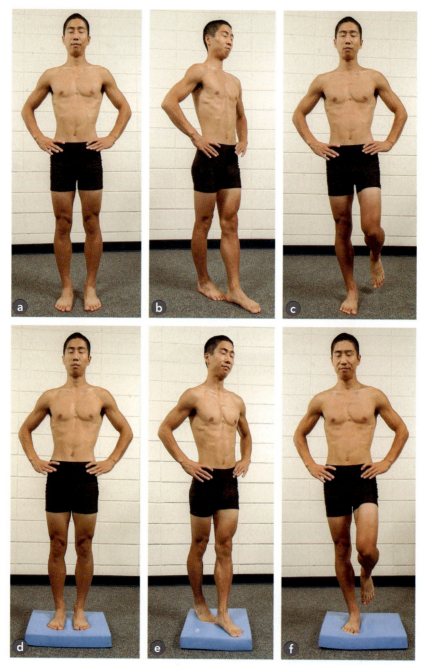

FIGURE 11.13   The Balance Error Scoring System (BESS) is one method of assessing balance after concussion.

Oculomotor Testing

Oculomotor function is another dimension of vestibular function that should be assessed following a concussion. The cranial nerve assessment that is included as part of the neurologic evaluation should enable the clinician to evaluate visual acuity, saccades, smooth pursuits, eye motion, and vergence (convergence and divergence) (Valovich McLeod and Hale 2015; Mucha et al. 2014). Recently, two clinical assessments have been introduced that can supplement the clinical examination and provide objective measures of oculomotor function: the Vestibular/Ocular Motor Screening (VOMS) and King-Devick test. The VOMS is a clinical examination that evaluates smooth pursuits, horizontal and vertical saccades, convergence, horizontal vestibular–ocular reflex testing, and visual motor sensitivity, along with self-report symptom assessment following each test to determine the presence of headache, dizziness, nausea, and fogginess (Mucha et al. 2014). The King-Devick test is an evaluation of horizontal saccadic eye movement, processing speed, and attention (Galetta et al. 2011). This test is a timed rapid number reading assessment in which the difficulty increases as the patient progresses through the three cards. The test is scored as the total time required to read the three test cards, and the examiner also records the number of errors made during the testing time (Galetta et al. 2011; Galetta et al. 2015).

Multifaceted Testing

Although each of the previously described assessment categories is important, a multifaceted approach to concussion assessment has been advocated by several consensus and position statements (Giza et al. 2013; Broglio et al. 2014; McCrory, Meeuwisse, Aubry, Cantu, Dvorak, Echemendia, et al. 2013) and supported by research (Broglio and Puetz 2008; McCrea et al. 2005). These multifaceted concussion plans have been shown to increase diagnostic accuracy when compared with individual tests of neurocognition, postural stability, or self-report symptoms (Van Kampen et al. 2006; Broglio and Puetz 2008; McCrea et al. 2005). McCrea and colleagues (2005) reported increased sensitivity up to 93% with a protocol consisting of a GSS, the SAC, and BESS, compared with the sensitivity of each individual tool: GSS (89%), SAC (80%), and BESS (34%). Similarly, the sensitivity of a PCSS increased from 64% to 83% with the addition of ImPACT (Van Kampen et al. 2006). Finally, higher sensitivity values were found with the addition of postural stability measures and a GSS to ImPACT (91.7%), the HeadMinder Concussion Resolution Index (CRI) (89.3%), and pencil-and-paper neurocognitive batteries (95.7%) (Broglio, Macciocchi, and Ferrara 2007).

Clinicians may benefit the most by using a multifaceted assessment paradigm that includes a PCSS, the SAC, and a measure of postural stability during their initial assessment within the first 48 h postinjury, followed by the use of a PCSS, postural stability measure, and a pencil-and-paper or computerized neurocognitive battery, which may provide more useful information, once the athlete is asymptomatic, in making return-to-play decisions.

Management and Return to Activity

An initial period of physical and cognitive rest, followed by a gradual return-to-activity progression is recommended for managing concussion (Broglio et al. 2014; McCrory, Meeuwisse, Aubry, Cantu, Dvorak, Echemendia, et al. 2013). During this time, the patient should remain out of sport participation and other exercise, such as physical education classes. The patient may also be prescribed a period of cognitive rest that may include academic adjustments in the classroom.

Cognitive rest involves avoiding or limiting activities that produce mental exertion that could result in neurometabolic processes and stressors that may delay recovery (Valovich McLeod and Gioia 2010). Many concussion-related symptoms may follow cognitive activity, and patients should reduce mental challenges to levels that are tolerable during the initial postinjury stage (Valovich McLeod and Gioia 2010). Cognitive rest may include a reduction in activities of daily living, scholastic stressors, time spent using technology, and school attendance and activities. However, bed rest or strict rest from all cognitive activities may actually worsen symptoms and result in a longer recovery (Thomas et al. 2015). Clinicians need to balance rest with light activity and progressively increase mental demands as the patient's symptoms resolve.

The progression of cognitive activities is also termed the *return to learn* progression, and it helps the patient to achieve a full return to the classroom (Halstead et al. 2013), which should precede any return to sport participation (Halstead et al. 2013; Broglio et al. 2014; McCrory, Meeuwisse, Aubry, Cantu, Dvorak, Echemendia, et al. 2013; Giza et al. 2013). Every patient will be different, and some may progress rapidly, while others may require a more gradual progression that may include formal academic accommodations, such as a 504 plan or an Individualized Education Plan (Sady, Vaughan, and Gioia 2011; Gioia 2015). It has been suggested that the patient should not return to even a modified school day until he or she can concentrate for at least 30 min without an increase in symptoms (Gioia 2015). The progression should then move from partial attendance with academic adjustments, to full attendance with academic adjustments, to full attendance without additional support (DeMatteo et al. 2015). Academic adjustments are determined based on the types of symptoms the patient is experiencing. Successful return-to-learn progressions require collaboration and communication between the patient's health care providers and school personnel.

Similarly, return-to-play guidelines follow a specific progression that begins when the athlete reports asymptomatic, has returned to baseline values on all assessments, and is fully integrated back into the classroom. A stepwise progression (McCrory, Meeuwisse, Aubry, Cantu, Dvorak, Echemendia, et al. 2013; Broglio et al. 2014; DeMatteo et al. 2015) calls for a 24 h symptom-free period between steps. The progression allows the athlete to begin performing exercises of increasing intensity, beginning with a subexertional exercise protocol of 10 to 15 min (i.e., stationary bike intervals) to determine whether symptoms return with the onset of exercise and the associated increase in heart rate and blood pressure. The next day, the athlete can then participate in sport-specific exercises for a set duration of 20 to 30 min, followed by on-field practice with no contact, on-field practice with body contact, and then return to full competition. A recurring suggestion in many recommendation and consensus statements is that in the absence of objective balance or neurocognitive assessments, once the athlete reports symptom free, a 7 d waiting period is observed before beginning the stepladder return-to-play progression. In this progression, a level is not begun until the athlete is symptom-free for 24 h after completing the previous step (McCrory, Meeuwisse, Aubry, Cantu, Dvorak, Ruben, et al. 2013; Broglio et al. 2014).

Prognosis

The prognosis for most patients after SRC is good. In general, symptoms tend to resolve in the first week after injury, cognition returns to baseline levels in 5 to 7 d, and postural stability impairments return to preinjury levels within 3 to 5 d (McCrea et al. 2003). However, there is some evidence to suggest that athletes with certain modifying factors may have a prolonged recovery or require a more conservative return-to-play progression (McCrory Meeuwisse, Aubry, Cantu, Dvorak, Echemendia, et al. 2013; Scopaz and Hatzenbuehler 2013; Makdissi et al. 2013). These modifying factors include <18 years of age, history of migraine, depression, or other mental health disorders, attention deficit hyperactivity disorder, learning disabilities, and sleep disorders. Furthermore, patients with a prior concussion history—especially those with past injuries that occurred close together or that took longer for symptoms to resolve—should be managed more conservatively (McCrory Meeuwisse, Aubry, Cantu, Dvorak, Echemendia, et al. 2013).

Prevention

There is currently no evidence that any piece of athletic equipment (helmet, mouth guard, headgear) can effectively reduce the incidence or severity of SRC (McCrory, Meeuwisse, Aubry, Cantu, Dvorak, Echemendia, et al. 2013; Broglio et al. 2014; Benson et al. 2009; Benson et al. 2013; McCrory, Meeuwisse, Aubry, Cantu, Dvorak, Ruben, et al. 2013). Awareness and education currently serve as the best means of prevention by informing athletes, coaches, parents, and health care providers about the signs and symptoms of SRC so that these injuries can be reported appropriately. Several educational programs have been advocated, including the Centers for Disease Control and Prevention's concussion tool kits (Sarmiento et al. 2010) and Canada's Think First program (Sarmiento et al. 2010; Williamson et al. 2014).

Stroke

A stroke, also called a **cerebrovascular accident (CVA)**, is a condition caused by lack of oxygen to the brain that may lead to reversible or irreversible paralysis and other neurological damage. Such damage to a group of nerve cells in the brain is often caused by interrupted blood flow from a blood clot or aneurysm in which the blood vessel bursts. Depending on the area of the brain that is damaged, a stroke can cause coma, paralysis, speech problems, dementia, or death. An often overlooked category of stroke is the transient ischemic attack (TIA). Because the episode is momentary, often lasting only a few minutes, the TIA does not leave permanent damage to the brain, but that does not diminish the gravity of the event. The cause, presentation, and risk factors are the same in TIAs and in strokes. Any damage is less noticeable because the blockage is temporary. Nonetheless, TIAs are warnings that full blood flow to the brain is not occurring. As with a stroke, the TIA is a medical emergency.

The American Heart Association states that stroke is the fifth leading cause of death in the United States, and African-American men have twice the risk of stroke that other racial groups or gender affiliations do (American Heart Association 2015). The main risk factors for stroke are dyslipidemia (38%), smoking (34%), hypertension (20%), and diabetes mellitus (11%) (Ruijun et al. 2013). Other risk factors for a stroke are obesity, high cholesterol (total cholesterol greater than 200 mg/dl), family history of stroke or cardiovascular disease, and lack of vitamin D.

Although rare, approximately 10% to 14% of ischemic strokes occur in persons between the ages of 18 and 45, but children can sustain them as well (Ruijun et al. 2013). In recent years, a 14-year-old football player sustained a stroke secondary to a concussion, a 15-year-old was misdiagnosed with a migraine, and a 27-year-old girl's basketball coach thought she had a dizzy spell, but all were eventually diagnosed with a stroke, and all recovered (Dorksen 2015; Janes 2013; Comer 2015). In athletes, a primary cause of stroke may be head injury. Head injury often causes intracranial bleeding, with common sites including intracerebral areas, especially the inferior frontal and temporal lobes, and the subarachnoid, subdural, and epidural spaces (see figure 11.2). Another cause of stroke associated with intracerebral hemorrhage in young adults is drug abuse, specifically the designer drugs amphetamine, cocaine, and ecstasy (Ruijun et al. 2013). In such cases, evaluation may be hindered when a cause is not readily apparent. A careful clinical history from the athlete or especially close friends and acquaintances is vital.

Signs and Symptoms

Health care providers working with physically active people need to recognize the signs and symptoms of a possible stroke, and they should not rule it out simply due to the age or fitness of the patient. The National Stroke Association has a simple mnemonic to help you to quickly recognize a suspected stroke (National Stroke Association 2016). Speedy identification and access to medical care improve stroke recovery. The mnemonic is "Act **FAST**":

F Face: Ask the person to smile. Does one side of the face droop?

A Arms: Ask the person to raise both arms. Does one arm drift downward?

S Speech: Ask the person to repeat a phrase. Is their speech slurred or strange?

T Time: Time is of the essence. If any of these signs are observed, call the emergency medical service (9-1-1).

Knowledge of the cranial nerves and their functions is also helpful in determining the extent of neurological involvement. Awareness of Brodmann's areas of the brain is very helpful in diagnosing where a problem may lie (see figure 11.4).

In the athletic setting, a differential diagnosis for a stroke may include epileptic seizure with postictal Todd's paresis, a focal weakness after generalized or focal motor seizures that is uncommon in persistence for more than a few hours. Other differential diagnoses include tumor, migraine, metabolic encephalopathy caused by fever or infection, hyperglycemia, or hypercalcemia (Ferri 2016). In addition, drug interactions, overdose, or abuse should not be overlooked.

Referral and Diagnostic Tests

A stroke is a medical emergency. Emergency treatment is crucial because every minute lost from the onset of symptoms to the time of emergency contact limits the window of opportunity for intervention. Many patients do not go to the emergency department until 24 h or more after the onset of symptoms. The longer the delay, the greater the damage and loss of potential for recovery.

Diagnosis requires a complete medical history, physical and neurological examination, complete blood count (CBC) including electrolyte levels, and a battery of specific diagnostic tests. The tests fall into four categories: imaging tests, including CT scan and MRI; **electroencephalogram (EEG)** and evoked potentials test to record electrical activity and sensory response patterns; Doppler blood flow studies to reveal the patency of the arteries at the base of the skull or in the neck; and arteriography (in which dye is injected into the vessels) combined with radiography to reveal blood flow through the vessels in the brain and to show the size and location of any blockages (Ferri 2016).

Treatment and Return to Participation

Acute treatment is designed to reverse or lessen the amount of tissue death. The goal is to have the patient stabilized, imaged, and have compete laboratory studies within 60 min of the onset of the stroke (Jauch 2015). This involves medical support to optimize tissue perfusion and to prevent complications such as infection, deep vein thrombosis (DVT), and pulmonary embolism (PE). Administration of pharmaceutical agents through intravenous or intraarterial lines may be combined with anticoagulant and antiplatelet agents, heparin or aspirin, and possibly hypothermia to mitigate cell destruction secondary to ischemia (National Stroke Association 2016; Jauch 2015).

Poststroke rehabilitation starts in the hospital as soon as possible after the stroke. Stable patients can begin rehabilitation within 2 d after the stroke has occurred and

---

🚩 **RED FLAGS FOR STROKE**

Signs and symptoms of a possible stroke include sudden occurrence of the following:

- Numbness or weakness of the face, arm, or leg, especially on one side of the body
- Confusion, trouble speaking or understanding
- Vision difficulties in one or both eyes
- Problem with speaking, slurred speech
- Trouble walking, dizziness, loss of balance or coordination
- Severe headache with no known cause

continue as necessary after release from the hospital. The choice of rehabilitation options after stroke depends on tissue damage and severity and includes the following:

- Rehabilitation unit in the hospital
- Subacute care unit
- Rehabilitation hospital
- Home therapy
- Home with outpatient therapy
- Occupational therapy
- Speech–language therapy

The goal of rehabilitation is to improve function so that the stroke survivor can continue an independent lifestyle. Such training must be accomplished in a way that preserves dignity and motivates the patient to relearn basic skills for the activities of daily life that may have been lost, including communicating, eating, dressing, and walking.

It is not fully understood how the brain compensates for the damage caused by stroke. A slight interruption in the flow of oxygenated blood may damage a few brain cells temporarily that later resume functioning. In some cases, because different areas of the brain overlap in function, the brain can reorganize, with one area taking over for the area damaged by the stroke. Because of this organ fluidity, stroke survivors sometimes experience remarkable and unanticipated recoveries.

For an athlete, return to full athletic participation after a stroke depends primarily on the level of recovery and residual impairment as well as the type of sport (i.e., contact or collision sports vs. noncontact sports). An athlete who has incurred a stroke as a result of a head injury may be ruled medically ineligible to participate even when recovery has been complete. Any athlete who has sustained a stroke related to a medical issue that could be exacerbated by activity should refrain from dangerous activity in the future. Further, the risk of additional injury may be too great to continue participation in sports such as hockey, football, or lacrosse.

Regarding participation in physical activity and exercise, studies have documented the positive effects of physical training on the recovery and rehabilitation process after a stroke. In addition to the obvious physical benefits of a training and reconditioning program, a return to physical activity may also boost the athlete's psychological recovery. Activities' intensity, duration, and volume are best chosen with the guidance of the medical team and the athletic trainer supervising the athlete's recovery. A recent systematic review found that stroke survivors expend more energy during walking than healthy people. The take-home message is that typical low-intensity exercises may be moderate-level exercises for stroke patients, and the focus should be on patient

efforts (Kramer et al. 2015). Recovery is generally slow and tedious and may take many months.

Prevention

Stroke prevention has two major components: lifestyle risk factors and trauma prevention factors. Lifestyle risk factors such as obesity, diabetes, hypertension, and smoking may not be issues for physically active young people, but athletes should understand their significance for cerebrovascular disease later in life. Death from stroke is the fifth leading cause of fatalities in the United States.

In addition, hypertension in the athlete cannot be underestimated as a risk factor for stroke. Athletes who are hypertensive on the preparticipation examination should have serial blood pressures taken before and after exercise for several weeks to see if the high readings continue. If blood pressures continue to be hypertensive, the athlete needs to be referred to a physician for further evaluation and possible medications.

Trauma protection is key in the prevention of stroke for an athlete involved in collision sports; this may include proper helmet fitting and compliance. Stroke caused by intracranial hemorrhage from head trauma is considered one of the most severe sequelae.

According to the American Heart Association, prevention strategies include increased physical activity; a diet high in fruits, vegetables, and whole grains; and a lowering of saturated fats in the diet. The moderate consumption of alcohol (one or two glasses of red wine a day) may lower the risk for stroke, but the negative effects of alcohol may negate the positive. The once-popular daily dose of aspirin to thin the blood also has negative consequences for the gastrointestinal system (American Heart Association 2015).

Guillain-Barré Syndrome

Guillain-Barré syndrome (GBS) is an acute, diffuse demyelinating disorder of the spinal roots and peripheral nerves. On rare occasions it also attacks the cranial nerves. This polyneuropathy is an autoimmune syndrome that is sudden, often severe, and rapidly progressive (Ferri 2016). Specific lymphocytes are thought to produce antibodies against components of the myelin sheath and may contribute to the destruction of myelin. As noted previously, without myelin, nerve conduction is interrupted.

GBS occurs year-round at a rate of approximately 1 case per 1 million people per month; there are approximately 3,500 cases per year in North America. The condition may occur in either gender and at any age but is uncommon in early childhood. Race is not a factor. The incidence increases with age, and about two-thirds of patients with GBS experience symptoms of viral respiratory or gastrointestinal infection 1 to 3 wk before the onset of neurological symptoms (Centers for Disease Control and Prevention 2015b). In 1976, there was a small increase in GBS following swine flu vaccination. Although the trend is to blame the vaccine on the illness, there are no confirmed data following that year that support this claim (Centers for Disease Control and Prevention 2015b; Toussirot and Bereau 2016). GBS is not contagious.

The health care provider must be able to recognize the symptoms of rapid onset of bilateral muscle weakness in the lower extremities with the absence of fever or other systemic symptoms and refer the athlete immediately to the appropriate medical facility, usually the hospital emergency department.

Signs and Symptoms

The major clinical symptom of GBS is distal muscle weakness and loss of deep tendon reflexes that occurs bilaterally. The pattern is typically an ascending paralysis initially noted in the legs. The weakness evolves quickly over several hours or days and may be accompanied by tingling and dysesthesias in all extremities. The trunk, intercostals, neck, and cranial muscles may be involved later. Weakness may progress to total motor paralysis with death from respiratory failure within a few days. Frequently, early symptoms will also include paresthesias and numbness. A varying degree of sensory loss occurs in the first days and in a few days is barely detectable. When sensory deficits are present, deep sensations such as touch, pressure, and vibration are likely to be more affected than superficial sensations to pain or temperature. Complaints of pain and an aching discomfort, especially in muscles of the hips, thighs, and back, occur in 50% or more of the patients (Andary 2015; Ferri 2016). GBS patients may also present with a facial droop similar to Bell's palsy, diplopia, and difficulty with speech or swallowing.

Differential diagnoses for GBS include metabolic myopathies, poliomyelitis, spinal cord compression, heavy metal intoxication, botulism, tick paralysis, and basilar artery occlusion (Andary 2015; National Institute of Neurological Disorders and Stroke 2015a).

Referral and Diagnostic Tests

A patient who experiences bilateral, rapidly evolving muscle weakness with absence of fever or other systemic symptoms and has a history of a recent viral upper respiratory infection (URI) or gastrointestinal illness must be referred to a physician immediately. GBS in its most severe form is a medical emergency. Most patients require hospitalization, and almost 30% require breathing assistance at some time during the course of the illness. Severe GBS may result in total paralysis and inability to

⚑ RED FLAGS FOR GUILLAIN-BARRÉ SYNDROME

Signs and symptoms of Guillain-Barré syndrome include the following:

- Progressive weakness beginning distally and moving proximally
- Areflexia
- Afebrile state
- Pain with slightest movement of affected area
- Nocturnal muscular cramps

breathe without the help of a ventilator. Thirty percent of patents complain of residual weakness 3 yr after recovery (National Institute of Neurological Disorders and Stroke 2015a; Andary 2015).

In addition to deficient deep tendon reflexes, key diagnostic and laboratory tests include an **electromyologram (EMG)** and CSF analysis via a lumbar puncture. An EMG records and measures the electrical activity produced by a specific skeletal muscle. The test is performed by applying surface electrodes or by inserting small needle electrodes into a muscle. This test is performed to determine whether there is any defect in the nerve associated with the muscle or whether the nerve is not responding normally because of disease or impingement. CSF findings are distinctive but conclusive only after the first week. They include an elevated CSF protein level (100 to 1,000 mg/dl) without an accompanying increase in cells. When symptoms have been present for less than 48 h, the CSF is often normal. Nearly 75% of those diagnosed reach their lowest point of clinical function within 1 wk, and the remainder reaches it within 1 mo (Ferri 2016).

Nerve conduction velocity (NCV) has also proven to be diagnostic, as the rate at which the nerve impulse travels to the muscle is often slower in a limb affected with GBS. The principal EMG findings are a reduction in the amplitudes of muscle action potentials, slowed conduction velocity, and conduction block in motor nerves (Andary 2015). GBS is described as a syndrome and not a disease because there is no specific disease-causing agent. Diagnosis is made by a physician carefully evaluating the athlete's symptoms and recognizing the pattern of rapidly evolving signs of paralysis, diminished or absent reflexes, lack of fever or other systemic symptoms, and the results of laboratory tests, EMG, NCV, and CSF analysis. If the diagnosis is strongly suspected, treatment is initiated without waiting for the occurrence of characteristic EMG and CSF findings.

Treatment and Return to Participation

Treatment is initiated as soon after diagnosis as possible. There is no cure for the syndrome, and although patients do get better, they rarely recover completely. Therapies are aimed at lessening the severity of the symptoms, accelerating the rate of recovery in most patients, and managing complications of the syndrome, such as fluctuations in blood pressure and heart rate, inability to breathe without respiratory assistance, and inability to chew and swallow. Plasmapheresis and high-dose immunoglobulin therapy have been demonstrated to be effective (Andary 2015).

Rehabilitation involves being prudent with respect to possible thrombophlebitis, urine retention, and airway management for the sickest of patients. Skin conditions such as bedsores and contractures can occur. These can be circumvented with diligent skin care and inspection and range-of-motion exercises.

Most people reach the stage of greatest weakness within the first week after symptoms appear, and by the fourth week of the illness, 98% of all patients are at their weakest (National Institute of Neurological Disorders and Stroke 2015a). The recovery period may be as short as a few weeks or as long as several years. Approximately 85% of patients with GBS recover completely or nearly completely, with mild motor deficits in the feet or legs. About 3% may suffer a relapse of muscle weakness and tingling sensations many years after the initial attack. Evidence of widespread axonal damage, as well as early and prolonged mechanical ventilatory assistance, occur to those with the most severe and rapidly progressing form of the disease. EMG findings are consistent predictors of residual weakness. The mortality rate is less than 5% (Porter and Kaplan 2011).

Return to participation will be determined by the level of symptom resolution and clearance by the medical team. It may take 1 yr or more for symptoms to resolve.

Paroxysmal Disorders

Paroxysmal disorders are neurological conditions that have symptoms that come and go and are episodic in nature. Typically, these conditions go away on their own, only to return without warning. Examples of paroxysmal disorders discussed here are headaches, seizures, and vertigo.

Headaches

According to the World Health Organization, a headache is the most common disorder of the nervous system (World Health Organization 2012). The National Institute of Neurological Disorders and Stroke (NINDS) identifies four types of headache: vascular, muscle contraction (tension), traction, and inflammatory (National Institute of Neurological Disorders and Stroke 2015b). Vascular headaches are caused by spasms of the vessels surrounding the brain and include migraines, fever-inducing toxic headaches, headaches as a result of high blood pressure, and cluster headaches. Tension headaches result from muscular tension on the cervical spine and cranium. Traction and inflammatory headaches result from other disorders that could include eye strain, hypoglycemia, stroke, or a sinus infection (National Institute of Neurological Disorders and Stroke 2015b). In general, headaches can serve as indicators of potentially critical underlying conditions. Ninety percent of headaches are classified as vascular, tension or muscle contraction, or a combination of the two. The remaining 10% consist of headaches associated with intracranial, systemic, or psychological disorders. A migraine is a type of vascular headache that may present with or without neurological symptoms. The neurological symptoms that occur depend on the location of the disturbance in the intracranial vascular system because the symptoms can be caused by either vasoconstriction or vasodilation.

Usually the onset for migraine headaches is during puberty or in the second to third decade of life (that is, between the ages 10 and 40) with a familial occurrence of 50% (Porter and Kaplan 2011). Migraines strike women more than men and may partially or completely remit after age 50. In many women, symptoms worsen with the use of oral contraceptives or vasodilating medications, and they improve in both frequency and intensity after menopause. Symptoms also appear to worsen during the spring months, when pollen is higher.

About 5% of children experience migraines during the grade school years, with an increase to 20% of adolescents during high school (Lewis 2002). A strong female predominance is also evident in this age group. When boys experience migraines, it usually occurs between ages 10 and 12. A study conducted with nearly 800 NCAA Division 1 basketball athletes concluded that although women have an increased prevalence of migraines, these athletes in general had a lower incidence of migraines than did the general population (Kinart, Cuppett, and Berg 2002).

Some preventive strategies for younger athletes include eating regularly, avoiding skipping meals, getting adequate sleep by keeping a regular sleep schedule, and being aware of things that might trigger an attack, such as particular foods. Other contributing factors are excessive exercise or physical activity, specific exercise regimens, physical or emotional stress, and a regular schedule of recreational exercise or organized sport.

Signs and Symptoms

Vascular headaches usually have a rapid onset and present with unilateral throbbing pain in the frontal or temporal area. The headaches may occur in an episodic pattern and often last for hours as opposed to days. Specifically, migraines tend to start in the morning, peak about 2 h later, and resolve after 1 d although they can recur on a daily basis. As with most vascular headaches, migraines consist of a vasoconstriction phase (consisting of painless sensory phenomena) and a vasodilation phase (i.e., a throbbing headache). Figure 11.14 demonstrates the typical anatomical location of pain related to specific types of headaches.

A migraine diagnosis is based largely on presenting symptoms. The classic migraine begins with an aura and is accompanied by extreme sensitivity to sound and light (World Health Organization 2012). The aura may consist of visual disturbances, usually unilateral, such as scotomas (areas of darkness in the visual field), flashes of light, and bright-colored or white objects. These phenomena commonly last for 20 min and usually resolve before any pain or intense throbbing begins. In contrast to the classic migraine, common migraines may be unilateral or bilateral and do not begin with an aura. These headaches generally last for days as opposed to hours, with associated symptoms including nausea, vomiting, diarrhea, weight gain, dizziness, and a prodromal period of endocrine dysfunction resulting in fluid retention. In addition, photophobia often accompanies these headaches. Cigarette smoking, sleep deprivation, stress, chocolate, and tyramine-containing cheeses are precipitating factors in the development of both the classic and common forms of migraines (Smith, Swartzon, and McGrew 2014).

Other types of migraines are associated with neurological deficits, such as the basilar artery migraine and the hemiplegic or ophthalmoplegic migraine. The basilar artery migraine is common in young women, occurring before their menstrual period; symptoms, which last for minutes to hours, may include facial or finger paresthesias, vertigo, ataxia, dysarthria, and tinnitus. The hemiplegic or ophthalmoplegic migraine is more common in young adults and can present in two ways. One condition involves extraocular muscle palsies (CN III) and ptosis, which may become permanent in recurrent cases. The other involves hemiplegia and hemiparesis that can persist even after the headache resolves.

Differential diagnoses include headaches associated with a head injury; facial pain such as temporomandibular joint (TMJ) pain, sinus headache, cluster headache, or trigeminal neuralgia; systemic conditions that include hypertension or infection whether viral, sinus, or influenza; side effects from medications such as mood-altering medications, antidepressants, analgesics, antibiotics, antihypertensives, caffeine, lack of caffeine if habitual user, steroids, or nicotine; and environmental factors including high altitude, hypercapnia, and hyperthermia. Headaches associated with hunger are also possible in the athlete who comes to practice without adequate caloric intake.

Referral and Diagnostic Tests

A detailed and thorough clinical history helps to differentiate migraines from other types of headache. Merely recognizing the key presenting symptoms of vascular headaches can help to exclude tension headaches. The location of pain may also be an indicator of the type of headache experienced (see figure 11.14).

Sinus

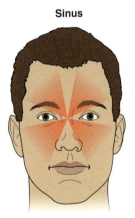

Pain is usually behind the forehead or cheekbones

Cluster

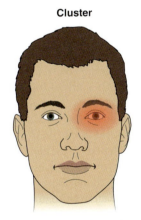

Pain is in and around one eye

Tension

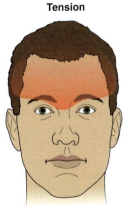

Pain is like a band squeezing the head

Migraine

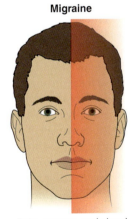

Pain, nausea, and visual changes are typical of classic form

FIGURE 11.14   Location of pain in the head for certain types of headaches.

Precipitating Factors for Migraine

Endocrine changes

    Premenstrual

    Menstrual

    Oral contraceptive pills

    Pregnancy

    Puberty

    Menopause

    Hyperthyroidism

Metabolic changes

    Fever

    Anemia

Rhinitis

Change in temperature or altitude

Change in activity

Alcohol, especially red wine

Foods

    Chocolates

    Cheese

    Hot dogs

    Nuts

Drugs

    Nitroglycerin

    Nitrates

    Indomethacin

Blood pressure changes

Sleep, too much or too little

Physical examination assesses commonly affected cranial nerves by testing visual acuity and visual fields, pupil reaction, extraocular muscle movements, and facial symmetry. A physician may also order a CBC, biochemistry profile, skull and cervical spine radiographs, CT or MRI of the brain, EEG, or lumbar puncture. In addition, treatment responses can help pinpoint the diagnosis (National Institute of Neurological Disorders and Stroke 2015b; Smith, Swartzon, and McGrew 2014). For instance, tension headaches caused by muscle contraction tend to respond positively to traditional nonsteroidal anti-inflammatory drugs (NSAIDs), whereas migraines generally do not.

It is important to distinguish whether an athlete's headache is associated with exercise. These types of headache include exercise-induced migraine, benign exertional headache (also referred to as weightlifter's cephalgia), and vascular headache resulting from prolonged exercise. All three of these headaches are classified as vascular but have definite distinguishing factors.

An effort or exercise-induced migraine is a unilateral retroorbital headache that presents with a visual aura and is more prominent at the end of activity. The symptoms are more likely in hot weather and accompany dehydration. In benign exertional headache, the symptoms are bilateral, have rapid onset and short duration, and occur at the beginning of activity. They are often associated with the increased intrathecal pressure associated with lifting weights with a closed glottis. Exertional headaches generally decrease in frequency over time. It is critically important that a physician evaluate athletes with this type of headache because 10% will have associated intra-

cranial pathology such as arteriovenous malformation, Arnold-Chiari malformation, subdural hematoma, brain tumor, aneurysm, or basilar impression (Smith, Swartzon, and McGrew 2014). The vascular headache with prolonged activity presents true to its name and may last for up to 24 h after exercise. It may also have associated transient or persistent neurological deficits depending on the presence and severity of cerebral ischemia (Lewis 2002; Smith, Swartzon, and McGrew 2014).

The health care provider also needs to recognize the features of headaches associated with intracranial hemorrhage and head trauma for on-the-field evaluation of the athlete. Headaches associated with intracranial hemorrhage usually present with more severe neurological signs, especially involving altered levels of consciousness, than those associated with exertion or dehydration.

After head trauma, two headaches of special concern include posttraumatic migraines and dysautonomic cephalgia. Posttraumatic migraines are common in soccer players secondary to heading a ball. This headache presents as a classic migraine with prominent visual symptoms and usually has a cervical muscle associated headache component. **Dysautonomic cephalgia** occurs with trauma to the anterior triangle of the neck and causes injury to the sympathetic nerve fibers near the carotid artery. Sympathetic nerve injury results in autonomic dysfunction presenting as Horner's syndrome, often with ptosis, hyperhidrosis, and a unilateral headache.

In addition, athletes with headaches should always be referred for medical evaluation if there is a history of head trauma or loss of consciousness, signs of a postconcussion syndrome, or an exertional headache

(Smith, Swartzon, and McGrew 2014). General headache symptoms that warrant further evaluation by a physician are the following:

- New or unusual headache
- Sudden onset of severe headache
- Change in the pattern of a headache
- Chronic headache with localized pain
- Headache that interrupts sleep during the night or in the early morning
- Headache that worsens over days
- Headache with severe nausea and vomiting leading to dehydration
- Visual disturbances
- Numbness, paralysis, or weakness of one side of the face or body
- Headache with associated stiff neck or meningeal signs
- Systemic symptoms, such as fever or weight loss
- Neurological symptoms
- Local extracranial symptoms

Treatment and Return to Participation

Treatment for migraines includes identifying the cause and appropriately treating the mechanism. Health care providers need to help the athlete learn to recognize the precursors of an episode and how to avoid them.

Persons with migraines may be discouraged from specific athletic activities, such as scuba diving, where the diving environment itself can induce migraines that are often of increased severity. Typical stresses experienced in the diving environment include anxiety, associated sinus barotrauma, cold exposure, and possible saltwater aspiration.

Prevention

The key to prevention is to identify and avoid precipitating factors such as stress, smoking, sleep deprivation, red wine, chocolate, and tyramine-containing cheeses. In addition, good control of blood pressure and monitoring medication side effects are important. Supportive psychotherapy can also assist in headache prevention by teaching techniques to reduce and relieve stress and tension.

Two preventive treatment protocols are specific to exercise-related headaches. Exercise-induced migraines brought on because of effort may be prevented by a graded warm-up period before exercise, which primes the sympathetic nervous system. In addition, avoiding training in hot weather and ensuring adequate hydration may also reduce the occurrence of these migraines. Rarely, in cases of severe unrelenting headache, the offending activity needs to be significantly reduced or discontinued (Smith, Swartzon, and McGrew 2014). Benign exertional headache is generally successfully treated with NSAIDs, neck massage, and hydration, and it may be prevented by the administration of acetaminophen or ibuprofen before exercise (Smith, Swartzon, and McGrew 2014; National Institute of Neurological Disorders and Stroke 2015b).

Simple treatment options for migraines include placing the athlete in a quiet, dark room and encouraging sleep, which will often neutralize the headache. Pharmacological treatment is often necessary. Medical therapy for migraines consists of two classes of drugs: abortive and preventive medications.

Seizure Disorder and Epilepsy

A seizure is caused by abnormal discharges of electrical activity in the brain, and it may arise from a number of pathologies. The outward manifestation of a seizure is altered awareness, involuntary movements, and convulsions. Seizures may occur because of brain injury/insult, heatstroke, hypoglycemia (low blood sugar), hyponatremia (too little salt in the blood due to overhydration), alcohol consumption, drug withdrawal, meningitis, encephalitis, drug interaction, or fever. Febrile seizures can occur in children younger than age six who have a body temperature greater than 38 °C (100 °F). Complex febrile seizures are those that last longer than 15 min or occur in a series. These require medical attention. There are genetic tendencies toward febrile seizures, and the overall risk of recurrence is 35% (Ferri 2016). The most common chronic seizure disorder is epilepsy, which is discussed below.

Although an estimated 10% to 30% of people will have a seizure at some time, epilepsy is a chronic condition consisting of unprovoked, randomly recurring seizures that occur in approximately 2% of the population (Centers for Disease Control and Prevention 2015a). Epilepsy is diagnosed before age 21 in 75% of these cases and shows a prevalence of 0.5% in children under age nine (Ko 2015). The diagnosis of epilepsy is based on the occurrence of more than two seizures; therefore, single-seizure episodes during a person's lifetime, including infantile febrile seizures, do not meet the clinical definition.

As stated previously, a seizure is abnormal electrical activity in the brain that causes involuntary systemic convulsions, depending on the area of brain involvement. There are many underlying causes of seizures, although more than one-half of the cases are idiopathic. In fact, more than 75% of seizures in young adults and a smaller percentage in children under age three have no identifiable cause (Centers for Disease Control and Prevention 2015a). The etiology is presumed to be some form of inherited neuronal abnormality. In general, most idiopathic seizures develop between the ages of 2 and 14. Other seizures occurring in children younger than 2 are usually related to developmental defects, birth trauma, or metabolic diseases of the brain. In people over age 25, the etiology is usually identified (Ko 2015). In addition to the causes listed previously, some identifiable causes of seizures include recent or old brain injury, brain tumor, stroke, infection, metabolic disturbances, inherited disorders, sleep deprivation, and extreme emotional and physical stress.

Exercise-induced seizures occur very infrequently and present during or immediately after exercise. In sports of prolonged activity, such as marathons and triathlons, the underlying cause may be metabolic imbalance (such as hyponatremia) as opposed to the exercise itself. The best diagnostic approach for seizures that occur during or immediately after activity, outside of the history and physical examination, is an EEG performed during exercise.

Signs and Symptoms

Seizures result in systemic activity that can affect the level of consciousness and manifest as motor activity, sensory phenomena, psychic disturbances, or inappropriate behavior. With this in mind, the classification of seizures is based on the clinical manifestations of the abnormal electrical activity. Seizures are divided into two major categories: generalized seizures and partial or focal seizures.

Generalized seizures involve electrical activity in both cerebral hemispheres. These types of seizures may have bilateral cerebral hemisphere involvement from the onset, or they may evolve from a partial seizure to involve both cerebral hemispheres. Generalized seizures are further classified as **tonic–clonic seizures**, such as those seen in intermittent or status epilepticus, absence seizures, or any of a varied array of less common seizures. Intermittent tonic–clonic seizures are among the most common types of seizures. They are associated with an aura of smells or sounds that alert the person to impending seizure; tongue biting caused by uncontrolled muscle contraction; incontinence; and a postictal state of disorientation, confusion, exhaustion, or lethargy. The postictal state is a 5 to 30 min period of altered consciousness resulting from an epileptic seizure (Ferri 2016). These seizures are generally of short duration and are self-limited, at times requiring no medication. Continuous tonic–clonic seizures are called status epilepticus and are medical emergencies. These are defined as continuous tonic–clonic convulsions lasting more than 30 min or recurrent tonic–clonic convulsions without regaining consciousness between attacks. These seizures require immediate intervention with monitoring and support of the airway, breathing, and circulation and prompt administration of medications to abort the continued pattern.

Absence seizures are another type of generalized seizure and are characterized by brief episodes of loss of attention or awareness lasting between 3 and 15 s without an aura or postictal state. Associated automatisms may include chewing, lip smacking, swallowing, or facial twitching. As many as 15 other types of generalized seizures occur, including myoclonic seizures and febrile seizures.

A partial seizure starts with a focal presentation of a motor, sensory, autonomic, or psychic disturbance that manifests on the basis of the area of its origin in one cerebral hemisphere. Examples of these disturbances include involuntary motor activity of the face, limbs, or head; somatosensory symptoms of tingling, numbness, or pins and needles; special sensory phenomena such as visual, auditory, olfactory, or **gustatory hallucinations**; autonomic dysfunction including diaphoresis (sweating) and flushing; and psychic phenomena such as feelings of **déjà vu**, **jamais vu**, paranoia, or fear. In simple partial seizures, consciousness is not impaired, and the manifestations are usually restricted to one anatomical area on only one side of the body. In complex partial seizures, consciousness is impaired, and this impairment may occur alone or in association with integrated purposeful movements or experiences such as automatisms or psychic disturbances. Automatisms may be simple, such as chewing, lip smacking, and swallowing, or complex, such as walking into a room or getting dressed. Both types of partial seizure can evolve into generalized seizures. There are also obvious partial seizures that cannot be further differentiated as simple or complex, and these account for approximately 7% of all seizures (Ko 2015).

Convulsive activity caused by seizures must be differentiated from that prompted by other disorders, such as concussive convulsions and convulsive syncope. Concussive convulsions are brief periods of tonic posturing that are expressions of the concussion event. They are benign and require no specific treatment outside of that for the underlying concussion. Convulsive syncope involves generalized convulsive movements, tongue biting, and incontinence during a syncopal or fainting event. Both entities involve convulsive movements related to reflex phenomena rather than abnormal cerebral electrical activity.

Referral and Diagnostic Tests

Any athlete who experiences a seizure, whether of new or established onset, needs to be referred for neurological assessment to ensure appropriate diagnosis and management in new cases and to review medical management for effective control in established cases. Also, any athlete with a syncopal event needs to be referred for medical examination.

General evaluation of an athlete with a seizure disorder involves a detailed medical history, including occurrences and precipitating factors, and a physical examination thoroughly reviewing the neurological system. Laboratory tests include a CBC, chemistry panel, and urinalysis. Prolactin levels are determined immediately postevent to determine the etiology (epileptic vs. nonepileptic). Neurological testing may include an EEG, MRI, or CT of the brain; lumbar puncture in cases of suspected infection; and possibly a positron emission tomography (PET) scan. CSF is evaluated if meningitis or encephalitis is suspected (Ko 2015).

Treatment and Return to Participation

Acute management of a seizure includes protecting the athlete from further harm by ensuring all dangerous objects are out of the way during a seizure. This includes moving desks, chairs, and anything the athlete may hit while seizing. It is neither necessary nor indicated to restrain someone undergoing a seizure. After a seizure, the athlete is placed in the recovery position, on the left side with head resting on the left arm (figure 11.15).

Although it has been reported that 25% to 30% of patients with seizure activity do not respond to anticonvulsant medications, it is still the best option in the management of seizures (WebMD 2015). There are no pharmaceuticals that can cure epilepsy, but management of the symptoms is quite possible. Medical control of epilepsy follows some general guidelines. Initially, a single medication is used to control the seizures. A second agent is added only when maximal dosage of the first is attained, side effects or toxicity limits further dosage increases, or adequate seizure control is not attained with a single agent. Most medications prescribed for treating seizure activity have adverse effects. It is up to the practitioner and patient to weigh the benefits of a medication against its potential negative effects. It is important to monitor the serum levels of medications and the blood chemistry they may affect. Another consideration for treatment of epilepsy is the management of the disorder in the elderly population. Typically, senior adults have concomitant diseases and are prescribed medications for their other afflictions. Antiepileptic drugs tend to metabolize other drugs; therefore, patients must work closely with their physicians and pharmacists to ensure that no drug interactions will interfere with the seizure medications (WebMD 2015; Ko 2015; Centers for Disease Control and Prevention 2015a).

Other medical treatments include surgical intervention to the area of the brain most affected. Epilepsy surgery has grown rapidly in China in recent years, but the same trend has not yet occurred in the United States (WebMD 2015; Ko 2015).

The health care provider must also assess and treat underlying complications that can occur during seizures, such as fractures, dislocations, and head and neck injuries.

Participation by an epileptic athlete in sports or physical activity depends on a number of issues that include the type of sport, risk of injury, and presence of preexisting neurological injury or dysfunction. The following criteria must be carefully considered before an athlete with epilepsy returns to participation:

- Sport type: collision, contact, or noncontact
- Risk of severe injury or death if seizure occurs during the activity
- Preexisting brain injury and neurological dysfunction
- Risk of traumatic brain injury from athletic participation
- Seizure control: frequency, association with exercise, medications

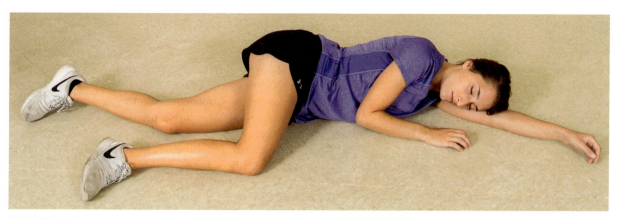

FIGURE 11.15   The correct recovery position for a person after a seizure.

- Effects of medications on performance: sedation and impaired judgment

The American Academy of Pediatrics maintains a document outlining the conditions under which youths with a given medical condition may engage in activity (Boyajian-O'Neill et al. 2004). In determining an athlete's ability to return to sport, the medical team considers the level of risk, which is lower when the athlete has been seizure-free for 1 yr on medications or for 2 yr without medications. High-risk sports, including gymnastics, high diving, sky diving, rock climbing, and motor sports, should be avoided (WebMD 2015). Noncontact sports that are still worrisome include archery, riflery, swimming, weightlifting events, and activities involving height.

Return-to-participation guidance is approached with caution and on an individual basis. One factor to consider is the athlete's ability to commute to practices and events; people with epilepsy commonly need to prove stable management of their seizures before they can obtain or reinstate their driver's license.

A person with epilepsy must meet certain additional legal obligations when operating a motor vehicle. The athlete and, as appropriate, the parents are alerted to this requirement. The actual reporting of epilepsy to an appropriate governing authority varies from state to state, and guidelines are available from the National Institutes of Health or Epilepsy Foundation websites as well as the local driver's license center. More stringent legal requirements exist for commercial licensing because the U.S. Department of Transportation has made it illegal to license anyone with a history of epilepsy for interstate trucking. Criteria for other professions, such as air traffic controllers, border patrol agents, FBI agents, law enforcement officers, firefighters, pilots, U.S. Postal Service mail carriers, and medical personnel, are also addressed on the Epilepsy Foundation website (Epilepsy Foundation 2015).

The main approach to preventing epileptic seizures is to avoid or promptly treat precipitating factors.

Vertigo

Vertigo is defined as a sensation of instability, loss of equilibrium, or rotation usually caused by a disturbance in the semicircular canals of the inner ear or vestibular nuclei of the brainstem (O'Toole 2013). Vertigo is described as either central or peripheral. Central vertigo arises when the cause of vertigo is due to brain or spinal cord anomaly; peripheral vertigo is due to problems with the inner ear (Taylor 2015). Vertigo associated with hearing loss is referred to as sudden sensorineural hearing loss (SSHL), and it is uncommon. The most common variety of vertigo falls under the peripheral category because it is associated with ailments of the inner ear. It is termed benign paroxysmal positional vertigo (BPPV), and it is what we focus on here. BPPV is a brief sensation of spinning accompanied by nystagmus. It usually lasts less than a minute, but it can continue episodically up to 4 wk (Ferri 2016; Li 2015; Taylor 2015). Typically, in BPPV, hearing is not affected. Dizziness should not be confused with vertigo, as dizziness is lightheadedness or unsteadiness, whereas vertigo involves sensations of spinning (O'Toole 2013; Taylor 2015).

Signs and Symptoms

Clinically, *subjective vertigo* is when one feels the body is spinning in space; *objective vertigo* is when one feels everything is spinning about the body (O'Toole 2013). Both are common in BPPV. BPPV is precipitated by changes in head position with respect to gravity, tends to affect women more than men, and has a peak onset between the ages of 50 and 60 (Li 2015). The motion sensation can be so severe that the patient is temporarily debilitated. Nausea or vomiting are not unusual. It should be noted that patients with BPPV do not typically feel vertigo all the time, and severe attacks are triggered by motion of the head. Persistent vertigo should be investigated as a pathophysiology other than BPPV (Li 2015).

Differential diagnoses for vertigo are many and varied. Stroke, Meniere's disease, migraine, otitis media with effusion, vestibular neuritis, tumor, migraine, hypoglycemia, fatigue, and dehydration can all present with dizziness, which some confuse with vertigo, or with true vertigo (Ferri 2016). Vertebral artery insufficiency is also a known cause of vertigo (Li 2015). Certain medications acting alone, or in combination with alcohol, can elicit vertigo-like sensations. A complete medical history is critical, including medication review. Acute head trauma can also present with vertigo symptoms.

Referral and Diagnostic Tests

Unrelenting or recurring vertigo should be referred to a neurologist or otolaryngologist for specialized evaluation to include ruling out BPPV. There is some evidence that vitamin D deficiency or osteopenia can contribute to BPPV (Buki et al. 2013), and assessing serum vitamin D and bone density may be indicated. The patient is given a thorough neurological exam, which should include assessment for uncontrollable lateral eye movement, or nystagmus. An otoscope is used to evaluate the tympanic membrane to look for swelling or effusion. If hearing loss is suspected, an audiometry may be ordered. Depending on the findings, the health care provider may perform a "roll" or a Dix-Hallpike test involving rapid repositioning of the patient to re-create symptoms or nystagmus (Taylor 2015). An MRI or CT scan may be ordered to rule out central causes of vertigo. Thirty-nine percent of those presenting with vertigo have no known etiology (Li 2015).

Treatment and Return to Participation

BPPV usually spontaneously resolves, but there are intermittent treatments that can retard the symptoms (Ferri 2016). There are several physical maneuvers that mitigate the spinning sensation. The most well-known treatment is the Epley maneuver, where specific head movements are performed to loosen the canaliths in the inner ear; this is reported to be 90% effective (Guo and Li 2015; Taylor 2015; Li 2015). The purpose of these maneuvers is to reposition the canaliths (crystals) in the semicircular canals of the inner ear, which in turn alleviates symptoms. Initially, these movements may worsen vertigo, and they should be first be performed by an experienced health care provider or physical therapist (Taylor 2015). There are also many head and eye exercises that the patient can perform to decrease symptoms. Medications, if prescribed, are antinausea and benzodiazepine (Valium). Both of these have side effects that include significant drowsiness, and they are not recommended if the athlete wishes to participate in sport.

Caution should be exercised when determining the patient's ability to operate machinery and to physically train. Sports with rotational components, such as swimming, diving, wrestling, gymnastics, and cheerleading, should be considered off-limits until the patient's symptoms are fully resolved. Sports that involve rotating head motions, such as volleyball and tennis, where the athlete is constantly moving and looking up to follow the ball at every play, can exacerbate BPPV symptoms. Patients who report vertigo to the point of falling should not be allowed to participate in activities where they can sustain more harm.

Neuromuscular Disorders

Neuromuscular disorders are conditions that affect voluntary muscle via the nerves that control them. Muscles that do not receive adequate nerve impulses atrophy and become useless. Two of the neuromuscular conditions discussed here are multiple sclerosis (MS) and amyotrophic lateral sclerosis (ALS). Both of these strike healthy people with little warning, and both have serious sequelae.

Multiple Sclerosis

Multiple sclerosis (MS) is a neurodegenerative, lifelong chronic disease diagnosed primarily in young adults. It is characterized by the gradual accumulation of focal plaques of demyelination in the brain. Peripheral nerves are not affected. The pathophysiology of MS involves myelinated cells being destroyed and replaced by hard sclerotic tissue. The result may be permanent disability in the affected nerves. In Western societies, MS is second only to trauma as a cause of neurological disability arising in early to middle adulthood (Wingerchuk and Carter 2014; Leray et al. 2015).

Current evidence indicates that MS is an autoimmune disease. The precise cause of MS remains unknown, but a number of epidemiological facts have been clearly established. MS develops in genetically susceptible individuals who reside in certain permissive environments. It affects approximately 400,000 Americans and 2.3 million people worldwide and is approximately two to three times as common in females as in males (National MS Society 2015). In both genders, the incidence rises steadily from adolescence to age 35 and declines gradually thereafter. About two-thirds of cases have an onset between ages 20 and 40, and there has been recent research that links the risk factor for MS to genetics. MS can be found in most racial groups, but it is more common in Caucasians. Environmental factors such as vitamin D deficiency have been linked but not confirmed, and those who smoke have a slightly higher incidences of MS. Epstein-Barr virus contracted after childhood has a relatable association to increased risk (National MS Society 2015; Leray et al. 2015). In contrast, vaccines, stress, allergies, and traumatic events have shown no evidence of increasing the risk of MS (Leray et al. 2015).

There are four distinct forms of MS that differ in their presentation but are similar in signs, symptoms, and treatment (National MS Society 2015):

Relapsing–Remitting MS

- Cyclic episodes of worsening neurological function, followed by complete recovery periods (remissions). Attacks are termed relapses, flare-ups, or exacerbations.
- 85% of people with MS have this form of the disease.

Primary–Progressive MS

- Gradually worsening neurological function without distinct remission.
- 10% of people with MS have this form of the disease.

Secondary–Progressive MS

- After a period of relapsing–remitting MS, these patients develop a secondary progressive decline in neurological function.

Progressive–Relapsing MS

- Progressive worsening of neurological function occurs, punctuated by occasional attacks of accelerated deterioration; no remission occurs.
- A rare form of MS, 5% of people have this form of the disease.

Manifestations of MS vary from a benign illness to a rapidly evolving and incapacitating disease requiring profound adjustments in lifestyle and goals for patients and their families. Complications from MS affect multiple body systems (Ferri 2016; Porter and Kaplan 2011).

Signs and Symptoms

The following are common signs and symptoms of multiple sclerosis (National MS Society 2015):

- Problems with balance and coordination
- Spasticity
- Fatigue
- Visual problems
- Dizziness
- Pain
- Numbness
- Bladder or bowel dysfunction
- Emotional behavior changes
- Cognitive function changes

Symptoms of MS may be mild or severe, may be of long or short duration, and may appear in various combinations. Most frequently, the disease is a relapsing–remitting disorder with symptoms that may come and go over time. Weakness or numbness in one or more extremities is the initial symptom in about one-half of patients. The initial presentation in about 25% of all patients with MS is an episode of optic neuritis (Luzzio 2015). Optic neuritis is a syndrome in which partial or total loss of vision, usually in one eye, evolves rapidly over several hours to days. Some patients may experience pain within the orbit that may be made worse with eye movement or palpation of the globe 1 or 2 d before visual loss. Other visual symptoms may include blurred or double vision or red-green color distortion. About one-third of patients with optic neuritis recover completely, and others generally improve significantly even when the initial visual loss was profound.

Systemic fatigue is also a common complaint associated with MS. Sixty percent of people with MS judge fatigue to be the worst symptom of their disease (Luzzio 2015; Ferri 2016). This symptom makes diagnosis challenging in the active population, in whom fatigue is common.

Patients with MS who experience muscle weakness in their extremities will have difficulty with coordination and balance. Most people with MS exhibit paresthesias, transitory abnormal sensory feelings such as numbness or "pins and needles." Some may also experience pain or loss of feeling. About one-half of people with MS experience cognitive impairments such as difficulties with concentration, attention, memory, and judgment. Such impairments are usually mild and rarely disabling, and intellectual and language abilities are generally spared (Luzzio 2015).

Heat is a culprit for the worsening of many MS symptoms, and athletes with this disorder should be monitored carefully during warmer days (National MS Society 2015).

A number of other diseases produce symptoms similar to those seen in MS. The possibility of an alternative diagnosis must be considered and eventually ruled out. Initially MS may mimic stroke, lupus, a progressive myelopathy, migraine, spinal cord tumor, arteriovenous disorders, Lyme disease, arthritis, Guillain-Barré syndrome, vitamin D deficiency, autoimmune conditions, and syphilis, among other conditions (Ferri 2016; Luzzio 2015).

Referral and Diagnostic Tests

The symptoms of MS are often vague, insidious, and nonspecific. However, anyone who experiences fatigue, numbness and tingling in the arms, legs, or elsewhere in the body, or vision irregularities must be referred to a physician. These are among the early indications of MS. Often the symptoms will be unilateral and will occur without trauma. Static tremors may be present, and a physician will determine whether a neurological condition such as MS may be the cause.

Physicians perform a neurological examination and take a medical history when they suspect MS. Imaging technologies include MRI, which provides an anatomical picture of lesions, and magnetic resonance spectroscopy (MRS), which yields information about the biochemistry of the brain. Other tests include a spinal tap to obtain a CSF sample to study the immunoglobulin G antibody, an EEG, sensory evoked potential (EP) studies, and an EMG (National MS Society 2015; Luzzio 2015). EP tests record the nervous system's electrical response to stimulation (e.g., visual, auditory). People with MS have slower response times than do people without MS. No single test unequivocally detects MS.

Other tests performed to diagnose MS include testing deep tendon reflexes, which are generally increased in the disease. Many times the challenge is to rule out other conditions, resulting in a diagnosis of MS. There are three criteria for diagnosing MS, according to the National MS Society: the presence of damage in at least two separate areas of the CNS; evidence that the damage took place a minimum of 1 mo apart; and exclusion of all other conditions (National MS Society 2015). Diagnostic criteria were further delineated in the revised McDonald criteria in 2010 to include visual evoked potential (VEP) and CSF analysis (Polman et al. 2011). These additional tests can confirm the diagnosis after only one attack.

Treatment and Return to Participation

There is no cure for MS. Approximately 85% of people with MS have the relapsing–remitting form of the disease, in which they experience acute exacerbations or relapses with near or complete recovery (National MS Society 2015). Treatment is divided into two categories: treatments designed to modify the course of the disease and symptom management. Several disease-modifying medications are available for relapsing–remitting MS: interferon β-1a (Avonex, Rebif), interferon β-1b (Betaseron), and glatiramer (Copaxone). All require daily or weekly self-injection of the medication, which in turn reduces the number of exacerbations. There have been recent and remarkable advances in treatment options for MS in the disease-modifying category, 10 of which have significantly changed the short- and intermediate-term natural progression of the disease (Wingerchuk and Carter 2014; Leray et al. 2015). Those referring athletes for referral would be wise to align with progressive physicians who are informed of current and emerging MS therapies that are effective and have few side effects.

MS may also be progressive. Medications to relieve symptoms in progressive MS include corticosteroids, muscle relaxants, and medications to reduce fatigue. Many medications are used for the muscle stiffness, depression, pain, and bladder control problems often associated with MS. Drugs for arthritis and medications that suppress the immune system may slow MS in some cases.

In addition to medications, other treatments may relieve MS symptoms. These include physical and occupational therapy with the goal of preserving independence by performing flexibility, strengthening, and proprioceptive exercises and the use of assistive devices to ease daily tasks.

Counseling for individuals or in group therapy sessions may help both the athlete and family cope with MS and relieve emotional stress (Wingerchuk and Carter 2014; National MS Society 2015; Luzzio 2015). Exercise is an excellent treatment for patients with MS when performed in moderation; the benefits of mild to moderate exercise for MS patients include the following:

- Decreases fatigue
- Allows more independent functioning
- Helps overcome depression
- Improves the following:
  Stamina
  Strength
  Muscle tone
  Balance
  Coordination
  Overall mood
  Sense of well-being

Exercise may also have some adverse effects, particularly if prolonged or practiced in hot environments; these bad effects include increased fatigue, weakness, pain, and spasticity. MS or medications used to control some symptoms can alter the body's ability to dissipate heat. Overheating will increase MS symptoms. In addition, muscle weakness around joints can leave MS patients unstable and vulnerable to injury, which causes pain that makes spasticity worse and promotes more weakness.

Because the exact cause of MS remains unknown, the clinical course and prognosis are as variable as the symptoms. Whereas one patient may present with the disease and have a virtually benign course, another may rapidly progress to dependency on wheelchairs and catheters for voiding.

Most people with MS have a normal, if not slightly shorter, life expectancy. The remission–exacerbation components of the disease make it challenging to predict future disability. Untreated, there is significant physical disability in 30% of patients, and males with primary progressive MS have the worst prognosis (Luzzio 2015). Those who experience a disease course that is progressive from the start are more likely to experience progression of disability. In the worst cases, MS can render a person unable to write, speak, or walk.

A young athlete who develops this chronic, debilitating disease can be particularly devastated. One of the first questions may be, "Can I continue to exercise or train?" The answer is "yes, but"; research has shown that although exercise does not change the impairment, physical exercise does help the patient feel better, both mentally and physically.

Because MS strikes people in different ways, some athletes who have completely or almost completely recovered from an exacerbation may be able to run 5 or 10 miles or bicycle 75 miles per day. Others may be severely disabled and need to use a powered wheelchair. Finding the optimal exercise management program requires a team effort among the physician, athletic trainer, physical therapist, and athlete. The best program combines elements of cardiovascular training, strength, flexibility, balance, coordination, and appropriate functional exercises and is designed with independence and quality of life in mind.

Amyotrophic Lateral Sclerosis

Amyotrophic lateral sclerosis (ALS) is also known as Lou Gehrig's disease, named after the famous New York Yankee baseball player who was stricken with ALS at age 36 and succumbed to it in 1941. It is a fatal, progressive neurological disease that slowly attacks neurons responsible for voluntary muscular actions. Both upper and lower neurons are affected, as they progressively degenerate and die. Without input from neurons, muscles begin to atrophy, leading to complete loss of all voluntary muscular movement. ALS does not affect other senses (sight, smell, taste, hearing) or cognitive thought. So, the patient is quite aware of his or her surroundings but is eventually unable to communicate by voice or to move. Patients with ALS progress in the disease to such a point that they are wheelchair bound. Neurons of the diaphragm eventually weaken, leading to the necessity of a respirator to maintain breathing.

According to the CDC's Morbidity and Mortality Weekly Report on ALS in 2011, about 12,000 Americans have ALS. As one of the most common neuromuscular diseases worldwide, it strikes all races, but it affects Caucasian men under age 60 more than any other group (Centers for Disease Control and Prevention 2015c). There is a heredity component, although it is small (5%–10%). Studies have shown that a mutated enzyme (superoxide dismutase 1, or SOD1) may account for the genetic tendency toward ALS (Ilieva, Polmenidou, and Cleveland 2009). Recent research has demonstrated robust evidence that long-term occupational exposure to lead has a strong association with ALS (Belbasis, Bellou, and Evangelou 2016; Wang et al. 2014).

Interestingly, veterans of the Gulf War (1990–1991) have demonstrated an increased incidence of ALS. Deployed veterans had both a greater postwar risk of ALS and a significantly more rapid progression than those veterans with ALS who were not deployed to the Gulf War (Karsarskis et al. 2009; Horer et al. 2003). Because past deployment to Vietnam was also related to a more rapid progression, researchers suggest a war-related environmental trigger for ALS.

The typical ALS patient survives 3 yr from the onset of muscle weakness but approximately 15% survive 5 yr or longer, with an additional 5% surviving 10 yr or more (Armon 2015). Researchers are working on medications and combinations of treatments to extend the quality of life for the patient with ALS. Because no definitive cause of ALS has been identified, there are no prevention strategies available.

Signs and Symptoms

The earliest symptoms of ALS may be attributed to being tired or clumsy, as 75% to 80% of patients report an increase in stumbling, tripping, or difficulty with small motor functions (e.g., buttoning a shirt, turning a key) (Armon 2015). Symptoms often begin in one limb—a hand or leg, for example—and patients complain of a gradual awkwardness in motor skills. Difficulty in swallowing (dysphagia) or with speech has also been noted. Because upper motor neurons are involved, there may be spasticity or hyperreflexia, and an exaggerated gag reflex. Twenty to 25% report slurred speech, hoarseness, and choking during meals as initial complaints that caused them to seek medical attention (Armon 2015). Patients report muscular twitching and weakness. Weight loss, fatigue, and difficulty controlling facial expressions or tongue movements are all additional indicators of ALS (National Institute of Neurological Disorders and Stroke 2016).

As the disease progresses, muscular atrophy spreads throughout the body. A person's intelligence, memory, and personality are typically not impaired. There are some reports of a small percentage of patients who experience memory loss and difficulty with decision making. Because most do not experience a loss of cognitive abilities, anxiety and depression are common.

Multiple sclerosis, HIV, multifocal motor neuropathy, spinal disc insult, myasthenia gravis, progressive strokes, and certain vitamin deficiencies (e.g., B_{12}) may all be differential diagnoses of ALS.

Referral and Diagnostic Tests

There is no definitive diagnostic test for ALS. Patients must experience signs and symptoms in both upper and lower motor neurons that cannot be linked to any other cause (table 11.1). To rule out MS and other potential causes of the symptoms, physicians may order a brain MRI, electromyography (EMG) and nerve conduction velocity (NCV) analysis, and blood work to determine whether other diseases or conditions are present. The EMG determines electrical activity in normal muscles; the NCV denotes the speed at which nerve impulses travel to a given muscle (Armon 2015). When all other organic explanations for the symptoms have been dismissed, ALS is considered the culprit.

Treatment and Return to Participation

There are no effective treatments that prevent, stop, or reverse the progression of ALS, but there is an FDA-approved drug (Rilutek) that prolongs life 2 to 3 mo (National Institute of Neurological Disorders and Stroke 2016). Rilutek does not relieve symptoms. Although baclofen or diazepam are prescribed to control muscular spasms, trihexyphenidyl or amitriptyline can address dysphagia. Patients with ALS often receive a gastros-

TABLE 11.1 **Signs and Symptoms of Upper Versus Lower Motor Neuron Disorders**

Feature	Upper lesion	Lower lesion
Reflexes	Increased	Decreased or absent
Atrophy	Absent*	Present
Fasciculations	Absent	Present
Tone	Increased (spastic)	Decreased or absent (flaccid)

*May appear with prolonged limb disuse.

tomy to facilitate nutritional intake without swallowing (Armon 2015). The patient and family should be informed about risks with unproven treatments and clinical trials and whether they should participate in life-extending decisions such as long-term ventilation or gastrostomy (Eisen and Krieger 2013).

Several studies promote a multidisciplinary approach to the care of the patient with ALS (Armon 2015; Eisen and Krieger 2015; National Institute of Neurological Disorders and Stroke 2016). Critical components include health care providers who can address both the physical and emotional symptoms of the disease, including end-of-life decisions and care.

Bell's Palsy

Unlike other conditions in this chapter, Bell's palsy is a disease that typically affects one nerve—the facial cranial nerve (CN VII)—resulting in unilateral or bilateral facial weakness or paralysis. It has a rapid onset and most always spontaneously resolves. Bell's palsy affects all ages and both genders equally, but it occurs most often in young people, teenagers, and those in their early 20s. The etiology of Bell's palsy is most likely secondary to an immune reaction or inflammatory response. Herpes simplex is thought to be the most common trigger (Ferri 2016). Patients have a quite visible presentation, as their faces appear to be distorted, and they cannot perform bilateral facial expressions (figure 11.16). Corticosteroids are the treatment of choice. Most recover completely within 1 to 8 wk but some suffer from permanent contractures. Other complications are blindness, corneal ulcers, and impaired nutrition (inability to chew on one side). Other conditions to consider that could present with facial neuropathies include a stroke, Lyme disease, parotid tumor, HIV, syphilis, or trauma (Ferri 2016).

Rabies

Rabies is a preventable infection of the central nervous system (a viral encephalitis) acquired from the saliva of infected bats and other mammals. Although it is not

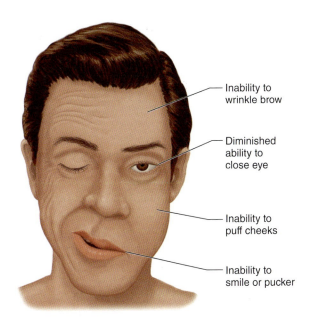

Inability to wrinkle brow

Diminished ability to close eye

Inability to puff cheeks

Inability to smile or pucker

FIGURE 11.16 Bell's palsy.

common in the United States, there are still approximately 15 deaths annually (Gompf 2015). The chief culprits are infected bats, raccoons, skunks, and foxes. However, rabies has been found in dogs, cats, ferrets, and several types of rodents, which include mice, rats, hamsters, squirrels, gerbils, chipmunks, rabbits, and guinea pigs. Death is almost always certain and occurs within 3 to 10 d after the onset of symptoms. There is an incubation period of 20 to 90 d when the infected person is asymptomatic. Following this period is a 2 to 10 d period when the virus enters the CNS and vague symptoms of malaise, headache, fever, anorexia, nausea, insomnia, and pharyngitis may present themselves (Gompf 2015). Patients who survive are identified early as possibly infected and receive immunoprophylaxis before developing symptoms. As the infection progresses, the patient experiences excessive salivation and encephalitis-related issues (hallucination, confusion, agitation, restlessness). It may be difficult to connect the injury (bite) to the symptoms, given the long incubation period of up to a year.

Pain Disorders

Complex Regional Pain Syndrome

Complex regional pain syndrome (CRPS) is a condition involving overactivity of the sympathetic nervous system that can occur after minor injury due to trauma to a nerve or, more commonly, a condition of unknown etiology. CRPS type I was at one time termed reflex sympathetic dystrophy (RSD); it traditionally follows an injury such as one in which soft tissue is damaged, crushed, or immobilized mechanically or pathologically (a too-tight cast or a frozen shoulder). CRPS type II is the new term for the condition causalgia, which is a documented injury to a nerve (Wheeler 2015). Both conditions present with sympathetic nervous system overactivity. The incidence of CRPS I is 21 per 100,000, and that of CRPS II is 4 per 100,000. It effects all races but is more common in women. Whereas adolescents are more affected than are children, the mean age of onset appears to be in the range of 40 to 49 (Wheeler 2015). Strains or sprains are the most common cause of CRPS, followed by surgical wounds, fractures, and crush injuries. It is extremely unusual, but some cases have presented following lacerations, burns, electric shock, venipuncture, inflammatory processes, and spinal cord injuries (Wheeler 2015).

Both types of CRPS present with the hallmark symptom of pain out of proportion to the severity of injury. It generally appears posttraumatically with underlying ligament, bone, or nerve injury. The presentation in children is quite different from that in adults. For example, CRPS in adults has a higher incidence of upper extremity involvement, especially the shoulder, compared with a predominance of lower extremity involvement in children and adolescents, where ankle or foot sprains are the likely trigger. The prognosis and outcomes of CRPS treatment are generally better for children than for adults.

Signs and Symptoms

The pain symptoms are typically completely out of proportion to the signs of injury. Patients report regional pain, not specific pinpoint pain or that which follows a dermatome. The onset of CRPS I can begin in a distal extremity in days or weeks following a seemingly benign injury. It is unusual to have an onset months after the original insult. The vasomotor disturbances encompass vasodilation responses of warmth and erythema and vasoconstrictive responses of coolness, cyanosis, and mottling. The signs and symptoms of CRPS could be attributed to disuse, due either to immobilization or to cognitive disuse, where patients avoid using the injured area (Wheeler 2015). CRPS may progress through three

---

> ⚑ **RED FLAGS FOR COMPLEX REGIONAL PAIN SYNDROME**
>
> Signs and symptoms of a patient with complex regional pain syndrome (CRPS) include the following:
>
> - Severe burning pain
> - Hyperhidrosis
> - Pain beyond what would be expected for the injury
> - Local edema
> - Pathological changes in skin
> - Radiographic changes in bone
> - Extreme sensitivity to pressure or touch

distinct phases of deteriorating function: acute within less than 3 mo, dystrophic over 3 to 6 mo, and atrophic after more than 6 mo (Blake 2010).

Often, the most notable findings for the clinician are reduced joint range of motion, complaints of acute pain with movement of the affected limb, and delayed injury recovery. Of interest is the high incidence of associated anxiety and depression with CRPS, which is probably a function of and proportional to the chronic nature of the pain.

Referral and Diagnostic Tests

To delineate the difference between the false positives and those patients with true CRPS, a respected group of international physicians with experience in these types of disorders put forth a more statistically significant means of clinically diagnosing it. The four criteria are the following:

1. Continuing pain, disproportionate to the inciting event
2. At least one symptom, reported in at least three of these categories:
   - Sensory: Complains of hyperesthesia and/or allodynia
   - Vasomotor: Complains of temperature asymmetry and/or skin color changes and/or skin color asymmetry
   - Submotor/edema: Complains of edema and/or sweating changes and/or asymmetrical sweating
   - Motor/trophic: Complains of decreased range of motion and/or motor dysfunction and/or trophic changes (hair/nail/skin)

3. At least one sign at time of evaluation, in two or more of these categories:

   - Sensory: Evidence of **hyperalgesia** (to pinprick) and/or allodynia (to touch and/or temperature sensation and/or deep somatic pressure and/or joint movement)

   - Vasomotor: Evidence of temperature asymmetry (>1 °C) and/or skin color changes with asymmetry

   - Submotor/edema: Evidence of edema and/or sweating changes and/or asymmetrical sweating

   - Motor/trophic: Evidence of decreased range of motion and/or motor dysfunction (weakness, tremor, dystonia) and/or trophic changes (hair/nail/skin)

4. No other diagnosis that can better explain the signs and symptoms

Reprinted, by permission, from R.N. Harden et al., 2007, "Proposed new diagnostic criteria for complex regional pain syndrome," *Pain Medicine* 8(4): 326-331.

Following these criteria, a clinical diagnosis of CRPS had a 0.70 sensitivity and a 0.94 specificity for the condition (Harden et al. 2007).

Often the best diagnostic tool for identifying and confirming CRPS is the clinical response to a coordinated comprehensive rehabilitation program. It is not uncommon for the therapeutic clinician to initially refer the patient to a physician for further evaluation. As the rehabilitation course progresses, recovery that is slower than expected is one of the first clues that CRPS may be developing. This finding alone may warrant referral back to the physician for assessment as to whether early CRPS changes are occurring or whether there are other injuries that were not initially identified.

CRPS is primarily a clinical diagnosis that is made after a thorough medical history and examination and after other, more common, conditions that prompt a high level of suspicion have been excluded. Physical examination can be helpful in the accurate identification of CRPS and may even assist in determining its severity and chronic prognosis. Findings may reveal a warm, swollen joint with reduced and painful range of motion. The overlying skin may be sweaty and erythematous with dense hair growth and accelerated nail growth. These findings may change depending on the stage of CRPS at the time of presentation (Harden et al. 1999). Over time, fat atrophy leads to thin, waxy, pale skin, muscle atrophy is prominent, nails become brittle and fractured, muscle spasms ensue, and extremity pain and stiffness progress. At the end stages of CRPS, irreversible changes to the extremity result in a nonfunctional atrophic extremity with joint contractures, lost mobility, and severe pain.

Diagnostic tests are generally nonspecific. Radiographs taken early may be negative; however, within 2 to 3 mo, patchy juxtaarticular demineralization or osteoporosis may develop. Nuclear bone scans, although not very helpful, can also show changes of increased uptake in the juxtaarticular areas of bones, often involving joints distal to the actual site of injury. Yet again, the expected results will vary depending on the stage of the disorder, with

CONDITION HIGHLIGHT

Complex Regional Pain Syndrome

Patients with CRPS usually experience intense, unrelenting pain at a joint. The pain is generally worse with any weight bearing or loading of the affected extremity, and it is relieved by rest and joint immobilization in severe cases. This pain is accompanied by varying degrees of autonomic dysfunction, including vasomotor disturbances or dystrophic changes. In addition, the affected area may exhibit edema, sweating, nerve hypersensitivity (allodynia) in 90% of cases, and dermatographia.

Delayed recovery in the presence of pain disproportionate to the degree of injury, reduced joint motion, or hypersensitivity to touch and movement requires prompt referral back to the physician for further evaluation for definite CRPS.

CRPS is often a diagnosis of exclusion. It is vital to rule out other conditions that have a similar clinical presentation as well as underlying conditions that could actually be the cause of the presenting CRPS. In the latter case, if these conditions are not identified and treated, the CRPS may never resolve or improve. Diagnoses to exclude include Raynaud's phenomenon, systemic lupus erythematosus, polymyositis, gout, myofascial pain syndrome, heterotopic ossification (myositis ossificans), compartment syndromes, and thrombophlebitis. Demonstrated underlying causes of CRPS are peripheral nerve entrapment such as carpal tunnel syndrome and tarsal tunnel syndrome, nerve injury caused by laceration or neuroma, ligament sprain or tear, and fracture.

these variations being much more common in children and adolescents. Nerve conduction studies and electromyography are useful in determining only if a nerve is actually damaged, as it is in CRPS II; it is not helpful in diagnosing CRPS I (Wheeler 2015).

Another diagnostic approach tests the function of the sympathetic nervous system compared with the uninvolved side by skin wheal assessment, thermography, and sympathetic nerve blocks. Dermatographia is an abnormally prolonged wheal and erythematous response that can develop in CRPS after lightly scratching the skin of both extremities. An abnormal test suggests sympathetic nervous system dysfunction. Thermography is often used in pain centers to assist in the diagnosis of CRPS. Because it also depends on the stage and severity of the condition, thermography is often inconsistent, nonspecific, and inconclusive (Ferri 2016; Blake 2010).

One procedure that can be therapeutic as well as diagnostic is a sympathetic anesthetic block. This block may be performed at the cervical level of C6 for upper-extremity conditions, at the celiac plexus for upper abdominal area conditions, or at the lumbar level of L2 for lower-extremity conditions.

Treatment and Return to Participation

The mainstay in the treatment of CRPS is early motion and pain control. Prompt initiation of a physical rehabilitation program is critical. The goals of rehabilitation for CRPS are to do the following:

- Desensitize the extremity
- Increase joint and extremity range of motion
- Reduce pain
- Effect control of the extremity
- Restore strength and function

Desensitization techniques for hypersensitivity consist of challenging the area with increasingly abrasive textured materials and stress loading the affected extremity. Range-of-motion activities are the central focus of rehabilitation, and they may be facilitated by the use of ultrasound, transcutaneous electrical nerve stimulation (TENS), muscle stimulation, or hydrotherapy. Contrast baths and range-of-motion exercises (figure 11.17) may both help to reduce edema in the extremity. In addition, biofeedback may allow the patient to gain some control over the autonomic nervous system functions of sweating, skin temperature variations, and blood flow. Supportive psychotherapy can offer these patients various skills to help them accept, cope with, and treat their pain. Some of these skills include relaxation training, biofeedback, and distraction techniques.

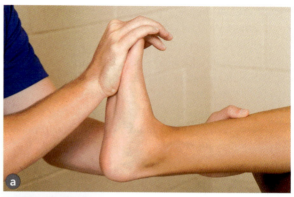
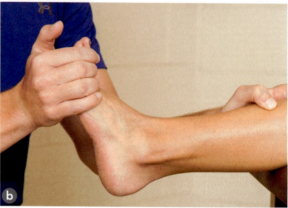

FIGURE 11.17 (a) Maintaining range of motion, shown here as passive dorsiflexion, and (b) for training light resistance, shown here as eversion after an injury, are treatments for complex regional pain syndrome (CRPS).

Pharmacological treatment is available for the management of pain with CRPS. Traditional treatment with NSAIDs may be used, but the relief is often incomplete or ineffective. Narcotic medications may also be given, but they should be prescribed judiciously because of the risk of addiction in patients with CRPS and other chronic pain conditions. NSAIDs and narcotic medications may successfully reduce the pain's intensity, but the actual course of CRPS is not changed (Blake 2010; Wheeler 2015). Other medications available for the treatment of CRPS include tricyclic antidepressants such as amitriptyline and the anticonvulsants gabapentin (Neurontin), phenytoin, and phenobarbital. In addition, either oral methylprednisolone or injected steroid preparations may give pain relief in some cases.

Chemical blockade, as mentioned earlier, consists of sympathetic anesthetic blocks to the cervical, celiac, or lumbar ganglia and may be the most effective form of treatment. If a therapeutic response is obtained with this technique, three to six blocks may be performed during a 2 to 3 mo period. The blocks are almost always successful in relieving the pain. In fact, if a person does not respond to a block, the diagnosis of CRPS is questioned (Blake 2010).

A program of range-of-motion activities and stress-loading exercises for the affected joint or extremity amplifies the potential for a good response to treatment. Exercise provides a way to continue desensitizing the affected extremity. For example, in CRPS of the hand, a stress-loading protocol may consist of household chores that include scrubbing a 3-foot-square area of floor for 20 min three times daily or lifting and carrying books several times each day. In some cases, the pain recurs during rehabilitation so intensely that a somatic block such as an epidural block or brachial plexus block may be necessary to calm down the noxious stimuli coming from the muscles and joints in the affected extremity.

At the far end of the spectrum of treatment options, permanent interruption of the sympathetic pathways either by a sympathetic neurolytic blockade or by surgical sympathectomy may be accomplished, but these treatments remain controversial (Blake 2010). The patient must realize that the goal of surgical blockade is to treat the pain and that surgical blockade has less benefit in restoring impaired function, especially in more severe conditions. In addition to the potential for unsatisfactory functional outcomes from surgery, there is often incomplete pain relief. Although surgical procedures are a viable treatment option in the face of other treatment failures, they are to be avoided if at all possible because, in some cases, the procedure itself can reactivate the CRPS. Further, the changes in vascular flow that occur after sympathectomy could affect bone and limb growth in children.

Prognosis in CRPS depends on the degree of severity and the progression of the condition. Most changes associated with CRPS are reversible in the early stages of the disease, within the first 4 to 6 mo, but they can become irreversible with time, often after 8 to 9 mo (Blake 2010). In most athletes, the condition is identified and treated early because of the limitations that it places on their performance. Athletes will seldom stay quiet for long when they cannot perform in sport. This propensity for early recognition and initiation of treatment in athletes is beneficial to both their recovery potential and their return to participation.

Given that recovery will vary depending on CRPS severity, the nature of the underlying injury, the extremity affected, and the athlete's sport, only general guidelines can be given for return-to-participation schedules. An athlete with CRPS can return to participation in sports when the following occur:

- Affected extremity and joint have full and pain-free range of motion.

- Flexibility is symmetrical to that of the unaffected extremity.
- Strength is at least 80% of that of the unaffected limb.
- Coordinated firing patterns of the supporting muscles and muscular groups have been re-established.

The athlete must be able to perform challenging agility tasks that simulate sport activity with sound biomechanics and appropriate skill. The return to participation can be expedited if the affected extremity is not critical in the performance of the sport. In these cases, modification of the athletic activity may assist in the athlete's return given adequate protection of the affected extremity.

In essence, the mainstay in the prevention of CRPS is early rehabilitative intervention for traumatic injuries. The athlete must progress through a complete rehabilitation course focused on restoring mobility, attaining strength, and regaining function.

Special Concerns in the Adolescent Athlete

A high level of suspicion for CRPS in active adolescents is always wise because they will often hide or downplay the severity of their symptoms in order to return to play sooner or to avoid missing any activity at all. Precautions also need to be taken in prescribing medications for this age group. The physician and athletic trainer must persist in encouraging compliance with therapy and maintenance programs in young athletes to ensure their recovery and to prevent chronic limitations, deformities, or disabilities.

Special Concerns in the Mature Athlete

The major concern with mature athletes is the tendency for stiffness to develop faster and to a greater degree than in younger people. Therefore, prompt initiation of joint and extremity mobilization in these athletes is critical.

Summary

Neurological disorders are alarming in the athletic population because they may be overlooked as symptoms of a benign condition. Without trauma, headaches are not typically a cause for concern in healthy people. This chapter describes conditions ranging from sport-related concussion to chronic disabling or fatal diseases, CRPS, epilepsy, and stroke that can all begin with a simple headache.

Two critical points in recognizing neurological disorders are (1) identifying symptoms that may seem benign, such as stumbling or chronic muscular twitching, and (2) understanding that strokes do occur in apparently healthy people. Rehabilitation of seemingly minor injuries that present with exaggerated pain should prompt the health care provider to consider CRPS. Having the knowledge to consider atypical neurological conditions in otherwise healthy athletes is critical to their future health.

 Apply It! The case study for this chapter looks at a 29-year-old judo participant suffering from problems with his eyesight. Read the scenario and answer the questions at www.HumanKinetics.com/MedicalConditionsInTheAthlete.

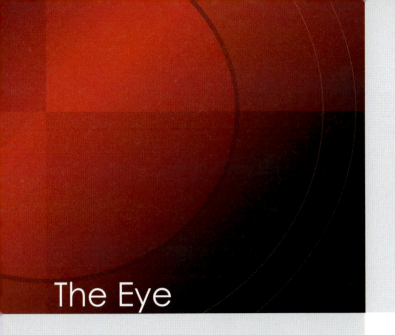

The Eye

OBJECTIVES

At the completion of this chapter the reader should be able to do the following:

- Describe the basic anatomy and physiology of the eye.
- Perform a basic eye examination.
- Describe appropriate initial management of common conditions and injuries of the eye.
- Recognize conditions of the eye that require referral.
- Recognize conditions of the eye that may preclude the athlete from participation.

Acute vision is vital to athletic success, and even minor eye disorders will sideline most athletes. An athletic trainer must understand the basic anatomy and physiology of the eye, be able to perform a basic eye examination, and know the common sport-related eye conditions and injuries for which referral to an eye care specialist is appropriate. This chapter discusses the structures of the eye, examination techniques for both healthy and injured eyes, and the pathological eye conditions that many athletic trainers might encounter.

Overview of Anatomy and Physiology

The anatomy of the eye consists of external and internal structures. All structures are contained within the bony eye socket. The eye socket, anatomically known as the bony orbit of the eye, comprises four walls made up of seven different facial bones of the skull, connective tissue, fat, blood vessels, and nerves (figure 12.1). Anteriorly, the orbit rim is created by the frontal, zygomatic, and maxillary bones (see figure 11.1). The sphenoid, lacrimal, ethmoid, and maxillary bones form the posterior and medial aspects of the orbit. The palatine, zygomatic, and maxillary bones create the floor of the orbit, and the zygomatic and sphenoid bones form the lateral aspect. The orbit provides protection for the eyeball (globe) and contains the lacrimal gland, which produces the tears that lubricate and rinse the surface of the eye. The bony orbit also provides anchorage for the six small extraocular muscles that move the eye. The optic nerve passes through the posterior aspect of the orbit. The visual cortex is located in the occipital lobe of the brain.

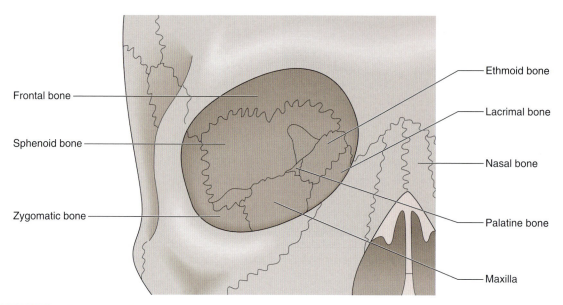

FIGURE 12.1   The eye socket, anatomically known as the bony orbit of the eye.

The external eye includes the eyelid, the conjunctiva, and the lacrimal gland (figure 12.2). These structures protect the eye from foreign objects and distribute tears evenly across the eye. The eyelids provide protection for the external surface of the eye. They help lubricate the ocular surface with their blinking action. The eyelid skin is the thinnest skin of the body. Within each eyelid is a relatively rigid tarsal plate containing meibomian glands, which secrete the oily component of the three-layered tear film. The conjunctiva is a thin, essentially transparent, highly vascular mucous membrane that covers the anterior sclera and the posterior surfaces of both the upper and lower eyelids.

The internal eye consists of many structures including the sclera, cornea, iris, lens, retina, choroid, optic disk, and macula (figure 12.3). The sclera is the dense white connective tissue that makes up more than 90% of the outer layer of the globe and provides structure for the contents of the eyeball. The cornea serves as the barrier between the environment and the aqueous humor. The cornea is made up of several layers and is the clear window of the eye through which light passes. The iris creates the color of the eye. The pupil is the round, central opening in the iris that creates a pathway for light to reach the retina. This aperture dilates or constricts to regulate the amount of light that enters the eye. Between the cornea

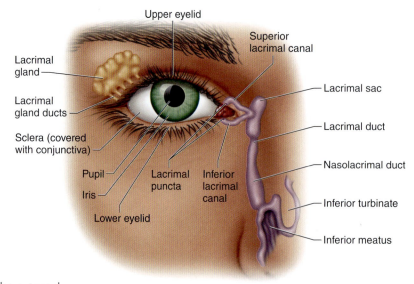

FIGURE 12.2   The external eye.

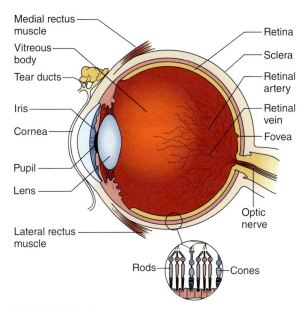

Medial rectus muscle
Vitreous body
Tear ducts
Iris
Cornea
Pupil
Lens
Lateral rectus muscle
Retina
Sclera
Retinal artery
Retinal vein
Fovea
Optic nerve
Rods
Cones

FIGURE 12.3 The internal eye.

and the iris is the anterior chamber. This space is filled with a clear fluid known as aqueous humor.

The crystalline lens is a round, transparent tissue located directly behind the iris. Tiny filaments called zonules, which are attached to the ciliary body, suspend the lens and control its thickness by contracting or relaxing it, allowing an image to be focused onto the retina. The ciliary body is responsible for production of the aqueous humor that fills the anterior chamber of the eye. The large space behind the lens is filled with the transparent gelatinous fluid of the eye known as the vitreous humor (Jarvis 2012).

The retina is the thin, transparent membrane lining the back of the eye that receives light and sends the initial visual signal through the optic nerve to the brain, where it is processed and interpreted. Between the retina and the sclera is the vascular tissue called the choriocapillaris. The choriocapillaris supplies blood and nourishment to the outer layers of the retina. The "red eye" seen in a photograph is caused by the reflection of the camera flash through a dilated pupil against the choriocapillaris. As the nerve fibers from the retina exit the eye through the optic nerve, they bunch together at the origin of the optic nerve to form the optic disk. The optic disk is the visible portion of the optic nerve that can be seen when examining the eye. The other structure that can be seen during examination with an ophthalmoscope is the macula and its center point, the fovea, which is considered the site of central vision and color perception of the eye. The majority of color receptors are found in the macula (Ball et al. 2014).

Evaluation of the Eye

After taking a thorough history, the clinician will examine the anatomical structures of the eyes and surrounding areas and will also test visual acuity, pupillary responses, the motility of the extraocular muscles, and peripheral vision. After the external structures are examined, the clinician may then examine the internal structures of the eye using an ophthalmoscope. The following sections describe a thorough examination of the eye.

Testing Visual Acuity

The most important part of an eye examination is the testing of visual acuity. The ability of the eye to focus clearly on distant or near objects is directly related to the structural integrity of all its parts. Visual acuity is assessed while the patient wears his or her glasses or contact lenses for distance vision. The Snellen chart is a quick and easy-to-use screening tool for far vision (figure 12.4a). The chart contains graduated sizes of letters with standardized acuity numbers at the end of each line. The patient is asked to read the lines of the chart while standing 20 ft away and covering one eye. The Snellen visual acuity is recorded as a fraction comparing the patient's performance with the standard or "normal" person's performance. The first number, or numerator, represents the patient's distance from the eye chart, which should be 20 ft, and the second number, or denominator, represents the distance at which a normal person can read the same-size letter or letters on the same line of the chart. For example, if a patient can read down to the 20/40 line (from 20 ft away), this indicates that the patient can see a letter at 20 ft that a person with normal visual acuity can see at a distance of 40 ft, thus revealing that the athlete has suboptimal acuity (Jarvis 2012) One must remember that this is a screening tool for distance vision only; it does not measure near vision or dynamic visual acuity. It may be necessary to refer a patient to an optometrist or ophthalmologist for a complete visual assessment. Each eye is tested independently while the other eye is covered with the palm of one hand or an opaque object. When testing acuity in children or nonreaders, an illiterate E or C or picture chart is used (figure 12.4b).

If a standard eye chart is not available, a near-vision card can be used to assess visual acuity (figure 12.5). These small cards can be easily added to a standard first-aid kit. If near vision is tested, then the patient should wear reading glasses or bifocals if he or she typically requires corrective lenses to read. A common alcohol prep pad may be used in lieu of a near vision card or Snellen eye chart when held at 14 in.

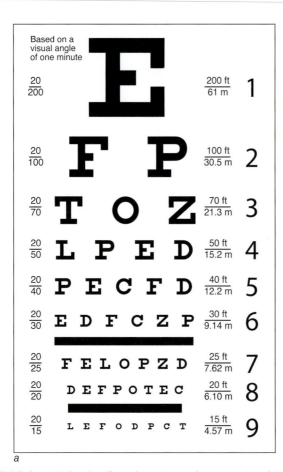
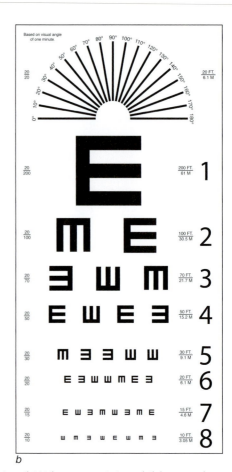

FIGURE 12.4 *(a)* The Snellen chart is used to test visual acuity. *(b)* When examining children or those who do not read, an illiterate E or C or picture chart may be used to test visual acuity.

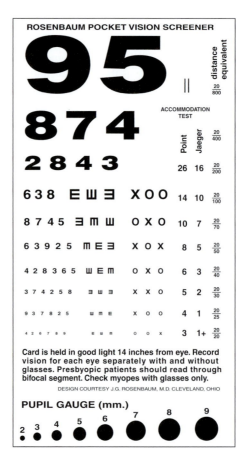

FIGURE 12.5 The Rosenbaum chart for testing near vision.

Visual Acuity

Normal visual acuity is 20/20. The top number indicates the distance at which a person is standing from the chart. The bottom number is the distance at which a normal eye can read that same line. The larger the denominator is the poorer the vision.

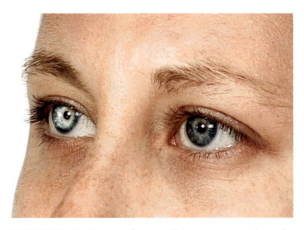

FIGURE 12.6 To test the pupillary response, the athlete looks into the distance while a light is moved in toward the eye from the side and shone directly into the pupil. The speed of the pupillary constriction is compared with that of the other eye.

© Micki Cuppett

When a patient cannot see the largest letters of an eye chart, the clinician may hold up some of the fingers of one hand and ask the patient to count them at progressively closer distances to the eye. This is documented as "count fingers vision at [for example] 2 ft." If the patient cannot count the fingers, the examiner can wave a hand in front of the eye and ask if the patient can detect the motion. This is documented as *hand motion vision*. If the patient cannot detect hand motion, any bright light source (e.g., a penlight) can be used to determine the patient's ability to detect light. This is documented as *light perception vision*. Reduction of visual acuity in an injured eye is a serious ocular emergency. Immediate referral to an eye care specialist is warranted.

Testing Pupillary Responses

The pupil's ability to react to light is a basic feature of a normally functioning ocular system. Brisk pupil constriction in response to a bright light also suggests the presence of vision in the absence of any standard eye chart. While the patient is looking into the distance, a light is moved in toward the eye from the side and shone directly into the pupil (figure 12.6). The speed (briskness) of the pupillary constriction is noted. Each eye is examined separately and should be similar to the other.

After examining each eye for its light reactivity and responsiveness, the examiner performs a swinging light test by swinging a light from the normal eye to the injured one. This test is based on the fact that the same quantity of light (i.e., from the same light source) should constrict each pupil by the same amount. When internal ocular damage or optic nerve damage occurs in one eye, the pupil of the injured eye will appear to dilate when the light is moved from the normal eye to the injured eye, indicating that the same amount of light is not being transmitted through the optic nerve in the injured eye (Cass 2012). This is known as an **afferent pupillary defect** and represents a potentially severe ocular emergency. Immediate referral to an eye care specialist is warranted.

A pupil that is larger in the injured eye or that does not react to light (**traumatic mydriasis**) or a pupil that is no longer round (e.g., it is peaked or oval) may represent significant intraocular trauma (e.g., traumatic iritis). The athlete should be immediately referred to an eye care specialist. The athletic trainer should know if the athlete has a previously existing or congenitally larger pupil on one side, or **anisocoria**, because this may confuse the findings of the examination.

Testing Extraocular Muscle Motility

Part of the basic assessment of a patient's eye is the examination of ocular motility. The inability of one or both eyes to move into the cardinal fields of gaze (figure 12.7), especially after an eye injury, indicates a severe eye injury with possible eye socket pathology or entrapment of the extraocular muscles (figure 12.8). The examiner asks the patient to follow an object or a fingertip up, down, left, and right with both eyes together. The examiner assesses the patient for smooth, uninterrupted movements of both eyes in all fields of gaze. There should be no restriction of gaze in either eye; movements of the two eyes should be harmonious and parallel. Any change of extraocular movements after an injury may also represent a neurological condition, and it requires immediate medical attention (Mishra and Verma 2012).

Testing Peripheral Vision

Although arguably not as crucial as central visual acuity, peripheral vision allows athletes to view the entire field of sport around them and to see where their teammates or competitors might be while they focus their vision centrally. Before any injury occurs, the range of an athlete's peripheral vision should be known from preparticipation vision testing.

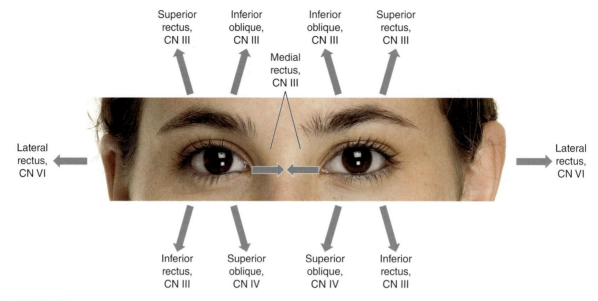

Superior rectus, CN III

Inferior oblique, CN III

Inferior oblique, CN III

Superior rectus, CN III

Medial rectus, CN III

Lateral rectus, CN VI

Lateral rectus, CN VI

Inferior rectus, CN III

Superior oblique, CN IV

Superior oblique, CN IV

Inferior rectus, CN III

FIGURE 12.7 Eye motility should be tested in all cardinal fields of gaze. CN = cranial nerve.

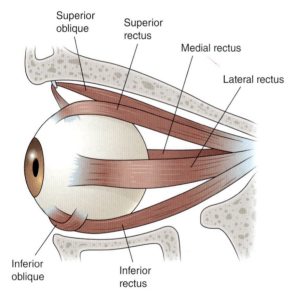

Superior oblique

Superior rectus

Medial rectus

Lateral rectus

Inferior oblique

Inferior rectus

FIGURE 12.8 Extraocular muscles of the eye.

The method most often used to grossly test peripheral vision is called confrontation visual field testing (figure 12.9). The examiner tests the patient's peripheral vision one eye at a time. To test the right eye, the examiner stands approximately 3 ft directly in front of the patient. The patient, left hand over left eye, focuses only on the examiner's left eye. The examiner's right eye is closed. This allows the examiner to watch his or her own open hands during the examination while fixating on the patient's right eye.

The examiner holds up one, two, or three fingers on each hand, equidistant between the examiner and the patient and equidistant on either side of the direct line of sight between the patient's right eye and the examiner's left eye. Examiners must be able to see their own fingers during this kind of examination. The patient is asked to add the total number of fingers seen while fixating only on the examiner's left eye and without looking at the examiner's fingers. The examiner will be able to detect whether the patient looked away from the examiner's left eye. It is best not to hold up the same number of fingers on each hand at the same time. This will allow the examiner to know exactly which field of vision was defective. Next, the other eye is examined in a similar fashion. All the cardinal fields of vision—right, left, above, below, above and to the right, above and to the left, below and to the right, and below and to the left—need to be tested. Any finding of the patient's inability to see in a particular field of vision should be referred to an eye care specialist before participation.

Examining the Anatomical Structures of the Injured Eye

A good assessment of the eye can usually be made by simply having the patient open his or her eyes and examining them directly. On occasion, the eyelids may have to be held apart by either the patient or the examiner. Eyelid swelling is a common consequence of direct trauma to the eye. Therefore, the eye must be examined as soon as possible before swelling of the eyelid makes direct assessment impossible.

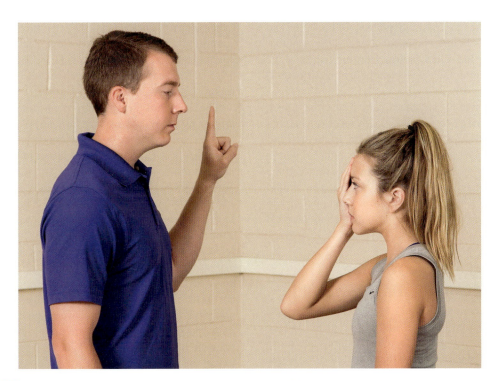

FIGURE 12.9   To test peripheral vision, confrontation visual field testing is used.

The examiner can use room lighting or a directed source of light (e.g., a flashlight or penlight) to assess the anterior portion of the eye. Inspection of the lids and palpation of the bony orbital rim can reveal serious trauma after a blunt injury. If there is any suspicion that the trauma was severe enough to penetrate or rupture the eyeball, then no external pressure should ever be placed on the eye or eyelids.

A light is directed toward the patient's opened eye; the patient is asked to look up while the examiner retracts the lower lid (figure 12.10*a*) and to look down while the examiner retracts the upper lid (figure 12.10*b*). This facilitates examination of the entire anterior aspect of the globe, including the conjunctiva, sclera, cornea, and iris. Foreign bodies are commonly found in the conjunctival fornices (Riordan-Eva and Cunningham 2011). The

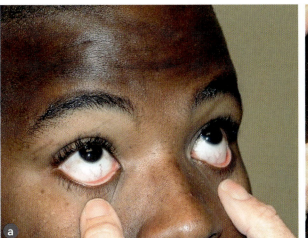 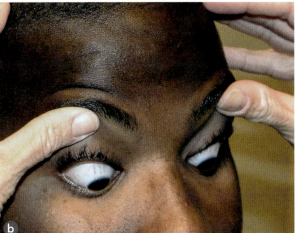

FIGURE 12.10   *(a)* Examining the anterior aspect of the globe with the lower lid retracted. *(b)* Examining the anterior aspect of the globe with the upper lid retracted.

fornices are the most posterior portions of the upper and lower portions of the conjunctiva, where the conjunctiva overlying the sclera (**bulbar conjunctiva**) and the conjunctiva lining the eyelids (**palpebral conjunctiva**) join together.

Obscuration of the structures behind the cornea, such as the iris or lens, because of a cloudy anterior chamber is an ominous sign of potential blood in the anterior chamber (hyphema). This can often be detected with a penlight, and it indicates a very serious eye injury. If the eye is anatomically distorted or bleeding, you should discontinue any further palpation or examination and seek emergency medical attention and ophthalmological referral.

Examining the Eye With the Ophthalmoscope

The ophthalmoscope (figure 12.11) is an instrument used to view the internal structures of the eye. The head of the instrument contains a light source that allows the examiner to visualize the inner eye through a series of lenses and apertures to allow for near or far focusing. The most commonly used aperture projects a large, round beam.

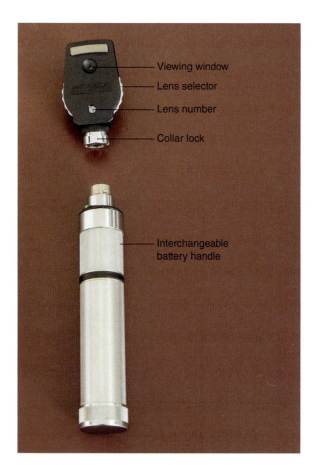

FIGURE 12.11   The parts of an ophthalmoscope.

Other apertures include the small aperture, the slit-lamp aperture to examine the anterior eye, the red-free filter aperture that shines a green beam to check the optic disk, and the grid aperture used to estimate the size of fundal lesions (Bickley 2012).

The diopter of the ophthalmoscope, that is, the magnifying power of the lens, may be changed by turning the lens selector disk to the desired magnification (Ball et al. 2014; Jarvis 2012). The black numbers indicate positive magnification, and the red numbers indicate negative. Turning the wheel clockwise selects positive lenses, and rotating it counterclockwise selects negative lenses. Lens numbers range in magnification power from ±20 to ±140. The range of plus and minus lenses can compensate for myopia or hyperopia in both the examiner and the patient (Bickley 2012). The diopter is set at zero (clear glass) when both the patient's and the examiner's eyes are normal. The globe in a hyperopic eye is shorter than normal. The black numbers (convex lens) on the ophthalmoscope lens selector wheel are used to place the focal point on the retina. In the nearsighted person, the globe is longer than in the normal eye, so the lens selector wheel is moved to the red numbers (concave lens) to adjust for myopia in either the patient or the examiner.

The heads of both the ophthalmoscope and the otoscope (used to view the ear and nose) typically share a common handle containing a rechargeable battery. The heads are interchangeable so one can easily convert from one instrument to the other. To change from an otoscope head to an ophthalmoscope head, the examiner pushes down on the head that is currently on the handle while turning to unlock the attachment, inserts the other head, and fastens it to the handle in the same manner.

Both instruments are turned on in the same way, namely, by pushing the on/off switch while turning the black rheostat clockwise to the desired intensity of light.

To examine a patient's eye with the ophthalmoscope, the athletic trainer turns on the ophthalmoscope and selects the large aperture. This should project a large, round light on the examiner's hand or the wall. Next the room is darkened. The examiner holds the handle of the ophthalmoscope in the right hand (to examine the patient's right eye) with the index or middle finger on the lens selector wheel. To examine the left eye, the left hand is used. The ophthalmoscope is held firmly against the bony orbit of the examiner's eye (right eye for examining the patient's right eye and left eye for the patient's left eye) with the handle tilted laterally. This will prevent the athletic trainer and the patient from bumping noses during the examination.

The patient is instructed to look up over the shoulder of the athletic trainer. The examiner should start about 15 in. away from the patient, shining the light into the eye to visualize the reddish orange glow (red reflex) from the light reflecting off the highly vascularized retina of the eye. The athletic trainer should approach the patient from the side at about a 15° angle. Shining the light directly into the patient's eye must be avoided because it will cause the pupil to constrict, making it more difficult to visualize the internal eye through an undilated pupil. While keeping the light focused on the red reflex, the athletic trainer moves in close to the eye, almost touching the patient's eyelashes. Absence of a red reflex is often the result of an improperly positioned ophthalmoscope.

To view the internal structures of the eye, such as the optic disk, arteries, veins, and retina, the athletic trainer may need to turn the lens selector wheel to focus on various structures. The fundus or retina will appear as a yellow or pink background with blood vessels branching away from the optic disk (figure 12.12). It is often easier to find the blood vessels and follow them back to the optic disk than to try to locate the optic disk by itself. The arterioles are smaller than the venules and reflect brighter light. The vessels should be followed as far as possible in each of the four quadrants of the eye (superior, inferior, nasal, and temporal) as they go away from the optic disk. When the optic disk is visualized, it should appear yellow

to creamy pink, but it may be darker in dark-skinned people (Bickley 2012). The borders of the disk should be sharp and well defined. Moving in a temporal direction from the optic disk, the macula (fovea centralis) may be visualized (Richardson 2013). To bring the fovea into the field of vision, the examiner asks the patient to look directly at the light of the ophthalmoscope. It will appear as a yellow dot surrounded by a deep pink periphery and will not have any blood vessels running through it (Ball et al. 2014). Considerable practice is needed to visualize the macula, and it may be impossible to view without the pupil being dilated.

Refractive Error

For clear vision, both near and distant images must be sharply focused onto the retina, which lines the back of the eyeball. The ability of the eye to focus these images is directly related to the length of the eye, the curvature of the cornea, the clarity of the ocular media, and the flexibility of the crystalline lens (figure 12.13). The first two parameters, length of eye and curvature of cornea, determine the refractive error of an eye. **Myopia**, or near-sightedness, is produced by a longer-than-normal eye. A distant object is focused in front of the retina instead of on it. **Hyperopia**, or farsightedness, is produced by a shorter-than-normal eye. A distant object is out of focus when it reaches the retina and, theoretically, focuses behind the retina (Wu, Liu, and Zhang 2015). The shape of the cornea is typically spherical (just like a tennis ball) on its anterior curvature. When this curvature is not spherical and has multiple curvatures (such as an egg or football), the eye is considered astigmatic. After age 40, the crystalline lens inside the eye begins to lose its flexibility and thus its ability to focus on nearby objects. This is known as **presbyopia**. Presbyopic patients eventually require reading glasses for near vision.

Signs and Symptoms

Mild degrees of refractive errors can remain undetected for years until very clear distance vision is needed, such as when an adolescent first begins an athletic season. In other cases, patients may complain of slowly declining visual acuity. Impaired visual acuity may be confirmed by

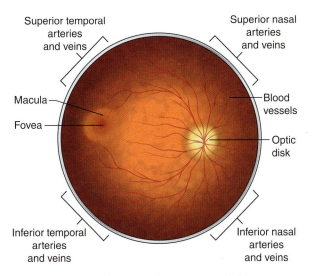

Superior temporal arteries and veins

Superior nasal arteries and veins

Macula

Fovea

Blood vessels

Optic disk

Inferior temporal arteries and veins

Inferior nasal arteries and veins

FIGURE 12.12 The retinal structures of the eye.

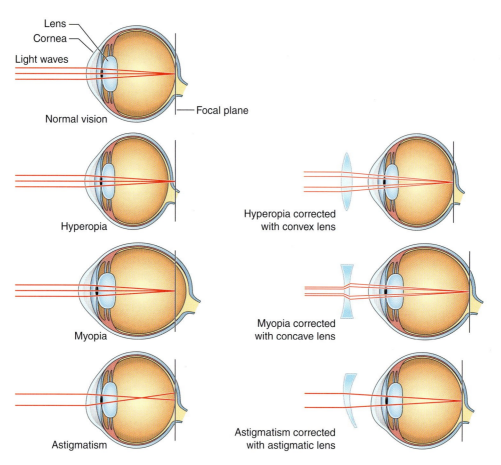

FIGURE 12.13 Common refractive disorders and their corrections.

testing with a Snellen chart. The vision should improve with pinhole testing. Pinhole testing is a method to distinguish a refractive error (correctable with lenses) from organic eye disease. Pinhole testing is performed by punching several pinholes in a card. The patient looks through a pinhole in the card one eye at a time. If vision improves, the condition is refractory.

Referral and Diagnostic Tests

Patients who complain of poor vision, either at a distance or close up, need to be referred to an eye care practitioner who will determine the refraction of their eyes and perform other ocular tests. The refraction determines the refractive error of an eye. The refractive error will change

Common Misconceptions About Vision and the Eye

The following statements are often passed along as advice, but all are false.

- Reading in the dark is harmful to the eyes.
- Children will outgrow crossed eyes.
- A cataract is a film growing over the surface of the eye.
- One should avoid reading to save eyesight when vision is failing.
- Children must be cautioned not to sit too close to the television.
- Wearing someone else's glasses may damage your eyes.
- Misuse of the eyes in childhood results in the need for glasses later in life.
- Emotional stress increases intraocular pressure.

over time as the shape and length of the eye change up to the ages of 23 to 25. After that the refractive error tends to stabilize.

Treatment and Return to Participation

The refractive error can be corrected with glasses or contact lenses. Refractive surgery, such as laser-assisted *in situ* keratomileusis (LASIK), is also an option for treatment. LASIK is performed to correct myopia, hyperopia, or astigmatism. In LASIK, a small, partial-thickness flap is made from the top of the cornea. A laser is used to reshape the corneal tissue under the flap and remove any refractive error present. The corneal flap is repositioned onto the lasered cornea surface. This procedure takes approximately 15 to 30 min, with many patients capable of seeing an immediate improvement in their vision. Not everyone is eligible for LASIK. The success of the operation depends on the degree of initial refractive error and on the thickness of the cornea (Kuryan, Cheema, and Chuck 2014). In one study, 36.4% of patients interviewed cited the desire to pursue sports and leisure activities as one of their main reasons for having LASIK (Liu et al. 2016). Many athletes consider having LASIK to avoid wearing glasses or contact lenses while playing sports as these may fog or dislodge during play. There have been no studies to date showing any improvement in the performance of players who have had LASIK. Although generally viewed as a safe procedure, there have been multiple case reports of dislodged flaps due to sport-related eye trauma (Liu et al. 2016). LASIK should not be performed until the refraction has been stable for at least 2 yr, especially in the adolescent or young adult.

The prognosis for the vast majority of refractive errors is excellent. Return to participation can be immediate after the athlete has received correction for the refractive error.

Conjunctivitis

Conjunctivitis is a general term for an inflammation of the conjunctiva, the transparent vascular tissue covering the anterior sclera and the posterior surface of the eyelids. It is commonly caused by bacteria, viruses, allergies, or dry eye or occurs in response to a corneal injury or irritation.

Signs and Symptoms

The symptoms of conjunctivitis, sometimes called pink eye, are not specific to the causative agent and can include all or some of the following: redness, burning, itching, tearing, irritation, and foreign body sensation. Allergic conjunctivitis is classically characterized by itching. Viral conjunctivitis is often associated with recent cold or flu symptoms or recent contact with someone with a red eye (Ferri 2016). The most obvious signs of conjunctivitis are redness or vascular engorgement (figure 12.14). There may be a discharge, ranging from watery to mucoid to frank purulence (pus). Redness of the conjunctiva in the space between the eyelids associated with a burning sensation is common after exposure to sun, wind, or dusty conditions, which are all common to outdoor athletics.

A few basic features can help differentiate bacterial, viral, and allergic conjunctivitis, especially if a **slit-lamp** biomicroscope is available. A watery or mucous discharge can be seen in both allergic and viral conjunctivitis (Ferri 2016). Typically, the discharge in bacterial conjunctivitis is purulent (figure 12.15). Patients with an allergic

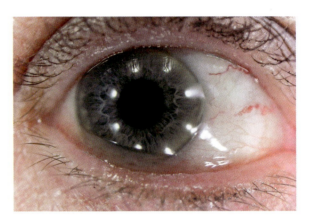

FIGURE 12.14 This photograph of allergic conjunctivitis shows the redundant conjunctiva rising over the edge of the lower lid margin in addition to redness and vascular engorgement of the sclera.

Photo courtesy of Charles B. Slonim

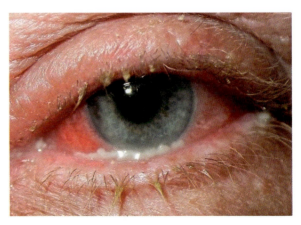

FIGURE 12.15 The discharge in bacterial conjunctivitis is typically purulent when compared with the watery discharge seen in allergic conjunctivitis in figure 12.14.

Photo courtesy of Charles B. Slonim

conjunctivitis typically complain that their eyes itch. Viral conjunctivitis often involves the cornea, which is difficult to visualize without high magnification. Viral conjunctivitis often presents with **preauricular lymphadenopathy**, a small, tender lymph node located just in front of the tragus of the ear.

Referral and Diagnostic Tests

Viral conjunctivitis is highly contagious, and therefore referral to an eye care practitioner for diagnosis is important in most cases of conjunctivitis. Without the benefit of a slit-lamp biomicroscope used by the ophthalmologist or optometrist, determining the exact cause of conjunctivitis may be difficult. Follow these steps to assess the need for referral of a patient with red eye:

1. Check the patient's visual acuity.

2. Inspect for a pattern of redness. A diffuse pink color is quite different from a deep localized redness.

3. Observe for the presence of discharge.

4. Use a fluorescein stain and blue cobalt light to observe for corneal defects if an abrasion is suspected.

5. Use an ophthalmoscope to observe the inner structures of the eye for irregularities.

6. Refer a patient with any abrasions, foreign bodies, hyphemas, or irregularities in the shape of the pupil to an eye care specialist immediately.

CLINICAL TIP

The Cause of Red Eye

Many patients present with a chief complaint of a "red eye." An engorgement of the conjunctival vessels causes the eye to be red. It may be associated with a subconjunctival hemorrhage that requires no treatment, or it may be a manifestation of a serious eye disorder that requires immediate attention. Common disorders involving red eye include the following:

- *Conjunctivitis:* Bacterial, viral, allergic, and irritative
- *Herpes simplex keratitis:* Inflammation of the cornea caused by a herpes virus
- *Scleritis:* Inflammation of the sclera
- *Subconjunctival hemorrhage:* Accumulation of blood in the potential space between the conjunctiva and the sclera
- *Abrasions and foreign bodies:* Hyperemic response

Treatment and Return to Participation

Standard treatment for mild acute bacterial conjunctivitis includes topical antibiotic eyedrops or ointments, such as fluoroquinolone ophthalmic drops (e.g., ofloxacin, ciprofloxacin, levofloxacin, moxifloxacin, gatifloxacin, besifloxacin), aminoglycoside ophthalmic drops (e.g., gentamicin, tobramycin), or erythromycin or bacitracin ophthalmic ointments. Viral conjunctivitis usually resolves spontaneously within 2 wk and cannot be treated effectively with topical antibiotics (Ferri 2016). Typically, the worst signs and symptoms occur on the third to fifth days. Because antiviral therapies are not effective in treating viral conjunctivitis, treatment is directed at relieving symptoms such as redness and burning. This may involve the use of over-the-counter vasoconstrictors (i.e., whiteners), topical antiallergy drops (e.g., ketotifen), or simply artificial tears to lubricate the ocular surface. Allergic conjunctivitis is often self-treated with a variety of over-the-counter topical ophthalmic antihistamine or decongestant products. There are also prescription antiallergy ophthalmic products that can be prescribed by the eye care practitioner. These include topical ophthalmic antihistamines (e.g., emedastine), mast cell stabilizers (e.g., cromolyn sodium), mast cell stabilizer and antihistamine combinations (e.g., olopatadine, azelastine, epinastine), nonsteroidal anti-inflammatories (e.g., ketorolac), and steroids (e.g., loteprednol, fluorometholone) (Geissler and Borchers 2015).

Viral conjunctivitis is highly contagious. Therefore, any athlete with acute watery conjunctivitis should not be in close contact with others until the condition is resolved. A persistent or worsening conjunctivitis may be secondary to more aggressive bacteria or a moderately severe allergy. In such a case, the athlete should receive an ophthalmic assessment. After 2 or 3 d, the athlete can return to participation. Some extremely virulent strains of viral conjunctivitis can cause corneal clouding that can persist for weeks to months. This can adversely affect the patient's vision. Bacterial conjunctivitis, although contagious, is not as easily spread from one person to another as is viral conjunctivitis. After 1 or 2 d of topical antibiotic therapy, the athlete can return to participation (Roat 2014).

Appropriate hygiene and hand washing, and isolating the patient with a red eye until it is properly diagnosed, can prevent the spread of viral conjunctivitis. Team members are advised not to share cosmetics or other products used around their eyes.

Hyphema

Blood in the anterior chamber of the eye is known as a **hyphema**, and it is a common complication of blunt trauma to the eyeball (figure 12.16). It is often associated with other types of orbital or ocular damage, such as corneal abrasions, orbital fractures, eyelid contusions, and open globe injuries (Andreoli et al. 2012; Bansal et al. 2016; Chang, Huynh, and Borboli-Gerogiannis 2012; Logothetis, Leikin, and Patrianakos 2014; Sbicca and Hatch 2012). The blood often comes from a damaged blood vessel in the iris or ciliary body. The appearance of blood in the anterior chamber of the eye begins as a crescent shape inferiorly and may progress until the entire anterior chamber is filled with blood. Spontaneous hyphemas in the absence of trauma are rare and are associated with a variety of rare ocular syndromes.

Signs and Symptoms

The two main symptoms of a hyphema are pain and blurred vision. The pain is associated with both the initial trauma and the inflammatory effect that the blood has on the anterior structures of the eye. The blurred vision is associated with the interruption of the clear aqueous humor in the anterior chamber by the opaque blood. The blood can often be seen by close examination with an external light source. With a vertical head position, the blood will form a layer in the anterior chamber with the heavier blood settling to the bottom and the lighter aqueous humor rising to the top (Andreoli et al. 2012; Bansal et al. 2015). On occasion, the blood creates a very thin, microscopic layer at the bottom of the anterior chamber. This may be imperceptible to the naked eye of the examiner.

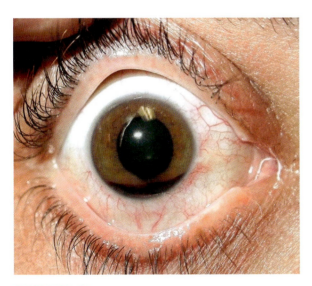

FIGURE 12.16 A hyphema most often is caused by trauma to the eye, as in this racquetball player's injury. This injury points out why it is important always to wear eye protection.

Photo courtesy of Charles B. Slonim

In the presence of trauma, blood in the anterior chamber can represent only a hyphema. On occasion, the source of the bleeding can be visualized. Hyphemas are associated with a number of other sight-threatening conditions and complications. The differential diagnoses are aimed at looking for other potential ocular damage that may have occurred in association with the hyphema. These conditions include a ruptured globe, corneal abrasion, dislocated lens, traumatic **cataract**, bleeding in the vitreous cavity, increased intraocular pressure (e.g., secondary glaucoma), and retinal tear or detachment (Andreoli et al. 2012). The presence of a hyphema may make it difficult to examine the more posterior structures of the eye, such as the retina.

Referral and Diagnostic Tests

A hyphema represents a serious, sight-threatening condition that requires immediate referral to an eye care specialist. During transport, the patient should keep the head elevated in order to allow the blood to settle to the bottom of the anterior chamber. This will give the eye care specialist a better opportunity to visualize the rest of the ocular structures.

Treatment and Return to Participation

Protective eyewear can prevent the vast majority of hyphemas caused by direct trauma to an eye. The athlete must wear protective eyewear after sustaining a hyphema to prevent a recurrence. An uncomplicated hyphema is typically managed with bed rest and the administration of topical steroids (e.g., prednisolone, loteprednol, dexamethasone), pupil-dilating drops known as mydriatics (e.g., **atropine**, **homatropine**), and, if required, eye pressure-lowering (antiglaucoma) agents (Bansal et al. 2015). The patient should sleep with the head of the bed slightly elevated. A significant late risk of hyphema is a rebleed that typically occurs between the third and fifth day after the initial injury. This rebleed can completely fill the anterior chamber with blood. This is commonly referred to as an eight-ball hyphema (Chang, Huynh, and Borboli-Gerogiannis 2012). This can produce elevated intraocular pressure and permanent blood-staining of the inside of the cornea. Both of these conditions are sight-threatening. On occasion, systemic medication may be needed to control the bleeding and the high intraocular pressure. In cases of very high intraocular pressure or severe bleeding in the front of the eye, the patient may require hospitalization or surgical evacuation of the blood.

The prognosis for an uncomplicated hyphema is excellent. Depending on the size of the hyphema and the intraocular pressure measurement, daily follow-up by an eye care specialist may be needed until the blood starts to resorb. The athlete can return to participation 2 to 3 wk after the blood has completely resolved. Less frequent examinations by the eye care specialist over the following months may be required to rule out late complications such as secondary glaucoma. Undetected high intraocular pressures can cause irreversible damage to the optic nerve. Blood-staining of the cornea may require months to resolve.

Subconjunctival Hemorrhage

Bright red blood appearing acutely in a sector of the eye under the clear conjunctiva and in front of the white sclera is termed a **subconjunctival hemorrhage** (figure 12.17). Although striking in appearance, this condition is benign. It represents a broken blood vessel under the conjunctiva and is analogous to a subcutaneous hematoma.

Signs and Symptoms

Subconjunctival hemorrhages can be caused by trauma, coughing or straining, high blood pressure, breath-holding or Valsalva maneuver, bleeding disorders, and ingestion of blood thinners. They can occur spontaneously without a known cause and are usually without symptoms; however, other people observing the eye can easily detect the blood. Rarely, more serious conditions such as conjunctival tumors can emulate a subconjunctival hemorrhage.

Referral and Diagnostic Tests

Unless there has been blunt trauma, subconjunctival hemorrhage does not require ophthalmic evaluation as long as no other signs or symptoms are present and vision is unaffected.

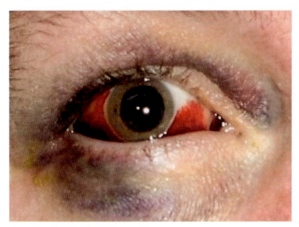

FIGURE 12.17 Eyelid contusion with subconjunctival hemorrhage.

Photo courtesy of Charles B. Slonim

Treatment and Return to Participation

Because of the nature of its pathophysiology, with the exception of direct trauma, there is no way to prevent a subconjunctival hemorrhage. Protective eyewear should prevent subconjunctival hemorrhage caused by direct trauma to the conjunctival surface. For mild irritation, artificial tears can be given. A simple subconjunctival hemorrhage usually clears within 2 or 3 wk; it may change color as the blood resolves, similar to a bruise.

Prognosis is excellent. Athletic participation is not restricted because of subconjunctival hemorrhage. If there are recurrent bleeding episodes, visual symptoms, pain, or persistence of blood, an ophthalmic referral should be sought.

Corneal Abrasions

A corneal abrasion results from a scratch to the surface of the cornea that causes a defect in the most superficial layer of cells, called the epithelium (Ahmed, House, and Feldman 2015). The most common cause of a corneal abrasion is direct trauma with a foreign object.

Signs and Symptoms

The most common symptom of a corneal abrasion is the sensation of having something in the eye, referred to as a foreign body sensation. Other symptoms include decreased vision, tearing, sensitivity to light, **blepharospasm** (abnormal blinking), and reactive conjunctivitis (Design et al. 2012).

Some corneal infections can have a similar presentation to a corneal abrasion, and it is important to distinguish between them by staining and magnification. Often a corneal abrasion is caused by an embedded foreign body that remains stuck to the ocular surface or possibly stuck onto the surface of the conjunctiva under the eyelids. Persistence of a foreign body sensation in the absence of an abrasion requires looking for a retained foreign body somewhere on the eye.

Referral and Diagnostic Tests

Most corneal abrasions should be referred to an eye care specialist in order to rule out an injury that might be deeper into the cornea than just the epithelial surface. A corneal abrasion can be difficult to see in a penlight examination. It is best visualized by a special ophthalmic vital dye staining technique. This technique involves placing a water-soluble orange dye, called fluorescein, on the ocular surface. Fluorescein dye is commercially available as individually wrapped, sterile paper strips that have been impregnated with the orange fluorescein dye

(Richardson 2013). To administer a fluorescein dye test, the clinician follows these steps:

1. Wet the tip of a fluorescein strip with sterile saline or eyewash.

2. Pull the lower lid down and away from the eye.

3. Touch the tip of the strip to the lower lid conjunctival cul-de-sac; do not place the strip directly on the eye.

4. Ask the athlete to close his or her eye for a few seconds in order to spread the dye.

5. Darken the room.

6. Use a cobalt blue light to illuminate the eye.

7. Observe the eye; the dye fluoresces as a bright yellowish green color under the cobalt blue light and pinpoints abrasions (figure 12.18).

Treatment and Return to Participation

The treatment of a simple corneal abrasion is lubrication with artificial tears and occasionally a topical antibiotic drop (e.g., fluoroquinolone or aminoglycoside) or ointment (e.g., bacitracin or erythromycin) if the potential for a corneal infection exists. The antibiotic preparation should be administered as directed, and follow-up should be with the eye care practitioner as prescribed. Some patients are also treated with a topical nonsteroidal anti-inflammatory drop (e.g., ketorolac) for pain management (Mishra and Verma 2012). Corneal abrasions are occasionally patched for 24 to 48 h to prevent the eyelid from rubbing over the abrasion during blinking. Multiple studies investigating the utility of early patching of corneal abrasions, however, have shown no evidence of improvement in level of pain or rates of healing (Design et al. 2012). Patching also results in a loss of binocular vision with subsequent loss of depth perception. Most of these studies were performed on corneal abrasions less than 10 mm in size. Therefore, routine patching of small corneal abrasions is not recommended, and the decision should be left up to an eye care practitioner (Ong et al. 2012).

Under the patch, the eye continues to move and rub against the posterior surface of the eyelid and lid margin. The epithelial defect continues to be traumatized by this movement, and the patient may continue to feel uncomfortable until the epithelial defect is completely healed. With the advent of soft bandage contact lenses, patching has become much less common. A soft contact lens with no refractive power, referred to as a *bandage contact lens*, can be placed over the corneal abrasion, which not only serves as a protective barrier to the movements of the eyelid but also aids in reepithelialization. Patients treated with soft bandage contact lenses along with a nonsteroidal anti-inflammatory drop were able to return to normal activity much more quickly than those who were patched (Ferri 2016). The addition of the anti-inflammatory drop significantly decreased the pain associated with the abrasion. Contact lenses should not be worn until the eye care specialist decides it is appropriate.

Simple noninfected corneal abrasions usually resolve clinically within 24 to 72 h (Design et al. 2012). After healing (reepithelialization) of the uncomplicated corneal abrasion, the area where it occurred is typically undetectable during future examinations, and it will not pose future problems for the patient. The athlete can return to participation as soon as the foreign body sensation is gone. Larger abrasions may require more time for reepithelialization and resolution of symptoms.

Corneal or Scleral Lacerations

One of the most serious traumatic eye injuries is a corneal or corneal–scleral laceration, also known as an open globe (Sridhar et al. 2015; Sbicca and Hatch 2012; Cass 2012). An open globe is an eyeball that has been ruptured after blunt or sharp trauma or injury with a projectile foreign body (figure 12.19). Lacerations allow leakage of intraocular fluid or extrusion of intraocular tissues and contents. They also allow the introduction of infectious pathogens from the environment into the intraocular spaces.

Signs and Symptoms

The symptoms of an open globe are decreased vision and pain after trauma. The patient often has a hyphema, dense subconjunctival hemorrhage, decreased eye movements, or bloody tears. An open globe should be considered after

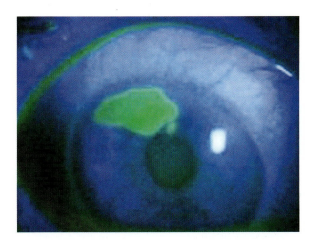

FIGURE 12.18 A corneal abrasion stained with fluorescein dye and "excited" with a cobalt blue filter.

Photo courtesy of Charles B. Slonim

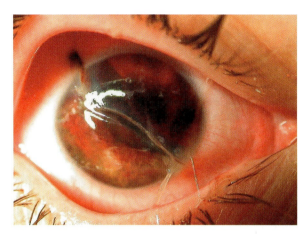

FIGURE 12.19 A corneal laceration (open globe) caused by a paintball injury.

Photo courtesy of Charles B. Slonim

any ocular trauma. Corneal lacerations can be penetrating, identified as open globe lacerations, or nonpenetrating (Sridhar et al. 2015). Some penetrating or perforating injuries may or may not have an extrusion of intraocular contents. The differential diagnosis is left to the eye care specialist.

Referral and Diagnostic Tests

If a rupture is suspected, it is imperative that the eye not be touched and that the patient be immediately transported to the nearest emergency room.

Treatment and Return to Participation

The treatment of a lacerated eye is prompt surgical repair, often followed by several days of intravenous and topical antibiotics. Infection of the eye after an open globe can be catastrophic and can cause loss of vision or even loss of the eye.

Visual rehabilitation of an eye with a corneal laceration is prolonged. Even after prompt diagnosis and appropriate treatments, the eye may still develop a cataract or a permanent scarring of the cornea. Scar tissue inside the eye often requires several eye surgeries to restore vision. Often the level of pretrauma vision cannot be regained, even after the most heroic efforts to restore the normal eye structure.

Corneal and Conjunctival Foreign Bodies

Any object embedded in or adhering to the conjunctiva or cornea is defined as an ocular foreign body (figure 12.20a). The patient may or may not recall getting something in the eye. Most ocular bodies are washed off the surface of the eye by the rinsing lubrication of the tear film or brushed off by the blinking action of the eyelids. Those foreign bodies that remain on the eye can cause the patient significant discomfort.

Signs and Symptoms

The symptoms of a foreign body are typically immediate. The patient may complain of a sensation of "something in the eye" or of "scratchiness." There is often an associated reflex tearing as the eye reacts to the foreign body and tries to relieve the eye by lubricating it. The foreign body may not be visible to the examiner depending on its size, shape, and color.

A corneal or conjunctival abrasion without a foreign body can mimic the symptoms of a foreign body as the blinking eyelids continue to rub over the abraded surface.

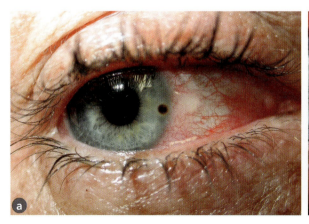
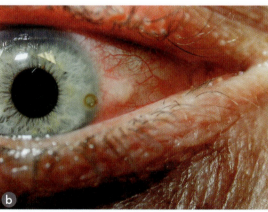

FIGURE 12.20 *(a)* A metallic corneal foreign body in the eye. *(b)* The same eye with a residual rust ring after the foreign body was removed.

Photos courtesy of Charles B. Slonim

Frequently, the patient will feel as if the foreign body is under the upper eyelid even if the foreign body or abrasion is in the middle or lower part of the eye.

Referral and Diagnostic Tests

Most foreign bodies lodged on the less sensitive conjunctival surface can be removed on site. Those on the extremely sensitive corneal surface may require referral to an eye care specialist if they cannot be removed with a few simple maneuvers (Ahmed, House, and Feldman 2015).

Treatment and Return to Participation

A loose foreign body on the ocular surface can often be rinsed off the eye with additional lubrication such as an eye rinse or just a few drops of an artificial tear supplement. A contact lens in the affected eye should be removed before treatment. It is appropriate to wash an eye with a foreign body at an eyewash station if available. If the foreign body sensation persists after irrigation, the upper eyelid can be gently pulled away from the eyeball by grasping the upper lid eyelashes and pulling the upper eyelid down over the lower eyelid lashes. The lower eyelid lashes will then act as a "brush" against the back (conjunctival) side of the upper lid and potentially dislodge a loose foreign body from under the upper eyelid.

If the foreign body sensation persists after the brushing maneuver, the upper lid can be everted to allow a direct inspection of its conjunctival surface (Bickley 2012). The examiner can pull the upper lid away from the eye by gently grasping the upper lid lashes and having the patient look down. When a small cotton-tipped applicator is placed against the upper eyelid crease (found approximately 0.5 in. above the margin of the eyelid), the eyelid can be rotated around the applicator (figure 12.21a). The

examiner's finger can keep the lid everted by pressing the lashes against the brow. If the foreign body is located, the same applicator can be used to gently lift the foreign body off the surface of the conjunctiva.

The cornea should never be touched. No attempt to remove a foreign body from the cornea should be made because inadvertent pressure on a sharp corneal foreign body could potentially push it deeper or even perforate the thin cornea. If the foreign body cannot be removed and remains embedded on the conjunctival or corneal surface, the patient needs to be referred to an eye care specialist.

Topical antibiotics (e.g., fluoroquinolone, aminoglycosides, erythromycin) are sometimes prescribed to prevent infection. Residual foreign body sensation, such as that caused by an abrasion from the foreign material, can be treated with artificial tears.

The prognosis for simple conjunctival foreign bodies is excellent. The athlete can typically return to participation immediately after the foreign body has been removed. Sometimes the maneuvers to remove the foreign body may create an additional ocular surface abrasion. Although the foreign body is gone, the foreign body sensation may remain for another 24 h. The prognosis for removing corneal foreign bodies depends on their depth and size. The recovery time is usually a little longer and may require 24 to 48 h for the symptoms to completely resolve.

Orbital Fracture

Among the seven bones that make up the walls of the bony orbit are some of the thinnest bones of the body. When there is a blunt injury to the eye, the forces against the orbit create a sudden increase in pressure within the orbit. The orbital contents, including the eyeball, are displaced posteriorly, toward the back of the orbit. This pressure

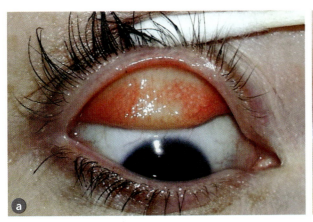 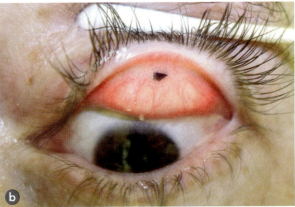

FIGURE 12.21   *(a)* The upper eyelid is everted with a cotton-tipped applicator. *(b)* A foreign body (plastic) on the upper eyelid.

Photos courtesy of Charles B. Slonim.

can break the thin orbital walls, causing an orbital wall fracture that is often referred to as a blow-out fracture. Often the nearby orbital contents, such as the extraocular muscles and orbital fat, can be forced through the fracture site and become incarcerated in the space behind the fractured wall. The two orbital walls that most commonly fracture during blunt trauma are the inferior wall (orbital floor) and the medial wall. The spaces behind these two walls are the maxillary and ethmoid sinuses, respectively.

Signs and Symptoms

Depending on the severity of the injury and fracture, the symptoms of an orbital fracture can include pain with attempted eye movement, double vision (**diplopia**) when orbital contents are trapped in the fracture site, and numbness, or hypesthesia, in the distribution of the infraorbital nerve, which gives sensation to the cheek, upper lip, and upper teeth (Cass 2012). The double vision resolves when the patient covers one eye. The patient may show signs of restricted eye movements in up- or down-gaze, decreased sensation in the cheek or upper lip on the same side as the injury, misalignment of the orbital rim on palpation along with point tenderness, and sometimes a "crunchy" sensation under the skin of the orbit (Aerni 2013) (figure 12.22). This latter condition, called **orbital emphysema**, is a result of air from the sinus that has become trapped beneath the skin. Eyelid ecchymoses are often seen.

RED FLAGS FOR ORBITAL FRACTURES

An orbital fracture often causes the patient's eye on the affected side to have restricted upward movement due to trapping of the inferior rectus muscle through the orbital floor. Any patient with unilateral restricted eye movement must be referred for further examination.

Blunt head trauma can damage certain cranial nerves associated with extraocular movements (e.g., cranial nerves III, IV, and VI), and the athlete can present with diplopia (Kriz et al. 2015). Localized swelling over the infraorbital nerve can cause temporary hypesthesia along its sensory distribution. Retrobulbar (behind the globe) hematomas can cause irreversible optic nerve damage.

Referral and Diagnostic Tests

A patient with a suspected orbital fracture requires orbital imaging studies. The most important diagnostic test is a computerized tomography (CT) scan of the orbit with both coronal and axial views. It is also important to examine the eye for potential intraocular injuries (e.g., retinal detachment, hyphema, open globe injury, foreign body).

Treatment and Return to Participation

Not all orbital fractures require surgical repair. Depending on the size and location, and on whether there is tissue entrapment, an orbital fracture may be monitored to determine whether the patient's signs and symptoms spontaneously resolve with time. An orbital fracture technically represents an open fracture because the normally closed orbital space can allow sinus air to enter through the fracture site. For this reason, systemic antibiotics are administered. Iced compresses for the first 24 to 48 h can help reduce the periorbital swelling. No compresses are used until the eyeball has been cleared of any injuries. Patients with suspected orbital fractures are instructed not to blow their noses because this can force bacteria-laden air from the paranasal sinuses under the eyelids or into the orbit and cause a secondary infection. For large fractures or persistent diplopia in primary or down-gaze, surgical repair of the fracture is often required. The patient may be observed for up to 2 wk before any surgical intervention to determine whether the signs and symptoms resolve

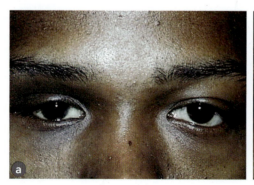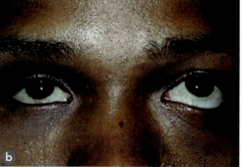

FIGURE 12.22 This right orbital floor fracture injury seen in a basketball player is assessed by (a) having the athlete look straight ahead, and (b) noting the restricted upward gaze of the right eye, which is on the reader's left.

Photos courtesy of Charles B. Slonim.

spontaneously. Ophthalmologists, otolaryngologists, plastic surgeons, and maxillofacial surgeons perform this surgery.

The prognosis for complete resolution of the signs and symptoms of an orbital fracture depends on the spontaneous resolution of symptoms or the success of the surgical outcome. Persistent diplopia may require further extraocular muscle surgery. Shrinkage of the orbital fat after orbital trauma may cause delayed **enophthalmos** (movement of the eyeball deeper into the orbit). Infraorbital nerve hypesthesia may be transient or permanent, depending on the extent of injury to that nerve. Athletes may return to sport participation in approximately 2 to 4 wk, with facial and eyewear protection for approximately 4 to 6 mo.

Retinal Tear and Detachment

The retina is the delicate transparent tissue lining the back of the eye. Light-sensitive retinal fibers receive images projected through the lens and send them to the brain through the optic nerve for interpretation as a visualized image. When the retina is damaged, the transmission of the images is distorted or absent. Retinal tears and retinal detachments (figure 12.23) may occur through illness, injury, or heredity or as the result of normal aging. These conditions are most typically found in people who are nearsighted, have undergone previous eye surgery, have experienced eye trauma, or have a family history of retinal detachments. Middle-aged and older people are at higher risk than the younger population. Retinal tears and detachments are also likely to recur in athletes with a history of a previous retinal tear or detachment. Athletes with risk factors associated with retinal tears or detachments should avoid contact sports in which head

or eye trauma is possible. Protective eyewear can prevent direct trauma to the eye that can cause retinal tears or detachments; however, blunt head trauma without direct eye trauma can also cause these conditions.

Retinal detachment typically begins with one or more small holes or tears in the retina. These holes are caused by shrinkage (e.g., during the aging process) or sudden movement (e.g., in trauma) of the vitreous humor that is intimately attached to the retina. Once a tear has occurred, more liquid vitreous humor may flow through the hole or tear, causing the retina to elevate and detach.

Signs and Symptoms

A retinal tear or detachment typically occurs in only one eye. The most common symptoms of a tear in the retina are brief flashes of light (**photopsia**) in the peripheral visual field or an abrupt increase in vitreous floaters. *Floaters* are the perception of images caused by opacity in the vitreous; they are common but typically few in number, and they only appear occasionally. The most common symptoms of a retinal detachment are the same as for a retinal tear, plus a curtain or shadow moving over the field of vision. Sometimes central visual acuity may be lost. The signs of a retinal tear or detachment are essentially limited to the direct visualization of the elevated or torn retina by an eye care specialist (American Academy of Pediatrics 2003).

As people age, the vitreous begins to liquefy. Eventually, it becomes so liquid that it collapses into itself and peels away from the retina. This phenomenon is called **posterior vitreous detachment (PVD)** or posterior vitreous separation. People who have had a PVD often notice floaters in their vision caused by small opacities in the vitreous that cast shadows on the retina. They may also experience a split-second flash of light in the corner of their vision. These symptoms are similar to those of a retinal tear.

Referral and Diagnostic Tests

Patients with a new onset of flashes or floaters, or what appears to be a curtain moving over their vision, especially after trauma, must be immediately referred to an eye care professional. These patients are often referred to retinal specialists. Proper examination requires pharmacological dilation of the pupil along with a detailed examination of the retinal periphery with specialized ophthalmic instruments.

Treatment and Return to Participation

Retinal detachments caused by traumatic breaks or tears to the retina are treated surgically. Ophthalmologists use

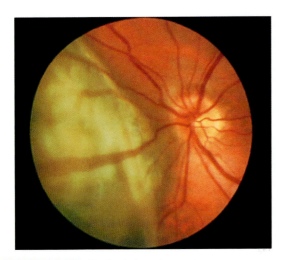

FIGURE 12.23   Retinal detachment.
Photo courtesy of Charles B. Slonim

lasers or cryoprobes to create adhesions between the detached retina and the back surface of the eye (Vinger 2012). Silicone oil, filtered air, or special gases are sometimes injected into the vitreous cavity to push the retina against the back of the eye during the healing process.

The prognosis for a retinal tear or detachment is based on the number of tears or holes or the size and location of the detachment. Early diagnosis and treatment are critical factors in successful surgical outcomes. If the central retina (macula), which is responsible for central 20/20 acuity, is not detached, successful surgery can preserve excellent central vision. However, complications of surgery, infection, redetachment, or a primary detachment of the central part of the retina can drastically decrease vision. Once a patient has had retinal surgery, the eye requires several weeks to heal. The risk of redetachment is higher in a patient with a previous history of one (Joondeph and Joondeph 2013). Return to participation depends on the extent of the retinal injury and the success of the repair. It also depends on the sport involved (e.g., contact vs. noncontact). Lengthy discussions between the athlete and the retinal specialist are necessary to determine the athlete's safety and the risk of future visual loss when returning to sports.

Dislocated Contact Lens

More than 30 million Americans wear contact lenses as a substitute for glasses to correct refractive errors and to improve their visual acuity. Contact lenses are categorized by the flexibility of the plastic material from which they are manufactured. Soft contact lenses are relatively large, soft, and pliable. They are designed to cover the entire corneal surface and extend approximately 1 to 2 mm beyond the cornea onto the conjunctiva and sclera. Rigid contact lenses, whether hard or gas permeable, are relatively small, hard, and less flexible. They are designed to fit only on the corneal surface. Contact lenses can be moved from their normal central location over the cornea when the eye is subjected to a shearing force, such as a tangential trauma from a ball or a hand (Zimmerman, Lust, and Bullimore 2011). Protective eyewear can prevent shearing forces from displacing contact lenses. The use of prescription safety goggles eliminates the risks associated with contact lenses and simultaneously protects the eyes from other trauma.

Signs and Symptoms

The symptoms of a displaced contact lens include loss of visual acuity and the presence of a foreign body sensation. Most currently available contact lenses have a visible tint for easy handling. This makes it easier for the examiner to identify a dislocated lens against the background of the white sclera. Nontinted lenses may be more difficult to see. Soft lenses may become rolled up and lodged in the upper limits of the conjunctiva under the upper eyelid.

Other acute conditions associated with contact lens wear can present with decreased acuity and a foreign body sensation, including corneal abrasions, corneal foreign bodies, some corneal infections, an inside-out contact lens, and hypersensitivity to a new or overused contact lens cleaning solution.

Referral and Diagnostic Tests

If the dislocated lens is located but cannot be removed by either the athlete or the athletic trainer, then a referral to an eye care specialist may be necessary. If no lens is found but a foreign body sensation remains, the patient may need the services of an eye specialist to rule out a possible corneal or conjunctival abrasion and to further examine the eye for the dislocated lens. If an athlete believes that a contact lens has become dislocated, the athletic trainer should help find it. Often the athlete can manipulate the lens and reposition it.

Treatment and Return to Participation

Pulling the upper and lower lids away from the eye to inspect the conjunctiva will often reveal the dislocated contact lens.

Before a displaced contact lens is removed, the eye should be lubricated with saline eyewash, an artificial tear solution, or contact lens rewetting solution. If the contact lens is dislodged under the upper lid, the lid must be everted. Once the lens is located, the eyelid is allowed to assume its normal position by simply asking the patient to look up. The lens can be moved to the lower portion of the eye by applying gentle, direct pressure through the eyelid. The athletic trainer must avoid excessive pressure on the contact lens. If the contact lens is dislodged under the lower lid, the conjunctiva is exposed by pulling the lower eyelid away from the eye. The lens can be repositioned by gentle finger pressure through the eyelid or removed from the eye. Applying a small contact lens suction cup, which should be included in the athletic trainer's kit, to a rigid lens can assist in lifting the lens out. The suction cup technique is not effective with soft contact lenses, and the suction cup should never be placed on the cornea.

A rigid lens may be reinserted on the cornea, if necessary. A soft lens should not be reinserted until it has been disinfected. Once good acuity is achieved, either through replacement contact lenses or corrective glasses, the athlete may return to sport.

Chemical Burns

Any chemical substance that comes into contact with the ocular surface has the potential to cause a serious chemical burn. Common chemicals that can produce serious, vision-threatening conditions and that are found in athletic training facilities include cleaning solutions or solvents, detergents, and aerosol hygiene products. Chemical compounds typically found around an athletic facility should be well labeled and kept away from areas where accidental spills and splashes can occur. Protective eyewear can prevent some splash injuries.

Signs and Symptoms

The symptoms of a chemical burn are the rapid onset of pain, a foreign body sensation, and frequently, loss of vision after contact with a chemical substance. The signs of a chemical burn of the ocular surface range from defects on the corneal surface to corneal opacification with pronounced swelling and blanching of the cornea or conjunctiva (Mittal et al. 2015) (figure 12.24). Burns to the surrounding skin of the face may also occur where the substance touches it.

A radiation burn to the cornea can present with symptoms similar to those of a chemical burn. The differential diagnosis is based on the presence or absence of a history of contact with a noxious substance.

Referral and Diagnostic Tests

Any chemical burn to the eye should be evaluated by an eye care professional. Treatment must be initiated before transporting the patient to the nearest emergency facility.

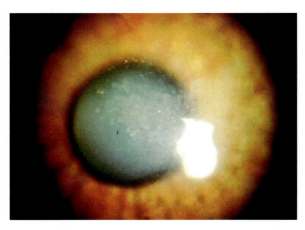

FIGURE 12.24 A chemical burn to the cornea; note the tiny white dots, which are irregularities on the corneal surface. Each dot represents a tiny corneal abrasion.

Photo courtesy of Charles B. Slonim

Evaluation of the eye with a chemical burn requires biomicroscopic (slit-lamp) examination, occasional assessment of the pH of the eye with test strips, and fluorescein staining of the cornea (Coronica and Murty 2015).

Treatment and Return to Participation

The most important treatment for a chemical burn to the ocular surface is immediate irrigation of the eye with copious amounts of any available clean fluid or liquid. These include saline eyewash, sink or shower water, a very low-pressure water fountain or hose, or noncarbonated sports beverages. Irrigation should be performed from the nasal corner of the eye to the temporal (lateral) side of the eye whenever possible to avoid flushing the chemical into the other eye. Irrigation should continue until the eye can be assessed at an emergency facility. A cooperative patient should have the conjunctival pockets under the upper and lower eyelids swept with a moistened cotton swab and have the upper eyelid everted and irrigated. Irrigation is continued at the emergency facility until the pH of the eye has returned to normal. The patient should then be treated by aggressive lubrication with an ointment, possibly one containing a topical steroid (e.g., prednisolone, loteprednol, or fluorometholone), if significant inflammation is present (Coronica and Murty 2015). Topical antibiotics should be considered if an abrasion is present. Associated complications, such as corneal damage or opacification and elevated intraocular pressure, may require further treatment.

Prognoses for chemical burns to the eye can vary widely depending on the severity of the burn and the type of chemical causing the injury. Alkali burns tend to create more serious ocular injuries than do acid burns. Most chemical burns create large corneal or conjunctival abrasions. A rapid resolution, with a rehabilitation course similar to that for a corneal abrasion, is common when irrigation is promptly initiated. However, if irrigation is delayed, vision-threatening ocular surface damage can result. Return to sport depends on the severity of the chemical burn.

CLINICAL TIPS

Chemical Burns

A chemically injured eye must be immediately irrigated with copious amounts of clean water or saline solution. Irrigate from the nasal side to the temporal side of the eye whenever possible to avoid flushing the chemical into the nonaffected eye.

Periorbital Contusion

Direct trauma to periorbital structures (e.g., eyebrows, eyelids, cheeks) can result in localized swelling and subcutaneous hemorrhages. Periorbital contusion is commonly referred to as a *black eye*. The dark purple, or "black and blue," appearance beneath the skin of the tissues around the eye is due to damaged blood vessels in the skin and muscles (ecchymoses) of the eyelids and face. These hemorrhages may extend to the subconjunctival space. The collection of blood and fluid produces the discoloration as well as the swelling within the surrounding ocular tissues.

Signs and Symptoms

Anyone who suffers a periorbital contusion can present with localized pain from the initial traumatic event. Diplopia may occur. The swelling and hemorrhages can be so severe that the eyelids may be swollen shut and may prevent access to the eyeball for an appropriate examination (figure 12.25). The external signs of a periorbital contusion with hemorrhage are usually obvious to the examiner. They include facial and eyelid ecchymoses with or without tissue edema and swelling (Aerni 2013). Extraocular muscle motility may be reduced as a result of severe periorbital swelling that prevents the eye from moving in all fields of gaze. An increase in the pressure around the eye or inside the anterior orbit may give the appearance that the eyeball is being pushed forward (proptosis).

The typical appearance of a black eye with bruising and swelling often worsens within 1 to 2 d after blunt periorbital trauma. Prolonged increased pressure within the orbit can damage both the optic nerve and extraocular muscle functions.

Any orbital or ocular injury resulting from blunt trauma may present with mild to severe periorbital contusions. Therefore, all potential orbital or ocular injuries (e.g., open globe, hyphema, orbital fracture) must be ruled out.

Referral and Diagnostic Tests

In the absence of any intraocular or visual damage, periorbital contusions can be treated without a referral to an eye care specialist. If there are any visual symptoms or evidence of intraocular injury, the patient is referred to an eye care specialist for a complete ophthalmic examination.

Treatment and Return to Participation

In the absence of intraocular or visual damage, conservative therapy consisting of ice compresses for the first 48 h followed by warm compresses until the ecchymoses have resolved will typically result in resolution within 1 to 2 wk. Pain can usually be controlled with non-aspirin-containing analgesics.

Most periorbital contusions resolve spontaneously and uneventfully. Most athletes without visual complaints or increasing or persistent pain can return to sport participation as long as the swelling of the periorbital tissue does not compromise their vision.

Traumatic Iritis

Traumatic iritis refers to an inflammation of the iris secondary to blunt traumatic injury to the eye. The term is

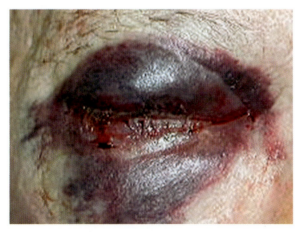

FIGURE 12.25 A severe periorbital contusion. An examiner would not be able to do an appropriate examination of the eye because the eyelids are swollen shut.

Photo courtesy of Charles B. Slonim.

RED FLAGS FOR CONDITIONS FOR IMMEDIATE REFERRAL

- Persistent blurred vision
- Diplopia
- Restricted eye movement
- Hyphema
- Distorted pupil
- Unilateral pupil dilation or constriction
- Foreign body protruding into the eye
- Large lacerations of the eyelids
- Lacerations that involve the margins of the eyelid
- Persistent floaters

often used to refer to an inflammation within the anterior chamber of the eye. The many nontraumatic causes of iritis are related to various medical and ocular conditions.

Signs and Symptoms

Inflammation of the iris or anterior chamber of the eye is associated with a dull, deep, aching pain when either the iris or pupil moves. The most common symptom of traumatic iritis is **photophobia** or pain when light is shone into the eye. This is due to the constriction and movement of the pupil and iris when stimulated by a direct light source. A traumatic iritis can occur 1 to 7 d after the initial trauma (Borrione et al. 2015). In addition to a mild to marked sensitivity to light, the patient may also complain of decreased vision, different-sized pupils (traumatic mydriasis), or a red eye with the redness forming a ring just outside the edge of the cornea. Definitive diagnosis is difficult without a slit-lamp biomicroscope.

In the presence of blunt ocular trauma, light sensitivity is caused by traumatic iritis until proven otherwise. Other ocular injuries associated with blunt trauma (e.g., corneal abrasion, hyphema, retinal detachment) need to be ruled out through a complete ophthalmic examination (Aerni 2013).

Referral and Diagnostic Tests

An eye care specialist must evaluate for suspected traumatic iritis. The diagnosis of iritis can only be made under the high magnification of a slit-lamp biomicroscope. In iritis, microscopic inflammatory white cells can be seen floating in the aqueous humor within the anterior chamber of the eye. These cells can plug the outflow tract of the aqueous humor, causing the intraocular pressure to rise (secondary glaucoma).

Treatment and Return to Participation

The treatment of traumatic iritis involves preventing the iris from moving and reducing the internal ocular inflammation. Dilation and temporary paralysis of the pupil with mydriatic drops (such as cyclopentolate) will typically alleviate the photophobia. Topical ophthalmic steroid drops, such as prednisolone and loteprednol, are used to reduce the anterior chamber inflammation. Depending on the severity of the inflammation, the treatment may last 2 to 4 wk. The topical steroid must be tapered to prevent a rebound of the inflammatory response. On occasion, additional drops (e.g., brimonidine, timolol) to treat secondary glaucoma may be necessary (Ahmed, House, and Feldman 2015).

The prognosis for traumatic iritis is excellent. Improvement of symptoms begins as soon as the pupil is dilated. Reduction of the internal inflammation often occurs within 5 to 7 d. Eyedrops are discontinued once the inflammation is resolved. The patient should receive a thorough eye examination within 1 mo of resolution of symptoms to check for other, subtle signs of anatomical damage from the blunt trauma. Athletes can return to sport participation once the inflammation has subsided.

Proptosis

Direct trauma to the orbit can result in deep orbital swelling and hemorrhages. Swelling that occurs behind the eye can push the eyeball forward, causing a bulging of the eye from between the eyelids (figure 12.26). This is called **proptosis**, or **exophthalmos**. Swelling and hemorrhages behind the eyeball can cause direct damage to the optic nerve by compromising its blood supply. This same swelling can put pressure on the outside of the eyeball, which can subsequently increase the pressure inside the eye (secondary **glaucoma**) (Borrione et al. 2015; Sbicca and Hatch 2012; Riordan-Eva and Cunningham 2011). The hemorrhages may extend to the subconjunctival space.

Signs and Symptoms

Patients who suffer from traumatic proptosis will often present with a bulging eye. The patient may complain of diplopia. Often the patient will also complain of pain and may be nauseous. Extraocular movements may be significantly reduced or absent. The eyelids may not close all the way (**lagophthalmos**), or there may be a severe subconjunctival hemorrhage that protrudes between the eyelids. Eyelid ecchymoses are not uncommon. These may not be evident for a day or two after the injury. Prolonged increased pressure within the orbit can damage both the optic nerve and extraocular muscle functions.

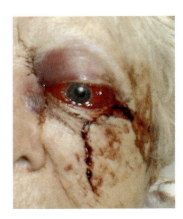

FIGURE 12.26 A retrobulbar hemorrhage with proptosis.

Photo courtesy of Charles B. Slonim.

In the presence of blunt trauma, proptosis may also be caused by significant orbital ecchymoses originating from a sinus as a result of an orbital fracture. All potential orbital or ocular injuries, including open globe, hyphema, and orbital fracture, must be ruled out.

Referral and Diagnostic Tests

Protrusion of the eye after blunt trauma must be referred immediately to an eye care specialist. A patient with a suspected orbital hemorrhage requires orbital imaging studies. Either CT scans or magnetic resonance scans of the orbit with both coronal and axial views should be performed. It is also important to examine the eye for potential intraocular injuries such as retinal detachment, hyphema, and open globe injury.

Treatment and Return to Participation

In the absence of any intraocular or visual damage, conservative therapy consisting of ice packs for the first 24 to 48 h, ocular lubricants to protect the cornea from drying out, and careful observation may be all that is required. Pain can usually be controlled with non-aspirin-containing analgesics. In the presence of any intraocular or visual damage, orbital decompression surgery may be required to preserve vision (Chang, Huynh, and Borboli-Gerogiannis 2012). Systemic (e.g., acetazolamide) and topical medications (e.g., brimonidine, timolol) to reduce intraocular pressure may be needed.

Traumatic proptosis has a guarded prognosis depending on the severity of the proptosis and damage to the ocular structures. Many cases resolve spontaneously and uneventfully, whereas others require surgical intervention. Most patients without visual complaints or increasing or persistent pain can return to sport participation after the proptosis has completely subsided.

Eyelid Lacerations

The eyelids and periorbital skin are very susceptible to both blunt and sharp trauma. The eyelid skin is the thinnest skin in the body. The thicker periorbital skin overlies a relatively solid orbital rim. These tissues are readily vulnerable to direct trauma.

Signs and Symptoms

In the presence of trauma, eyelid lacerations will present as an open wound of the eyelids or surrounding tissues. As with any tissue laceration, the presence of a foreign body needs to be ruled out. An examination for other evidence of ocular damage must be performed.

Referral and Diagnostic Tests

Lacerations that are not amenable to adhesive strip bandages and require suturing need to be referred to the appropriate oculofacial surgeon or ophthalmologist. Complete examination of the eyeball remains the highest priority before closure of the wounds.

Treatment and Return to Participation

Although the eyelids are not amenable to adhesive strips for closure of lacerations, for small wounds around the periorbital area, such as to the eyebrows, adhesive strips usually work well. Tissue adhesives (e.g., Dermabond; Ethicon, Somerville, NJ) can be used to close small eyelid or periorbital wounds. Suturing the wound closed is the most effective way to close an eyelid wound. During wound cleaning and antisepsis, care must be taken to avoid getting nonophthalmic antiseptic solutions, rinses, and ointments into the eye.

Most eyelid and periorbital lacerations heal nicely and uneventfully. Most athletes without visual complaints or increasing or persistent pain can return to sport participation as long as the swelling of the eyelid or periorbital tissue does not compromise their vision.

Protective Eyewear

More than 100,000 sport-related eye injuries are reported each year, and the overwhelming majority of such injuries occur in athletes under age 25. Baseball and basketball are the highest-risk sports for eye injuries, followed by water sports, racquet and court sports, and football (Armstrong et al. 2013; Castle 2012; Ellis and Falcons 2013; Farrington et al. 2012; Kriz et al. 2015; Ong et al. 2012; Peck et al. 2013; Stacey et al. 2012). Many eye injuries sustained in athletics are permanent and are associated with serious vision loss. Appropriate eye protection reduces the risk of eye injuries by at least 90% during any sport (Farrington et al. 2012).

The American Academy of Ophthalmology recommends specific protective lenses for both low-eye-risk and high-eye-risk sports: American Society for Testing and Materials (ASTM) standard F803 recommends *strap-fit* and sport goggles with polycarbonate lenses stronger than CR-39 plastic, respectively (Castle 2012). The NCAA (Parsons 2014) recommends protective eyewear for all sports that involve a projectile when the size of the projectile or its speed could potentially damage the eye. For athletes who are functionally monocular, such as those with a history of **amblyopia** (*lazy eye*) or a history of a prior eye injury, wearing protective eyewear should be mandatory at all times during any sport participation

CONDITION HIGHLIGHT

Cataract

Although not common in young athletic patients, cataracts are very common, and the athletic trainer may come across a patient or patient's family with a cataract. A cataract is a clouding of the lens of the eye; it is the leading cause of blindness among people older than 55. Cataracts are generally painless and usually start out as a small opaque spot. Vision is not usually affected until a larger area of the lens becomes opaque. Other symptoms include blurred vision, impaired night vision, light sensitivity, or changes in eyewear prescription. The diagnosis is determined by slit-lamp examination and retinal exam. Surgery is the only cure for cataracts, although some never need treatment. The surgical procedure involves removing the clouded lens and replacing it with a lens implant (Riordan-Eva 2011).

(Farrington et al. 2012). Athletes with functional vision in only one eye should consider sports other than contact sports and should not participate in sports involving high-velocity projectiles such as ball sports and hockey.

Contact lenses offer no protection from eye injuries, and protective eyewear without a refractive correction should be worn over contact lenses. Here are tips for choosing protective eye guards:

- Fit an athlete who wears prescription glasses with prescription eye guards.
- Purchase nonprescription eye guards at sport specialty stores or optical stores.
- Only "lensed" protectors are recommended for sports use.
- Fogging of lenses can be a problem for an active athlete. Some eye guards are available with anti-fog coating; others have side vents for additional ventilation.
- Look for an indication on the eye guard's packaging that it has been tested and approved for the athlete's sport. Polycarbonate eye guards are the most impact resistant.
- Make sure the eye guard is padded or cushioned along the brow and bridge of the nose. Padding will prevent the eye guard from cutting the athlete's skin during rugged sport activity.
- Adjust the eye guard straps to be secure on the face but not so tight that the eye guard is uncomfortable.

As athletes (and coaches) spend considerable time in the sun, special consideration should be given to wearing sunglasses to decrease the effects of ultraviolet (UV) rays on the eyes. Prolonged UV exposure can contribute to cataracts, macular degeneration, and growths on the eyes. Ophthalmologists recommend wearing 99% (and higher) UV-absorbent sunglasses and a brimmed hat when in the sun for prolonged periods of time. Just as chapter 16 discusses the importance of applying sunscreen, protecting the eyes with sunglasses is equally important (Cass 2012). The color and darkness of the lenses do not indicate their ability to block UV light. Even clear lenses can be coated to block UV. Wraparound frames are shaped to keep light from entering the eyes from the side, and sunglasses with such frames seem to be most effective in reducing the amount of UV light reaching the eyes (Vinger 2012).

Summary

Athletic trainers must recognize those eye conditions that require immediate attention and referral to an eye care practitioner. This chapter describes how to perform a basic examination of the eye, including tests for visual acuity and eye motility. If blurred vision is prolonged or eye motility is hindered, the patient should be referred. The patient who presents with an abnormally shaped pupil or diplopia also needs to be immediately referred. The athletic trainer should be skilled in the basic visualization of the internal structures of the eye and should be able to recognize abnormal conditions. The skilled use of an ophthalmoscope is necessary to visualize the internal structures of the eye. Protective eyewear is the athlete's best defense against periorbital and ocular trauma.

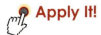 **Apply It!** The case study for this chapter looks at a 30-year-old male complaining of eye issues after a softball tournament. Read the scenario and answer the questions at www.HumanKinetics.com/MedicalConditionsInTheAthlete.

13

Ear, Nose, Throat, and Mouth

At the completion of this chapter the reader should be able to do the following:

- Describe the basic anatomy of the ear, nose, mouth, and throat.
- Perform a basic examination of the ear, nose, mouth, and throat, identifying normal and pathological conditions.
- Properly use an otoscope to examine the ear and the nose.
- Recognize common pathological conditions of the ear, nose, mouth, and throat, including signs and symptoms, differential diagnoses, and knowing when to refer the patient to a physician.
- Know the common diagnostic tests and standard medical treatment for conditions of the ear, nose, mouth, and throat.
- Identify the implications for participation in athletics with various conditions of the ear, nose, mouth, and throat.

This chapter covers nontraumatic conditions of the ear, nose, mouth, and throat. Many of these conditions are common occurrences in physically active people, and the athletic trainer may have ample opportunity to see them. Clinicians must understand the anatomy and physiology discussed in this chapter and feel comfortable performing an examination of the patient. Diagnosis of these conditions can usually be made on the basis of the patient's history, signs and symptoms, and the caregiver's observations.

Overview of Anatomy and Physiology

This section gives an overview of the anatomy and physiology of the ear, nose, throat, and mouth. Each body part is discussed independently, but the clinician must be aware of the interaction among the ears, nose, throat and mouth, and the history and examination must address all of these areas.

Ear

The ear serves two main functions: (1) to identify, locate, and interpret sound and (2) to maintain equilibrium. It consists of three distinct parts: the external, middle, and inner ears (figure 13.1). The external ear consists of the pinna, or auricle, the external auditory canal, and the lateral surface of the tympanic membrane. The pinna has a cartilage framework that is covered in skin, whereas the earlobe is fat covered in skin. The shape of the pinna is designed to gather or channel sound into the canal. The approximately 2.5 cm long canal is lined with epithelial cells, hairs, sebaceous glands, and ceruminous glands (Ball et al. 2014). The ceruminous glands produce

cerumen, or earwax, which lubricates the ear canal and tympanic membrane while serving as a protective barrier against foreign matter and bacteria. The outer third of the canal is flexible where it attaches to the pinna but is rigid for the last two-thirds as it enters the skull.

The external ear and the middle ear are separated by the tympanic membrane. The translucent tympanic membrane permits visualization of the middle ear, which is an air-filled cavity in the temporal bone that contains the ossicles: the malleus, incus, and stapes. These bones transmit vibrations from the tympanic membrane mechanically to the inner ear, where the mechanical vibrations are changed to electrical signals. The middle ear is connected to the **nasopharynx** by the **eustachian tube**. This passage opens briefly to equalize pressure in the inner ear when that pressure changes with swallowing, sneezing, or yawning (Bickley 2012; Jarvis 2012).

The inner ear consists of the vestibule, semicircular canals, and cochlea. The cochlea encodes the mechanical vibrations as electrical impulses that are then sent to the eighth cranial (vestibulocochlear) nerve. The vestibule is directly responsible for balance as the fluid in the semicircular canals shifts with head movement. Feedback from this movement is provided to the brain, helping to maintain upright posture and balance (Bickley 2012; Jarvis 2012).

Hearing is an interpretation of sound waves received through an air conduction path. The most efficient and normal hearing pathway is through the air conduction pathway, which produces sound from the tympanic membrane to the stapes to the basilar membrane of the cochlea. Bone also conducts sound by transmitting the vibrations of the skull directly to the inner ear and the vestibulocochlear nerve (figure 13.2).

Nose and Nasopharynx

The external nose consists of bone in the proximal third of the nose and cartilage in the lower two-thirds covered by skin. The nasal bones arise from extensions of the frontal and maxillary bones, forming the nasal bridge. The hard and soft palates form the floor of the nose, and the frontal and sphenoid bones form the roof. The external nose humidifies, filters, and warms inspired air and serves as a passageway for expired air (Ball et al. 2014; Bickley 2012).

The internal nose is divided into two anterior cavities, or vestibules, by the septum (figure 13.3). Air enters the nose through the nostrils and passes posteriorly to the nasopharynx through one of the **choanae**, separated by one of three turbinate bones. The **cribriform plate** that is part of the ethmoid bone on the roof of the nose houses the sensory endings of the olfactory nerve (cranial nerve I). A group of small, fragile arteries and veins is located on the anterior superior portion of the septum. This group of arteries and veins is called **Kiesselbach's plexus** and is often responsible for epistaxis. The **adenoids** lie on the posterior wall of the nasopharynx.

Three turbinate bones form the lateral walls of the nose. Covered by vascular mucous membrane, the turbinates separate the nose into a superior meatus, medial meatus, and inferior meatus. The turbinates help to increase the surface area for warming, filtering, and humidifying air.

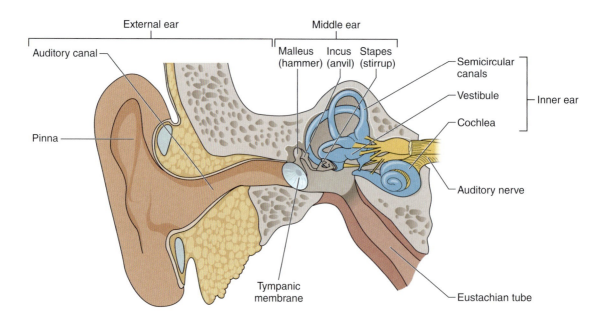

FIGURE 13.1 Anatomy of the ear.

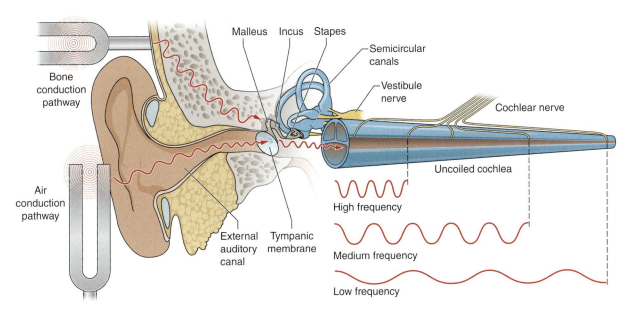

FIGURE 13.2 Pathways of hearing.

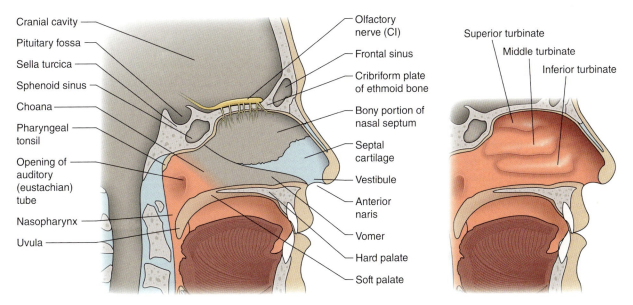

FIGURE 13.3 The nose and nasal septum.

The paranasal sinuses are a group of four paired air-filled spaces within the cranium (Jarvis 2012). They are generally named for their location in relationship to the eyes: the maxillary sinuses are under the eyes; the ethmoid sinuses are between the eyes; the frontal sinuses are above the eyes; and the sphenoidal sinuses are behind the eyes. The sinuses drain into their respective nasal cavities. The sinuses lighten the weight of the skull bones and serve as resonators for sound production. They also produce mucus from the membranes that line the sinus cavities, and this mucus drains into the nasal cavity.

Because the sinus openings are narrow and occlude easily, they are a common site for inflammation.

Mouth, Oropharynx, and Throat

The oral cavity consists of the lips, cheeks, tongue, teeth, and salivary glands (figure 13.4). It functions in several capacities, including serving as a passage for food as well as the initiation of digestion by mastication and salivary secretion. The mouth and oropharynx also emit air for vocalization and expiration.

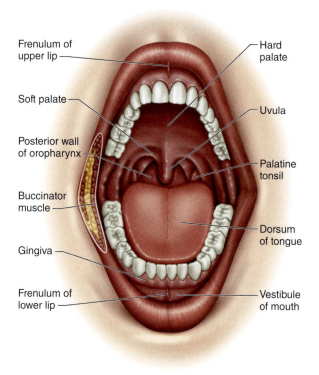

FIGURE 13.4 The anatomical structures of the oral cavity.

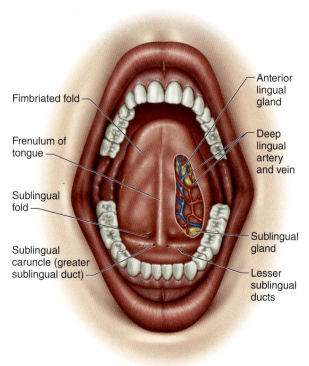

FIGURE 13.5 The ventral surface of the tongue showing anatomical landmarks.

The oral cavity may be divided into the mouth and vestibule. The vestibule is the area between the buccal mucosa and the outer surface of the teeth and gums (Ball et al. 2014). The roof of the mouth, which is formed by the hard and soft palates, separates the oral cavity from the nasal cavity. The soft palate is muscular tissue covered by mucous membrane that plays an active role in swallowing and vocal resonance. The soft palate, the tonsillar pillars, tonsils, base of the tongue, and posterior pharyngeal walls make up the oropharynx. The tongue is a skeletal muscle covered by mucous membrane, which helps to form the floor of the mouth, and is anchored to the floor of the mouth by the frenulum (figure 13.5) (Ball et al. 2014; Bickley 2012). Papillae cover the surface of the tongue to assist in the movement of food. Taste buds are contained within the papillae, and they allow people to taste what they are eating.

Three pairs of salivary glands are located in the mouth. The parotid, submandibular, and sublingual glands secrete saliva to moisten and lubricate food and to begin the digestion process (figure 13.6). A parotid gland lies within each cheek, just anterior to the ear, and for each gland a duct, known as Stensen's duct, extends to an opening on the buccal mucosa opposite the second molar. The submandibular glands lie beneath the left and right mandibles at the angle of the jaw. For each, a duct runs

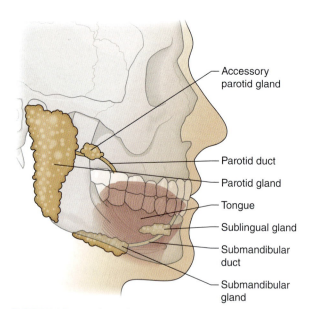

FIGURE 13.6 The salivary glands.

to the floor of the mouth, with the opening on either side of the frenulum. The sublingual glands are the smallest of the three pairs and are located under the tongue.

The teeth are embedded in the alveolar ridges and are protected by **gingivae** that cover the neck and roots of each tooth. The teeth and the gums are inspected during any evaluation of the mouth. Adults typically have 32 permanent teeth that are divided into upper and lower rows (figure 13.7). Each tooth consists of enamel, dentin, and pulp (figure 13.8). The enamel is an extremely hard surface that covers the dentin. The periodontal ligament that surrounds the root of the tooth helps keep the tooth stable. The pulp chamber contains the pulp, nerves, and blood vessels (Ball et al. 2014).

The pharynx consists of the combined upper parts of the respiratory and digestive tracts: the nasopharynx, oropharynx, and laryngopharynx (see figure 7.1). The larynx functions in respiration, prevents food and saliva from entering the respiratory tract, and produces sound. It is protected anteriorly by the thyroid cartilage and inferiorly by the cricoid cartilage (Bickley 2012).

Evaluation of the Ear, Nose, Mouth, and Throat

The examination of the ear, nose, mouth, and throat is most commonly done as a single examination because many conditions affect more than one anatomical area. For example, sinusitis may affect not only the sinuses but also the nose, ears, and throat. Often the patients with sinusitis will complain of pain in their teeth. Examination of each anatomical area may reveal important signs and symptoms from which to determine a diagnosis.

Examination of the Ear

When examining the ears, the examiner begins with a general inspection of the auricle, or pinna, noting its general size, shape, and symmetry. The clinician notes any deformities or discoloration that may indicate trauma to the external ear. The examiner also looks for lesions or nodules. The ear examination includes an inspection of the external auditory canal for obvious discharge or odor. Straw-colored fluid draining from the ear after a head injury could be cerebrospinal fluid (CSF), which is indicative of a brain injury. The auricles and mastoid areas are palpated for point tenderness, swelling, and nonvisible nodules. The auricle should be firm and mobile without nodules.

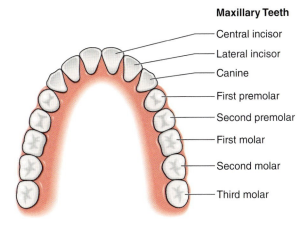

Maxillary Teeth

- Central incisor
- Lateral incisor
- Canine
- First premolar
- Second premolar
- First molar
- Second molar
- Third molar

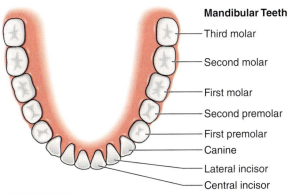

Mandibular Teeth

- Third molar
- Second molar
- First molar
- Second premolar
- First premolar
- Canine
- Lateral incisor
- Central incisor

FIGURE 13.7 Permanent adult teeth.

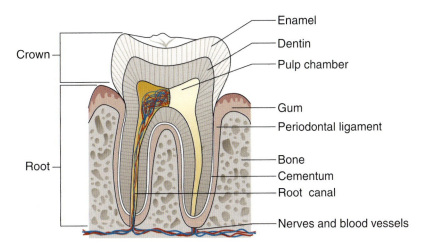

- Crown
- Root
- Enamel
- Dentin
- Pulp chamber
- Gum
- Periodontal ligament
- Bone
- Cementum
- Root canal
- Nerves and blood vessels

FIGURE 13.8 Anatomy of a tooth.

CLINICAL TIPS

Ear Examination

- Use the largest speculum that can comfortably fit in the ear.
- Pull the pinna up and back to straighten the canal.
- Do not insert the speculum too deep.
- Expect the normal ear canal to look pink, without scaling or discharge.
- Expect the normal tympanic membrane to be pearly gray, with no perforations, bulging, or redness.

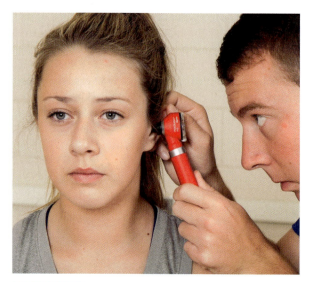

FIGURE 13.9 To view the inner structure of the ear with an otoscope, the ear canal must be straightened by pulling the pinna up and back.

The clinician conducts a gross determination of hearing when hearing loss is suspected. The patient's response to questions or directions may give a good indication of gross hearing ability. To distinguish between sensorineural and conductive hearing loss, the Weber and Rinne tests may be used (see the sidebar).

An otoscope with a disposal speculum is used to inspect the ear canal. Specula come in different sizes to conform to different-sized ears. The largest speculum that can be comfortably fit into the ear is used to allow the best view of the canal and the tympanic membrane. The otoscope is turned on by rotating the dial on top of the handle. The examiner asks the patient to tip the head slightly toward the opposite shoulder and to avoid moving during the examination.

Because the canal slopes inferiorly and forward toward the eye, the external auditory canal must be "straightened" from its S shape by pulling up and back on the pinna (figure 13.9). Otitis externa is suspected if the patient experiences pain while the examiner is pulling on the pinna. The speculum is inserted gently and slightly down and forward approximately 0.5 in. into the ear canal. The examiner places a finger or side of the hand against the cheek to guard against inserting the speculum too far into the ear.

The canal lining is lubricated with cerumen that is secreted by the sebaceous glands in the distal one-third of the canal. Cerumen often builds up in the external canal; impacted cerumen may be a cause of **otalgia** or hearing loss, and it will make examination of the tympanic membrane difficult. The skin in the external auditory canal is examined; it should be smooth and somewhat pink or "fleshy" colored. The examiner looks for and notes any scaling or increased redness in the canal as well as any discharge, lesions, or foreign bodies. A reddened canal with discharge signifies inflammation or infection.

To visualize the tympanic membrane, the otoscope must be slowly moved in a circular direction as if looking at a large area through a small window. The tympanic membrane appears translucent and pearly gray in color (figure 13.10). The translucent nature of a healthy tympanic membrane allows visualization of the middle ear cavity, including the malleus. The tympanic membrane is concave because it is pulled in at the center, or umbo, by the malleus, allowing a light reflex to be visible when

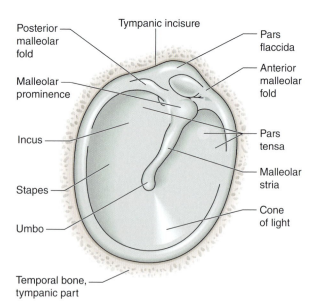

FIGURE 13.10 Anatomic landmarks of the tympanic membrane.

Weber Test and Rinne Test to Distinguish Between Sensorineural and Conductive Hearing Loss

Weber Test for Lateralization of Sound

1. Hold the tuning fork at its base, and tap it lightly against the palm of the hand to start its vibrations.
2. Place the tuning fork at the vertex of the patient's head.
3. Ask the patient if the sound is heard better in one ear or equally in both.

Results

- Normal finding: sound heard equally in both ears
- Conduction hearing loss: sound heard best in impaired ear
- Unilateral sensorineural hearing loss: sound identified only in normal ear

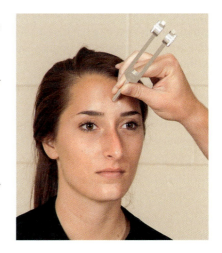

Rinne Test

1. Hold the tuning fork at its base, and tap it lightly against the palm of the hand to start its vibrations.
2. Place the stem of the tuning fork against the patient's mastoid process *(a)*.
3. Ask the patient to say when the sound is no longer heard. Count the seconds until the sound is no longer heard (by bone conduction), and note the number of seconds.
4. Quickly, place the still-vibrating tines 0.5 to 1 in. from the ear canal *(b)*.
5. Ask the patient to say when the sound is no longer heard. Count the seconds until the sound is no longer heard (by air conduction), and note the number of seconds.
6. Compare the number of seconds the sound is heard through the air and when in contact with the bone.

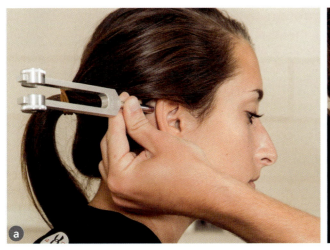
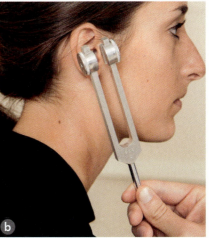

Results

- Normal finding: air-conducted sound heard twice as long as bone-conducted sound
- Conduction hearing loss: bone-conducted sound can be heard longer
- Sensorineural hearing loss: sound reduced and heard longer through the air

it is inspected with an otoscope. The light reflex occurs as a result of the otoscope's light beam reflecting off the semitransparent tympanic membrane. It can be seen as a wedge-shaped bright spot originating from the umbo. The tympanic membrane should be free from holes or breaks and should not be bulging or bloody. These signs may indicate a tympanic membrane puncture. Abnormal findings of the tympanic membrane and their possible indications are as follows:

- Pink or red, bulging: inflammation of the tympanic membrane
- Bluish or dark color: blood behind the tympanic membrane
- White color: pus behind the tympanic membrane
- Perforations or scarring: current or previous tympanic membrane rupture

A pneumatic otoscope (which can deliver a small puff of air to the tympanic membrane) may be used to confirm the flexibility of the tympanic membrane. A tympanic membrane that is bulging because of inflammation or infection will not be flaccid but will be rigid when the puff of air strikes it. This is indicative of otitis media.

Examination of the Nose and Nasopharynx

Nasal disorders may present with local symptoms, or they may result from disorders of other structures such as the paranasal sinuses. The major nontraumatic problems related to the nose are nasal obstruction, drainage, facial pain or headache, epistaxis, and change in smell or taste. A thorough history of symptoms will help the examiner to determine the nature of the nasal disorder.

> **CLINICAL TIPS**
>
> ### Nose Examination
>
> - Use universal precautions when bleeding or discharge is present.
> - Stop the epistaxis before performing an examination.
> - Look for deformity of the external nose.
> - Compare the sizes of the **nares** bilaterally.
> - Determine the characteristics of any discharge.
> - Determine the nature of any obstruction: unilateral or bilateral.
> - Use a short speculum to examine the septum and nasal cavity.

The examiner asks the patient about the onset and duration of the symptoms. In the case of nasal obstruction, it is important to determine whether trauma was involved or whether the onset was insidious. It is also important to determine whether the obstruction is bilateral or unilateral and whether it is constant or intermittent. Assessment of inspiratory and expiratory airflow is done by occluding one nostril at a time while the patient inspires (figure 13.11).

Unilateral obstruction may indicate an anatomical problem, such as a deviated septum or polyp, whereas bilateral obstruction could arise from a simple cold (Domino et al. 2016). If drainage is present, it is helpful to determine its characteristics. Is it unilateral or bilateral? Is it clear or discolored? Clear drainage suggests **rhinitis**, either allergic or nonallergic, whereas yellow, green, or brown drainage suggests bacterial or viral infection (table 13.1). Straw-colored drainage occurring after a head injury could be CSF and an indicator of possible brain injury. If discharge is present, the examiner should wear gloves for the examination.

The patient may also experience facial pain and headache. Many nasal or sinus disorders will present with headaches but these should be differentiated from headache or face pain caused by migraine, tension headache, or temporomandibular joint (TMJ) pain. Dental disorders may also cause diffuse facial pain. When pain

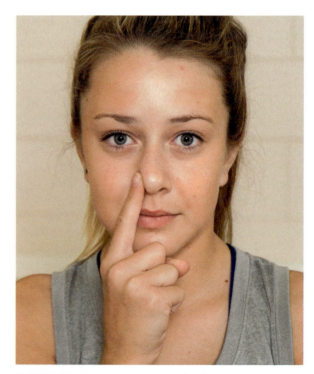

FIGURE 13.11   Determining whether an obstruction is unilateral or bilateral may be done by occluding one nostril at a time during inspiration and expiration.

TABLE 13.1   **Differential Diagnoses of Nasal Conditions With Drainage**

Drainage characteristics	Typical other symptoms	Conditions
Watery discharge	Sneezing, watery eyes, sore throat, facial pain, itchiness, lower airway symptoms, congestion	Allergic or nonallergic rhinitis
Purulent yellowish or greenish discharge	Sinus or upper respiratory infection	Sinusitis (bacterial or viral)
Bloody discharge	Traumatic or dry nasal mucosa	Epistaxis

and swelling occur over the sinuses accompanied by purulent drainage, sinusitis may be suspected.

During or after the history, the clinician visually examines the external nose, noting its shape, size, and color. The athlete is asked whether there are subtle changes in shape. Sometimes standing behind the patient and looking down the nose while the patient is sitting allows better visualization of whether the nose is straight. Next, the nares are examined for discharge as well as any unilateral flaring or narrowing.

Palpation may reveal swelling, tenderness, or masses, as well as any displacement of bone or cartilage. The patency of the nares is evaluated by gently squeezing them together. Unilateral variations may indicate a deviated septum or polyp in the nose. One must remember that recent trauma may cause ecchymosis and edema of the nose and surrounding areas as well as localized tenderness.

The examiner palpates the facial bones and the sinuses to determine any areas of tenderness, swelling, or defor-mity. The facial areas over the frontal sinuses are palpated by pressing upward beneath the athlete's supraorbital ridge (figure 13.12*a*). The maxillary sinuses are palpated by pressing with thumbs up under the zygomatic process (figure 13.12*b*). Healthy sinuses are not generally tender to the touch, and pain with palpation of the facial bones over the sinuses often indicates inflammation from infection or allergy.

Transillumination

The sinuses also may be transilluminated. This is often performed by the physician, but the athletic trainer may want to try the technique. Transillumination is done in a darkened room, using a penlight or an otoscope. The frontal sinus may be transilluminated by placing a light against the medial aspect of each supraorbital rim while looking for a slight red glow of light just above the eyebrow (Ball et al. 2014; Jarvis 2012). The absence of a glow in the sinus indicates that the sinus contains secretions. Likewise, the maxillary sinus may be illuminated

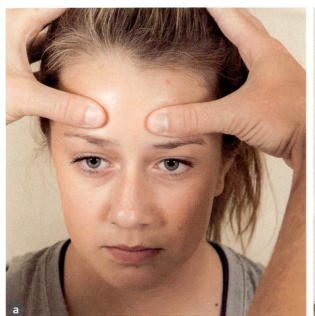 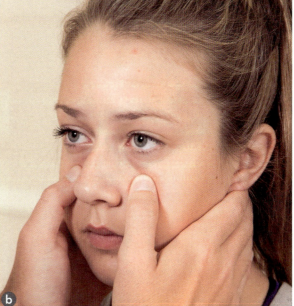

FIGURE 13.12   Palpation. (*a*) Frontal sinuses. (*b*) Maxillary sinuses.

by placing the light lateral to the athlete's nose beneath the medial aspect of the eye while asking the athlete to open the mouth. If the sinus is clear, the hard palate will be illuminated.

Speculum Examination

To view the septum and turbinates, the examiner tips the patient's head slightly backward. The nares may be dilated and viewed by the use of a speculum and a light, or the speculum on an otoscope may be used. The speculum is held in one hand while the other guides the patient's head.

The septum may be visualized by tipping the speculum toward the midline (figure 13.13). The septum is normally pink and glistening, and it should be thicker anteriorly. The examiner checks for any discoloration, perforations, bleeding, or crusting and notes differences such as polyps, holes, swelling, or abnormal coloring (Jarvis 2012). The

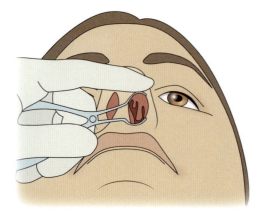

FIGURE 13.13   The septum is examined with an otoscope equipped with a nasal speculum.

© Micki Cuppett

septum should be straight and positioned close to the midline. To determine the position of the septum, it is best to compare sides bilaterally, ensuring that the space between the lateral wall of the nose and the septum is the same in both nostrils.

After the integrity of the septum is determined, the vestibule and the turbinates can be visualized with the patient's head fairly erect. The examiner tilts the patient's head backward to see the middle meatus and middle turbinates (figure 13.14). The turbinates should be pink, moist, and free of any lesions or discolorations.

Examination of the Mouth and Throat

The assessment of the mouth and oropharynx starts with an inspection of the face, head, and neck. The face, ears, and neck are observed, noting any asymmetry or changes on the skin. The neck is palpated, with the examiner paying special attention to the hyoid bone, thyroid and cricoid cartilages, and the thyroid gland. Special attention should be paid to the size of the various glands in the face and neck, including the parotid glands in the cheeks over the mandible, the submandibular glands that lie beneath the mandible at the "angle" of the jaw, and the thyroid gland. During palpation, the examiner should also note swelling or tenderness of the lymph nodes in the neck and along the jaw. Examination continues with evaluation of the lips with the mouth both open and closed, noting the texture, color, and any surface abnormalities (figure 13.15a).

The examiner asks the athlete to open the mouth and visually examines the labial mucosa and the maxillary and mandibular vestibules, noting the color and texture as well as any swelling of the mucosa or gingivae. The buccal mucosa is examined, extending from the labial commissure back to the anterior tonsillar pillar. A tongue depressor or gloved finger may be used to pull the buccal

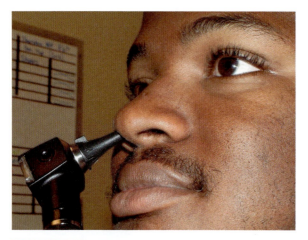

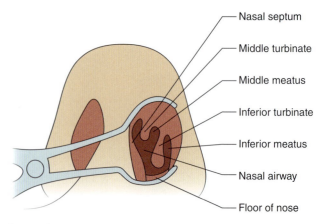

- Nasal septum
- Middle turbinate
- Middle meatus
- Inferior turbinate
- Inferior meatus
- Nasal airway
- Floor of nose

FIGURE 13.14   The patient's head is tilted backward in order to view the nasal mucosa and middle turbinate through a nasal speculum.

Mouth and Throat Examination

- Inspect the lips, noting color and lesions.
- Note any cracking of the lips that may indicate dehydration.
- Note the condition of the teeth and gums as an overall indicator of general health.
- Inspect the tongue and buccal mucosa for color, lesions, and presence of white plaque.
- Inspect the sides of the tongue for lesions.
- Use a tongue depressor to hold down the tongue to visualize the tonsils, uvula, and pharynx; redness, swelling, exudates, or spots indicate inflammation or infection.
- Palpate the mouth when indicated, being sure to wear gloves.
- Palpate the cervical lymph nodes for swelling.

mucosa away from the teeth (figure 13.15*b*). The examiner notes pigmentation, color, texture, mobility, and other abnormalities of the mucosa.

The examiner inspects the buccal and labial aspects of the gingivae and alveolar ridges (processes) by starting with the right maxillary posterior gingivae and alveolar ridge and then moving around the arch to the left posterior area (Jarvis 2012). The inspection continues with the left mandibular posterior gingivae and alveolar ridge and moves around the arch to the right posterior area. The examiner looks for any abnormal lesions, especially white or dark pigmented areas. Stensen's duct, the opening of the parotid gland, will look like a small dimple opposite the upper second molar (Ball et al. 2014).

With the patient's tongue at rest and mouth partially open, the dorsum of the tongue is inspected for any swelling, ulceration, coating, or variation in size, color, or texture. The examiner visualizes the papillary pattern on the surface of the tongue, asks the athlete to stick out the tongue, and notes any abnormality of mobility or positioning. Then the tip of the tongue is grasped with a piece of gauze to assist in its full protrusion and to aid in the examination of the more posterior aspects of the tongue's lateral borders. The ventral surface of the tongue is examined along with the floor of the mouth.

The examiner is looking for changes in color, texture, swelling, or other surface abnormalities. With the mouth wide open and the patient's head tilted back, the base of the tongue is gently depressed with a tongue blade. The hard palate is examined, followed by the soft palate and oropharyngeal tissues. Movement of the soft palate may be evaluated by asking the athlete to say "ah." This also tests cranial nerves IX and X, the glossopharyngeal and vagus nerves, respectively.

Next, the oropharynx is inspected while keeping the tongue depressed with a tongue blade. The tonsillar pillars should be pink and should blend in with the integrity of the retropharyngeal wall. Hypertrophied or reddened tonsils that may be covered in exudates indicate a viral or bacterial infection. The posterior wall is normally pink and smooth, although some irregular spots of lymphatic tissue may be present. A yellowish film may indicate postnasal drip. The examiner may elicit the gag reflex at this point in the examination, which also tests the glossopharyngeal and vagus nerves.

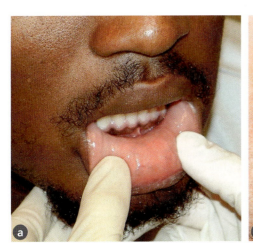
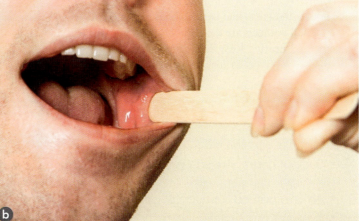

FIGURE 13.15   Inspection. *(a)* Inner oral mucosa. *(b)* Retraction of the buccal mucosa.

(a) © Micki Cuppett

Pathological Conditions of the Ear

Hearing Loss

Hearing loss may include the inability to hear a specific pitch or the inability to detect any sound. Hearing loss affects approximately one-third of adults ages 61 to 70 and 80% of those over 85 (Walling and Dickson 2012). It is estimated that 10% to 15% of the population under age 60 has some degree of hearing impairment. The inability to detect any sound is referred to as deafness. The most efficient and normal hearing pathway is through air conduction; however, bone also conducts sound. In bone conduction, the vibrations of the skull are transmitted directly to the vestibulocochlear nerve (cranial nerve VIII) (Ball et al. 2014; Bickley 2012).

Hearing loss may be divided into conductive hearing loss and sensorineural hearing loss. In conductive hearing loss, the sound conduction pathway is blocked, and sound does not pass through the external and middle ear to reach the inner ear. It is considered a mechanical dysfunction because the person can hear if the sound is amplified enough. A buildup of impacted wax, injury, foreign body, or infection in the external ear can cause conductive loss. Otitis media, sinus infections, small or blocked eustachian tubes, and allergies can also cause conductive loss (Kosaner Kliess et al. 2015).

Sensorineural loss is more serious and involves the inner ear, where sensory receptors convert sound waves into neural impulses that are transmitted to the brain for translation. Most people who are born deaf have this type of loss. Causes of this type of loss are generally idiopathic. Other identified causes include hereditary factors, meningitis, measles, scarlet fever, mumps, and encephalitis. Hearing loss caused by gradual nerve degeneration, known as **presbycusis** (Araujo and Iorio 2015), often occurs with aging and may cause the person to be unable to understand words. Simple amplification of sound will not increase the ability to hear in cases of sensorineural hearing loss. Balance problems may also accompany this type of loss. A combination of both conductive and sensorineural hearing loss in the same ear is called a mixed hearing loss. If hearing impairment is suspected, the athlete should be referred as soon as possible for proper diagnosis and treatment. Treatment depends on the cause of the hearing loss.

Signs and Symptoms

The patient experiences difficulty in hearing in either general or specific situations. Often the athlete will complain of hearing loss after bathing or swimming; he or she may also note hearing loss associated with upper respiratory infection. It should be noted whether the athlete has any pain, dizziness, or **tinnitus**.

Referral and Diagnostic Tests

Quick tests for hearing may be performed while taking the patient's history. These include observing the responses to questions spoken at different intensities. Comparing the athlete's ability to hear sounds with whispering, normal conversational intensity, and shouting gives rough estimates of the amount of hearing loss. Additional tests include the Rinne test and the Weber test to differentiate between conductive and sensorineural hearing loss (Ball et al. 2014; Bickley 2012). Audiometry may be performed by an audiologist to determine the extent of the hearing deficit.

Treatment and Return to Participation

The prognosis and return to sport after hearing loss are usually determined by the cause of the hearing deficit. Treatment of the condition responsible for the hearing loss may return the hearing to normal.

Prevention of hearing loss largely depends on preventing those things that may cause damage to the ear: sharp objects in the ear that may perforate the tympanic membrane, extremely loud noises, blows to the ear, and excessive buildup of cerumen. Because some hearing loss is congenital or occurs with age, there is no definitive method of prevention.

Otitis Externa

Otitis externa is an inflammation or infection of the external auditory canal and tympanic membrane (figure 13.16). Subgroups include acute localized otitis externa, or furunculosis; acute diffuse bacterial otitis externa, or swimmer's ear; chronic otitis externa; eczematous otitis externa; fungal otitis externa, or otomycosis; and rarely, invasive or necrotizing otitis externa (Ferri 2016). Otitis externa occurs in 4 of every 1,000 Americans each year, with the incidence being higher during the

RED FLAGS FOR HEARING LOSS

- Blood or pus coming from the ear
- Sudden onset or rapidly progressive hearing loss
- An unexplained conductive hearing loss
- Evidence of traumatic deformity of the ear or ruptured tympanic membrane
- Dizziness

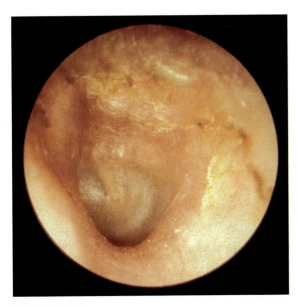

FIGURE 13.16 Otitis externa.

Phototake RM / ISM

summer months. It is more prevalent in people who have narrow inner ear canals or in someone whose canals slope downward more than normal. Because prolonged water exposure causes tissue swelling and oozing, otitis externa is a common malady seen in swimmers and others involved in water sports. Eczema, seborrhea, or psoriasis may also be present. Excessive cleaning of the external auditory canal may also contribute to otitis externa by removing the protective cerumen from the canal (AAO-HNSF 2014). A normal acidic balance in the external canal maintains the level of *Pseudomonas aeruginosa* that is present in virtually all auditory canals. When the epidermal barrier is compromised, the pH protection is lost, and the *Pseudomonas* organisms proliferate, causing serous exudates (AAO-HNSF 2014).

Signs and Symptoms

Signs and symptoms include pain, itching, or burning with possible drainage. The external auditory canal will be edematous and erythematous, perhaps causing narrowing of the canal. Scaling or crusting of the epithelial cells of the canal and an apparent absence of cerumen may be noted. Pulling on the pinna will increase pain in a person with otitis externa. The athlete may present with inflammation outside the ear canal as well. This is typically cellulitis and not otitis externa. With otitis externa, the middle ear is generally not involved, and the athlete will not have systemic symptoms, such as fever or chills. Acute otitis externa should be distinguished from acute otitis media, impacted cerumen, cellulitis, and ruptured tympanic membrane. The telltale symptom of otitis

externa that is not present with middle ear problems is the pain the patient experiences when the pinna is pulled. Other conditions to consider are herpes zoster and foreign bodies in the ear (Ferri 2016).

Referral and Diagnostic Tests

A thorough history and physical examination are typically the primary diagnostic tests. Cultures are generally ordered only when the patient is not responding to treatment.

Treatment and Return to Participation

Treatment typically includes the application of ear drops, three or four times daily, which may contain an acidifying agent, such as aluminum acetate or vinegar, and a drying agent that is often isopropyl alcohol. Many ear drops also contain broad-spectrum antibiotics or topical steroids. The efficacy of topical antibiotics and steroids in the treatment of otitis externa has been debated; however, oral antibiotics may be appropriate for swimming athletes (AAO-HNSF 2014). Treatment with ear drops will usually cure acute otitis externa in 1 to 2 d. Chronic conditions will take much longer, that is, weeks or even months. Oral analgesics may be used for pain. Some physicians advocate a hot pack applied to the side of the face for its soothing properties.

Athletes, other than those in water sports, may participate as symptoms allow, provided the head stays dry. Aquatic athletes with otitis externa are kept out of the pool until completing at least 24 h of antibiotics. Persistent or recurrent otitis externa may require that the swimming athlete discontinues in-pool training for longer. When the patient is restricted from the pool, on-land exercises, such as weight training or conditioning, may be continued. Mild infections may be treated with rubbing alcohol or a mixture of alcohol and vinegar. Creating a more acidic atmosphere will prevent the growth of bacteria (Domino et al. 2016).

Prevention

Although recurrent otitis externa is not completely preventable, several measures may help reduce its occurrence. Swimming in potentially contaminated waters, such as lakes or rivers, increases the incidence of otitis externa compared with swimming in a chlorinated pool. The ear canals should be emptied of water and dried carefully after swimming or bathing. Self-inflicted trauma to the ears, such as using cotton swabs or inserting objects into the canal, should be avoided. Frequent washing of the ears with soap may leave an alkaline residue in the ear canal, thereby reducing the normally acidic pH of the ear canal. Using an acidifying ear drop after swimming to help dry and acidify the ear is helpful in the patient who is susceptible to recurrent otitis externa.

Otitis Media

Otitis media (OM) is the presence of fluid in the middle ear accompanied by signs and symptoms of infection (figure 13.17). It is the second most common childhood disease (following upper respiratory infection), with a peak incidence between 6 and 36 mo and between 4 and 6 yr. Otitis media is a recurrent disease, with more than one-third of children experiencing more than six episodes before age 7 (Chhetri 2014; Dinc et al. 2015). The incidence of otitis media dramatically decreases with age, and it occurs infrequently in adults.

Otitis media often occurs simultaneously with an upper respiratory infection and can be caused by a virus or bacteria. Common bacterial sources for otitis media are *Streptococcus pneumoniae* and *Haemophilus influenzae* (Ferri 2016). Although otitis media is any inflammation of the middle ear without reference to pathology, the most important factor in recurrent OM is a dysfunctional eustachian tube.

Signs and Symptoms

Common signs and symptoms of otitis media include **otalgia** (earache), fever, a feeling of fullness in the ear, dizziness, tinnitus, headache, and diminished hearing (AAO-HNSF 2015). Typically, children are febrile, but adults may not be febrile and may not feel sick (Chhetri

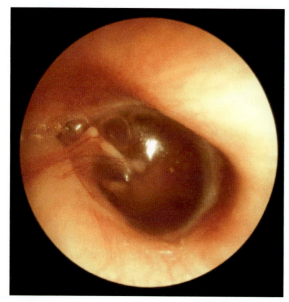

FIGURE 13.17　Otitis media.

Phototake RM / ISM

2014; Dinc et al. 2015; Wasson and Yung 2015). The young child will often pull or rub the affected ear(s), with the otalgia increasing when the child is lying down. There may be discharge from the middle ear; however, this is rare in normal OM.

The primary differential diagnoses for otalgia are otitis media, otitis externa, and temporomandibular joint (TMJ) dysfunction. People with TMJ problems typically do not have hearing difficulties, and physical examination should rule out otitis externa. The location of patient-reported ear pain is a clue to its cause:

External Auditory Canal

- Otitis externa
- Auricular hematoma
- Foreign body in the ear
- Obstructive cerumen

Middle Ear

- Acute otitis media
- Chronic otitis media
- Ruptured tympanic membrane

Referred Pain

- Temporomandibular joint dysfunction
- Inflammation from nasopharynx, larynx, or pharynx

Referral and Diagnostic Tests

Otitis media may be confirmed by physical examination with an otoscope. Visualization of the tympanic membrane may be difficult and painful in the otalgic ear, but the tympanic membrane will appear erythematous, bulging, and perhaps more opaque than normal. Pneumatic otoscopy will reveal less mobility in the tympanic membrane and is considered the standard examination technique for patients with suspected OM. When performed correctly, this technique is 90% sensitive and 80% specific for the diagnosis of OM (Chhetri 2014; Laine et al. 2015). Three criteria are necessary to confirm the diagnosis of acute otitis media: acute onset, presence of middle ear effusion, and signs or symptoms of middle ear inflammation (Wasson and Yung 2015). A Weber test will confirm conductive hearing loss in the affected ear. The patient is referred to a physician for treatment as soon as possible.

Treatment and Return to Participation

The physician will often prescribe a broad-spectrum antibiotic such as amoxicillin; however, with the growing concern about antibiotic-resistant strains of bacteria, the treatment currently recommended by the American Academy of Pediatrics is to treat the pain on the first visit and to observe the condition to determine that it meets the criteria for acute otitis media (AOM) before prescribing antibiotic therapy. If all three conditions for acute otitis media are present (acute onset, presence of middle ear effusion, and signs or symptoms of middle ear inflammation), then the recommendation for any patient over age 2 is antibiotic therapy. Amoxicillin is still the most commonly used antibiotic for AOM, but for patients who are allergic to penicillin, a cephalosporin or erythromycin may be used (Chhetri 2014). Chapter 5 gives more information about antibiotics. Antihistamines and decongestants have not proven beneficial for managing otitis media.

After dealing with the discomfort that accompanies otitis media, the patient who is afebrile may participate in sport. Air travel should be avoided until the middle ear has returned to normal appearance and function because of the increased risk of ruptured tympanic membrane from pressure changes on ascent and descent. If antibiotic treatment does not improve symptoms within 72 h, then high-dose antibiotics are indicated. Complications of acute otitis media are uncommon but are best recognized early and treated aggressively (Wasson and Yung 2015). These complications may include meningitis, facial nerve paralysis, and neck infections.

Prevention

Avoidance of situations that will introduce bacteria into the ear may help decrease the occurrence of otitis media. Aggressive treatment of upper respiratory infections may also reduce the risk. The efficacy of prophylactic antibiotic treatment for upper respiratory infections for those who are susceptible to otitis media is debatable.

Ruptured Tympanic Membrane

A ruptured tympanic membrane, or tympanic membrane perforation (TMP), may occur when there is a sudden change of air pressure caused by blunt trauma or an infection that inhibits the ability to regulate inner ear pressure (Kraus and Hagen 2015). Infection is the principal cause of TMP. The increasing pressure in the middle ear often causes extreme pain before the rupture. Sticking a sharp object, even a cotton swab, in the ear may also rupture the membrane, as can incorrect irrigation of the ear canal.

Signs and Symptoms

Signs and symptoms of TMP include audible whistling sounds and decreased hearing. Purulent fluid or bleeding may be noted leaking from the ear. TMP may be painless if not accompanied by infection, typically otitis media. The hearing loss is more severe if the ossicular chain is disrupted or the inner ear injured. Vertigo may be present if the inner ear is injured.

Other causes of hearing loss, otalgia, and **otorrhea** should be ruled out, including otitis media, impacted cerumen, otitis externa, or infectious myringitis. A TMP can usually be visualized with an otoscope, thus differentiating it from other ear conditions.

Referral and Diagnostic Tests

Radiography and magnetic resonance imaging (MRI) are usually of no use in uncomplicated TMP and are typically not performed. TMP is usually diagnosed on the basis of simple history, physical examination, and otoscopy. The presence of a hole or perforation in the tympanic membrane is often visible on examination (figure 13.18). A **tympanogram** is often performed to determine the integrity of the tympanic membrane. Audiometry is typically performed by the physician to determine the amount of hearing loss and is particularly relevant before any attempt at repair.

Treatment and Return to Participation

The tympanic membrane tends to heal itself, and even eardrums that have been perforated multiple times often remain intact. Larger perforations may take 3 to 6 mo to heal. The patient with a small perforation will tend to heal quickly, but the injury must be protected from water and debris (Hong, Bance, and Gratzer 2013). Over-the-counter analgesics may be needed during the

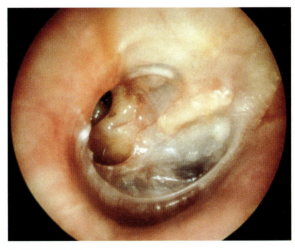

FIGURE 13.18 View of a large tympanic membrane perforation.

Prof. Tony Wright / Inst. of Laryngology & Otology / Science Source initial healing stages if the patient is in pain. If the TMP was caused by an infection, the physician will generally prescribe drying agent drops, as well as topical and oral antibiotics.

Larger or complicated ruptures may require surgery by an **otolaryngologist** and involve a graft of surgical paper, fat, muscle, or other material (Bilge et al. 2016; Lee et al. 2015). These procedures are usually done in the office with the patient under local anesthesia.

The prognosis for small, uncomplicated perforations of the tympanic membrane is good and should result in minimal time lost, especially in the nonswimming athlete. Larger or multiple perforations may cause scarring of the tympanic membrane and some resultant hearing loss (Park et al. 2015; Zakaria, Othman, and Lih 2016). Divers may be held out of activity longer than swimmers because of the combination of water and pressure changes associated with the sport. Patients with TMP are more susceptible to middle ear infections and thus must take special care to keep the ear dry until it heals.

Prevention

Prevention of TMP includes keeping foreign objects out of the ear, such as sharp objects or cotton-tipped applicators, that are inserted too deeply. Treating otitis media aggressively to reduce the pressure on the tympanic membrane will also reduce the chances of TMP. The patient with otitis media also needs to avoid sudden altitude changes resulting in pressure from air or water. A TMP from a blow to the external ear may be unavoidable unless head or ear protection is worn.

Pathological Conditions of the Nose

Allergic Rhinitis

Allergic rhinitis is an immunoglobulin E-mediated response to nasally inhaled allergens that causes sneezing, **rhinorrhea**, nasal pruritus, and congestion (Sur and Plesa 2015). It affects 10% to 20% of the U.S. population (Ferri 2016). Seasonal allergic rhinitis occurs in the spring, summer, and fall and is triggered by pollens, ragweed, or grasses. Perennial rhinitis occurs daily and is typically triggered by dust, animal allergens, smoke, detergents, or soaps. Although a common disease, its effect on performance and daily activities should not be underestimated.

Signs and Symptoms

Allergic rhinitis presents with clear nasal discharge and sneezing, nasal congestion, cough, and sensation of plugged ears accompanied by itchy, watering eyes. The mucosa of the turbinates may appear pale from venous engorgement. The throat may appear erythematous from postnasal drip (Goldman and Schafer 2011).

Allergic rhinitis must be distinguished from viral, bacterial, or fungal rhinitis as well as influenza. Septal obstruction must also be ruled out as a cause of nasal congestion. In addition, rhinitis medicamentosa from cocaine use or excessive nasal drop use should be considered.

Allergic rhinitis can be associated with a number of comorbid conditions including asthma, atopic dermatitis, and nasal polyps. Uncontrolled allergic rhinitis can actually worsen the inflammation associated with these disorders (Settipane and Kaliner 2013).

Referral and Diagnostic Tests

Diagnostic tests are often unnecessary; however, a detailed medical history is useful in identifying the irritating allergen. A temperature may be taken to confirm that the patient is afebrile. The patient with chronic symptoms that affect athletic performance should be referred to the physician, especially if over-the-counter medications have not been effective in the past (Ferri 2016). The patient should be referred to a physician if the symptoms persist for more than 7 d. Some patients may benefit from allergy testing.

Treatment and Return to Participation

Optimal treatment includes allergen avoidance and pharmacotherapy. Second-generation antihistamines (loratadine, fexofenadine, or cetirizine) are readily available over the counter, generally control symptoms, and have fewer adverse effects than first-generation antihistamines. Intranasal corticosteroid (now available over the counter) is also used as a first-line treatment for allergic rhinitis with symptoms affecting the patient's quality of life. Targeted symptom control with immunotherapy should be considered for patients with moderate or severe persistent allergic rhinitis that is not responsive to the usual treatments. Chapter 5 gives a more complete description of antihistamines.

One must not underestimate the effectiveness of eliminating or reducing the allergen. Dust allergens may be the easiest to control as several types of filters are readily available. Studies have not found any benefit to using mite-proof impermeable mattresses or pillow covers (Sur and Plesa 2015). Most patients experience considerable relief by avoiding the allergens and properly using medications. Patients may participate in sport as they are able. Avoidance of the irritating allergens is the best form of prevention for patients with allergic rhinitis. The use of air conditioning and maintaining indoor humidity below 50% may also be helpful. The use of humidifiers and air filters may also be helpful.

Nonallergic Rhinitis

Nonallergic rhinitis is a syndrome resulting from nasal inflammation that encompasses several distinct diagnoses. There are several causes, including infection, vasomotor, occupational, hormonal, drug-induced, and gustatory (Settipane and Kaliner 2013). Regardless of the cause, rhinitis causes excessive production of mucus, resulting in nasal congestion and mucous discharge. Infectious rhinitis is most commonly caused by rhinovirus, adenovirus, and parainfluenza virus. Vasomotor rhinitis symptoms are exacerbated by changes in temperature and humidity or exposure to hot and cold foods. Drug-induced rhinitis is termed *rhinitis medicamentosa* and results from cocaine use or excessive nasal drop use. Patients may also experience rhinitis only at work. This is deemed occupational rhinitis and is caused by an inhaled irritant. Patients may also exhibit rhinitis only during hormonal changes such as puberty, pregnancy, or the introduction of hormone therapy. Gustatory rhinitis occurs after eating, particularly with hot and spicy foods.

Signs and Symptoms

Nonallergic rhinitis is similar to perennial allergic rhinitis, with symptoms of nasal obstruction, clear rhinorrhea, sneezing, watery eyes, and pruritus of the nose, eyes, and palate, but it fails to show responses on allergy testing. Nonallergic rhinitis is differentiated from allergic rhinitis, sinusitis, nasal obstruction, nasal polyps, and noninflammatory rhinitis. Many nasal conditions result in rhinorrhea. A yellow or brown discharge accompanied by a fever indicates a bacterial condition and not rhinitis (see table 13.1). Rhinitis will typically resolve in 7 to 10 d if viral.

Referral and Diagnostic Tests

The patient is referred to a physician for further evaluation if the symptoms persist for more than 7 d. The patient's temperature may be taken to rule out a fever. Allergy tests may be performed to rule out allergic rhinitis.

Treatment and Return to Participation

Rhinitis is usually treated symptomatically with over-the-counter medications. With athletes, second-generation antihistamines should be used because of their nonsedating properties. Decongestants and intranasal steroid spray are also used for the management of symptoms. Adequate hydration should be ensured if the patient is taking antihistamines because of the drying effects of the medication. Rhinitis is self-limiting, and typically patients can participate in sport with few limitations.

Sinusitis

Sinusitis is an inflammation of the mucous membrane lining of the nasal cavity or one or more of the paranasal sinuses. Sinusitis may be acute, subacute, recurrent, or chronic and may result from bacterial or viral exposure. Sinusitis occurs when mucus or other infectious materials cause blockage within the passageways connecting the sinuses to the nasal cavity. It may follow upper respiratory tract infections; however, less than 1% of upper respiratory tract infections result in the clinical syndrome of acute sinusitis (Wald et al. 2013). Most cases of sinusitis are caused by bacterial infections. Besides upper respiratory infections, sinusitis (typically in the maxillary sinus) may be caused by dental infections or by swimming in contaminated water (Taschieri et al. 2015). It is almost always accompanied by inflammation of the nasal mucosa and thus may be more correctly termed rhinosinusitis. Acute viral infection may be preceded by infection with the common cold or influenza. This is typically followed by mucosal edema and sinus infection. The drainage of thick secretions is decreased, resulting in obstruction of the sinus (Ferri 2016). This may result in the entrapment of bacteria in the sinuses, resulting in a secondary bacterial infection.

Signs and Symptoms

The patient typically presents with a history of previous upper respiratory infection with postnasal drip lasting more than 7 to 10 d. Patients may experience a purulent nasal discharge, facial tightness, nasal obstruction, and headache (Goldman and Schafer 2011). They may also complain of point tenderness over the infected sinus and toothache if the maxillary sinus is involved. On occasion, patients will present with a cough that is often worse at night.

Because of the facial pain associated with sinusitis, it should be differentiated from migraine headaches and dental infections. Sinusitis should also be differentiated from viral or bacterial rhinitis and influenza.

Referral and Diagnostic Tests

Clinicians should refer patients with suspected sinusitis to a physician so that the diagnosis can be confirmed and pharmacological treatment started. Diagnosis is typically done through history and examination. Transillumination

Sinusitis

Sinusitis is a very common condition in the United States; there are more than 31 million cases per year. Most commonly, the maxillary sinus is involved, but the frontal sinus can also be involved in adults, whereas children tend to experience sinusitis in the ethmoid sinus. Sinusitis may be acute, subacute, chronic, or recurrent. The risk factors include allergens, smoke exposure, and air pollutants, as well as anatomical anomalies such as nasal polyps and septal deviation. Most sinusitis is viral and is called rhinovirus because it is mainly in the nasal passages. Other common viruses involved in sinusitis are influenza and adenovirus. Bacterial etiology includes *S. pneumoniae* and *H. influenzae* (Goldman and Schafer 2011). The clinician should watch for fever over 39 °C (102.2 °F) or visual complaints (diplopia) and severe facial or dental pain. These conditions require referral.

of the sinuses may help to confirm that the sinuses are indeed blocked. For chronic conditions that do not improve with medication, radiological examination may be performed, but it is helpful only to rule out, not to confirm, sinusitis (DeMuri et al. 2016).

Treatment and Return to Participation

Symptomatic treatment can be initiated for patients with mild symptoms using analgesics, antipyretics, decongestants, or mucolytics. Saline nasal spray may help clear nasal crusts and thick mucus. The use of topical decongestants, if necessary, should be short term only. Systemic decongestants may also be used to help dry up the sinuses. Because most cases of acute sinusitis have a viral etiology, they will resolve within about 2 wk without pharmacological treatment. Antibiotics are reserved for severe or chronic cases (DeMuri et al. 2016). Non-pharmacological treatments include air humidification, hydration, and application of hot compresses over the sinuses to help promote sinus drainage. Acute sinusitis is often self-limiting due to nasal obstruction, facial pain, headache, and fever and comes to full resolution in 3 to 4 wk (Akhlaghi, Esmaeelinejad, and Safai 2015). The patient who is afebrile and feels well enough may be allowed to participate in athletics. Chronic sinusitis represents a persistent low-grade infection involving the paranasal sinuses with persistent mucosal thickening (Goldman and Schafer 2011). More aggressive treatment is often required for chronic sinusitis to prevent long-term complications, and surgical procedures may be needed to relieve the obstruction.

Prevention

Seventy percent of cases of acute sinusitis are caused by *Streptococcus pneumoniae* or *Haemophilus influenzae* (DeMuri et al. 2016). Frequent hand washing is one of the best lines of defense when in contact with people who are known to be affected with the pathogens, and it may drastically reduce the incidence of infection. Rapid treatment of upper respiratory tract infections may decrease the incidence of sinusitis. Not swimming in contaminated water will also reduce the incidence.

Deviated Septum

A deviated septum typically occurs from trauma, often a blow to the side of the nose. It may present with epistaxis and is often associated with nasal fracture. A deviated septum often is discovered well after the initial trauma has healed and may present with only a minor deformity or complaints of chronic nasal obstruction (figure 13.19).

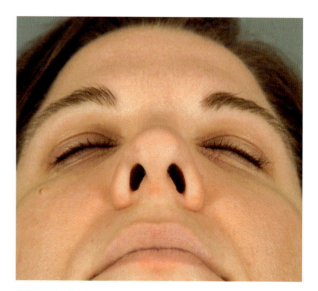

FIGURE 13.19   A septal deviation may be recognized by the difference between the spacing in the nares and the angulation of the septum.

Signs and Symptoms

The patient with a deviated septum will typically present with a history of trauma to the nose and initially will have swelling and pain throughout the nose. There may be external nasal deformity. The patient may complain of a unilateral nasal obstruction often confirmed on examination by visualization of the space between the septum and the lateral nasal wall on the affected and the nonaffected sides. The nasal passage will appear narrow on the side to which the septum is deviated.

Referral and Diagnostic Tests

A deviated septum may be diagnosed on the basis of the history and physical examination. Visualization of the nasal passage will usually reveal the deviation; radiographs are inconsequential. When a deviated septum is suspected, both nasal fracture and septal hematoma should be ruled out. Other causes of unilateral nasal obstruction, such as polyps or a foreign body, must also be eliminated.

Treatment and Return to Participation

The acute treatment of nasal trauma involves stopping the epistaxis and minimizing the swelling. If considerable swelling occurs, it may be more difficult to correct the deviation by a minor surgical procedure. The patient must be seen quickly to prevent long-term complications from septal deviations (Wang et al. 2015). Correction of a deviated septum is typically a minor elective surgical procedure that is performed with the patient under local anesthesia. If an external nasal deformity is also present, then a **rhinoplasty** may also be performed to improve both function and cosmetic appearance.

Early recognition and treatment of the deviated septum may prevent long-term complications, and the patient should be able to return to play as soon as the septum has been reduced and healed. The physician may allow the patient to go back sooner if the nose is adequately protected with a mask. If the septum is not treated expediently, the patient may have chronic unilateral nasal obstruction later in life. The incidence of deviated septum by trauma is drastically reduced in athletes who wear facial protection. Many collision sports require facial protection; however, a large number of traumatic nasal injuries occur in the noncollision sports, where the unprotected athlete is still at risk from contact with another athlete or with a ball, bat, or tennis racket.

Epistaxis

Epistaxis, commonly known as nosebleed, is a common occurrence among athletes. It is typically associated with trauma to the nose; however, it may occur without trauma.

Epistaxis can be divided into anterior bleeds and posterior bleeds, depending on where the bleeding originates. More than 90% of all epistaxes occur anteriorly, where Kiesselbach's plexus forms on the septum (Ferri 2016; Fox et al. 2016; Andreeff 2016). The cause is often an erosion of the mucosa that causes the vessels to become exposed. Anterior bleeds from capillaries and veins provide a constant ooze rather than the profuse pumping of blood observed from an artery.

Posterior epistaxes are usually more profuse and often have an arterial origin. A posterior bleed is a more serious hemorrhage that presents a great risk of airway obstruction and difficulty in controlling bleeding.

Signs and Symptoms

Epistaxis will present with blood coming from the nostrils. The patient will generally complain of swallowing and spitting up blood. Epistaxis may result from local or systemic factors. Local causes generally occur in young children and are usually spontaneous events. Epistaxes resulting from local events are often related to nose picking, excessive blowing, sneezing, or rubbing of the nose. Recurrent bleeding may occur if a scab forms at the bleeding site and becomes dislodged. In adults, bleeding tends to be caused by external trauma to the nose (Andreeff 2016), or it may be caused by the previously mentioned local factors, especially in very dry or high climates, in which nasal membranes tend to dry.

Systemic epistaxis may be caused by intrinsic coagulopathies such as hemophilia, or by acquired coagulopathies such as the use of blood thinners or long-term aspirin use (Fox et al. 2016). Hypertension is not a cause of epistaxis but may impede clotting.

It is important to determine the cause of the epistaxis. If it is caused by trauma, a deviated septum, nasal fracture, and septal hematoma must all be ruled out. If the epistaxis is recurrent, a thorough history may reveal information leading to its cause.

Referral and Diagnostic Tests

Typically, the diagnosis of epistaxis is made through the history and physical examination. A nasal speculum is used to visualize the site of bleeding once the

🚩 RED FLAGS FOR NASAL CONDITIONS

- Unilateral blockage following trauma
- Visualization of polyps
- Visualization of deformity
- Loss of smell
- Unexplained epistaxis

active bleeding is slowed. Sinus radiographs are done only when tumors are suspected as the cause of the bleeding.

Treatment and Return to Participation

The management of epistaxis depends on the site of bleeding, the severity, and the etiology. If the patient presents with active bleeding, necessary treatment may precede the normal history and palpation of a nasal examination. As in all cases, in which the clinician is handling body fluids, universal precautions must be followed.

Most anterior epistaxes will stop spontaneously with direct pressure applied to the nose. The patient should be encouraged to sit with the head elevated but not hyperextended, which may cause bleeding into the pharynx. Digital compression or pinching of the nose should be done for 4 to 5 min. In traumatic situations, ice should also be applied. A cotton or gauze plug may be inserted into the nose to absorb the blood (Williams, Kamhieh, and Cohen 2015).

If direct pressure proves inadequate to treat an anterior bleed, gauze moistened with phenylephrine (Neo-Synephrine) or pseudoephedrine (Afrin) may be placed in the affected nostril to help promote vasoconstriction (Fox et al. 2016).

For recurrent nosebleeds, conservative treatment, such as improving the humidity of inspired air, using saline nasal drops, and applying antibiotic ointments to the affected area (Perez and Rada 2016), may be beneficial. Further evaluation by a physician should be sought to determine the etiology of the epistaxis.

Most cases of anterior epistaxis from Kiesselbach's plexus can be stopped by nasal compression and local vasoconstriction. If there is no indication of nasal fracture, septal deviation, or septal hematoma, the patient may return to participation once the nose has stopped bleeding. Because minimal aggravation can restart the bleeding, it is important to protect the athlete from trauma to the nose. If possible, strenuous physical activity should be avoided when bleeding is active.

Prevention

The incidence of epistaxis may be decreased by ensuring proper humidity and hydration, especially for patients in dry environments or at high altitudes. Saline nasal drops may be helpful in reducing dryness in the nose. Additional humidification through the use of humidifiers and vaporizers may be needed. Repeated trauma to the nose should be avoided, including foreign bodies, nose picking, and trauma in sports. Those patients susceptible to epistaxis may need to wear facial protection during athletic participation.

Pathological Conditions of the Mouth and Throat

Pharyngitis and Tonsillitis

Pharyngitis is an inflammation of the pharynx and is commonly known as a sore throat. Tonsillitis is an inflammation of the tonsils. Both may be caused by bacteria or a virus. Pharyngitis is initially viral in most cases, but it may be followed by a bacterial infection (figure 13.20a). Tonsillitis is most commonly caused by beta-hemolytic *Streptococcus* (figure 13.20b). When caused by *Streptococcus*, pharyngitis is called strep throat (Liu, Yan, and Zhang 2015). Pharyngitis may be secondary to sinusitis, tonsillitis, smoking, or alcoholism. Because many of the symptoms are identical, pharyngitis and tonsillitis are discussed together. Pharyngitis and tonsillitis occurs

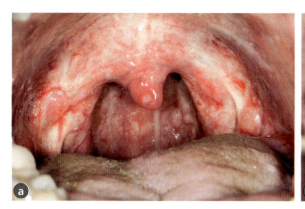 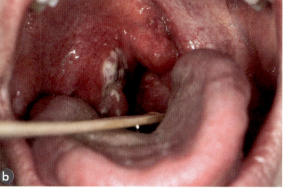

FIGURE 13.20   Examination of the mouth and throat may reveal the following: *(a)* acute viral pharyngitis; *(b)* pharyngitis caused by *Streptococcus* (strep throat).

(a) Dr P. Marazzi / Science Source; *(b)* Scott Camazine / Science Source

equally in males and females, with the peak incidence occurring in late winter to early spring.

Signs and Symptoms

Common signs and symptoms of pharyngitis and tonsillitis include sore throat, pain with swallowing, hoarseness, and possibly chills or fever. In both viral and bacterial pharyngitis, the mucous membranes may be inflamed mildly to more severely and may be covered with purulent exudates. If the pharyngitis is viral, it is usually accompanied by rhinorrhea, conjunctivitis, and a cough. Bacterial infections will normally present with a much higher fever and systemic signs of infection (Ebell 2014). Tonsillitis (either viral or bacterial) will present with red and swollen tonsils, possibly covered in white exudates. Fever and swollen neck lymph nodes are common.

When diagnosing pharyngitis or tonsillitis, other conditions that cause throat pain and fever must be ruled out. These include upper respiratory infection, laryngitis, and influenza. Viral infections may present with rhinorrhea, conjunctivitis, and cough, whereas patients with bacterial infections will not have these symptoms.

Referral and Diagnostic Tests

The health care provider should monitor the temperature of the patient. The patient with a persistent fever or symptoms for more than 5 d should be referred to a physician. If the tonsils or pharynx presents with exudates on observation, the patient must be referred. It is difficult to tell from physical examination alone whether pharyngitis is viral or bacterial. A throat culture, often conducted to determine whether the pharyngitis or tonsillitis is indeed caused by a *Streptococcus* strain, may be done by the use of a rapid streptococcal antigen test (Ebell 2014). A mononucleosis spot test (monospot test) may also be performed to rule out mononucleosis. Laboratory tests may also include a complete blood count with differential (CBC); a high leukocyte count supports the diagnosis of bacterial infection.

Treatment and Return to Participation

The physician will typically prescribe antibiotics (usually penicillin or erythromycin) for a 10 d course for strep pharyngitis or tonsillitis to prevent complications from the disease (Sanchez and Hicks 2014). Because viral pharyngitis is not treated with antibiotics, the throat must be cultured if there is any question about the etiology of the disease. Nonpharmacological treatment includes plenty of fluids and saltwater gargles. Acetaminophen is often given for discomfort and reduction of fever (Shy and Strayer 2014). The patient should be afebrile and must be able to tolerate fluids before participation in vigorous athletic activities. Full recovery typically occurs in 7 to 14 d (Cots et al. 2015). Several serious complications, such as rheumatic fever, can arise from untreated streptococcal infections.

Recurrent streptococcal infections are common and may represent reinfection from others in the living or working environment. As with other bacterial and viral conditions, frequent hand washing when in contact with people who are known to be infected with the pathogens may drastically reduce the incidence of infection.

Laryngitis

Inflammation of the larynx is termed **laryngitis**. It often occurs simultaneously with the common cold, bronchitis, pneumonia, or influenza, and it can be acute or chronic. Laryngitis may also be caused by direct trauma to the throat, gastroesophageal reflux disease (GERD), allergies, cigarette smoke, or excessive use of the voice. It is especially common in the athletic population and has been termed **cheerleader's nodules**.

Signs and Symptoms

The patient will typically experience a hoarse or weak voice and in some cases may be unable to speak. A constant urge to clear the throat or a tickling may also occur. In more severe cases, fever, **dysphagia**, malaise, and throat pain may occur (Ferri 2016). Edema of the larynx may cause dyspnea. Other conditions that can cause throat pain and dysphagia should be considered, including viral or bacterial pharyngitis, mononucleosis, or candidiasis. In chronic laryngitis, laryngeal tumors and papillomatosis must be ruled out.

Referral and Diagnostic Tests

The patient should be referred to a physician if symptoms do not resolve within 5 to 7 d. The physician may perform an indirect laryngoscopy that may disclose mild to marked erythema of the mucous membrane. Laryngeal cultures and biopsies may be performed if an etiology other than viral infection or irritation is suspected.

Treatment and Return to Participation

Voice rest and increasing humidification through a vaporizer may help to relieve symptoms. Alcohol and caffeine should be avoided because of their diuretic effect, and decongestants should be avoided because of their drying effect. Acetaminophen or other analgesics for pain may be helpful, as may other supporting treatments, such as throat lozenges or sprays. Guaifenesin may be useful as a mucolytic agent. Elimination or treatment of the irritating cause of chronic laryngitis (e.g., GERD, inhaled smoke) may decrease the symptoms dramatically. Most cases of laryngitis are viral, and antibiotics are usually indicated only if a specific pathogen is isolated. Most symptoms of uncomplicated laryngitis usually resolve within a few days. Athletes with laryngitis may participate in sport as long as they are afebrile and otherwise feel well. Chronic laryngitis is typically the result of overuse or exposure to irritants. The patient susceptible to chronic laryngitis caused by these irritants should try to avoid smoke, air pollution, and straining the voice as in cheerleading or singing.

Oral Mucosal Lesions

Lesions on the mouth and lips are common in athletics and may be caused by local trauma, infectious disease, autoimmune disorders, neoplastic disease, and toxic reactions. Identification of atraumatic oral lesions is especially important because it may allow early recognition and referral for oral cancer or infectious disease (table 13.2). Oral lesions are often the first clinical evidence of human immunodeficiency virus (HIV) infection and acquired immunodeficiency syndrome (AIDS).

Oral lesions may be categorized and described on the basis of clinical appearance, similar to skin disorders. They are often described as white or pigmented and as vesicular or ulcerated. Many oral lesions will present as a white plaque and can be differentiated depending on their location. White lesions that are easily removed by wiping them off suggest candidiasis, whereas a defect that cannot be wiped away is consistent with precancerous leukoplakia or squamous cell carcinoma.

Brown- or black-pigmented macules on the oral mucosa may be caused by something as benign as localized melanin production, or they may be the sign of something much more significant, including malignant melanoma.

Oral Candidiasis

Oral candidiasis is caused by the yeast-like fungus *Candida albicans*. It is called thrush in infants and is the most common white lesion of the oral cavity (figure 13.21).

Signs and Symptoms

Oral candidiasis presents as a white, cheesy, curd-like patch on the tongue and buccal mucosa. It is seen most commonly in newborns, and it also may occur after the use of antibiotics, in immunosuppressed patients, and in association with corticosteroid treatment.

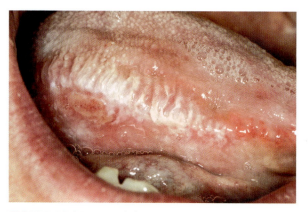

FIGURE 13.21 Candidiasis.
Dr P. Marazzi / Science Source

Referral and Diagnostic Tests

The white, curd-like patch characteristic of oral candidiasis can be scraped from the tongue or buccal mucosa with a tongue depressor and typically bleeds easily. If the plaque does not easily scrape off the surface, other oral lesions should be considered. In the adult with oral candidiasis, tests should be conducted for HIV infection.

Treatment and Return to Participation

Candidiasis is typically treated with an oral rinse of nystatin and oral antifungal medications. Antifungals such as fluconazole (Diflucan) are administered for 2 wk or until symptoms resolve (Ferri 2016). Candidiasis can often be persistent, requiring treatment for several weeks. The patient with oral candidiasis who is otherwise in good health may participate in athletics.

Oral Cancers

Oral cancer is a very serious condition and often involves the tongue, lips, and gums. This form of cancer accounts for about 3% of cancers in men and 2% in women. Oral cancer occurs more often in African-Americans than in Caucasians. The many predisposing risk factors include any type of tobacco use, excessive alcohol use, poor oral hygiene, over age 40, and a family history of oral cancer. At least 75% of head and neck cancers are caused by tobacco and alcohol use (American Cancer Society 2016). Men have twice the risk of women. Smokeless tobacco use increases the risk of oral leukoplakia to 5% for tobacco chewers and ranges from 29% to 63% for snuff users. The variation in the increased incidence is based on the amount used per day. Each year approxi-

TABLE 13.2 **Differential Diagnoses of Conditions Affecting the Oral Cavity**

Disease	Cause	Signs and symptoms	Appearance
Basal cell carcinoma of the lips	Prolonged exposure to sunlight	Lesion ulcerates, heals over, and then breaks down again; history of ultraviolet light exposure	Crusted ulcer with heaped or rolled borders
Candidiasis	*Candida albicans*	White to yellow lesions in the cheeks, at folds, and on tongue	Soft, white to yellow, slightly elevated plaques; milky curds
Gingival cyst	Developmental	Typically found on oral exam; present as a bump	Painless nodule; normal in color; should be biopsied to rule out other lesions
Herpes simplex	Herpes simplex virus type 1	Itching, complaints of neuralgiform symptoms in prodrome, changing to pain when lesions form	Recurrent, episodic eruptions of yellowish, fluid-filled vesicles on upper or lower lip or nose
Herpes zoster infection (shingles)	Varicella-zoster virus	Extremely painful; burning pain, fever, and malaise; lesions may appear in mouth, depending on which cranial nerve is affected	Unilateral vesicles on buccal mucosa, tongue, uvula, pharynx, or larynx; erosions noted when vesicles rupture
Kaposi's sarcoma	HIV infection	Purplish, tender or painful nodules on mucous membranes	Purplish macules; can also be raised, nodular, or ulcerated
Leukoplakia	Multifactorial (tobacco use, trauma, lupus, irritative reactions)	Painless, white patch or plaque on surface of mucosa	White patch typically on lips, tongue, palate, floor of mouth, or buccal mucosa
Lymphoepithelial cyst	HIV infection	Presents as a parotid gland swelling	Small (less than 1 cm), well-circumscribed, yellow or white, soft tissue nodule located in the floor of the mouth or ventral-lateral surface of the tongue
Squamous cell carcinoma; oral cavity, floor of mouth, or anterior tongue	Lack of specific etiology; tobacco, alcohol, and poor oral hygiene are implicated as contributors	Usually painless ulcer unless nerves or periosteum is involved; fetid breath	Ulcerated lesion with raised borders
Thyroglossal tract cyst	Developmental	Mass or lump located at the midline of the neck	Nonpainful, movable, and fluctuant

mately 30,000 new cases of oral cancer are diagnosed. The overall survival rate of patients with oral cancer is greater than 50% (American Cancer Society 2016).

Signs and Symptoms

Patients will typically present with red or white lesions or other open wounds in the mouth. The lesions become

🚩 RED FLAGS FOR EARLY SIGNS OF LIP AND ORAL CANCER

- A sore in the mouth that does not heal in 2 to 3 wk
- Any sores that are painful or bleed easily
- Any unusual lumps in the mouth
- Numbness or pain in the mouth and throat
- Persistent red or white patches on the oral mucosa
- A change in voice not associated with a cold or allergies
- Difficulty chewing or swallowing

more opaque with increased tobacco use. Patients may experience tongue swelling and dysphagia as well as abnormal taste sensation. Crusting lesions of the lips or ulcerated lesions within the mouth are prime suspects for oral cancer. Ninety percent of all oral cancer cells arise on the floor of the mouth, the ventrolateral aspect of the tongue, or the soft palate (Burgess 2015). Treatment, prognosis, and return to athletic participation after oral cancer are discussed in general terms.

Leukoplakia (Keratosis)

Leukoplakia is a precancerous lesion of the mucosa and is usually found on the sides of the tongue (figure 13.22), the lower lip, and the floor of the mouth. It appears as a white patch that cannot be removed by scraping. The early keratosis caused by snuff is a ribbed, translucent white patch. The rate of occurrence of leukoplakia is approxi-

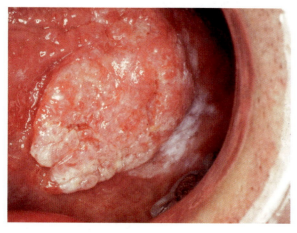

FIGURE 13.22 Oral leukoplakia on the lateral border of the tongue.

Biophoto Associates / Science Source

mately 1.5% to 12% in nonsmokers and more than 16% in smokers. The lesions can vary in appearance from a flat, almost translucent area to a raised, rough patch (Lynch 2014). The lesions will often resolve when the user quits using tobacco or moves the tobacco to another part of the mouth. There are several conditions that may present as leukoplakia on the buccal mucosa, so any suspicious lesion should be referred for biopsy. Leukoplakia, which is considered precancerous, can progress to squamous cell carcinoma if left untreated (Burgess 2015). The treatment for leukoplakia is based on the nature of the lesion and will vary depending on whether the lesion is benign or whether it exhibits malignant changes.

Squamous Cell Carcinoma

Squamous cell carcinoma is the most common type of malignant oral cancer, representing 90% of all oral cancers. It starts as a nonhealing, painless, red ulceration that may grow rapidly. Light-skinned people who do not tan well are susceptible to squamous cell carcinomas on the lower lip because of prolonged exposure to the sun. Other factors associated with oral squamous cell carcinoma are as follows:

- Use of smoking tobacco
- Use of smokeless tobacco
- Infections
- Human papillomavirus (HPV) infection
- Epstein-Barr virus (EBV) infection
- Human immunodeficiency virus (HIV) infection
- *Candida albicans* infection
- Chronic irritation (e.g., dental caries, overuse of mouthwash)
- Prolonged sun exposure
- Alcohol consumption

Squamous cell carcinomas that are detected early and removed almost always have a good result. Otherwise they may spread from the oral cavity to the cervical and submandibular lymph nodes.

Kaposi's Sarcoma

Unlike leukoplakia, **Kaposi's sarcoma** is a pigmented lesion that may be either flat or raised, and it is reddish to purple in color. It is found more often in males than females and is a common manifestation of HIV infection. Kaposi's sarcoma is initially asymptomatic, but it progresses to a painful lesion that interferes with eating and talking.

Referral and Diagnostic Tests

Other cancerous lesions, such as basal cell carcinoma and various melanomas, may also be found in and around the mouth. The reader is referred to chapter 16 for descriptions of these skin cancers. The health care provider should refer any patient with an unusual skin lesion in the mouth to the physician for biopsy. This includes any lesion that does not heal in a timely manner or that heals and then breaks down again (Stoopler and Sollecito 2014). One should be especially suspicious if multifactorial risk factors, such as alcohol, excessive sunlight exposure, and tobacco use, are present. Judicious use of sunscreen on the lips and face must be emphasized with athletic teams, coaches, and support staff who are exposed to sunlight over a prolonged period of time.

Treatment and Return to Participation

Early cancers of the lips and oral cavity are highly curable by surgery or radiation therapy. The choice of treatment, as well as the prognosis, often depend on the location of the cancer, how early it is detected, and anticipated functional and cosmetic results of treatment. Treatment options include excision, curettage, cryosurgery, radiation, and some topical medications.

The extent to which the athlete can participate depends largely on the treatment and not necessarily on the disease itself, often the disease goes undetected for a considerable time. For the patient being treated by radiation therapy or surgery, participation will be determined by the extent of treatment.

Dental Disease

Many conditions may fall under the category of dental disease, but for the purposes of this book, only gingivitis and periodontitis are discussed. **Gingivitis** is an inflammatory condition of the gums, caused by bacteria (figure 13.23). Bacteria, present in food and not removed because of inadequate brushing and flossing, will produce plaque

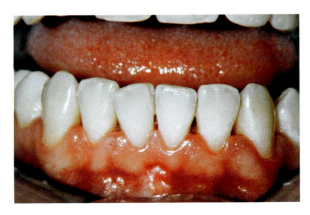

FIGURE 13.23   Gingivitis.
CNRI / Science Source

deposits leading to gingivitis. **Periodontitis** may occur if gingivitis is left untreated. Periodontitis results in a receding gum line and loss of alveolar bone.

Signs and Symptoms

In gingivitis, the gums will often appear red and swollen, and the patient will state that tooth brushing causes pain and bleeding gums (Lynch 2014). The patient may also have bad breath or complain of a bad taste in the mouth. If the disease progresses to periodontitis, the patient will experience tooth sensitivity; red, swollen gums; pain and bleeding with brushing; and possibly loosening of the teeth. Gingivitis and periodontitis should be differentiated from other conditions that may cause oral pain or sensitivity to hot or cold, including lacerations to the gums, oral lesions, or tooth decay.

Referral and Diagnostic Tests

Patients with swollen or bleeding gums are referred to a dentist or periodontist for evaluation. Radiographs and observation of the gums will reveal the extent of the disease.

Treatment and Return to Participation

Treatment of gingivitis includes an aggressive oral hygiene program to stimulate the gingivae. This may include flossing and the use of dental picks and oral stimulators (Martonffy 2015). Advanced gingivitis may require treatment with antibiotics, tooth scaling, and removal of plaque below the gum line (Stephen 2014). The patient with periodontal disease may participate in sport as able. If advanced periodontitis results in loosening of teeth, the athlete participating in contact sports must be cautious and use appropriate mouth guards.

Prevention

Dental disease continues to be a problem, and neglected dental hygiene may result in time lost from work or participation in athletics (Wojcik et al. 2015). Prevention of periodontal disease includes frequent brushing and flossing as well as the use of antibacterial mouth rinses. Regular dental hygiene visits allow periodontal disease to be detected at an early, reversible stage.

Dental Caries

Although dental caries are a common condition, the patient will typically seek the advice and treatment of a dentist for all dental problems. Dental caries represent a multifaceted disease that involves interactions among the teeth, the normal microflora, saliva, and diet. Tooth decay occurs when bacteria in the mouth accumulate on the enamel surface to form plaque, which collects on the teeth both above and below the gum line. The plaque then produces acids that cause tooth decay. Decay starts at the enamel and may extend into the dentin and even the pulp of the tooth. If the decay is caught early, only the enamel is affected, and the condition is fairly easily remedied. If the bacteria reach the pulp, the tooth will die, and an abscess may form near the root (Martonffy 2015).

Good dental hygiene and annual dental checkups will help catch dental decay in the early stages, when it can be easily treated. New dental treatments, such as early childhood fluoride and tooth-sealing treatments, have dramatically reduced the frequency of dental caries.

Signs and Symptoms

Decay will initially look white and chalky and later turn brown or black (figure 13.24). Clinically, dental caries can be classified as pit and fissure, smooth surface, cemental, or recurrent. Smooth surface caries are less common but appear as a white, "chalky" demineralization of the enamel (Martonffy 2015). The dental decay is often asymptomatic in the early stages; however, in advanced stages, the patient's teeth may be sensitive to hot or cold. Later stages of dental decay may also be accompanied by red, swollen gums. The patient may note a roughness on the tooth when feeling it with the tongue. If an abscess forms, the area around the tooth will be painful, and the tooth will be sensitive to heat. There will be a fluctuant mass on the buccal side of the tooth.

Referral and Diagnostic Tests

Everyone needs to practice good dental hygiene. A patient with poor dental hygiene needs to be educated about annual dental health visits and the importance of proper nutrition. A patient who presents with tooth decay can be referred to a dentist for treatment. Other conditions that may cause oral pain or sensitivity to hot or cold include gingivitis, periodontitis, fractured teeth, and oral lesions.

Treatment and Return to Participation

Treatment depends on the severity of the decay. Cavities caused by mild tooth decay are repaired with fillings, whereas more severe tooth decay requires repair with a crown. If the pulp is involved, a root canal treatment may be needed, or in extreme cases, the tooth may need to be extracted. The athlete with dental caries has no restrictions, and participation is self-limited.

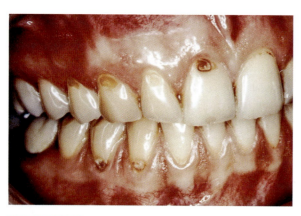

FIGURE 13.24 Teeth with decay.

CNRI / Science Source

Summary

The athletic trainer will commonly see injuries and conditions of the ears, nose, mouth, and throat as a result of athletic participation, as well as from causes not related to athletics. This chapter reviews the anatomy and evaluation of the ear, nose, mouth, and throat and highlights nontraumatic medical conditions common to these areas. The clinician must be able to recognize normal and abnormal conditions in the ear, nose, mouth, and throat and know when to refer the patient to a physician for more definitive diagnostic testing and treatment.

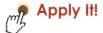 **Apply It!**   The case study for this chapter looks at a 16-year-old swimmer with complaints of pain, itching, and burning of the ear. Read the scenario and answer the questions at www.HumanKinetics.com/MedicalConditionsInTheAthlete.

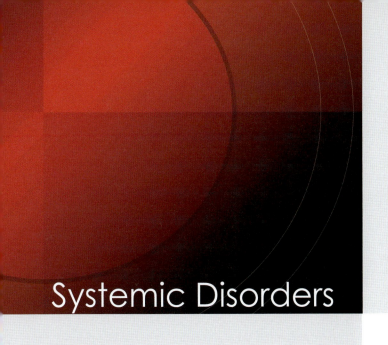

Systemic Disorders

14

OBJECTIVES

At the completion of this chapter the reader should be able to do the following:

- Appreciate the complexity of systemic disorders.
- Recognize signs and symptoms of common systemic ailments.
- Identify conditions that warrant referral to a physician.
- Relate the warning signs of malignancies involving the lymphatic system and blood.
- Describe prevention strategies for Lyme disease and type 2 diabetes mellitus.
- Determine and understand diabetic emergencies.
- Recognize and refer those with signs and symptoms of a malfunctioning thyroid.

Systemic disorders have shortened the careers of many athletes. The importance of the athletic trainer as a gate-keeper to the health care system for athletes cannot be overlooked because early detection often can prevent permanent disability or deadly consequences. Many systemic conditions can affect an athlete's general health. These range from vector-borne infections to life-threatening malignancies. Typically, systemic disorders cross several body systems and present in multiple fashions.

Because the discussion of systemic conditions covers all body systems, the organization of this chapter differs slightly from that of other chapters. The chapter begins with a review of the anatomy and physiology of the lymphatic system. The anatomy and physiology of the respiratory, cardiovascular, gastrointestinal, genitourinary, gynecological, and neurological systems are discussed in earlier chapters, and the integumentary system is covered in chapter 16.

The description of specific pathological conditions begins with lymphatic disorders, the lymphomas. A discussion of Lyme disease, a vector-borne illness, and two cancers with systemic implications follows. Several chronic systemic conditions and endocrine disorders are also covered in this chapter.

Most chronic systemic conditions are treatable, but they require special care both to ensure the athlete's safety and to optimize athletic performance. The conditions discussed here are typically not preventable; however, prevention is discussed when applicable.

Overview of Anatomy and Physiology

The anatomy and physiology of the lymphatic system are discussed because this system facilitates the spread of some pathological conditions, especially the lymphomas. The role of the lymphatic system is to maintain internal fluid balance and assist with immune functions in the body. It is a collection of vessels, ducts, nodes, organs, and tissue that transports fats, proteins, and lymphatic fluid throughout the body (figure 14.1). The system restores most of the fluid that filters out of the blood during normal homeostasis. It does this by collecting fluid that leaks from capillaries into surrounding tissues and returning it to the blood. The lymphatic system consists of lymph nodes, organs (spleen, thymus, and tonsils), and vessels that parallel veins. The lymph nodes are home to lymphocytes (T cells and B cells), the white blood cells that are largely responsible for producing antibodies to combat infections. A healthy node is typically round or kidney-shaped and up to 1 in. (2.54 cm) in diameter. Nodes cluster in the cervical region, axilla, and groin. Infections in these regions produce swollen nodes, which become enlarged and tender to palpation as the macrophage cells fight invading cells. In addition to lymphatic

system structures, many areas in the body support lymph tissue, such as bone marrow, the intestines, liver, skin, heart, and lungs.

The lymphatic system is not a closed circuit as is the circulatory system, but it does have access to all body organs and can facilitate the spread of disease throughout the body. Lymph is moved within this system through normal muscular movement and respiration. A malfunctioning lymphatic system can result in edema in the appendages.

The fluid in the lymphatic system is both lymph and interstitial fluid. Lymph is the clear fluid in the lymph vessels, whereas interstitial fluid is a by-product of lymph as it passes into surrounding cells. Lymph consists primarily of protein, salts, glucose, and urea. Lymph vessels collect interstitial fluid and return it to the circulatory system through the larger veins in the thorax. Compared with the cardiovascular system, lymphatic vessels are thinner and have more valves. Rarely are conditions of the lymphatic system preventable.

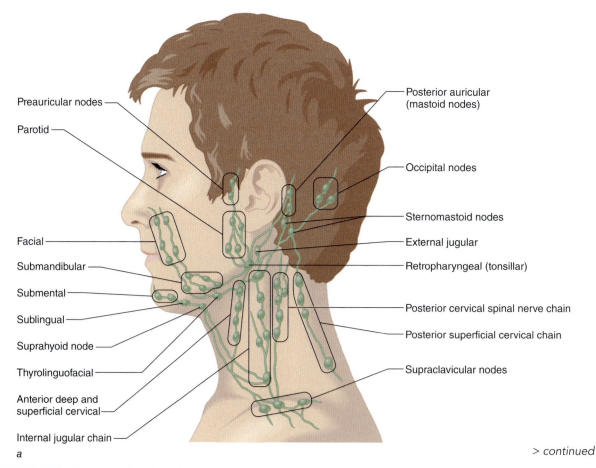

Preauricular nodes

Parotid

Facial

Submandibular

Submental

Sublingual

Suprahyoid node

Thyrolinguofacial

Anterior deep and superficial cervical

Internal jugular chain

a

Posterior auricular (mastoid nodes)

Occipital nodes

Sternomastoid nodes

External jugular

Retropharyngeal (tonsillar)

Posterior cervical spinal nerve chain

Posterior superficial cervical chain

Supraclavicular nodes

> continued

FIGURE 14.1 The complete lymphatic drainage pathways (a) from the head and neck and (b) through the trunk and extremities. The shaded area is drained through the right lymphatic duct, and lymph from the remainder of the body drains through the thoracic duct. The limbs have an extensive drainage system that follows venous return to the heart.

Malignancies

Cancer is another name for malignant entities, especially carcinomas and sarcomas. As a group, cancers represent the second leading cause of death in adults (Centers for Disease Control and Prevention 2015c). By their nature, malignant cells migrate to adjacent tissues, or they use the blood or lymph to transport cells to distant regions of the body. Once there, they infiltrate healthy cells and spread the cancer.

Because the cause of specific malignancies is largely unknown, it is difficult to prevent the condition. Cancer occurs when a cell mutates and no longer performs the function for which it was intended. These cells are abnormal in appearance, function, and growth. As the malignant cells divide and multiply, the cancer grows and potentially spreads. The lymphatic and circulatory systems are especially well suited to facilitate the spread of cancer throughout the body, and thus they are associated with the **metastasis** of lymphomas. Cancers discussed in this chapter have systemic ramifications because they present with vague symptoms and can have whole-body sequelae. Cancers of specific regions of the body are discussed in the chapters devoted to those regions. For example, lung cancer is discussed in the respiratory chapter, colon cancer in the gastrointestinal chapter, and breast and testicular cancers are discussed in the genitourinary and gynecological chapter. The malignancies discussed here involve both the lymphatic system and blood. Both are similar in presentation: a swollen lymph node, fatigue, and vague symptoms that can present systemically.

Non-Hodgkin's Lymphoma

Non-Hodgkin's lymphoma (NHL) is a group of malignancies of the **lymphoreticular system**. The lymphoreticular system is a collection of lymph nodes and lymphoid tissues formed by several types of immune system cells from both the lymph and reticuloendothelial systems that fight primarily against infection. Although it does

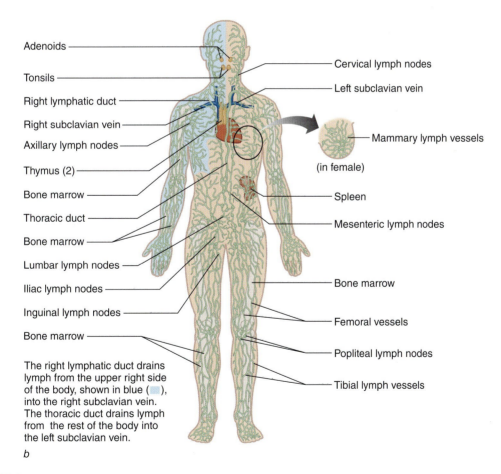

Adenoids

Tonsils

Right lymphatic duct

Right subclavian vein

Axillary lymph nodes

Thymus (2)

Bone marrow

Thoracic duct

Bone marrow

Lumbar lymph nodes

Iliac lymph nodes

Inguinal lymph nodes

Bone marrow

Cervical lymph nodes

Left subclavian vein

Mammary lymph vessels

(in female)

Spleen

Mesenteric lymph nodes

Bone marrow

Femoral vessels

Popliteal lymph nodes

Tibial lymph vessels

The right lymphatic duct drains lymph from the upper right side of the body, shown in blue ( ), into the right subclavian vein. The thoracic duct drains lymph from the rest of the body into the left subclavian vein.

b

FIGURE 14.1 *> continued*

occur in childhood (5% of adolescent cancer is NHL), the median age at diagnosis is 50 (Ferri 2016). There are several types of NHL and several different classifications. In 2015, about 73,000 new cases of NHL were diagnosed in the United States, and about 20,000 patients died of the disease (American Cancer Society 2016). Some evidence links pesticide and herbicide exposure to a greater incidence of NHL (Vinjamaram 2015; Schinasi and Leon 2014).

Signs and Symptoms

Because NHL is a group of lymphatic cancers, patients can present with a variety of symptoms depending on the site affected. The most common sites are the abdomen, mediastinum, and neck. If the abdomen is affected, the patient can experience nausea, vomiting, or diarrhea, usually accompanied by abdominal pain and weight loss. The patient may also have an enlarged spleen or liver or a palpable mass in the abdomen. Other general signs include excessive sweating, including night sweats, weight loss, fatigue, and unexplained fevers (Vinjamaram 2015). When the mediastinum is affected, the disease generally progresses more rapidly. Presenting symptoms can range from chest pain to severe shortness of breath on exertion. Neck masses and enlarged lymph nodes can also present as NHL. Figure 14.1*a* showed the location of specific cervical lymph nodes.

In patients with enlarged lymph nodes, the differential diagnoses are extensive. Hodgkin's disease, bacterial infections, human immunodeficiency virus (HIV), infectious mononucleosis, and sarcoidosis are just a few that need to be considered. Patients with chest pain or dyspnea would have differential diagnoses of hypertrophic cardiomyopathy, coronary artery disease, gastrointestinal–esophageal reflux disease, asthma, or influenza.

Referral and Diagnostic Tests

Athletes who have enlarged lymph nodes without apparent cause, such as infection distal to the gland, inexplicable chest pain, or dyspnea should be referred to a physician for further evaluation. When NHL is suspected, imaging by computed tomography (CT) or ultrasound can help confirm the presence and size of enlarged lymph nodes. The diagnosis is confirmed by sampling tissue from these lymph nodes by fine-needle biopsy or by removing them for analysis by pathologists. If the diagnosis is confirmed by biopsy, the athlete should be referred to an oncologist for specific treatment.

Patients suspected of having NHL will undergo a complete history and physical examination followed by laboratory work. Initially, patients may present with mild anemia and an elevation of lactate dehydrogenase (LDH) (Ferri 2016). A battery of other blood tests is performed to help stage the disease, as well as laparoscopic lymph node biopsy, bone marrow evaluation, PET scan, and other more common laboratory evaluations. Lymphoma and leukemia cancers are staged differently from most other cancers that use the TNM classification maintained by the American Joint Committee on Cancer (AJCC, see table 3.4). Lymphomas are staged according to the Ann Arbor system. The original Ann Arbor system has four stages (I–IV); the Cotswold modification (table 14.1) maintains these four stages and adds two sections for prognosis (X and E) and one for symptoms (A/B) (Lister et al. 1989).

Treatment and Return to Participation

The treatment depends on the histological type as well as the stage of NHL. Radiation therapy, chemotherapy, or both can be implemented as treatment and are performed by oncologists.

Prognosis varies widely and depends on the stage, size, and histological type of the disease. Patients with low-grade lymphoma, despite long-term survival of 6 to 10 yr, are rarely cured and usually die of lymphoma. Those patients with high-grade or metastasized NHL tend to do better and may achieve a cure with aggressive

TABLE 14.1 **Cotswold Modification of Ann Arbor Staging for Lymphomas**

Stage	Classification
I	Cancer affects a single lymph node group or organ
II	Cancer affects two or more lymph node groups; cancer is either above or below the diaphragm
III	Cancer affects lymph node groups on both sides of the diaphragm
IV	Cancer cells are widespread outside of the lymph system in other tissues or organs
X	Bulk > 10 cm
E	Extranodal extension or single, isolated site of extranodal disease
A/B	Presence or absence of symptoms B symptoms are weight loss of > 10%, fever, drenching night sweats

chemotherapy. The success rate for cure in this case is 35% to 50% (Lash 2015; Vinjamaram 2015).

A decision to return to athletic competition must be made once treatment has ended. Obviously, with NHL's poor prognosis and the risks involved with the treatments, athletes should remain out of competition while being treated, and any return to competition must be made after consultation with physicians.

Hodgkin's Lymphoma

Hodgkin's lymphoma is a malignant condition of lymphoreticular origin, different from NHL because of the existence of **Reed-Sternberg cells** (multinucleated giant cells) (Ferri 2016). The incidence of the disease increases throughout childhood and into the late teenage years, but peaks from ages 15 to 34 and again after age 50. It is less prevalent than NHL, with predictions of roughly 8,500 new cases annually. The disease is more common among Caucasians, higher socioeconomic groups, and males; of teens with Hodgkin's, 80% are male. The five-year survival rate has increased from 72% (1971) to 88% (2011) (American Cancer Society 2016). There are five types of Hodgkin's lymphoma, but all present similarly and have like initial signs and symptoms.

Signs and Symptoms

Although Hodgkin's lymphoma has several possible presenting signs, the most common initial sign is an enlarged lymph node, typically in the lower anterior neck region. It is usually nontender, discrete, firm, and rubbery; is not fixed to adjacent structures; and can vary in size (Lash 2015). Patients with mediastinal chest involvement can present with shortness of breath, chest pain, or cough. On occasion, enlarged lymph nodes are present in the axillary or inguinal region. Splenomegaly or **hepatomegaly** is not uncommon. Figure 14.2 illustrates the common sites of Hodgkin's lymphoma. Intense itching and intermittent fevers associated with night sweats are classic symptoms of this disease. Other systemic signs and symptoms are fatigue, fever, weight loss, **pruritus**, and CNS signs or symptoms (Lash 2015).

In patients who present with enlarged lymph nodes, the differential diagnoses are extensive. Non-Hodgkin's disease, bacterial infections, HIV, infectious mononucleosis, and sarcoidosis are just a few diagnoses that should be considered.

Referral and Diagnostic Tests

Athletes with persistent neck masses, any enlarged lymph node (figure 14.3), or constitutional symptoms, such as night sweats, intermittent fevers, and a weight loss greater than 10% of total body weight, should be evaluated by

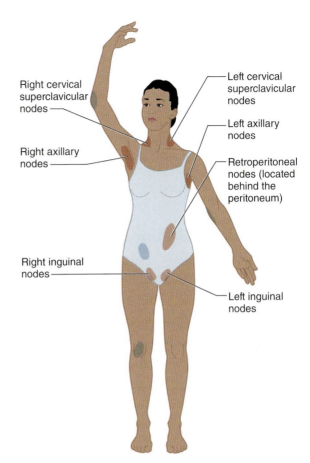

FIGURE 14.2 Sites common to Hodgkin's lymphoma. Note that red areas represent common sites and blue areas represent uncommon sites.

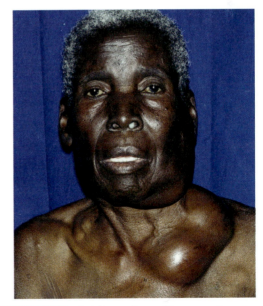

FIGURE 14.3 Sublingual swelling consistent with malignant Hodgkin's lymphoma.

Dr M.A. Ansary / Science Source

a physician. If the diagnosis is confirmed, the athlete is referred to an oncologist for further treatment.

If a patient presents with a persistent neck mass that does not respond to antibiotics or is not associated with an infection, an excisional or fine-needle lymph node biopsy is performed. This tissue can then be sent for histological diagnosis. If a persistent cough or other chest symptoms are found, a chest radiograph is taken. Blood work is performed as well, including complete blood count, LDH, and an erythrocyte sedimentation rate (ESR). Imaging studies are vital for staging the disease and include CT scans of the chest, abdomen, and pelvis (Ferri 2016).

Treatment and Return to Participation

Treatment revolves around the histological diagnosis as well as the staging, but Hodgkin's lymphoma generally requires radiation therapy as well as chemotherapy. With advances in chemotherapy, Hodgkin's disease can be cured in most patients with both localized and advanced disease. Surgery may be indicated if the disease is extensive.

The overall survival rate for Hodgkin's disease is 60% to 99% at 10 yr, depending on the type and involvement, but it comes with significant sequelae. Recent data show that long-term survivors have an increased risk of cardiovascular disease and a nearly 49% increase in the risk of developing a second cancer after 40 yr of surviving Hodgkin's lymphoma (Schaapveld et al. 2015). Awareness of the possibility of a second cancer and practicing a healthy lifestyle are important for Hodgkin's lymphoma survivors. Return-to-play decisions are made by the athlete's physician. It is best to avoid competition during the acute illness, as well as during the treatment phase, because the immune system response to the additional stress of competition may be detrimental to a timely recovery.

Leukemia

The several different types of **leukemias** have different treatments and prognoses. In general, leukemias are characterized by uncontrolled proliferation of white blood cells in the bone marrow, which accumulate and replace normal blood cells in the marrow. It can then spread to different parts of the body, including the lymph nodes, liver and spleen; occasionally gonads, kidneys, and the CNS can be affected (Porter and Kaplan 2011). As a group, there were more than 60,000 new diagnosis of leukemia in 2016 in the United States and about 24,400 deaths (American Cancer Society 2016). The five-year survival rate for all forms of leukemia rose from 33% in 1975 to 62% in 2011 (American Cancer Society 2016).

Cancers that start from other places and then spread to the bone marrow are not leukemias. It was thought at one time that lymphomas arose only from the lymphatic system, and leukemias from bone marrow, and that these two malignancies were distinctly different. This is no longer supported, as the distinction between these two is often vague.

Leukemia is among the top eight types of cancer in adults, but it is the most common malignancy in children, at 30% of all childhood cancers (American Cancer Society 2016). In adults, the most common leukemias are acute myeloid leukemia (AML) at 33% and chronic lymphocytic leukemia (CLL) at 31%. Chronic myeloid leukemia (CML) is about half as common as CLL at 13%, affects mostly adults, and is very rare in children (American Cancer Society 2016).

The specific etiology of leukemia is unknown; however, several different risk factors are associated with an increased incidence of leukemia. These include prior chemotherapy with certain agents, history of prior radiation therapy, infection with a virus (such as Epstein-Barr), genetic syndromes such as Down syndrome, and a family history of leukemia (Porter and Kaplan 2011).

Signs and Symptoms

The diagnosis of leukemia is challenging because the initial symptoms can be nonspecific and can mimic the symptoms of a common viral infection. Patients with chronic forms of leukemia may be asymptomatic (Wu 2015). Adults and children can present with generalized fatigue, loss of appetite, fevers, enlarged lymph nodes, and weakness. Additional findings include pallor, **petechiae**, ecchymoses, frequent nosebleeds, and weight loss. An enlarged liver or spleen noted on physical examination can be the explanation for a patient's abdominal pain. If leukemia spreads to the central nervous system, it may cause seizures, blurred vision, headaches, and loss of balance. Some patients are diagnosed on the basis of abnormal findings on a routine complete blood count (CBC) even though their symptoms may be very mild or absent. There are no screening tests for leukemia (Wu 2015).

> ## 🚩 RED FLAGS FOR ENLARGED LYMPH NODES
>
> The athletic trainer or health care provider should always be suspicious of any enlarged lymph gland. It could indicate a distal infection (enlarged groin lymph gland may be due to an infected knee turf burn), but it could also be a warning sign of many cancers.

In children and adults, the differential diagnoses are similar. This includes infectious mononucleosis caused by the Epstein-Barr virus, infiltrative diseases of the bone marrow, and aplastic anemia. The most significant among the differential diagnoses is leukemia in its various forms, which can usually be proven by bone marrow biopsy or a peripheral blood smear.

Referral and Diagnostic Tests

Athletes suspected of having leukemia should be referred to a hematologist or oncologist as quickly as possible to allow for initiation of treatment.

Several different findings evident on a CBC are helpful in the diagnosis of leukemia. Patients can have a very low (<5,000/mm^3) or very high (>100,000/mm^3) white blood cell count. See table 3.3 for normal blood values. The CBC may also reveal a low platelet count or anemia, which would explain easy bruising and fatigue, respectively. The key for identifying the type of leukemia is a peripheral blood smear or a bone marrow biopsy, which will show the type of abnormal white blood cells that predominate. Other abnormal laboratory findings include elevated LDH and uric acid levels. Chest radiographs are routinely performed to rule out mediastinal masses. CT, magnetic resonance imaging (MRI), or ultrasound of the abdomen is used to check for hepatomegaly or splenomegaly.

Treatment and Return to Participation

Treatment varies depending on which type of leukemia has been diagnosed. In general, the treatments include radiation, chemotherapy, blood and platelet transfusions, and possibly bone marrow or stem cell transplantation.

Avoidance of activity during treatment is essential, and return-to-participation decisions are made under the supervision of the oncologist. Follow-up examinations, laboratory work, CT and positron emission tomography (PET) scans are essential in the years after treatment to check for recurrence of disease.

Vector-Borne Disease

A vector-borne disease is one that is carried by an infected organism (such as a tick or mosquito) to a healthy person. This group of diseases is largely preventable by avoiding the habitats where these organisms live or by applying repellent. Here we discuss Lyme disease, a condition brought about by an infected tick bite. In chapter 15, we will cover other vector-borne conditions from mosquitoes that are infectious.

Lyme Disease

Lyme disease, the most common tick-borne illness in the United States, was first described in the late 1970s in Lyme, Connecticut. It is a multisystem disorder that, when left untreated, can lead to serious arthritic and neurological symptoms that become increasingly difficult to treat because of permanent tissue damage (DuPrey 2015; Lantos 2015). The culprit responsible for Lyme disease is *Borrelia burgdorferi,* a spirochetal bacterium that is transmitted to humans from infected ticks, usually the common blacklegged tick, also known as the deer tick (*Ixodes scapularis*), and by the western blacklegged tick (*Ixodes pacificus*) (DuPrey 2015; Wormser et al. 2006). These ticks reside in wooded areas and on the tips of grass, bushes, and shrubs. Athletes active in these areas, such as mountain bikers, hikers, and runners, are susceptible to infections from ticks.

People most affected by Lyme disease are those who spend a large amount of time outdoors and are bitten by ticks between May and September. Ninety-six percent of cases arise from 10 states (table 14.2). In 2014, an estimated 32,000 infections were reported in the United States (Centers for Disease Control and Prevention 2015d). The environment is also a factor with infected ticks. In general, ticks thrive in areas that have milder winters, ample rainfall, and warmer temperatures (Rapaport 2016).

Signs and Symptoms

Lyme disease can be broken down into three different categories based on the longevity of symptoms. In 70%

TABLE 14.2 Top Ten States to Report Lyme Disease

State	Number of cases 2010	Number of cases 2014
Pennsylvania	3,298	6,470
Massachusetts	2,380	3,646
New York	2,385	2,853
New Jersey	3,320	2,589
Connecticut	1,964	1,719
Maine	559	1,169
Virginia	911	976
Wisconsin	2,505	991
Maryland	1,163	957
Minnesota	1,293	896

From Center for Disease Control. Available: http://www.cdc.gov/lyme/stats/tables.html.

to 80% of patients, early localized Lyme disease begins as a red, circular rash called **erythema migrans** that enlarges over days (figure 14.4). This rash, which can stretch to 12 in. (30 cm), can appear anywhere from 3 to 30 d after a tick bite and generally occurs on the trunk of the body (DuPrey 2015). The rash is usually accompanied by a viral-like illness, with symptoms that can include headaches, muscle aches, fevers, joint aches, fatigue, and occasionally a stiff neck (Meyerhoff 2016).

A disease that is not treated at the onset of the rash can lead to early disseminated Lyme disease within weeks to months. Patients may present with Bell's palsy or even meningitis, carditis, or adenopathies (Meyerhoff 2016). Patients who develop lymphocytic meningitis generally have only neck pain and stiffness, but they may not have the typical findings associated with meningitis on physical examination, such as positive **Brudzinski's sign** and **Kernig's sign** (see figure 15.8).

Early disseminated Lyme disease can also present with cardiac manifestations occurring anywhere from 1 wk to 7 mo after the bite and peaking at 1 to 2 mo. Affected patients may have a variety of symptoms, including chest pain, palpitations, weakness, fatigue, or shortness of breath. The cause of these symptoms can be a conduction abnormality in the heart, leading to irregular rhythms or abnormal findings on an electrocardiogram. The heart muscle may also become inflamed because of infection of the heart tissue.

Late Lyme disease is characterized by manifestations involving the musculoskeletal system or central nervous system. Patients may experience intermittent attacks of brief swelling of the joints followed by chronic pain and arthritic changes. This can occur from weeks to years after the initial tick bite, and its incidence approaches 50% among those who were untreated at the time of infection (Lantos 2015). Tertiary neuroborreliosis is the name given to a syndrome of progressively worsening cognitive function, which is thought to be caused by infection of the central nervous system by the spirochete that is passed on from the infected tick, *B. burgdorferi*.

Differential diagnoses for Lyme disease include depression, fibromyalgia, cellulitis, and **chronic fatigue syndrome**. In athletes with no trauma and a joint effusion, autoimmune, infectious, neoplastic, and other inflammatory processes must also be considered (Centers for Disease Control and Prevention 2015d; Meyerhoff 2016).

Referral and Diagnostic Tests

Patients who have recently visited wooded areas and have a rash that looks like erythema migrans are referred to a primary care physician. Once signs and symptoms of Lyme disease are identified, the diagnosis can be confirmed definitively only by laboratory testing. A positive test without the symptoms does not support the diagnosis of Lyme disease because 3% to 5% of those tested can have false-positive test results. The CDC recommends a two-step process: Blood tests routinely used include an enzyme-linked immunoassay (EIA or ELISA) to identify antibodies to *B. burgdorferi*. If this test is positive, it must then be confirmed by a Western blot test. These two sequential tests must both be positive for the diagnosis of Lyme disease to be affirmative (Meyerhoff 2016; Centers for Disease Control and Prevention 2015d).

Despite this information, routine serological testing of those with erythema migrans is not recommended because only one-third of those patients with a single lesion will test positive. If several erythema migrans lesions are noted, the number of positive tests jumps to 90%. Those persons with suspected Lyme disease without the rash should have samples taken immediately with repeated sampling in 4 to 6 wk. Regardless of the laboratory outcomes, if the symptoms are consistent with Lyme disease, treatment should be initiated. The diagnosis of Lyme disease that has spread to the central nervous system is confirmed by testing spinal fluid taken by means of a lumbar puncture.

If the athlete has a clinical history of a tick bite and central nervous system manifestations or a swollen joint, fluid from the affected area should be taken for analysis. The clinician should remember that not all swollen joints are necessarily caused by trauma or injury, and if the suspicion is high, Lyme arthritis needs to be ruled out to ensure appropriate treatment.

Treatment and Return to Participation

Early treatment of Lyme disease usually prevents any of the aforementioned complications. For early disease, oral antibiotics, including doxycycline (100 mg twice a

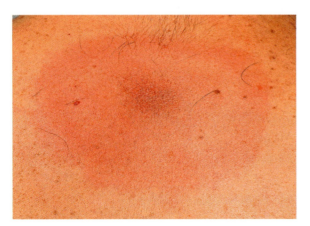

FIGURE 14.4 Erythema migrans rash consistent with Lyme disease.

Paul Whitten / Science Source

day), amoxicillin (500 mg three times a day), or cefuroxime axetil (500 mg twice a day) are used. In pregnant or nursing mothers, or children under eight years old, amoxicillin or cefuroxime axetil is suggested (Meyerhoff 2016). Cases diagnosed later or that involve the central nervous or cardiac systems typically require intravenous antibiotics. Giving antibiotics to symptom-free people who have been bitten by ticks has not been proven to lessen the incidence of the disease. The current recommendation is to monitor closely those bitten by ticks for findings of Lyme disease, including erythema migrans, and to treat those infected appropriately.

As with any acute illness, an individual assessment of the athlete must be made to determine clearance to play. Most patients can return to play when any aggravating symptoms have dissipated and proper treatment has been initiated. Transmission of Lyme disease from athlete to athlete cannot occur.

Prevention

With appropriate and expeditious treatment of Lyme disease, major late sequelae of the disease can be prevented, including central nervous system manifestations, carditis, and recurrent arthritis (Lantos 2015).

CLINICAL TIPS

Tick Removal

It is important to remove a tick as soon as possible to prevent Lyme disease. Follow these steps:

1. Cleanse the area with a povidone–iodine solution or antibacterial soap.
2. Grasp the tick as close to the skin as possible, using tweezers, forceps, or even gloved fingers.
3. Pull the tick up and perpendicular to the skin without twisting or jerking; such movements can break off parts of the insect's mouth and leave them embedded in the skin.
4. Remove the tick, taking care not to crush, squeeze, or puncture the body of the tick while it is attached to the skin, as it may release infectious fluid into the body.
5. Cleanse the area again as described previously.
6. To dispose of the tick, place it in a sealed container, wrap it tightly in tape, or flush it down a toilet. Never crush a tick with your fingers.

Primary prevention is obviously avoidance of ticks; wearing proper clothing, including long pants tucked into socks; using insect repellent; and routinely inspecting for ticks after possible exposure. Spraying skin and clothing with insect repellent containing the compound *N,N*-diethyl-3-methylbenzamide (DEET) has been shown to be especially helpful in deterring ticks, as has putting clothing in the dryer for 20 min following a workout session in areas indigenous to ticks (Rapaport 2016). Prompt and early removal of ticks is essential because transmission of *B. burgdorferi* is rare unless the tick has been attached to the human host for more than 36 h (Meyerhoff 2016). After marketing a vaccine for 4 yr, from 1998 to the beginning of 2002, the manufacturer (GlaxoSmithKline) announced that it would no longer be commercially available (Centers for Disease Control and Prevention 2015d).

Chronic Disorders

Raynaud's Disease

Raynaud's disease is a disorder characterized by vasospasm of the arteries, primarily in the hands, but it can also affect the feet, nose, and ears. The two presentations of Raynaud's disease are primary and secondary. Typically, the primary condition is referred to as Raynaud's disease if no other cause can be found beyond vasospasm. Secondary Raynaud's is caused by an underlying problem and is termed **Raynaud's phenomenon**. The many causes for Raynaud's phenomenon include medications such as oral contraceptives, systemic lupus erythematosus, rheumatoid arthritis, scleroderma, chemical exposure, smoking, arteriovascular disease, hyperthyroidism, pulmonary hypertension, and repetitive trauma from tools that cause vibration (Ferri 2016). Stressors, including cold temperatures and emotional trauma, exacerbate the phenomenon.

Raynaud's phenomenon is found in 3% to 5% of the population. Primary Raynaud's is more common than secondary Raynaud's and occurs more often in women and in people less than age 40.

Signs and Symptoms

Patients typically present with a **triphasic** color response to cold exposure:

- *Pallor:* The skin, most often of the fingers, will become pale, or pallid, because of vasospasm (figure 14.5).
- *Cyanosis:* The skin will then become blue because of the increase in venous, or deoxygenated, blood in the digits.

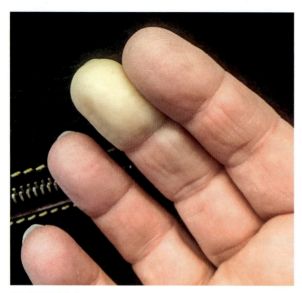

FIGURE 14.5 Raynaud's phenomenon, presenting initially as pallor of the digits when exposed to cold or stress.

© Katie Walsh Flanagan

- *Erythema:* The skin turns red when the vasospasm resolves and a rush of blood enters the digits causing pain and numbness.

As noted previously, these symptoms can happen in the hands, feet, nose, and ears and usually occur bilaterally. The symptoms generally resolve over minutes, but if they persist, they can lead to ulcerations, gangrene, and dead tissue (Hansen-Dispenza 2015).

The differential diagnoses of Raynaud's phenomenon include those secondary causes listed previously, as well as **CREST syndrome** (*c*alcinosis cutis, *R*aynaud's phenomenon, *e*sophageal dysfunction, *s*clerodactyly, *t*elangiectasia), scleroderma, carpal tunnel syndrome, thoracic outlet syndrome, peripheral vascular disease, and **Buerger's disease** (Ferri 2016; Hansen-Dispenza 2015).

Referral and Diagnostic Tests

If Raynaud's phenomenon is suspected, the appropriate referral should be made to determine the underlying cause. A rheumatologist should be involved for cases with underlying autoimmune diseases. The most common association with Raynaud's phenomenon are **scleroderma** (90%) and systemic lupus erythematosus (85%) (Hansen-Dispenza 2015).

A history of the symptoms is usually enough to diagnose Raynaud's disease. Once the diagnosis is made, a thorough history and physical examination should help in ruling out secondary causes of Raynaud's disease. If a secondary cause is suggested, the physician will order appropriate blood work. On occasion, the diagnosis can

be "seen" by having the patient expose the fingers to a cold environment, such as ice water, and monitoring the results. No blood tests assist in the diagnosis of Raynaud's, but a CBC, basic electrolytes, kidney and liver function tests, an ESR, and a urinalysis should be ordered to help differentiate this from other diseases.

Treatment and Return to Participation

The simplest of treatments is to avoid the triggers that propagate Raynaud's, such as avoiding medications that may cause it, staying out of the cold, wearing appropriate protective clothing, and avoiding other triggers such as caffeine and tobacco (Hansen-Dispenza 2015). For those with no relief from the nonpharmacological approach, medications can be used to decrease symptoms. Calcium channel blockers, such as nifedipine, have proven to be the most effective treatment for Raynaud's disease. Other medications that have proven helpful include α-blockers, and to a lesser extent, aspirin and topical nitrates.

Patients with primary Raynaud's can usually control their problems with nonpharmacological treatments. Unfortunately, for those with secondary Raynaud's caused by CREST syndrome, Buerger's disease, or scleroderma, symptoms may be so severe that the disease causes ulcerations, gangrene, and even autoamputations (Porter and Kaplan 2011).

Systemic Lupus Erythematosus

Systemic lupus erythematosus is a chronic autoimmune disorder potentially affecting many parts of the body: the musculoskeletal system, skin, kidneys, cardiac cells, and nervous system. In lupus erythematosus, the immune system makes autoantibodies, that is, antibodies to the body's own proteins, which then form complexes that cause injury and pain. It tends to be an exacerbation–remission disorder with long-term consequences. Of the four main types of lupus, systemic lupus erythematosus (SLE) is the most common, affecting approximately 7 to 9 per 100,000 people (Centers for Disease Control and Prevention 2015e). SLE affects predominantly women, especially during their childbearing years (ages 20 to 45), and is also more common in African-Americans and Asians (Dall'Era 2013). Children who are affected tend to have a more severe onset and follow a more aggressive clinical course.

The four main types of lupus are as follows:

- *Systemic lupus erythematosus:* Often called simply lupus, SLE can affect any part of the body.
- *Discoid lupus erythematosus:* This form is a chronic skin condition, can be localized or generalized, and can begin in childhood.

- *Drug-induced lupus erythematosus:* This form is caused by certain drugs (often hydralazine, procainamide, and isoniazid), and typically abates once the drug therapy is terminated.
- *Neonatal lupus erythematosus:* This form is passed *in utero* from mother to child. Infants with this form of lupus are born with a mild rash that typically disappears within 6 mo.

The exact cause of SLE is not known, but it may involve a genetic predisposition triggered by environmental factors. It is a chronic, progressive disorder that can affect several different systems at various times through the course of the disease. The effects of the condition range from mild to life-threatening, and there is no cure.

Signs and Symptoms

SLE is a multisystem disease process, so the patient often presents with multiple complaints. At some point during the course of their disease, 90% of patients with SLE will have musculoskeletal complaints. Typically, patients will have muscle aches and pains as well as arthritis or swelling of several joints (Porter and Kaplan 2011). Because of the long-term use of corticosteroids to treat many patients with SLE, they have a much higher risk of osteoporosis, as well as a high risk of avascular necrosis, typically presenting in the hip. Several large studies have reported that approximately 22% to 47% of patients with SLE will also present with fibromyalgia (Staud 2006).

The skin is often affected in patients with SLE. The hallmark sign is a red rash over the malar eminence of the face, with sparing of the nasolabial folds (the area between the nose and upper lip); it is called a *butterfly rash* because of its typical appearance (figure 14.6). Patients can also present with hair loss, red and scaly patches that turn to plaques, and oral ulcers, as well as photophobic skin responses to sunlight.

Cardiovascular risks to patients with SLE are high. There is a significant relationship between autoimmune diseases and increased atherosclerosis. In women with SLE, this raises the risk of myocardial infarction by 50% compared with the same sex and age population without SLE. Blood clots forming in the circulatory system also occur in SLE because of the production of specialized **antiphospholipid antibodies**. Patients with SLE also commonly develop anemia and a low platelet count that, at times, can be severe and require transfusions (Lisnevskaia, Murphy, and Isenberg 2014).

In addition, the kidneys can be affected, with approximately one-half of patients with SLE developing lupus nephritis. Although the treatment for lupus nephritis can keep the kidneys functioning well, kidney problems are a major cause of morbidity and mortality among patients with SLE.

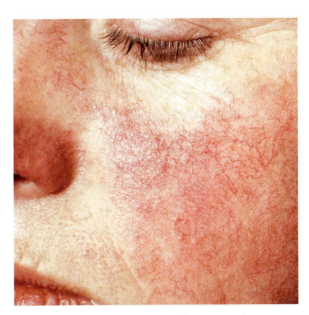

FIGURE 14.6 Butterfly rash of systemic lupus erythematosus.
BSIP / Science Source

The central nervous system effects of SLE are many and widely varied. Patients can present with seizures, psychosis, decreased cognitive function, stroke, or even coma.

Referral and Diagnostic Tests

Certified athletic trainers who see athletes with unexplained joint pain and swelling, especially if accompanied by a butterfly rash, should refer these athletes to a physician for further testing. Referrals depend on the severity of the disease and the organ systems involved. In addition to a primary care physician, patients with SLE need a rheumatologist to oversee their care. Nephrologists should be involved for patients with kidney disorders, hematologists for those with blood manifestations, and if needed, orthopedic surgeons for those with avascular necrosis.

The American College of Rheumatology (ACR) has developed criteria to aid in the diagnosis of SLE (table 14.3). Four of the 11 criteria must be met for a positive diagnosis (American College of Rheumatology 2016). In addition to the criteria, several blood tests can be performed to help in the diagnosis of SLE. The presence of antinuclear antibody (ANA), anti-Smith antibody, and antidouble-stranded deoxyribonucleic acid (anti-dsDNA) antibody are all helpful in the diagnosis. Other laboratory examinations include determination of the erythrocyte sedimentation rate, which indicates the level of inflammation in the body, and a urinalysis to determine whether protein or blood is present. Chest X-rays and electrocardiograms

TABLE 14.3   **ACR Diagnostic Criteria for Systemic Lupus Erythematosus**

Criterion	Definition
Malar rash	Flat or raised rash on the zygoma
Discoid rash	Erythematous-raised rash with scaling and possible older rash scars
Photosensitivity	Skin reaction as a direct response to sunlight; reported by patient and validated by physician
Oral ulcers	Oral or nasal ulcers, often painless; validated by physician
Arthritis	Arthritis on two or more peripheral joints, with tenderness or swelling
Serositis	1. Pleuritis (convincing history of pleural effusion) *or* 2. Pericarditis (documented by ECG or pericardial effusion)
Kidney disorder	1. Persistent proteinuria (protein in the urine) greater than 0.5 gm/day *or* 2. Cellular casts
Neurological disorder	1. Unexplainable seizures *or* 2. Unexplainable psychosis
Blood disorder	1. Hemolytic anemia *or* 2. Leukopenia (less than 4,000/mm total on 2+ occasions) *or* 3. Lyphopenia (less than 1,500/mm total on 2+ occasions) *or* 4. Thrombocytopenia (less than 100,000/mm present without drugs)
Immune disorder	1. Positive LE cell preparation *or* 2. Anti-DNA (antibody to native DNA in abnormal titer) *or* 3. Anti-Sm (presence of antibody to SM unclear antigen) *or* 4. False-positive serologic test for syphilis known to be positive for at least 6 mo
Antinuclear antibody	An abnormal titer of antinuclear antibody by immunofluorescence or equivalent assay at any point (in the absence of drugs associated with lupus)

Adapted, by permission, from E.M. Tan et al., 1997, "The revised criteria for the classification of systemic lupus erythematosus," *Arthritis and Rheumatism* 40: 1725.

(ECGs) may be ordered to evaluate the level of possible lung and cardiac involvement (Bartels 2015).

Because of its effect on multiple systems, many other illnesses, including various infections and malignancies, such as lymphoma and leukemia, must be excluded in the differential diagnosis of SLE. Because of its musculoskeletal involvement, rheumatoid arthritis (RA) and mixed connective tissue disease (e.g., scleroderma, dermatomyositis) may also produce symptoms similar to those of SLE.

Treatment and Return to Participation

The goal of treatment of SLE is to reduce the acute symptoms while avoiding the progressive, damaging effects of the disease in the long term. Photosensitivity for those with skin manifestations can be controlled with the use of sunscreen, protective hats and clothing, and avoidance of sunlight. Patients with musculoskeletal symptoms can benefit from nonsteroidal anti-inflammatory drugs (NSAIDs) or steroids. Corticosteroids have been the mainstay of treatment for SLE symptoms affecting the renal, nervous, and hematological systems. Although cor-

ticosteroid treatment is extremely beneficial for patients with SLE, its many side effects complicate the disease itself. Patients taking long-term corticosteroids have a higher likelihood of infections, osteoporosis, avascular necrosis, steroid-induced diabetes, and several skin ramifications (see chapter 5). All of these side effects need to be monitored and treated appropriately while the patient continues to take corticosteroids. The key is to have the patient take the lowest dose that controls the disease while limiting the side effects. The drug methotrexate and the hormone dehydroepiandrosterone (DHEA) are also both optional treatment regimens used in between other treatment choices (Sakthiswary and Suresh 2014).

Because patients with SLE tend to experience remissions and exacerbations, the prognosis is often complicated. Infection resulting from immunosuppression, the result not only of SLE itself but also the chronic corticosteroid treatment, is the leading cause of death in patients with SLE. Other causes of death in patients with SLE include renal and neurological diseases. Systematic reviews of patients with SLE determine that they show less cardiovascular response to exercise than others without the disease (Balsamo and dos Santos-Neto 2011; Tench et al. 2002). Therefore, the overall challenge for returning patients with SLE to activity is to monitor the patient for exacerbations and new complications of the disease while balancing the potential side effects of treatment.

Fibromyalgia

Fibromyalgia is a chronic, noninflammatory, diffuse pain syndrome characterized by multiple areas of musculoskeletal pain, sleep disturbances, fatigue, and depression. Women diagnosed with the condition outnumber men 7:1, and the predominant age range at diagnosis is between the ages of 30 and 50 (Porter and Kaplan 2011; Ferri 2016). The overall prevalence of fibromyalgia in the United States is 2% to 8% (Ferri 2016). People with an autoimmune disease (such as SLE, rheumatoid arthritis, and **Sjogren's syndrome**) are at higher risk for fibromyalgia (Staud 2006).

The cause of fibromyalgia remains unknown, but genetics and environmental factors have been identified to predispose one to it (Ferri 2016). Although how this process is set in motion in some people and not others is unknown, it is thought that a precipitating event, such as injury, surgery, infection, or emotional trauma, is often involved (Jiao et al. 2015). Research has discovered that patients with fibromyalgia have an abnormal and exaggerated response to pain in the neuroreceptors in the brain (Sumpton and Moulin 2014).

Signs and Symptoms

Patients with fibromyalgia typically experience severe and diffuse musculoskeletal pain that is unrelated to a clearly defined anatomical lesion. The pain is located mostly in the neck and lower back, but it can also affect the extremities. This pain syndrome will wax and wane not only in severity but also in location and may be exacerbated by any stress, emotional or physical trauma (Porter and Kaplan 2011). If a patient has any findings consistent with another disease process or injury, such as a swollen joint, warmth or redness over the affected site, or abnormal X-ray findings, a diagnosis other than fibromyalgia should be investigated thoroughly. Complaints of fatigue, ineffective sleep (the ARC terms this "waking unrefreshed"), or impaired cognition are also used to determine the presence of fibromyalgia (Sumpton and Moulin 2014; Wolfe et al. 2010).

The differential diagnoses of fibromyalgia include many diseases with similar signs and symptoms. These include depression, chronic fatigue syndrome, myofascial pain syndrome, hypothyroidism, rheumatoid arthritis, and SLE (Porter and Kaplan 2011; American College of Rheumatology 2015).

Referral and Diagnostic Tests

Health care providers should watch for those whose symptoms last longer than usual for a given injury or illness. If an athlete has symptoms that are thought to be consistent with fibromyalgia, referral to a primary care physician is appropriate to help with the diagnosis. The athlete can be referred to a rheumatologist, psychiatrist, physical therapist, or a specialist in fibromyalgia as needed.

The diagnosis of fibromyalgia rests on a thorough history, a physical examination, and a set of criteria established in 2010 by the ACR (see the sidebar "Diagnostic Criteria for Fibromyalgia"). The criteria include

Diagnostic Criteria for Fibromyalgia

The following criteria have been established by the American College of Rheumatology (Wolfe et al. 2010):

- History of widespread pain over the four quadrants of the body, lasting more than 3 mo
- Presence of specific widespread pain points (WPI). The ACR has identified 19 specific areas; seven areas must be represented for fibromyalgia to be considered:

  Shoulder girdle (R/L)   Jaw (R/L)
  Upper arm (R/L)   Upper back
  Lower arm (R/L)   Lower back
  Hip (buttock, greater trochanter) (R/L)   Chest
  Upper leg (R/L)   Abdomen
  Lower leg (R/L)   Neck

- Symptom severity (SS)

  Fatigue
  Waking unrefreshed
  Cognitive symptoms

widespread, bilateral pain located above and below the waist and pain involving the axial skeleton that has been present for at least 3 mo. To meet the diagnosis of fibromyalgia, the patient must also have pain at 7 of 19 sites when the examiner applies pressure and have fatigue, cognitive issues, unrefreshed awakening, and no other health issue that would explain the symptoms (American College of Rheumatology 2015). Physicians evaluate patients on two scales: the widespread pain index (WPI), which is the number of places the patient has pain, and symptom severity (SS), which relates the level of severity to fatigue, sleep, and cognitive symptoms. Basic laboratory evaluations, including a CBC, creatinine kinase, thyroid-stimulating hormone, iron and vitamin B_{12} levels, and ESR, are performed to differentiate fibromyalgia from other diseases that have overlapping symptoms (Boomershine 2015).

Treatment and Return to Participation

The treatment for fibromyalgia usually incorporates a variety of disciplines. The key element is patient education, which can be done through lectures, handouts, videos, or validated sites on the Internet. Counseling is also an important part of treating fibromyalgia, especially for those patients with manifestations of depression or poor coping skills (American College of Rheumatology 2015). Exercise has proven to be beneficial because deconditioning plays a large role in fibromyalgia (Segura-Jimenez et al. 2015). Good sleep habits and mild exercise have a positive effect on mood disorders and depression (Boomershine 2015) (see chapter 17). Cardiovascular exercise and muscle strengthening seem to be of more benefit than stretching and flexibility exercises, although these work for some patients. After a 3 mo program, some patients can see benefits that last for up to a year. Water aerobics, swimming, biking, yoga, and other nonimpact exercises are appropriate. Exercise compliance can be difficult because some perceive exercise to be causing their pain and fatigue. However, counseling the patient to start out slowly and at a low intensity, gradually increasing their exercise tolerance, has been helpful (Sumpton and Moulin 2014).

The patient with fibromyalgia may also benefit from pharmacological treatment. Antidepressants, especially tricyclic antidepressants, such as amitriptyline (Elavil) at low doses, have been shown to help. Not only do they help with the possible underlying depression, but their sedative effect makes them ideal, especially when taken before bedtime. The Food and Drug Administration has approved the following drugs in the treatment of fibromyalgia: pregabalin (Lyrica), duloxetine (Cymbalta), and milnacipran (Savella) (Boomershine 2015). These medications are effective in altering the chemicals (serotonin and norepinephrine) that process pain perception, improving sleep, and reducing depression. Muscle relaxants such as cyclobenzaprine (Flexeril) have shown merit in helping patients with fibromyalgia, and they also have a sedating side effect. Selective serotonin reuptake inhibitors (SSRIs), such as fluoxetine (Prozac), paroxetine (Paxil), and sertraline (Zoloft), also have proven beneficial, but they should be monitored due to their potential for abuse (Boomershine 2015). NSAIDs have not proven to be beneficial for patients with fibromyalgia. It is important to note that all of these medications have side effects that may make them detrimental in specific cases.

Several other treatments that may help patients with fibromyalgia include hypnosis, chiropractic treatments, acupuncture, and herbal medications. These modalities need to be further studied to determine their true effectiveness. A study of 400 women with fibromyalgia showed that only a small percentage (16%) were engaged in the 10,000 minimum step recommendations compared to the same number of healthy women in the same age range (Segura-Jimenez et al. 2015). The suggestion from the authors was that engaging in more activity—at least minimum daily standards—might be a helpful treatment for those with fibromyalgia (Boomershine 2015).

The prognosis for patients with fibromyalgia is uncertain because the symptoms commonly come and go over the course of the disease. Although patients can show improvement, there is no known cure. An aggressive, multifaceted, organized approach to treatment will help lead to a substantial improvement and ideally a remission of symptoms. Participation in athletic events is determined on an individual basis. Most athletes can function as long as their symptoms are well controlled.

Chronic Fatigue Syndrome

Chronic fatigue syndrome (CFS) is often a disabling illness, with the primary symptom being severe fatigue persisting 6 mo or longer. This is often accompanied by several other symptoms, most often cognitive difficulties, but the musculoskeletal, immunological, and neurological systems can be affected. There is a recent push to rename the condition **systemic exertion intolerance disease (SEID)** (Cunha 2016). People of all races and ages can be affected; however, it most commonly occurs in 30- to 50-year-old women.

There is no known cause of CFS, and no specific diagnostic tests are available. It is likely a spectrum of illnesses sharing a common pathogenesis with varying degrees of fatigue and associated symptoms (Cunha 2016). Some studies indicate certain infectious diseases, Epstein-Barr virus or pneumonia, as well as infections, upper respiratory infection (URI), or diarrhea may be the culprit in CFS, but the research is not definitive (Cunha 2016).

Signs and Symptoms

The primary presenting symptom for CFS is fatigue continuing for 6 mo or longer and accompanying cognitive difficulties. Several other symptoms can be present as well; however, these vary widely and are used mainly to differentiate CFS from other causes of persistent fatigue. Other symptoms are listed in the CDC's criteria for diagnosis in the next paragraph.

Referral and Diagnostic Tests

The diagnosis of CFS is one of exclusion. Because of the overlapping symptoms CFS has with several other diseases, including depression, fibromyalgia, and infectious mononucleosis, to name just a few, several criteria must be met in order to diagnose a person with CFS. A complete history and physical examination are mandatory to help exclude other disease processes. The CDC has determined that the diagnosis of CFS includes chronic fatigue lasting more than 6 mo accompanied by four of the following symptoms (Centers for Disease Control and Prevention 2015a):

- Substantial impairment of concentration or short-term memory
- Muscle pain
- Headache (new type, pattern, or severity)
- Frequent or recurring sore throat
- Tender lymph nodes
- Multijoint pain without swelling or redness
- Unrefreshing sleep
- Postexertional malaise lasting more than 24 h

Laboratory tests include a standard CBC, thyroid function, ESR, and liver function tests, but other laboratory tests are ordered depending on the patient's symptoms (Cunha 2016). Patients are often referred to infectious disease specialists due to elevated immunoglobulin levels. In CFS, the results of laboratory examinations are within normal limits. A host of diseases needs to be excluded before allowing the diagnosis of CFS:

- Mononucleosis
- Anemia
- Leukemia
- Depression
- Systemic lupus erythematosus
- Human immunodeficiency virus
- Multiple sclerosis

- Myasthenia gravis
- Thyroiditis
- Hypothyroidism
- Hypopituitarism
- Lyme disease
- Chronic hepatitis B or C
- Rheumatoid arthritis
- Tuberculosis
- Fibromyalgia
- Diabetes mellitus
- Pregnancy
- Sleep apnea
- Narcolepsy
- Medication reaction

Treatment and Return to Participation

The optimal treatment of CFS includes a multifactorial approach aimed at managing the disease and its manifestations. Because there is no definitive cure for CFS, and it may be related to a viral infection, treatment needs to be tailored to the individual. The basic treatment in current use seems to have a beneficial effect in managing the disease. Most medications and vitamins have proven ineffective, as have antidepressives (Cunha 2016). Suggested management includes supportive treatment: a graded exercise program, proper nutrition, and improved sleep. Counseling is important in the athletic setting because CFS can hamper a person's performance substantially, making return to competition at any level quite challenging.

Treatment of any other coexistent disorders, such as depression, fibromyalgia, panic disorders, and irritable bowel syndrome, is also important in the overall approach to patients with CFS.

The prognosis for people with CFS is unknown because there is no definitive cure for the disease. The hope is that, with a multidisciplinary approach, the athlete will be able to return to the previous level of competition; however, this may take months to years to accomplish.

Endocrine Disorders

Endocrine glands secrete hormones directly into the bloodstream, allowing specific body functions to occur. The disorders discussed here are related to the pancreas, a gland with both exocrine and endocrine functions, and the thyroid. The pancreas lies with its ends laterally touching the spleen and the duodenum of the small intestine medially (figure 14.7). The chief functions of the pancreas

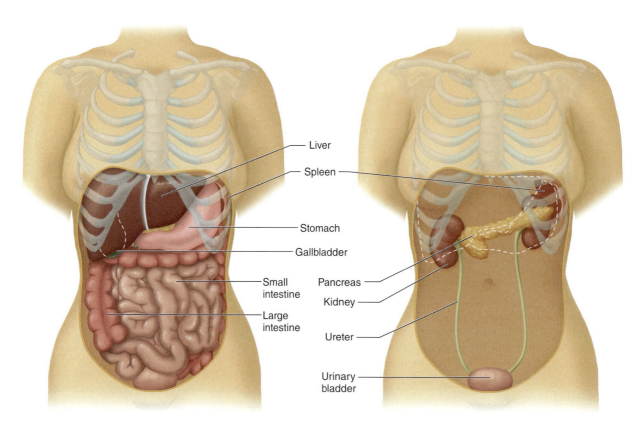

Liver
Spleen
Stomach
Gallbladder
Small
intestine
Large
intestine
Pancreas
Kidney
Ureter
Urinary
bladder

FIGURE 14.7   The pancreas is the primary gland secreting the hormones insulin and glucagon.

are to secrete bicarbonate to protect the duodenum from gastric acid and to produce insulin, glucagon, and somatostatin from the endocrine glands, called **islets of Langerhans**. The normal pancreas has between 500,000 and several million islets. The islets comprise four cell types, but only the two primary cells types, alpha and beta, are discussed here. Alpha cells produce glucagon, whereas beta cells secrete insulin.

When serum glucose (blood sugar) is high, the beta cells are stimulated to produce insulin. The secreted insulin then allows muscle, blood, and fat cells to absorb glucose out of the blood and store it in muscle and the liver as glycogen, effectively lowering blood sugar to normal ranges. The alpha cells of the islets of Langerhans secrete glucagon, which has the opposite effect from insulin. If blood sugar is low, glucagon is secreted where it has the most effect—the liver. Glucagon stimulates liver cells to break down stored glycogen into glucose and release it into the bloodstream, increasing serum levels of glucose. Glucagon also stimulates muscle to manufacture glucose from stored protein by means of gluconeogenesis. The human body functions best when glucose levels are relatively constant within the bloodstream. Because most body functions rely on glucose in some form, severely fluctuating levels can have profound sequelae.

Pancreatitis

Acute pancreatitis is an inflammatory process of the pancreas with intrapancreatic activation of enzymes. In 40% of cases, it is caused by blockage of the biliary tract by gallstone formation, but an additional 35% of acute cases can be attributed to alcohol abuse (Gardner 2015). In general, more males than females present with acute pancreatitis, but males tend to have the condition as a result of alcohol, whereas females tend to suffer from biliary-tract obstruction. Several medications have been implicated in pancreatitis as well. African-Americans tend to be at a higher risk than any other racial group (Gardner 2015).

Signs and Symptoms

Patients typically present with sudden onset abdominal pain in the epigastric area and occasionally radiating to the back. They may have severe nausea and vomiting. Some patients report weight loss as well. On examination, patients are typically guarding their abdomen because of the extreme pain associated with palpation of this area. Patients' bowel sounds will be hypoactive, and they may have signs of fluid or blood in their abdominal cavity, such as abdominal rigidity, distention, and guarding;

chapters 9 presents a basic assessment of the abdomen. These patients may also have fever, confusion, elevated heart rate, or jaundice. Tachycardia, hypotension, and dyspnea are not uncommon (Gardner 2015).

Several diseases can present with abdominal pain, and they should be considered when assessing for pancreatitis. These include peptic ulcer disease, intestinal obstruction, early acute appendicitis, pneumonia, and heart attack. The history, physical examination, and laboratory work will help differentiate these problems.

Referral and Diagnostic Tests

Athletes with acute nontraumatic abdominal swelling or pain accompanied by fever should be referred to a physician or the emergency department for further evaluation. Patients often require hospitalization for pain control and treatment of the pancreatitis.

History and physical examination are paramount in the assessment of these patients. Alcohol intake history is important to help elucidate a cause for the inflamed pancreas. Pancreatitis will present with elevated enzymes produced by the pancreas, including lipase and amylase. Of the two enzymes, lipase is more sensitive. Further testing, including blood count, liver enzymes, and glucose and serum calcium levels, is important in the initial workup. Abdominal radiographs, ultrasound, or CT scans are appropriate for diagnosis (Gardner 2015). They help to evaluate not only for inflammation of the pancreas but also for any potentially obstructing stones or cancers.

Treatment and Return to Participation

Pancreatitis is treated in the hospital. Food is avoided because it may irritate the pancreas and therefore slow healing. Maintenance of intravascular volume with intravenous fluids is critical because these patients tend to have a total body water deficit. Pain control is provided with medications such as meperidine (Demerol). Surgical consultation may be warranted if there is evidence of gallstone pancreatitis. Patients with severe acute pancreatitis typically require intensive care and may be intubated and sedated to manage pain.

The prognosis varies with the severity of the illness. The overall mortality for acute pancreatitis approaches 5% to 10% of patients (Ferri 2016). Individuals with a history of alcohol abuse commonly have recurrent bouts of pancreatitis, leading to chronic pancreatitis. People with chronic gallstone attacks are especially susceptible to pancreatitis and should be counseled to have the stones removed preemptively. There is also a documented higher risk of acute pancreatitis for patients with type 2 diabetes, and successful management of their disease may alleviate the chances of contracting pancreatitis (Noel et al. 2009).

Athletes with pancreatitis will need to refrain from competition until the acute phase has resolved. Because the pain associated with pancreatitis is so great, it will not allow the patient to make any sudden movements. Once the cause of pancreatitis is identified, it should be treated appropriately.

Diabetes Mellitus

Diabetes mellitus (DM) is a disease in which the body cannot produce or use insulin effectively. Diabetes mellitus affects 7.8% of the population, or roughly 29 million people, in the United States. An additional 86 million Americans have prediabetes, with 9 of 10 people unaware they have the condition. The risk for death among diabetics is nearly twice that of nondiabetics of the same age range (Centers for Disease Control and Prevention 2015b). Type 1 diabetes, formerly called insulin-dependent diabetes mellitus (IDDM), is characterized by the body's inability to produce insulin, which is needed for the proper use and storage of carbohydrates. Type 1 DM accounts for roughly 10% of the total number of cases, and its onset usually occurs in people under age 20. Type 2 DM, formerly called non–insulin-dependent diabetes mellitus (NIDDM), makes up the remaining 90% of cases (Ferri 2016). This form of DM is related to the body's inability to use insulin effectively because of a combination of resistance to insulin and an overall decrease in insulin production, not always but most often due to obesity.

The incidence of diabetes is known to increase with age. It is the leading cause of end-stage renal disease in the United States and is a primary cause of blindness and foot and leg amputations in adults. More than 75,000 people with diabetes will die annually due to complications of this disease (Centers for Disease Control and Prevention 2015c). It is also known to cause neuropathy (nerve damage) in up to 70% of diabetic patients. People with diabetes are twice as likely as those without diabetes to develop cardiovascular disease (Ferri 2016).

Type 1 DM is caused by autoimmune-mediated destruction of pancreatic beta cells, which are responsible for producing insulin. There appears to be a hereditary link in people with type 1 DM. Other factors have been postulated to induce type 1 DM, including viral infections, toxins, and other environmental factors. Although there is a genetic predisposition for developing type 2 DM, several physical factors also put a person at increased risk for the disease. Type 2 DM results more from an insulin resistance syndrome. In addition to environmental and physiological reasons for insulin resistance, the main cause is excess body fat (body mass index over 25) linked primarily to a sedentary lifestyle and an excess consumption of calories (Khardori 2015b). Women can also be affected by gestational diabetes, which usually occurs in the third trimester of pregnancy and typically resolves in the postpartum period. These women are more likely to develop type 2 DM later on in life. Uncontrolled high blood pressure and high cholesterol are also risk factors for type 2 DM, as is being over age 45. Certain racial populations are at increased risk for diabetes, including Native Americans, African-Americans, Asian-Americans, and Hispanic-Americans. Other causes of type 2 DM are Cushing's syndrome, pancreatic disorders such as pancreatitis, or prolonged medication usage, including glucocorticoids (Porter and Kaplan 2011).

Signs and Symptoms

There is usually a prolonged, albeit unknown, period of time when persons with type 2 diabetes have hyperglycemia but do not have any clinical symptoms. Later in the disease process, as the body can no longer compensate for the elevated sugar load, symptoms begin. The most common initial symptoms are listed in "Red Flags for Signs and Symptoms of Diabetes." All these symptoms are due to an elevated glucose level in the bloodstream. Overtreatment of diabetes or inadequate food intake can cause hypoglycemia, which is also dangerous.

Differential diagnoses of diabetes include diabetes insipidus, stress hyperglycemia, and diabetes secondary to medications, pancreatic disease, and possible hormonal excess.

Referral and Diagnostic Tests

Athletes with signs or symptoms consistent with diabetes or those who have risk factors are referred to a physician. Three tests of blood glucose levels can be performed to confirm the diagnosis of type 1 and type 2 DM (table 14.4). The random test, performed without regard to food intake, that yields a blood glucose level equal to or greater than 200 mg/dl, associated with weight loss, polyuria, and polydipsia, indicates DM. All three of these criteria can diagnose diabetes, but one positive test needs to be confirmed on the following day by another one of the tests (American Diabetes Association 2016). A fasting blood glucose level between 100 and 125 mg/dl is consistent with the diagnosis of prediabetes.

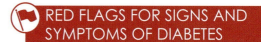

RED FLAGS FOR SIGNS AND SYMPTOMS OF DIABETES

Undiagnosed diabetes is dangerous because it can result in coma, convulsions, permanent brain injury, and possible death. Recognizing the following signs and symptoms, particularly when they present together, can lead to early diagnosis:

- Polyuria (increased urination)
- Polydipsia (excessive thirst)
- Polyphagia (persistent hunger)
- Tingling, pain, or numbness in hands or feet (type 2)
- Blurry vision
- Cuts or bruises slow to heal
- Fatigue
- Weight loss, even when eating more (type 1)
- Incoordination

Another common blood test is for glycated hemoglobin, or hemoglobin A1C (also HbA_{1c}). This test identifies the concentration of glucose in plasma over time, typically 3 mo. The American Diabetes Association's Standards of Medical Care for Diabetes–2016 recommends a level at or below 6.5% as a criterion for the diagnosis of diabetes (Cefalu 2016). Once diabetes is diagnosed, HbA_{1c} is also used periodically to monitor plasma glucose levels. For every percentage drop in HbA_{1c} value, diabetics have a 40% reduction in the occurrence of microvascular complications (including damage to nerves, kidneys, and eyes) (Khardori 2015b).

Once the diagnosis is confirmed, those caring for people with diabetes, especially athletes, need to be well versed in the signs and symptoms of hyperglycemia and hypoglycemia. See the sidebar "Comparison of Signs and Symptoms for Hypoglycemia and Hyperglycemia."

Although exercise is important to treating and controlling diabetes, there are also inherent risks for persons

TABLE 14.4　Normal Blood Glucose Levels

Time at which measurement is taken	Blood serum level (mg/dl)
After fasting for 8 h	60–80*
2–3 h after eating	100–140
Random and unplanned	<126

*mg/dl = Milligrams of glucose in 100 milliliters (1 deciliter) of blood; *hypoglycemia* is defined as less than 60 mg/dl and *hyperglycemia* is defined as greater than 180 mg/dl.

with diabetes who do exercise (Colberg et al. 2010). Hypoglycemia, or low blood sugar, defined as less than 60 mg/dl, usually presents several hours after exercise, but it can happen during competition or as a result of an overuse of insulin. People can have reactionary hypoglycemia, brought about by improper nutrition and exercise or fasting and exercise (Hamdy 2015). These athletes need to be counseled about making better nutritional choices. The treatment for hypoglycemia is to ingest glucagon or carbohydrates; the treatment for hyperglycemia is to receive a measured dose of insulin prescribed for that patient.

Treatment and Return to Participation

Patients with diabetes, whether type 1 or 2, need to be under the care of a physician because of the many complications that can arise if diabetes is not controlled. Diabetic athletes are more prone to tendinopathies, shoulder adhesive capsulitis, and articular cartilage diseases, and they have more surgical complications. Athletic trainers and others caring for diabetic athletes day to day must be aware of possible difficulties with routine healing and tendencies toward chronic musculoskeletal pathologies (Wolfson, Hamula, and Jazrawi 2013). Because there are so many people with diabetes in the United States, most primary care physicians can manage the disease without the assistance of specialists. If referral is needed, as may be true for most people with type 1 diabetes, an endocrinologist or diabetologist would be appropriate. The care of the person with diabetes requires a multidisciplinary approach. Patients may be referred for nutritional counseling, exercise prescriptions, yearly eye examinations, and routine podiatric care.

The overall goal in the treatment of diabetes is to decrease the end-stage effects such as renal disease and failure, coronary artery disease, blindness, and stroke. In addition to medications, diet, and exercise to improve glucose control, other conditions common to people with diabetes, including hypertension, elevated cholesterol and triglycerides, and tobacco abuse, need to be treated.

If further complications arise, nephrologists, cardiologists, podiatrists, or other appropriate specialists are called on.

The treatment for diabetes is multifactorial. At the cornerstone of therapy is education about the disease, sound nutrition, and increased physical activity. Lifestyle modification has been shown to delay or prevent the onset of diabetes (Harris and White 2012; Ferri 2016).

With intensive treatment of diabetes and its associated conditions, the development and progression of complications decrease immensely. If diabetes is not treated intensively, patients can expect many complications as the disease progresses. Neuropathy, or decreased and sometimes painful sensation in the extremities, is very common and can lead to eventual amputation. Infections are more common in diabetic patients and are much more difficult to control if blood sugars are not optimized. Surgical complications, such as delayed healing or grafting failure, can occur in patients who have not controlled their diabetes (Wolfson, Hamula, and Jazrawi 2013).

For athletes, a sound knowledge of their disease, medications, and dietary habits is a must in order to control blood sugar while training and competing. Wounds in persons with diabetes tend to heal more slowly than in those without diabetes; however, excellent control of blood sugars can almost negate this disadvantage. Common athletic wounds, such as blisters and calluses, need more diligent care in athletes with diabetes. These seemingly harmless lesions can lead to infections or chronic ulcers if not properly cared for. In the worst case, a person could have to undergo amputation because of an inability to

---

CONDITION HIGHLIGHT

Hyperglycemia and Hypoglycemia

Hypoglycemia can also affect the nondiabetic athlete, as many athletes show up to practice or events without having consumed the proper nutrition for the session they are about to endure. The symptoms of hypoglycemia are numerous and include sweating, palpitations, hunger, tremors, confusion, nausea, headaches, fatigue, slurred speech, inappropriate behavior, and incoordination (Khardori 2015b). Health care providers must recognize these symptoms in patients because if left uncorrected, hypoglycemia can result in coma, convulsions, permanent brain injury, and possibly death. Hyperglycemia is another risk factor for persons with diabetes; it has a variety of symptoms such as **polyuria**, **polydipsia**, fatigue, nausea, and elevated blood sugar. It has been reported that type 1 diabetic athletes will sometimes run chronically hyperglycemic to decrease the risk of exercise-induced hypoglycemia. This will increase their risk of infections. Athletic trainers should be aware of which athletes are diabetic and their increased risk of infection from cuts and abrasions.

Comparison of Signs and Symptoms for Hypoglycemia and Hyperglycemia

Hypoglycemia (<60 mg/dl)	Hyperglycemia (>180 mg/dl)
Palpitations	Weakness
Tachycardia	Polyuria
Anxiety	Altered vision
Hyperventilation	Weight loss
Blurred vision	Dehydration
Shakiness	Polydipsia
Weakness	Hyperventilation
Diaphoresis	Hypotension
Nausea	Cardiac arrhythmia
Confusion	Stupor
Behavior changes	Coma
Hallucinations	
Hypothermia	
Seizure	
Coma	

control ulcers caused by simple friction. These lesions must be meticulously cared for to avoid complications. Athletes with diabetes should inspect their feet daily and, if necessary, the athletic trainer should participate. Identifying and eliminating the underlying cause of lesions is important to preventing further damage; causes can include such things as shoe wear and gait variations. Education and a team approach between the athlete and the medical care team is essential to the athlete's longevity and safety, especially in the adolescent diabetic athlete (Draznin 2010; Cheadle 2015; Harris and White 2012).

Type 1 diabetes is not preventable. Type 2 diabetes, however, is a condition whose onset and severity can be greatly decreased, if not eliminated, with adequate exercise and a proper diet.

Type 1 Diabetes Mellitus

The goal of therapy is to have a normal blood sugar level and to prevent the complications that can occur when blood sugar remains elevated. This is achieved with insulin in persons with type 1 diabetes because of their decreased production of insulin. Many types of insulin are available. These include rapid-acting insulin (lispro or aspart), which begins to work in as little as 5 min and lasts up to 4 h. Regular, or short-acting insulin, will begin to work in 30 min and last up to 6 h, and intermediate-acting insulin (NPH) begins to work 2 h after injection and will last up to 18 h. There is also long-acting insulin (glargine or detemir) that has no peak of activity and will last up to 24 h. This allows the patient to have a basal level of insulin much like a nondiabetic. A newer medication is pramlintide (Symlin), which is a synthetic hormone that is injected and works in conjunction with insulin to maintain blood glucose levels (Khardori 2015b). The type of insulin used must be tailored to each person. This is commonly based on eating habits, exercise schedule, and convenience.

CLINICAL TIPS

Diabetes Insipidus

Although it has the word *diabetes* in its title, diabetes insipidus is a rare metabolic condition affecting the fluid balance in the body and resulting in excessive urination (polyuria) and thirst (polydipsia). Although diabetes mellitus (both 1 DM and 2 DM) can display with polyuria and polydipsia, these two condition affect glucose metabolism. Patients with diabetes insipidus display typical glucose ranges but pass copious amounts of urine daily and can easily become dehydrated.

Athletes with type 1 diabetes need to carry testing strips and a glucometer to measure their blood sugar levels (figure 14.8). They must also carry their own insulin at all times. The athletic trainer must be thoroughly familiar with the type of insulin the athlete uses, the regular schedule of injections and dosage used, and proper storage and disposal of insulin and needles. Insulin should never be stored in extreme heat, in direct sunlight, or in an area with high or low temperatures, such as the glove compartment of a car or a freezer. It is common for some athletic events to last an entire day and for athletes not to have access to proper nutrition. Athletic trainers must encourage their diabetic athletes to relay blood sugar levels to them on a daily basis and more often if the situation warrants it. It is also crucial to carry an emergency supply of appropriate food and glucagon for the athlete with diabetes in the event of an emergency.

Type 1 diabetics must be aware of their blood sugar level before competition. Ideally, preparticipation blood sugar levels should range from 120 to 180 mg/dl. Participation is postponed for athletes with blood sugar above 200 mg/dl and ketones in their urine or blood sugar is over 300 mg/dl and supplemental insulin is administered. If the athlete's blood sugar level is less than 100 mg/dl, a preparticipation snack is administered. The reasoning for this is that without insulin, skeletal muscle does not take up glucose, and it will burn fat for energy, leading to ketoacidosis. Also, a diabetic cannot control the amount of circulating insulin in the blood, and the exercising muscle will use the insulin to take up the glucose, leading to hypoglycemia. Persons who exercise should be familiar with their blood glucose concentrations and how they vary with different types of activity to prevent hyperglycemia or hypoglycemia (Colberg et al. 2010; Harris and White 2012; Cheadle 2015).

There are many types of insulin on the market; rapid, intermediate, and long-acting human insulin are all used to treat diabetes. Although all of these could be beneficial in athletes, the choice depends on the type, intensity, and duration of the activity. Many people using insulin on a regular basis prefer to use continuous glucose monitors (CGMs), also called insulin pumps. The pump is a pager-sized device that can be worn on a belt and is attached by a soft plastic catheter in the skin (see figure 4.5). CGMs use subcutaneous sensors that measure interstitial glucose levels every 1 to 5 min, and they send alarms to notify the wearer when glucose levels are at either end of the spectrum (Khardori 2015a). The pump can administer regular basal doses of insulin as well as insulin needed around mealtimes. CGMs allow insulin to be given with the push of a button, and they omit the need for individual injections. They are no longer cumbersome, and advances in pump technology have provided pumps that can be worn even while swimming if placed in a waterproof pack. Although they are convenient, CGMs have some drawbacks. There is a lag time between measuring blood glucose levels with the pump and measuring with a fingertip stick, which can lead to overtreatment of hypoglycemia. CGMs should not be worn in contact sports because they can be damaged and because they can also injure the athletes or their competitors. A pump can be reconnected after the competition is over (Harris and White 2012). The FDA approved a sensor-augmented insulin pump (MiniMed530G with Enlite) that can be used by type 1 diabetics ages 16 and older (Khardori 2015a). Should blood glucose fall below a specified level, and the patient fails to deliver insulin, the pump will stop insulin delivery, which will prevent blood glucose falling even further. While it is 69% smaller than other units, it is also more accurate than earlier sensors (Tucker 2013).

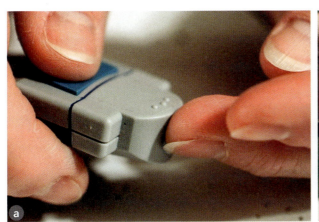
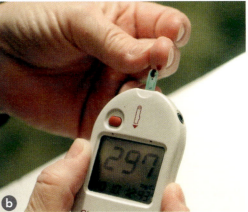

FIGURE 14.8 Using a glucometer, *(a)* the athlete pricks the distal side of his or her finger with a single-use needle and *(b)* places the resulting blood drop on a strip that inserts into the glucometer and registers the amount of glucose in the blood.

Type 2 Diabetes Mellitus

The treatment for type 2 diabetes is based on increased physical activity and proper nutrition. These two factors help everyone with the disease, and in the early stages, they may be the only treatment that is needed. If diet and exercise are not enough to control the patient's blood sugars, then medication is needed. Athletes with type 2 diabetes have access to an array of oral medications that can help control blood sugar levels. Medications called **sulfonylureas** are a first-line treatment for type 2 diabetes, but they may cause hypoglycemia, especially in those persons who are more active. These work by stimulating the beta cells of the pancreas to release insulin. Another class of agents is the **biguanides**, such as metformin, which decrease glucose production by the liver and reduce insulin resistance so that glucose is absorbed by the muscles (Khardori 2015b). Patients with impaired renal function are at risk for lactic acidosis, a potentially deadly side effect, when they take metformin, and it is therefore not recommended for them. The thiazolidinediones will increase insulin sensitivity in the muscle, liver, and adipose tissue, allowing for better deposition of glucose. Dipeptidyl peptidase (DPP)-4 inhibitors (Januvia) are a class of drugs that prevent the breakdown of glucagon-like peptide (GLP)-1, a gastrointestinal hormone that decreases blood glucose levels. GLP-1 is normally broken down quickly by DPP-4; DPP-4 inhibitors prevent this breakdown, thus decreasing blood glucose. A single agent or a combination of these agents may be needed to optimize treatment in each case. If these measures fail, insulin therapy may be needed (Khardori 2015b).

Although type 2 diabetes mellitus is rare in competitive athletes, it does happen in obese adolescents in shocking numbers. Athletic trainers caring for middle school and high school athletes should be aware of the treatment options for diabetics. Athletic trainers should also be aware of risky behavior that may occur in athletes engaging in certain sports. Some sports emphasize a certain body weight, and athletes may withhold insulin in order to decrease body weight rapidly to make their weight requirement; this can have deadly consequences (Harris and White 2012).

Thyroid Gland Disorders

The **thyroid gland** is an endocrine gland that lies anterior to the trachea in the neck and has an isthmus that joins two lateral lobes (figure 14.9). It is chiefly responsible for the synthesis of thyroxine (T_4) and triiodothyronine (T_3), reactions, which are stimulated by thyroid-stimulating hormone (TSH) from the anterior pituitary gland. The effects of thyroid hormones include protein synthesis in virtually every body tissue and increased oxygen consumption.

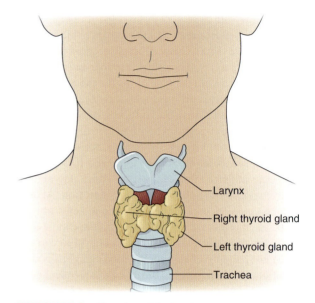

FIGURE 14.9   The thyroid gland.

Assessment of the thyroid gland involves palpation of the gland along the anterior aspect of the neck (figure 14.10). Correct finger placement is on the gland from an anterior approach while palpating for symmetry, swelling,

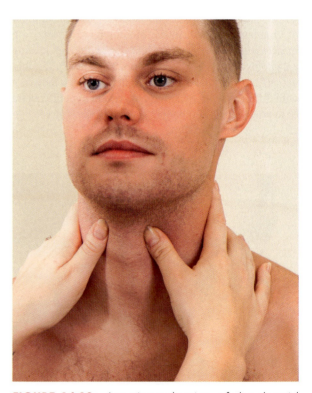

FIGURE 14.10   Anterior palpation of the thyroid gland; note that the right thumb displaces the trachea while the left is palpating for tenderness, swelling, or asymmetry.

edema, or pain. The trachea may be displaced laterally by one thumb while the other thumb assesses the gland. Typically, adults will not have a palpable thyroid gland. Abnormalities include enlarged lobes, tenderness, or lumps.

Hyperthyroidism

Hyperthyroidism is characterized by a hypermetabolic state that is caused by the excess production of thyroid hormones from the thyroid gland. It affects roughly 1 in 50 women and 1 in 500 men throughout their lifetimes, with a peak between ages 30 and 50 (Ferri 2016).

Hyperthyroidism is often called **Graves' disease** because Graves' disease is the cause of nearly 90% of all hyperthyroid cases (Ferri 2016). It is an autoimmune disorder characterized by a diffuse toxic **goiter**, or enlargement of the thyroid gland (figure 14.11). There is a familial predisposition to Graves' disease, but the exact etiology is unknown. It appears that an autoantibody forms and causes an imbalance in the production of TSH. Other causes of hyperthyroidism include a toxic multinodular goiter, toxic thyroid **adenoma**, subacute thyroiditis with transient hyperthyroidism, and factitious hyperthyroidism (Lee 2015).

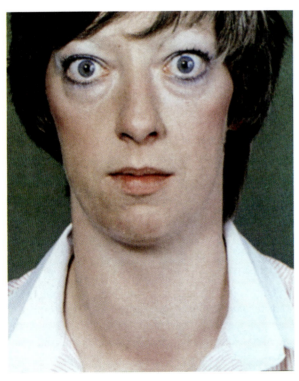

FIGURE 14.11   Hyperthyroidism is also called Graves' disease. Note the swelling in the thyroid region as well as the exophthalmos of the eyes.

Biophoto Associates / Science Source

Signs and Symptoms

The signs and symptoms of hyperthyroidism are vast. Common symptoms include an increased heart rate, heart palpitations, difficulty concentrating, shakiness, nervousness, gastrointestinal disturbances (excess gas, frequent normal bowel movements, or diarrhea), eyelid retraction, depression, menstrual irregularities, panic or anxiety attacks, weight loss despite a good appetite, and increased sweating (Ferri 2016). Athletes can also present with fatigue and muscle weakness leading to impaired performance.

The physical findings of hyperthyroidism include brisk reflexes, tremors, anxiety, reddening of the palms, an elevated heart rate, and occasionally an irregular heart rhythm such as atrial fibrillation. Patients will also usually have an enlarged or swollen thyroid gland. Because of swelling that accumulates behind the globe of the eye, patients may present with **exophthalmos** or a bulging out of the eyes (figure 14.12). Other eye symptoms include diplopia and blurred vision (Lee 2015).

The differential diagnoses of hyperthyroidism include anxiety, diabetes mellitus, myasthenia gravis, premenopausal state, metastatic neoplasms, and pheochromocytoma.

Referral and Diagnostic Tests

Athletes who appear to have an enlarged thyroid gland, bulging eyes, and symptoms associated with hyperthyroidism are referred to the team physician. Those with hyperthyroidism can be initially evaluated by their primary care physician and then referred to an endocrinologist who specializes in diseases of the thyroid if needed. A surgical referral may be needed if part of the

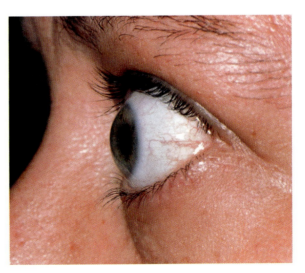

FIGURE 14.12   Exophthalmos associated with hyperthyroidism.

Dr P. Marazzi / Science Source

treatment would require removal of the thyroid gland. A patient who presents with an acute exacerbation of thyroiditis may need to be admitted to the hospital for further management.

The diagnosis of hyperthyroidism is usually made on the basis of a complete history, a physical examination, and a simple blood test to check the TSH level. If TSH is elevated, additional testing can be done, including a free T_3 index and a free T_4 index. These tests measure the thyroid hormone that is not bound to protein and is typically elevated in patients with hyperthyroidism. Because hyperthyroidism can be an autoimmune disorder, the autoimmune status of the patient is assessed via the enzyme-linked immunosorbent assay (ELISA) test (Lee 2015).

Imaging studies also can be performed to help differentiate types of hyperthyroidism. The test most often used is a 24 h radioactive iodine uptake (RAIU) scan (Ferri 2016). The radioactive iodine will be taken up by the thyroid gland and will have dissimilar appearances on the scan due to the differences in uptake by healthy and diseased tissues; it will help determine the underlying cause for the hyperthyroidism.

Treatment and Return to Participation

The treatment for hyperthyroidism centers on controlling the patient's symptoms and slowing the overactive thyroid gland. The three ways to manage the thyroid gland are medications, radioactive iodine, and thyroid surgery. To control symptoms, especially the increased heart rate and tremors associated with hyperthyroidism, patients are typically given β-blocker medications, also commonly used to treat hypertension. These medications are used in the acute presentation and are usually withdrawn after definitive treatment of the overactive thyroid (Lee 2015). Those taking care of athletes must know that β-blockers are banned substances in several governing bodies for sports such as archery and shooting.

Other medications typically used to treat hyperthyroidism include propylthiouracil (PTU) and methimazole. These medications inhibit the production of thyroid hormone. They are usually given for 6 to 24 mo and are typically used as adjunctive therapy before thyroid surgery or radioactive iodine treatment. While the patient is taking this medication, free T_3 and T_4 indexes are checked to determine how well the medication is working. Radioactive iodine ablation of the thyroid is common in the United States, and it is an effective and safe treatment for those patients who are not pregnant. A single dose of radioactive iodine will put roughly 80% of patients into a normal state (Lee 2015). Thyroid surgery is usually limited to those with very large goiters that may be causing obstruction, abnormal-appearing thyroid nodules, or pregnant women. It is rarely used in the United States because the other treatments are effective and, in general, have fewer adverse effects.

After successful treatment of hyperthyroidism, many people will need to take lifelong thyroid replacement therapy because the gland itself may be incapable of producing thyroid hormone. Patients with a history of treated hyperthyroidism must be checked annually with blood tests to determine the functional status of their thyroid. Return to full participation is generally not problematic.

Hypothyroidism

Hypothyroidism is a metabolic condition caused by thyroid hormone deficiency. It is more prevalent in women, has an increasing frequency with age, and occurs in about 1 of 300 people (Orlander 2015; Ferri 2016).

Of the many causes of hypothyroidism, 95% are classified as primary hypothyroidism, that is, the origin of the problem involves the thyroid itself. The most common cause of primary hypothyroidism is an inflammatory disorder of the thyroid gland called Hashimoto's thyroiditis. Hashimoto's is the most frequent cause of goiter in the United States and is characterized by a lymphocytic infiltration of the thyroid gland (Orlander 2015).

Another common cause of primary hypothyroidism is previous treatment for hyperthyroidism, such as radioactive iodine ablation or surgery to remove the thyroid. These treatments lead to intentional destruction of the thyroid gland; the patient then requires supplemental thyroid hormone replacement. In addition, medications such as lithium and interferon can cause hypothyroidism. The thyroid gland can be infiltrated by abnormal tissue caused by diseases, such as sarcoidosis and **amyloidosis**, which can then result in hypothyroidism.

Causes of secondary hypothyroidism include cancers of the pituitary or hypothalamus.

Signs and Symptoms

Hypothyroidism usually presents with signs and symptoms that develop over a prolonged period and represent a slowed metabolic state. The most common symptoms include weakness, fatigue, dry or coarse skin, cold intolerance, weight gain, and swelling of the tongue leading to thickened or slurred speech. Other symptoms include coarse, dry hair; hair loss; constipation; depression; a hoarse voice; carpal tunnel syndrome; and memory impairment (Orlander 2015; Porter and Kaplan 2011).

Active patients, especially those involved in athletics, may prove difficult to diagnose in the early stages of hypothyroidism because of common muscle fatigue and overuse injuries that may be attributed to delayed-onset muscle soreness.

Physical findings in hypothyroidism are nonspecific and include bradycardia (slow heart rate), low blood pressure, hair loss—especially the outer third of the eyebrows—dry skin, and decreased reflexes (Orlander 2015). The thyroid gland may feel enlarged on palpation.

The differential diagnoses for hypothyroidism are based primarily on the symptoms and includes depression, fibromyalgia, chronic fatigue syndrome, anemia, and viral infections such as infectious mononucleosis.

Referral and Diagnostic Tests

An athlete who has many musculoskeletal complaints, does not respond to typical treatments in the expected time frame, and experiences persistent, unexplained fatigue should be referred to a physician to rule out hypothyroidism.

Because of the vague symptoms of the initial stages of hypothyroidism, athletic trainers need to be suspicious of the possibility for this disease if no other plausible explanations exist. Evaluation for elevated TSH level is the first laboratory test for hypothyroidism. Determination of the free T_4 level can also help in the diagnosis and in differentiating between primary and secondary hypothyroidism (Orlander 2015). There are no imaging studies to aid in the diagnosis of primary hypothyroidism, but evaluation of the pituitary gland by MRI or ultrasound is appropriate when a secondary cause is suspected.

Treatment and Return to Participation

When the diagnosis is made, treatment can start by replacing thyroid hormone with levothyroxine. The starting dose is based on the patient's weight, age, and other medical problems. The dose can then be titrated, as needed, with the goal of returning TSH levels to normal ranges. Blood samples to check TSH levels should be drawn every 4 to 6 wk to help with the titration. The medication is generally safe but will need to be monitored, especially in older adults and in those with heart conditions because too much medication can elevate the heart rate and have deleterious effects on certain heart conditions (Orlander 2015).

The prognosis for patients with primary hypothyroidism and their prospects for a return to activity are excellent because the symptoms of the disorder improve immensely, if not completely, with medication. Follow-up to ensure the proper dosage of levothyroxine is imperative. The prognosis for patients with secondary hypothyroidism depends on the underlying cause.

Summary

Systemic disorders are not uncommon in the general population and are often accompanied by general maladies, such as body aches and fatigue. The challenge with active people is to distinguish exercise-related body aches from something more ominous. Persistent fatigue, body aches, weight loss, or slower-than-typical healing must alert the athletic trainer to conditions that may warrant referral to a physician. Many systemic disorders, once correctly diagnosed, can be effectively treated, allowing the athlete to continue participation in sports.

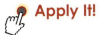 **Apply It!**   The case study for this chapter looks at a middle school cross country runner dealing with unexplained weight loss and constant thirst. Read the scenario and answer the questions at www.HumanKinetics.com/MedicalConditionsInTheAthlete.

15

Infectious Diseases

At the completion of this chapter the reader should be able to do the following:

- Explain how infections are commonly transmitted and how to prevent transmission.
- Justify the importance of maintaining immunity against those diseases for which there is vaccine.
- Describe the reporting rationales for communicable diseases.
- List the signs and symptoms of common infectious diseases.
- Recognize common childhood diseases and explain how to prevent them.
- Demonstrate universal precautions for the prevention and transmission of infectious disease.

Nearly every chapter in this text addresses an infectious condition: sinusitis in the chapter on disorders of the ear, nose, mouth, and throat; urinary tract infection in the chapter on genitourinary and gynecological system; and pneumonia in the chapter on respiratory disorders. This chapter provides an overview of the infectious disease process that includes common transmission mechanisms and routes, as well as preventive measures that can be used to stop the infectious cycle and protect athletes and the population at large. The conditions discussed in this chapter include many common childhood diseases in addition to hepatitis, streptococcal, staphylococcal, and neurological infections. Sexually transmitted infections (STIs) are discussed in chapter 10.

Transmission

Most infections arise from one of four transmission routes: airborne, direct contact, bloodborne, or water- and foodborne. Sick people can spread infectious organisms by these pathways, so sanitary precautions are the most important line of defense in preventing illness. Healthy humans live in harmony with microbial flora that protect against the invasion of disease-causing microorganisms (Porter and Kaplan 2011). These flora reside in specific organs of the body, such as the skin, respiratory system, and gastrointestinal tract, and they help to protect these organs' natural environments. Certain medications can disrupt this balance, as can repeated exposure to infectious organisms in an overtrained athlete. Many flora that protect humans can also do a turnabout and invade their hosts under certain conditions. Disease transmission routes are discussed with each disorder.

Nosocomial Infections

A **nosocomial infection** is one that is acquired in the athletic training facility or medical facility and is unrelated to the athlete's purpose for the visit. Many infections and illnesses discussed in this text can be acquired in the athletic training setting from other athletes or personnel. They include influenza, sinusitis, conjunctivitis, and certain staphylococcal and streptococcal infections.

Prevention

Preventing infectious conditions is largely common sense. There are many vaccines available that are dependable, effective, and have minimal, if any, side effects. There are no robust, data-driven published studies that tie vaccines to life-long sequelae, and people who do not get vaccinated are at risk for developing the condition the immunization was intended to prevent. Sometimes, well-meaning parents mitigate the vaccination's effectiveness by providing infants and children with Tylenol or a similar medication to alleviate side effects of the shot. Some evidence suggests that follow-up booster vaccinations may be required in certain circumstances.

Good personal hygiene is also critical in preventing the spread of disease. Often the simple practice of hand washing with soap and water can deter an infection or disease from spreading. Finally, proper nutrition and rest help to keep the body resistant to conditions that seek opportunities to infect those who may be worn down.

Vaccination

Practicing universal precautions and sanitation measures (see chapter 1) can prevent the transmission of most infectious diseases. In addition, immunization, such as the MMR vaccine for measles, mumps, and rubella, has deterred the spread of many adult and childhood diseases.

Researchers continue to provide new vaccines in the hope of preventing infectious diseases. In recent years, vaccines have been approved and distributed to prevent meningitis, human papillomavirus (HPV), and varicella (chicken pox). Colleges often require proof of meningitis vaccination before admission, and pediatricians are encouraging 12- to 15-year-old girls to take the three-shot series that may prevent future cervical cancer that can be caused by HPV. A varicella vaccine was approved in 1995, and studies indicate that a two-dose series was warranted in order for the vaccine to truly be effective. It was recommended in 1996 that all children receive the two-

dose immunization for full immunity (Porter and Kaplan 2011; Centers for Disease Control and Prevention 2016c). Adults are not exempt from immunizations. In addition to pneumonia vaccine for those over age 65 and annual influenza protection, the Food and Drug Administration (FDA) recommended in 2008 that adults over age 60 be vaccinated to prevent varicella-zoster (shingles) (Centers for Disease Control and Prevention 2016c; Porter and Kaplan 2011).

Some adults missed the window of opportunity for certain immunizations because they were born before these immunizations became available. For example, an effective vaccine for hepatitis B virus (HBV) was not established until 1982. Immunization against HPV is also an example, as 13- to 26-year-old females are encouraged to complete the series if they missed their window of opportunity (Centers for Disease Control and Prevention 2015a). Adults who were not immunized as children and who have no history of a particular disease should be vaccinated as adults, especially if they work in areas where they would be susceptible to the disease. Figures 15.1 and 15.2 provide the recommended schedules for vaccination for children and adults.

Children are no longer routinely vaccinated for smallpox because this disease has not been found in humans for more than a generation. Other communicable diseases, such as typhus, botulism, *Escherichia coli,* polio, and anthrax, are not common but are extremely dangerous if contracted (Sifton 2002). The danger with rare and dormant diseases is that they do still live in some laboratories, and terrorist attacks have made many people aware that releasing these organisms could initiate global germ warfare. Because few people are currently vaccinated against these dormant, yet deadly, diseases, their rapid spread is plausible (Sifton 2002). The same is true with vaccine-preventable diseases. Those who choose to forgo available immunizations put themselves at risk should the disease reoccur.

Due to the threat of germ warfare, there are vaccines for typhoid and yellow fever, but they are not widely used. These are typically available for persons traveling to countries where the contagion is more common than in the United States, and there are significant side effects,

Records of Immunization

Immunization records with proof of vaccination against communicable diseases are required for entrance into most public schools and colleges. Some colleges now require proof of vaccination against meningococcal infections, which tend to affect college students living in dormitories.

These recommendations must be read with the footnotes that follow. For those who fall behind or start late, provide catch-up vaccination at the earliest opportunity as indicated by the green bars in Figure 1. To determine minimum intervals between doses, see the catch-up schedule (Figure 2). School entry and adolescent vaccine age groups are shaded.

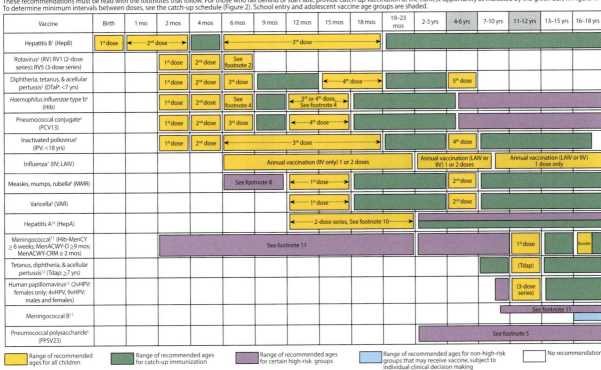

FIGURE 15.1 Recommended childhood immunization schedule.

Reprinted from Centers for Disease Control and Prevention, www.cdc.gov/vaccines/schedules/hcp/imz/child-adolescent.html.

especially for certain populations. Smallpox is another available vaccination that has many contraindications as well as tedious instructions for weeks following the immunization (Centers for Disease Control and Prevention 2016i).

U.S. public health officials established a goal through the Healthy People 2010 program to eliminate diphtheria, hepatitis B, measles, mumps, polio, rubella, varicella, and tetanus by the year 2010 (Healthy People 2016). However, immunity after vaccination is not always guaranteed. Of the 6,584 people who contracted mumps in the outbreak of 2006, 77% to 97% of the college students who acquired the illness had received the required two-dose MMR (mumps/measles/rubella) vaccine shots (Anderson and Seward 2008; Huang, Cortese, and Curns 2009). The updated Healthy People 2020 continues to promote healthier behaviors, including immunization and other more current issues (Healthy People 2016).

With prevention being paramount, health histories typically include immunization records. However, in a

study of the immune status of first-year medical students in New South Wales, Australia, it was discovered that immunity corresponded poorly with the self-reported histories. Tests were done to determine the students' antibody titers to certain vaccine-preventable diseases; results showed that their antibody titers were inadequate to protect them from future infection. Other articles provided evidence for what many parents already know: Giving an infant acetaminophen (Tylenol) to reduce fever caused by an immunization actually reduces the effect of the vaccine (Chen, Clark, and Halperin 2009; Oldfield and Stewart 2016). This research may shed light on why so many previously immunized people have had less than the desired benefit of the vaccine later in life.

Although there may be little debate among health care providers over recommended vaccines, not all agencies have adopted minimal standards for immunization, leaving it to institutional autonomy or state authority. Even the Commission on Accreditation of Athletic Training Education (CAATE) standards (number 66) only call

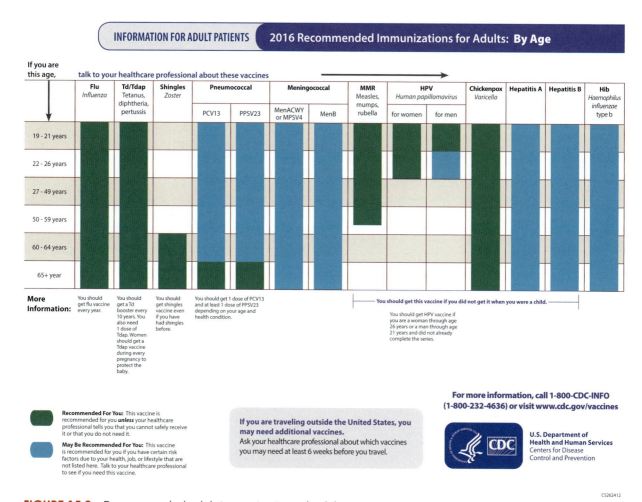

FIGURE 15.2 Recommended adult immunization schedule.

Reprinted from Centers for Disease Control and Prevention 2016c.

for "…documentation of immunizations appropriate for health care providers…" for athletic training students; they do not articulate from what diseases the students should be immune (CAATE 2015). Interestingly, according to the CDC, only 60% of health care workers in the United States have completed the three-series hepatitis B vaccine (Centers for Disease Control and Prevention 2016c; Shefer et al. 2011).

Annual Immunization

An annual influenza shot for health care workers, older adults, children, and those with weakened immune systems has become an important health care benchmark each fall (Centers for Disease Control and Prevention 2016d). The seasonal influenza shot is usually targeted for a specific type of influenza; it does not provide global immunity against all types of influenza. Typically, influenza A and B cause seasonal epidemics in the winter months in the United States (Centers for Disease Control

and Prevention 2016d). Each of these flus has subtypes and a slightly different physiological makeup. Vaccines are created annually to deter the viruses, but these illnesses have been known to alter themselves genetically to better fit a host. When this occurs, the vaccine becomes ineffective against the new strain. The two most common influenza vaccines are the inactivated influenza vaccine (IIV) and the live attenuated influenza vaccine (LAIV). The former is administered via an intramuscular injection, whereas the LAIV is a nasal spray that provides a small amount of a live virus. The "FluMist" nasal spray has some contraindications. Those with chronic respiratory conditions or sinusitis must receive the injectable version instead because of potential complications from the inhalation of the live virus. The live virus usually creates some flu-like symptoms within a few days of administration, whereas the injected variety does not. Because seasonal influenza most often strikes in the winter months (typically between October and March), it is recommended that patients receive their annual dose in

October to provide full-season coverage that lasts through mid-spring (Centers for Disease Control and Prevention 2016d; Grohskopf et al. 2015).

As was previously mentioned, airborne transmission and direct contact are two ways to infect others with communicable diseases. The close surroundings of athletic huddles, time-outs, locker rooms, and team buses present many opportunities to spread infections among team members (Howe 2003). However, common sense precautions can help prevent infections from being transmitted. The basic practices of personal hygiene are underappreciated in the fight against the spread of disease. Simple habits of frequent hand washing, covering one's mouth or nose when coughing or sneezing, showering with quality antibacterial soap, and protecting the skin, including good feet care, are all examples of personal responsibility in hygiene that can be practiced in all walks of life (Lam, Dawson, and Fowler 2015). Athletes with infections are isolated while they are contagious, and any equipment or clothing that they have worn is sanitized before the next use.

Methods of protection against disease that could affect the whole team include safeguarding the water source and containers and sanitizing surfaces that athletes have contact with, such as treatment tables, mats, and rehabilitation equipment. Certain states have regulations about the type of hose that may be used to draw potable (drinkable) water. These regulations may be found at the state's health website or at the U.S. Occupational Safety and Health Administration (OSHA) website. When sanitizing equipment, surfaces, and water containers, such as coolers, ice containers, and water bottles, a solution of 1:100 ratio of bleach to water is effective as a germicidal agent (Howe 2003).

It is not difficult to prevent the spread of many of the infectious diseases discussed in this chapter. Compliance with preventive immunization programs when available can be followed up with good hygiene, sanitation, and the practice of universal precautions.

Reporting Communicable Diseases

The health care provider has a legal obligation to report certain medical conditions to the public health authorities, such as some sexually transmitted infections (STIs) or tuberculosis. The rationale behind reporting these conditions is to protect the public from an outbreak of the disease; the courts have ruled that for certain medical conditions, the risks of exposure outweigh the patient's right to privacy. Local, state, and national agencies review the lists of reportable diseases and report them to the proper authority when diagnosed by physicians or in laboratories (U.S. National Library of Medicine 2016).

In the United States, the National Notifiable Diseases Surveillance System (NNDSS) is used to report commu-

nicable diseases from all public health agencies. When a physician has confirmed a certain infectious disease, the disease but not the person is reported to the appropriate agency (U.S. National Library of Medicine 2016; Centers for Disease Control and Prevention 2015d). NNDSS works in collaboration with agencies to monitor, control, and prevent the spread of communicable diseases. On rare occasions, such as with an STI, the infectious person is identified, and any partners who may have been infected are contacted.

The purpose of reporting communicable diseases is twofold: to isolate a given disease and retard its spread and to generate data about current disease trends so they may be prevented in the future. Our discussion of the reporting system will focus on the local level. Basic reporting involves both individual cases and epidemics.

Local health officials, in conjunction with state and federal agencies, decide which individual cases are to be routinely reported and develop policies for collecting, documenting, and reporting the information. Physicians and other health care workers with knowledge of a reportable illness are required by law to report it. Hospitals generally have a specific officer who handles such reports; smaller medical clinics often have similar protocols, policies, and procedures for reporting communicable diseases. Minimal data for these reports include the patient's name, address, diagnosis, age, gender, and date of report. The right to privacy is paramount, but so is the right of the community to prevent the spread of a communicable disease and to protect unsuspecting people. Collective reports can simply list the number of cases for a given disease in a specific time frame. Diseases and conditions that are considered reportable vary by state, and state public health organizations are encouraged to enter cases into NNDSS (Centers for Disease Control and Prevention 2015d).

Pandemic

The term *pandemic* refers to an illness that affects an exceptionally high proportion of the population in a wide geographic area. Pandemics in modern history

CLINICAL TIPS

Comparing an Epidemic to a Pandemic

An epidemic is a (usually sudden) increase in the number of cases of a disease or condition beyond what is expected in a given region; a pandemic is an epidemic that has spread to a multitude of countries or continents (Centers for Disease Control and Prevention 2015d).

include human immunodeficiency virus (HIV) and the "swine flu." Pandemics are infectious diseases that cross continents; seasonal flus are not included. Historically significant pandemics include cholera, typhus, smallpox, measles, tuberculosis, leprosy, malaria, and yellow fever. A disease must meet three criteria to be called a pandemic by the World Health Organization (WHO) (Kelly 2011):

- Nearly simultaneous transmission occurs worldwide or is rapidly spread worldwide.
- It infects humans, causing serious illness.
- It is easily spread and sustained among humans.

The reason some illnesses (e.g., avian flu) are not pandemics is that they do not have easily sustainable human-to-human transmission.

Influenza

In the United States, seasonal influenza has caused approximately 49,000 deaths and 200,000 hospitalizations each year. Ninety percent of the deaths and 60% of the hospitalizations are of adults over age 65 (Centers for Disease Control and Prevention 2016d). In 2015, approximately 83% of the U.S. population met the criteria to undergo vaccination to prevent the common forms of influenza, yet less than 40% received the influenza vaccine (Centers for Disease Control and Prevention 2016d). The percentage of deaths due to influenza and pneumonia exceeded epidemic levels for the years 2013 through 2015 (Appiah et al. 2015).

The two main human influenza viruses that cause epidemics each year are the A and B viruses, but influenza A is further broken down into subcategories. Influenza A is labeled for two proteins, hemagglutinin (H) and neuraminidase (N). Within each protein are subtypes that generate viruses named H1 though H18 and N1 through N11 (Centers for Disease Control and Prevention 2014b). Influenza B is not subdivided. The CDC adheres to internationally approved methods for naming influenza viruses. The name depends on the following:

- Antigen type (e.g., A, B)
- Host of origin (e.g., swine, bird, equine)
- Geographic origin (e.g., Taiwan, Denver)
- Year of isolation (e.g., 2009, 2014)
- Protein type for influenza A (e.g., H1N1, H3N2) (Centers for Disease Control and Prevention 2014b)

One popular influenza variant that has surfaced periodically throughout the world is swine flu. Originally detected in 1976, it was transmitted from pigs to humans, and in 2009, another outbreak occurred, this time attributed to the H1N1 influenza virus. H1N1 was labeled a pandemic by the WHO in June 2009, and by July, there were more than 94,000 confirmed cases in more than 100 countries (Cutler et al. 2009). H1N1 is different enough from the 1976 strain of swine flu that those who were vaccinated in 1976 were most likely not immune to the H1N1 virus of 2009 (Centers for Disease Control and Prevention 2015b).

Avian influenza (bird flu) was first discovered in 1997 in Hong Kong, and outbreaks in humans occurred in China in 2003. There are now three main varietals categorized with nine subtypes in each influenza A: H5, H7, and H9. Each is represented with H5N1 to H5N9, with the first number changing to represent varietal 7 or 9, as the proteins have changed slightly and create different strains. The bird flu is not easily transmitted between humans and therefore does not pose a threat for a pandemic. The purpose of identifying the strains of influenza is to determine which vaccine to create to protect against the projected virus for the coming season. Each February, WHO collaborates with over 100 countries to review the influenza viruses reported for the preceding year. From these data, laboratories create a vaccine to prevent the most common influenza strains identified. In 2016, a vaccine was created to protect against influenza A H1N1, H3N2 and influenza B/Phuket, but this vaccine may not be effective after that year due to changes in the influenza strains (Centers for Disease Control and Prevention 2015e).

Signs and Symptoms

Signs and symptoms of influenza include fever, cough, sore throat, body ache, headache, stuffy nose, chills, and fatigue. People are contagious from 1 d before the onset of symptoms until up to 7 d after they realize they are sick. For referral and diagnostic tests and treatment and return-to-participation guidelines for the flu, please see chapter 7.

Infectious Mononucleosis

Infectious **mononucleosis (mono)** has also been called the *kissing disease* because it is easily transmitted by oropharyngeal contact. Caused by the Epstein-Barr virus (EBV), mononucleosis is a common occurrence in college-aged athletes, but 50% of children have also shown serologic evidence of the infection by age 5 (Cunha 2015). There is some speculation that chronic fatigue syndrome is associated with a chronic EBV infection, but little evidence supports this theory (Porter and Kaplan 2011).

The EBV is a herpesvirus that attacks lymphocytes and nasopharyngeal cells. It is found in oropharyngeal saliva secretions of up to 25% of healthy, nonsymptomatic adults. Despite its reputation as the kissing disease, it is not a particularly contagious disease, as only 5% of patients have a recent history of contact with an infected person (Porter and Kaplan 2011). For reported direct exposure, the incubation period is 10 to 50 d. Nevertheless, athletes are warned to avoid sharing drinking cups and putting their mouths on common water bottle spouts.

Signs and Symptoms

The chief signs and symptoms of infectious mononucleosis are fatigue, pharyngitis, fever, and **lymphadenopathy**, but not all signs and symptoms are present in every patient. Often, the first complaint is of overwhelming fatigue and the inability to get enough sleep. The athlete will feel run down or will experience a sore throat. Other manifestations include tonsillitis, hepatomegaly, jaundice, and a **maculopapular rash** (Cunha 2015).

Splenomegaly (figure 15.3) is present in 50% of mononucleosis cases and is most prevalent in the second and third weeks of the disease (Porter and Kaplan 2011). A blow to the left ribs of an athlete with splenomegaly can rupture the spleen, causing a life-threatening emergency if the injury is not quickly recognized and treated.

Although 10% of patients experience hepatomegaly, or an enlarged liver, with infectious mononucleosis, it does not carry the severe ramifications that splenomegaly does in athletes. There are hepatic complications because hepatocellular enzyme levels are elevated two to three times normal in 95% of patients, and they can take as long as 1 mo to return to normal levels (Porter and Kaplan 2011).

Other potential complications due to mononucleosis are related to the central nervous system (CNS), including seizures, peripheral neuropathy, aseptic meningitis, meningitis, cranial nerve palsy, and Guillain-Barré syndrome (Porter and Kaplan 2011).

🚩 RED FLAGS FOR SPLENOMEGALY

Splenomegaly is a possible side effect of mononucleosis, which causes the spleen to enlarge and protrude out from under the normal protection of the lower left ribs. Unprotected, the spleen is susceptible to injury and rupture from athletic activity. An unrecognized ruptured spleen is life-threatening.

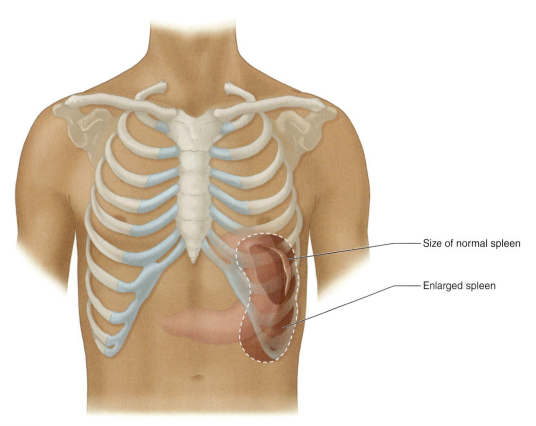

Size of normal spleen

Enlarged spleen

FIGURE 15.3 Splenomegaly, an enlargement of the spleen, is sometimes associated with acute infections such as mononucleosis.

Group A α-hemolytic streptococci, cytomegalovirus (CMV), hepatitis B, rubella, and primary HIV infection are all options to consider and rule out when diagnosing mononucleosis.

Referral and Diagnostic Tests

An athlete who presents with a history of malaise combined with a sore throat and a fever should be referred to a physician, especially if the symptoms are present for a number of days.

Athletes suspected of having infectious mononucleosis will often present with mild **leukocytosis**, which is also common in a number of other illnesses (Porter and Kaplan 2011). A strong indicator for EBV includes a blood count indicating **lymphocytosis**; a low or falling hematocrit is suggestive of splenic rupture (Ferri 2016). A more specific blood test, the heterophile antibody test, more commonly called a monospot, is based on agglutination, or clumping, of erythrocytes. This screening test is reliable in up to 90% of patients and is usually positive within 4 wk of onset. However, the monospot test may not be sensitive to the presence of Epstein-Barr virus in the early days after infection (Cunha 2015). False-positive monospot results can occur in the context of other diseases, such as lymphoma, autoimmune disease, HIV, and hepatitis (Porter and Kaplan 2011).

Treatment and Return to Participation

The standard treatment for mononucleosis is rest and hydration, although complete bed rest is not recommended. More than 95% of patients recover with symptomatic treatment alone.

Research has shown that there is no effective pharmacological treatment for infectious mononucleosis (Porter and Kaplan 2011; Cunha 2015). However, if the pharyngitis is such that it warrants medication, corticosteroids have been shown to relieve pain and prevent airway compromise from swelling. To assist in the management of body aches and fever, acetaminophen is preferred over aspirin because of aspirin's association with **Reye's syndrome** (Porter and Kaplan 2011). In addition, athletes would be wise to avoid prolonged use of nonsteroidal anti-inflammatory drugs (NSAIDs) during the illness because of the hepatic complications already associated with mononucleosis.

Athletes must be sure they are reconditioned for sport before they return to competition. Those in contact or collision sports may need 1 mo or more to recover enough to allow the spleen to again fit behind the rib cage for adequate protection. Physicians must consider the details of each case before allowing a full return to activity. A swimmer may return to full activity rather quickly, whereas a diver may still be in danger of spleen injury with a premature return.

Return to full participation depends on the type of sport (noncontact, contact, collision), the return to appropriate fitness levels, and control of symptoms. There is no strong evidence that either physical examination or ultrasonography can reliably determine if the spleen has returned to normal size, so these measurements should be used with caution (Becker and Smith 2014; Waninger and Harcke 2005). Serial ultrasonography, however, has been found to be useful in determining the spleen's gradual return to normal size following mononucleosis (O'Connor et al. 2011).

Mumps

Mumps is a contagious viral disease that manifests with enlarged parotid and salivary glands and on occasion involves the sublingual or submaxillary glands as well (figure 15.4). It presents as an acute epidemic that peaks in late winter or early spring and chiefly involves 5- to 15-year-old children. Children younger than 2 are typically immune (Porter and Kaplan 2011). A national immunization campaign was intended to eradicate the disease by 2010, but with a 2006 outbreak in the Midwest involving more than 6,500 people, it appears the disease is still present in the United States. The two-dose childhood vaccination was not sufficient to prevent the disease for many (Anderson and Seward 2008; Huang, Cortese, and Curns 2009).

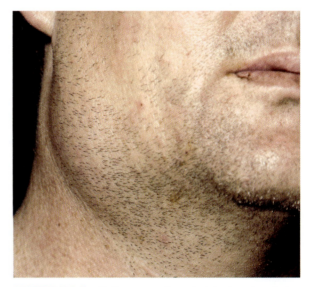

FIGURE 15.4 Salivary and parotid glands of the mouth and neck can become rapidly and painfully inflamed as a result of mumps; note the swelling anterior to the lower earlobe.

Dr P. Marazzi / Science Source

Mumps has a 2 to 3 wk incubation period and is spread through the air via infected droplets as well as through direct contact with contaminated saliva. It has been found in saliva 1 to 6 d before onset and up to 9 d after glandular swelling. The disease has been found in the urine 6 d before **parotitis** (inflammation of the parotid salivary glands) and 15 d afterward. In addition, the virus may be isolated in symptomatic patients' blood (Porter and Kaplan 2011).

Signs and Symptoms

The chief signs and symptoms of mumps include parotitis, headache, low-grade fever, malaise, anorexia, vomiting, and **nuchal rigidity** in the posterior neck. Common symptoms also include pain with chewing and swallowing, especially swallowing acidic drinks or foods such as orange juice, pickles, or lemons. Within 24 h of onset of these signs and symptoms, the parotid glands swell and become sensitive to palpation. Initially, it is not unusual for only one gland to become swollen, with the second following about 2 d later. An athlete generally presents with asymmetry in the face and jaw caused by the unilateral swelling of the parotid gland. The enlargement of the glands can extend from in front of to below the ear, and the associated skin can become tight and shiny because of the pressure of the swelling.

The complications of mumps include orchitis, oophoritis, **meningoencephalitis**, and pancreatitis. Postpubertal males may experience testicular inflammation, which is typically unilateral. Although this can occur in up to 50% of the adult males with mumps, it is rarely associated with infertility, but it can lead to testicular atrophy in 50% of the cases (Yohannes 2015). CNS involvement is relatively uncommon and most often manifests as meningitis or encephalitis, which occur in up to 15% of cases (Yohannes 2015; Defendi 2016). Encephalitis is thought to be an autoimmune response producing demyelination and has an onset 7 to 10 d after parotitis.

In females, oophoritis occurs in 5% of postpubertal women with mumps and is more difficult to diagnose; however, it rarely results in fertility issues (Ferri 2016; Porter and Kaplan 2011). Exposure to mumps within the first trimester of pregnancy may induce spontaneous abortion (Porter and Kaplan 2011; Yohannes 2015).

Because the patient with mumps has a headache, stiff neck, and sometimes low (20 to 40 mg/dl) cerebrospinal fluid (CSF) glucose levels, it is often mistaken for bacterial meningitis. Fifteen percent of patients with mumps experience CNS involvement but only 1% to 10% manifest symptoms. Although permanent damage, such as deafness or facial paralysis is unusual, it may result from mumps with CNS involvement.

The differential diagnoses for mumps include streptococcal throat infection, encephalitis, meningitis, dental caries, influenza A, leukemia, **lymphosarcoma**, malignant and benign tumors of the salivary glands, and an obstructed duct in the parotid gland. Epididymitis, orchitis, and ovarian torsion may also be considered (Yohannes 2015).

Referral and Diagnostic Tests

Patients who present with swollen salivary glands, malaise, or a low-grade fever are referred to a physician. The diagnosis is largely based on signs and symptoms coupled with a history of recent exposure. Atypical presentations require laboratory confirmation, usually by culturing the mumps virus or discovering the mumps immunoglobulin M (IgM) antibody (Yohannes 2015).

Treatment and Return to Participation

A person with mumps should be isolated from others until parotid swelling returns to normal. Treatment of the disease is based on the person's symptoms. Over-the-counter analgesics or antipyretics are used as necessary to alleviate headache and fever. Patients should avoid acidic foods and beverages and maintain a soft diet to lessen the need for **mastication**. Because mumps is typically a self-limited disease, most patients recover without pharmacological intervention (Yohannes 2015; Ferri 2016).

Because most of the symptoms (e.g., fever, malaise, vomiting, nuchal rigidity, parotitis) seem to resolve within 3 to 10 d, long-term absence from athletic participation is not typical. It is more important to prevent the spread of infection.

Prevention

A vaccine for mumps is available that causes little systemic reaction. The live virus vaccine, introduced in the United States in 1967, is administered alone or in combination with mumps, measles, and rubella (MMR) vaccine. It is generally administered any time after the first year of life but most typically between 12 and 15 mo of age. Current recommendations include a second dose between ages 4 and 6 (Centers for Disease Control and Prevention 2016c).

Rubeola

Also known simply as "measles" or "red measles," **rubeola** is one of the most highly communicable infectious diseases. Before immunization was available, more than 90% of the population was infected by the age of 20 (Chen 2015). Since immunization was introduced, measles cases have dropped 99%, with the residual in the United States attributed to unimmunized or underimmunized children who have had only one shot. By the year 2000, measles was said to be eliminated in the United States (Chen 2015; Centers for Disease Control and Prevention 2016e). There have been measles outbreaks in the United States since 2010, but they are largely attributed to travelers to the country spreading the virus to unvaccinated residents (Chen 2015; Centers for Disease Control and Prevention 2016e). There are also outbreaks elsewhere in the world, with China (131,441 reported cases in 2008) and Japan (11,015) leading Western Europe in outbreaks (Centers for Disease Control and Prevention 2008). The resurgence of measles has been attributed to living in remote communities, misinformation about the vaccine, cultural factors, and insufficient vaccine coverage.

Measles is spread through airborne droplets from nasal or throat secretions of infected people. A lesser means of transmission is through direct contact with soiled articles such as towels, which may contain secretions from those already sick. The incubation period is typically 10 d, but it can range from 7 to 17d. Measles is most contagious from the 3–5 d before the rash erupts through 4 d after eruption (Chen 2015).

Signs and Symptoms

Most often, a rash is the manifestation of rubeola, and it appears after a **prodromal** fever, most often in the third to seventh day of the disease. The erythematous rash begins on the face before spreading to the body proper and lasts approximately 4 to 7 d. Other signs and symptoms of measles include conjunctivitis, cough, **leukopenia**, headache, fever, and sore throat. Leukopenia will be present beginning with the onset of the rash largely because of a decrease in lymphocytes. Complications can occur as measles suppresses the immune system, allowing opportunistic conditions to take hold. Common infections arising from the disease include sinusitis, otitis media, pneumonia, encephalitis, diarrhea, and laryngotracheobronchitis, or keratitis, which can lead to blindness (Chen 2015; Centers for Disease Control and Prevention 2015c).

Differential diagnoses for rubeola are rubella, mononucleosis, influenza, Rocky Mountain spotted fever, and allergic rhinitis. Many childhood diseases have similar presentations and are often the differential diagnoses of each other. Table 15.1 compares several childhood diseases.

Referral and Diagnostic Tests

People with a rash indicative of measles are referred for further evaluation. Likewise, those with signs or symptoms of measles before the onset of the rash, such as sore throat, fever, cough, conjunctivitis, or recent exposure, must be referred to a physician. A recent history of measles vaccine does not preclude one from contracting measles. Therefore, a recently immunized person who shows signs or symptoms of the disease needs to be referred immediately to a physician.

A diagnosis of measles can be confirmed by the presence of a measles-specific IgM antibody in the blood, which presents itself 3 to 4 d after onset of the measles rash. A nasopharyngeal swab is also used to identify the antigen but is less commonly done than the blood test (Centers for Disease Control and Prevention 2015c).

Treatment and Return to Participation

Because no antiviral remedy for measles is currently available, the best treatment is supportive and symptomatic care. Rubeola is largely a self-limiting disease, but analgesics and antipyretics may help alleviate symptoms associated with the illness (Chen 2015). If the patient has accompanying bacterial complications, such as conjunctivitis, otitis, sinusitis, or pneumonia, antibacterial therapy may be warranted.

Mortality rates for measles are low, but pneumonia and encephalitis are complications of the disease in children under age 5. For athletes, activity during the contagious stages is discouraged.

Prevention and Public Health Implications

Measles is one of the most easily communicable diseases and one of the most deadly childhood illnesses, yet it is vaccine-preventable (World Health Organization 2015a). People born after 1957 are encouraged to be immunized

TABLE 15.1 Comparison of Childhood Infectious Diseases

Disease	Incubation (wk)	Mode of transmission	Duration of symptoms
Mononucleosis	2–3	Saliva, air droplets	Up to several months
Mumps	2–3	Saliva, air droplets	Up to 10 d
Rubeola	1–2	Airborne, direct contact	4–7 d
Rubella	2–3	Respiratory secretions, placental blood	3 d
Varicella	2–3	Direct contact, respiratory secretions	1 wk

for measles. A single injection of the live measles virus is often administered in conjunction with two other live viruses, mumps and rubella, and it reduces susceptibility to measles by 94% to 98%; a second dose may elevate immunity to 99% (Centers for Disease Control and Prevention 2009). The two-dose vaccine is recommended to offset the possibility of immunization failure. Most often, the MMR initial dose is given at age 12 to 15 mo, with the second dose administered at the onset of school (ages 4 to 6), although if exposure risk is high, the second dose can be delivered as soon as 4 wk after the first.

Measles is a reportable disease. Reporting to the local agency within 24 h of diagnosis can improve chances of controlling the spread of the disease. Typically, patients are not quarantined, but it is a good idea to isolate school-aged children and athletes while they are contagious.

Rubella

Rubella, once known as *German measles,* and also called *three-day measles*, is an acute contagious virus that has mild symptoms in children and adults but can cause death or profound congenital defects in infants born to mothers infected during the first trimester of pregnancy. In the United States in 1969, nearly 58,000 rubella cases were reported, but since 2001, there have been fewer than 20 per year, largely due to vaccination. Internationally, rubella still exists, as there were over 304,000 cases reported in Europe in 2003 (Ezike 2014).

Rubella is acquired through the upper respiratory tract or through placental blood exchange with a mother infected in early pregnancy. Exposure to rubella during pregnancy can cause spontaneous abortion, stillbirths, or can have other profound effects on the fetus. Babies born with congenital defects caused by maternal rubella are said to have congenital rubella syndrome (CRS) and number 100,000 annually worldwide (World Health Organization 2015b). Obviously, great care must be taken to ensure that pregnant women are safeguarded from exposure.

Signs and Symptoms

Rubella has a 12 to 24 d incubation period, and infected patients present with low-grade fever (less than 38.3 °C [101 °F]) that is often transient, a mild rash, lymphadenopathy, conjunctivitis, cough, headache, and joint pain (arthralgia). The rash usually lasts 2 to 3 d and is a blotchy eruption that has its origin on the face and spreads to the trunk and limbs (figure 15.5) (Ferri 2016; Mayo Clinic 2016; Ezike 2014). Mild rose-colored spots may appear on the palate, and although the pharynx may be bright red, the throat is not typically sore. Swelling of specific glands, including the suboccipital, postauricular, and postcervical glands, precedes the rash by 5 to 10 d and

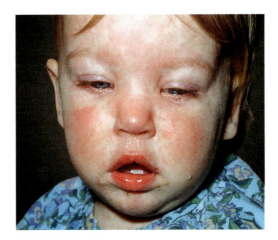

FIGURE 15.5   Rubella lesions.
Biophoto Associates / Science Source

may be first noted by the patient when washing his or her hair or as an athlete is putting on a helmet. On occasion, the patient has splenomegaly and hepatitis in conjunction with the rash. Arthritis can be involved as a complication, especially in adult females (Porter and Kaplan 2011).

Differential diagnoses of rubella include allergic reactions, scarlet fever, secondary syphilis, mononuclear viral infections, and Kawasaki's disease (see chapter 8).

Referral and Diagnostic Tests

Any unimmunized person with a history of exposure to rubella who presents with symptoms of the disease is referred to a physician for confirmation. Diagnosis of rubella is often made on the basis of the combination of glandular swelling and the onset of facial rash. A history

 RED FLAGS FOR RUBELLA

Rubella is profoundly dangerous to the unborn fetus of expectant mothers because exposure during the first trimester of pregnancy can cause the following to the fetus:

- Spontaneous abortion
- Intrauterine death
- Stillbirth
- Deafness
- Intrauterine growth retardation
- Mental retardation
- Behavior disorders
- Bone radiolucencies
- Diabetes mellitus
- Cardiac defects

of immunization or recent exposure may expedite disease confirmation or rule it out. Serological testing can confirm the disease by revealing a fourfold increase in specific antibodies (Porter and Kaplan 2011).

Treatment and Return to Participation

There is no known antiviral treatment for rubella after the disease is present. Most patients do well with supportive care.

Rubella is a mild illness, and symptoms rarely last more than 3 to 4 d. However, the person is contagious from the seventh day of exposure through the 21st day after the last known exposure and should be isolated from pregnant women.

Prevention and Public Health Implications

The MMR immunization provides protective antibodies to 90% to 95% of those immunized at age 1, with 99% protected by the second vaccination (World Health Organization 2015b). Also, adult women should practice birth control for at least 3 mo after administration of the vaccine. Congenital rubella has been a reportable disease in the United States since 1966.

Chicken Pox and Shingles

Varicella-zoster virus (VZV) causes varicella (chicken pox) and herpes zoster (shingles). Chicken pox is a viral, readily communicable disease (figure 15.6a). It was one of the most common childhood diseases in the United States, and children tend to contract the disease before beginning school. Ninety percent of cases of varicella occur within 10 to 20 d of exposure (Anderson 2015).

Shingles, also known as herpes zoster (see figure 15.6b), is a reactivation of varicella disease in the dorsal ganglia. The dorsal ganglia are a group of nerve cell bodies that exit the spinal cord posteriorly and provide sensation to specific regions of the body. Both diseases are problematic to the **immunosuppressed patient**. Ninety percent of unvaccinated contacts become infected, making varicella an extremely contagious disease to the unprotected person (Ferri 2016).

Although both varicella and herpes zoster have similar methods of transmission, varicella is much more contagious. These infections are spread by direct person-to-person contact, by respiratory secretions that are seen in varicella only, by direct contact with vesicle fluid, or indirectly by vesicle fluid on soiled articles such as towels or jerseys. Sports in which there are more opportunities for skin-to-skin contact, such as wrestling, carry a greater risk of transmission of infection. In a 15-year

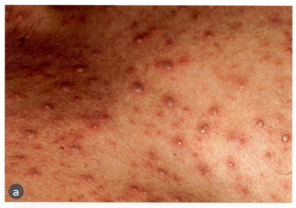
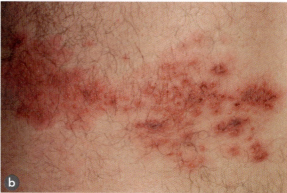

FIGURE 15.6 (a) Varicella, or chicken pox, lesions. (b) Herpes zoster, or shingles, lesions.

The Division of Dermatology at Brody School of Medicine, East Carolina University

study on collegiate wrestlers, 5% of the dermatological issues were attributed to VZV (Agel et al. 2007). Scabs themselves are not transmittable sources of the infection.

Signs and Symptoms

Chicken pox begins rapidly with a headache and a maculopapular rash that gives rise to vesicles within hours of onset. The lesion is described as a dew drop or a vesicle on an erythematous base. New lesions will develop over about 4 d and will start as erythematous papules progressing to vesicles. The subsequent vesicles last 3 to 4 d and represent the time of highest contagiousness. These lesions are of varying size, shape, and age and will quickly rupture to form crusts. The patient will usually have a combination of papules, vesicles, and crusts all at once. Lesions may occur anywhere on the body, but they tend to cluster on covered, rather than exposed, parts of the body. Lesions begin on the trunk and face, eventually spreading to the extremities, but it is also common to find lesions on the scalp, buccal mucous membrane, conjunctiva, and axilla. Other findings include intense itching, headache, fever, chills, malaise, and backache (Ferri 2016).

As with chicken pox, herpes zoster presents with a vesicular rash. However, in herpes zoster, these vesicles follow the track of one or more sensory nerve roots. They give rise to patterns following specific dermatomes and most often are unilateral (see figure 11.6). In patients with herpes zoster, severe pain and paresthesia along the rash increase with the age of the patient. Patients are typically contagious from a few days before the rash to until the vesicles have scabbed over.

The differential diagnoses for varicella and herpes zoster include impetigo, scabies, urticaria, smallpox, acute nerve root injury, and an allergic drug rash (Anderson 2015).

Referral and Diagnostic Tests

People who present with complaints associated with varicella or shingles are referred to a physician. Symptoms tend to be more severe in adults, and they may mimic myocardial infarction, pleurisy, acute abdomen, or migraine, depending on the location of the outbreak. In general, laboratory tests are not warranted, but a complete blood count (CBC) may reveal leukopenia and **thrombocytopenia**.

Treatment and Return to Participation

Although varicella is a self-limiting disease, the drug acyclovir (Zovirax) is often prescribed. Valacyclovir (Valtrex) and famciclovir (Famvir) are used to treat herpes zoster (Anderson 2015). If acyclovir is administered within 48 h of initial rash, it alleviates symptoms and shortens their duration, and it lessens recurrent outbreaks. Other treatments for varicella combat pruritus and superinfection. Simple calamine lotion is an excellent agent to diminish itching associated with this disease, as is a colloidal starch bath. Antibiotics also may be needed to help prevent secondary bacterial infections.

Collegiate athletes may return to participation when all lesions have a firm, adhered crust and there is no evidence of a secondary bacterial infection (see the sidebar "NCAA and NFSH Participation Regulations for Wrestlers With Bacterial Infections" in chapter 16) (Parsons 2014). Scholastic athletes follow the same return-to-participation guidelines as those with herpes simplex virus: 10 to 14 d of antiviral medication and no new lesions within 48 h (National Federation of State High School Associations 2013). Athletes may return to sport when fully asymptomatic, and they may engage in noncontact (and nonswimming) activities as long as they have no vesicles and feel good. Activities in the water should be avoided until patients are cleared by a physician.

Prevention and Public Health Implications

In 1995, the varicella virus vaccine (Varivax) was recommended as a single dose to protect children aged 12 to 18 mo and for immunization of children up to age 12. Studies have demonstrated that this one-time immunization has an effectiveness of 70% to 90% for complete prevention and 100% prevention of moderate to severe outbreaks (Porter and Kaplan 2011). Immunization within 3 d of exposure will lessen the symptoms and duration of the disease. Interestingly, the varicella vaccine is not a routine childhood prevention strategy in Europe, although studies are underway to determine whether this practice should continue (Bonanni et al. 2009).

The vaccine Zostavax is available for the prevention of herpes zoster but not for treatment. It is a one-injection drug that was approved by the FDA in 2011 for people over 50. Although Zostavax does not provide immunity from shingles, it lessens the risk of developing it by 70% (Lichenstein 2015).

Varicella is not a reportable disease. Affected children must be isolated from school, the public, and medical offices until the lesions have scabbed over. Likewise, adults must not have contact with others until their vesicles dry. Extra caution is maintained with athletes involved in contact or collision sports because vesicles can "unroof" and secrete fluid infected with the virus.

Hepatitis A to D

The liver is the largest organ in the body, and it functions primarily as the central organ of glucose homeostasis. It lies protected chiefly by the lower right ribs in the upper right abdominal cavity (figure 15.7). This four-lobe organ secrets bile to facilitate the digestion of fats, and it has metabolic functions as well. The liver also assists in amino acid and carbohydrate metabolism, fat-soluble vitamin storage (A, D, E, K), phagocytosis, and detoxification of potentially harmful substances. Damage to the liver has profound repercussions for many body functions.

Hepatitis, literally translated, means inflammation of the liver, and it is characterized by diffuse necrosis affecting the smallest secretory units of the liver (Porter and Kaplan 2011). The many varieties of the disease are differentiated by letters, mechanisms of acquisition, and lasting sequelae. Table 15.2 compares the common hepatitis viruses. The diseases are typically abbreviated to HAV (hepatitis A virus), HBV, HCV, and so on. The emphasis in this chapter is on hepatitis A, B, C, and D; hepatitis E and hepatitis G typically do not affect the healthy population, occurring more often in endemic countries or immunocompromised patients.

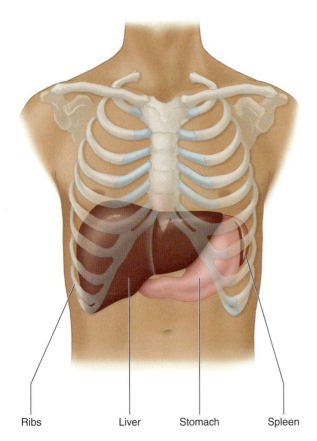

Ribs   Liver   Stomach   Spleen

FIGURE 15.7 The liver in its normal anatomical position is well protected by the lower right ribs.

In general, hepatitis can be caused by certain bacteria or viruses in addition to some drugs, toxins, and excessive alcohol abuse. Hepatitis A and hepatitis E are infectious and highly contagious forms of the disease associated with poor sanitation and oral–fecal transmission. Hepa-

titis B, hepatitis C, and hepatitis D are varieties of serum hepatitis and are transmitted via parenteral (blood) or sexual contact; these forms can lead to chronic conditions. In 2013, the CDC reported 1,781 new cases of HAV in the United States and 3,050 newly reported incidences of HBV. Whereas HAV and HBV showed small declines over the 2009–2013 reporting period, HCV rose from 781 to 2,138 new cases. Injectable drug use has been the culprit for up to 60% of the new cases of HCV, with most acute HBV cases from the same cause. Household contact and sexual contact had equal roles in the transmission of HBV (Ferri 2016; Centers for Disease Control and Prevention 2015f).

Signs and Symptoms

Viral hepatitis has an incubation period of 2 wk to 6 mo and has several phases, each marked by specific signs and symptoms, except phase 1, in which patients are asymptomatic. In the prodromal stage (phase 2), the patient could experience malaise, fatigue, upper respiratory infection (URI), anorexia, nausea and vomiting, mild abdominal pain, myalgia, or arthralgia (Buggs 2014). Some patients have accompanying headaches, fever, and a rash. When jaundice occurs, it typically manifests 5 to 10 d after the prodromal symptoms present and peaks within 1 to 2 wk. Phase 3—the icteric phase—is typically marked by patients presenting with pale stools and dark urine. Icteric means "pertaining to jaundice," and this phase is when jaundice appears. The chief complaints besides jaundice are gastrointestinal symptoms, malaise, and hepatomegaly (Buggs 2014). The final phase (4) is a 2 to 4 wk recovery and convalescent phase marked by a state of well-being, return of appetite, and disappearance of fatigue and pain. General recovery is based on the specific virus, but the acute illness typically subsides

TABLE 15.2 **Comparison of Hepatitis Viruses**

Disease	Incubation	Transmission	Notes
Hepatitis A (HAV)	30 d	Oral–fecal contact, crowding, poor sanitation, contaminated food or water	Clinical illness more severe in adults than children
Hepatitis B (HBV)	6 wk–6 mo (average is 12–14 wk)	Infected blood and blood products; sexual contact; virus is present in saliva, semen, and vaginal secretions	Chronic HBV creates a high risk for cirrhosis and liver cancer
Hepatitis C (HCV)	6–7 wk	Intravenous drug use, body piercing, multiple sex partners	High coinfection rate among patients with HIV; highest mortality
Hepatitis D (HDV)	30–150 d	In the United States, primarily by intravenous drug use	Best prevented via HBV vaccine

HAV = hepatitis A virus; HBV = hepatitis B virus; HCV = hepatitis C virus; HDV = hepatitis D virus; HIV = human immunodeficiency virus.

within 2 to 3 wk. Some patients have few of these signs but instead experience a lingering, unexplainable fatigue. Taking a good and thorough history is critical because each type is distinguished by its method of transmission.

Differential diagnoses may include EBV, herpes simplex, URI, cholecystitis (gallstones), pancreatitis, influenza, and infectious mononucleosis (Ferri 2016).

Referral and Diagnostic Tests

Patients with unexplainable fatigue are referred to a physician for further evaluation. Physical findings include an enlarged liver and jaundice, but if these occur, it is later in the progression of the disease. Blood and urine tests will reveal a normal to low white blood cell (WBC) count, mild proteinuria, and bilirubinuria in patients with jaundice (Porter and Kaplan 2011). Each type of hepatitis has its own antigen that will be assessed to ascertain the specific type of virus, and therefore the treatment plan.

Treatment and Return to Participation

Hepatitis typically resolves spontaneously within 4 to 8 wk but can have lasting sequelae. Until the patient has completely recovered, alcohol is avoided and sex partners are limited. To prevent the possible spread of the disease, household members receive immune globulin and initiation of vaccine as appropriate. Physician follow-up for hepatitis requires thorough management to ensure complete resolution of the disease; specialists in gastroenterology or hepatology are often involved.

Athletes who participate in collision sports may need additional laboratory tests to determine any residual effects of the disease before resuming full activity (Harris 2011).

Prevention and Public Health Implications

HAV and HBV can be prevented by vaccine and good personal sanitation measures, such as hand washing after bowel movements and after contact with contaminated linens, clothing, patients, or utensils. The athletic trainer must routinely adhere to universal precautions when working with athletes with open wounds or when cleaning up body fluid spills (Harris 2011). Hepatitis B and C can be transmitted via contact during competition, so return-to-play decisions must be made individually by athlete and type of sport (Anish 2004; Buxton et al. 1994). Sexually transmitted hepatitis can be prevented by using prophylactic barriers.

All cases of acute hepatitis need to be reported to local or state health agencies after diagnosis.

Hepatitis A

Hepatitis A virus (HAV) is caused almost exclusively by poor sanitation because it is transmitted via oral–fecal contact. Outbreaks occur most often in crowded areas and through contaminated food or water. Transmission of HAV through food is typically via milk, sliced meat, shellfish, and salads (Gilroy 2016). In HAV, patients present with mild flu-like symptoms. In the icteric phase, they acquire dark urine, pale stools, and jaundice. Jaundice is present in 70% to 85% of adults with acute-onset HAV (Gilroy 2016). Forty percent also have abdominal pain and pruritus (itching). Although the acute phase of the disease lasts up to 3 wk, the convalescence is prolonged, and relapsing HAV is common. Treatment consists of supportive care for the side effects. HAV is a self-limiting disease that rarely causes death. There has been a vaccine available for HAV since 1995, and it is nearly 100% effective after two doses (Gilroy 2016).

Hepatitis B

HBV is a worldwide health care problem. Nearly one-third of the earth's population has been infected with HBV, and about 400 million will have lifelong infection from it (Pyrsopoulos 2015). HBV reportedly causes 5,000 deaths a year in the United States.

Transmission of HBV is primarily by sexual activity, and high-risk activities include multiple sex partners, intravenous drug use, men who have sex with men, and piercing or tattooing. HBV is also spread by contamination with blood and body fluids (which are occupational hazards for health care workers) or from an infected mother to her unborn child. It is commonly contracted through exposure to blood, saliva, semen, vaginal secretions, urine, and feces (Pyrsopoulos 2015). This is a hardy virus that can live for an extended time outside the human host, including on inanimate objects such as toothbrushes, utensils, and medical supplies (Ferri 2016). HBV is approximately 100 times easier to contract than HIV (Buxton et al. 1994). HBV has been shown to be transmitted among football players and sumo wrestlers (Tobe et al. 2000; Kashiwagi et al. 1982; Ferri 2016). The 1982 licensure of the HBV vaccine has made a considerable difference in the spread of HBV; in 1996, the United

CLINICAL TIPS

Hepatitis B Immunization

Hepatitis B vaccine is given as a series of three shots over 9 mo and is highly recommended for all health care workers.

States recommended vaccination for adolescents who missed the immunization as a child (Arnot 1998; Centers for Disease Control and Prevention 2016c).

The signs and symptoms of HBV follow the other versions of hepatitis, and treatment is centered on preventing further sequelae from the disease. Although people can recover from HBV, it is a protracted recovery. The acute phase lasts approximately 6 mo, with potential for the chronic state to last years. Patients with either HBV or HCV are more susceptible to chronic infection, cirrhosis, and liver cancer than those with other types of hepatitis (Centers for Disease Control and Prevention 2015g).

Most athletes in noncontact sports who contract acute HBV are allowed to participate in athletics depending on clinical signs and symptoms. In the absence of fever or fatigue, there is no evidence that intense training is contraindicated. In close-contact sports, such as wrestling or boxing, however, athletes with acute HBV need to refrain from participation until they are not infectious (Howe 2003). The risk of transmission to others is limited, but it is a higher risk than with HIV (Ferri 2016; Porter and Kaplan 2011; Centers for Disease Control and Prevention 2015g). As a precaution against infecting others, athletes who develop chronic HBV should not participate in close-contact, combative sports. Chronic hepatitis B is a nationally reportable disease.

Hepatitis C

Although HCV is less prevalent than HBV, approximately 50% to 84% of the patients remain chronic carriers of the virus (Buggs 2014). HCV is a dangerous variety of the virus and is the cause of liver disorders. Close to 20% of chronic HCV carriers will develop cirrhosis over 20 to 30 yr; of these cases, up to 2.5% will also develop hepatocellular carcinoma (Dhawan 2015).

Common transmission routes for HCV involve intravenous or intranasal drug use (60%) or multiple sex partners (20%); the remaining transmission comes from needle sticks, maternal–fetus transmission, and unknown etiology (Buggs 2014; Ferri 2016). At present, there is no known prevention method for HCV other than avoiding risky behaviors. Hepatitis C is a nationally reportable disease.

HCV is the most likely hepatitis virus to fluctuate for several months or years, and HBV is likely to have a higher mortality rate than HAV or HCV. Chronic hepatitis occurs most often with HBV; 5% to 10% of patients have persistent inflammation and cirrhosis and are subclinical chronic carriers (Porter and Kaplan 2011).

Hepatitis D

HDV, or delta virus, is linked to HBV but is structurally dissimilar to HAV, HBV, and HCV. It is far less common than other hepatitis viruses (Roy 2015). Transmission is via sexual contact and injected drug use. Those at particular risk are the recipients of multiple blood products, but transmission is less efficient for HDV than for HBV (Buggs 2014). As a separate disease, HDV presents with symptoms similar to those of other hepatitis viruses, but it has a shorter incubation period, 21 to 45 d (Roy 2015). There is no vaccine for HDV, but HBV immunization also prevents HDV disease.

Streptococcal Infections

Streptococci (strep) are small, spherical, gram-positive chains of bacteria commonly found in human tissue. Various types of streptococci are typically found in the gastrointestinal tract, throat, respiratory system, vagina, and skin. The presence of streptococcal bacteria does not in itself indicate an infection, and it only poses a problem when these bacteria occupy areas outside of their usual habitat. Streptococcal infections are, however, among the most common, yet dangerous, infections known to humans (Porter and Kaplan 2011). Table 15.3 compares the various streptococcal bacteria, their normal habitats, and related illnesses.

Streptococcal infections are a group of microbially similar pathogens that have unique characteristics. They are categorized into groups A, B, C, D, and G, with groups A, B, and D being most common (table 15.4). Certain streptococci in groups C and G are resistant to bacitracin therapy and are naturally found in the human intestinal tract, skin, pharynx, and vagina. These can attack their host and cause a variety of problems, including pneumonia, cellulitis, impetigo, sepsis, and pharyngitis. This chapter provides an overview of groups A, B, and D; most of the common streptococcal infections are discussed in chapters covering the system related to infection.

Streptococcal infections can have a carrier or non-active state (Khan 2015). The term *carrier state* is used to refer to the presence of streptococci in tissues that have no sign of infection (Hill 2010). Those with acute infections show physical signs of streptococcal bacteria invading tissues, and the delayed state becomes apparent approximately 2 wk after an overt streptococcal infection. Streptococcal infections are communicable diseases and are primarily spread by person-to-person contact, but they have been also contracted from infected food or water (Khan 2015).

Group A Streptococcal Infections

Group A streptococcal infections (GAS) are caused by group A β-hemolytic streptococci *(Streptococcus pyogenes)* and fall into two categories: **suppurative** and **nonsuppurative**. Suppurative infections are derived from invading bacteria that produce necrosis and cause acute

TABLE 15.3   Comparison of Streptococcal Infections

Bacterium	Normal location	Diseases or illnesses caused
Streptococcus agalactiae	Raw milk	Meningitis in newborns, endometritis and fever in postpartum women
Streptococcus bovis	Alimentary tract of cattle	Endocarditis
Streptococcus equisimilis	Upper respiratory tract	Pneumonia, osteomyelitis, endocarditis, bacteremia
Streptococcus mutans	In dental cavities	Dental caries, endocarditis
Streptococcus pneumoniae	Upper respiratory tract	Pneumonia, meningitis, conjunctivitis, endocarditis, periodontitis, otitis media, septic arthritis, osteomyelitis
Streptococcus pyogenes	Upper respiratory tract	Scarlet fever, septic sore throat, impetigo, toxic shock syndrome, necrotizing fasciitis
Streptococcus viridans	Upper respiratory tract	Endocarditis

TABLE 15.4   Categories of Common Streptococcal Infections

Group	Common streptococcal infections
A	Pharyngitis, impetigo, pneumonia, cellulitis, otitis media, sinusitis, meningitis, rheumatic heart disease, necrotizing fasciitis
B	Neonatal, maternal, and cutaneous infections in persons with diabetes
C and G	Respiratory infections, pneumonia, cutaneous infections
D	Bacteremia associated with gastrointestinal cancer, urinary tract infection, endocarditis, meningitis, otitis media, pneumococcal pneumonia

inflammation, whereas nonsuppurative diseases occur in tissues remote from the original bacterial attack. Examples of the former are tonsillitis, streptococcal pharyngitis (strep throat), impetigo, myositis, pneumonia, toxic shock syndrome, and cellulitis. Toxic shock syndrome (TSS) became known in 1978 for its occurrence among women using highly absorbent tampons and keeping them in to long during their menstrual cycles. Fewer than 50% of TSS cases are due to tampon use, and this syndrome has been uncommon in recent years, but it still occurs. TSS is caused by either GAS or *Staphylococcus aureus* (see next section), and it is preventable by good hygiene in wound care and tampon replacement (Venkataraman 2015). Nonsuppurative infections include rheumatic fever and acute poststreptococcal glomerulonephritis (Khan 2015). *S. pyogenes* skin infections tend to occur more often in the summer or in climates where it is warm year-round, when more skin is exposed, and the likelihood of abrasions, cuts, or bites is higher (Khan 2015).

One form of group A streptococcus, group A β-hemolytic streptococcus (GABS), popularly referred to as "flesh-eating bacteria," causes a form of gangrene called **necrotizing fasciitis**, which has created interest because infection in previously healthy people can rapidly become critical, requiring hospitalization and surgical debridement of the infected skin. Other forms of streptococcal and staphylococcal infections also have been known to cause necrotizing fasciitis (Edlich 2015). Other names for this affliction are hemolytic streptococcal gangrene, acute dermal gangrene, suppurative fasciitis, and synergistic necrotizing cellulitis.

Necrotizing fasciitis is a rare and severe condition in which an infection progressively invades the skin, fascia, and blood supply. There has recently been a rise in the frequency of cases, most likely due to an increase in immunocompromised patients (Edlich 2015). It has a mortality rate of 20% to 80% and is related to age and overall heath at the time of infection (Khan 2015). Transmission occurs through a break in the skin and subsequent contact with a carrier of strep A. Inanimate objects are not likely to transmit strep A, and necrotizing fasciitis is not necessarily contagious between people as is methicillin-resistant *Staphylococcus aureus* (MRSA). The condition is progressive, and it rapidly spreads via the fascial tissues to contiguous areas of the body. It may begin in a region distant from the original insult, and it may be caused by a minor invasion of the skin, such as an insect bite, an injection site, or a boil or minor scrape,

🚩 RED FLAGS FOR NECROTIZING FASCIITIS

Necrotizing fasciitis has a mortality rate as high as 80%. Signs and symptoms include the following:

- Pain disproportionate to the severity of the injury or wound
- Rapid deterioration of the wound over the first 24 to 48 h
- Rapidly changing skin surface over the injury or wound (e.g., color, integrity)
- Fever
- Respiratory difficulty or failure
- Possible mental confusion

as well as surgical procedures or cauterizations. It has also been discovered when a seemingly minor wound is contaminated with salt water (Edlich 2015).

The main symptom associated with necrotizing fasciitis is disproportionate pain for the size and apparent severity of the wound or incision combined with a rapid degeneration within the first 24 to 48 h. Open wounds can be further inspected to reveal yellow-greenish necrotic fascia, and closed tissue will reveal the same result through an incision (Edlich 2015). Other key signs are putrid discharge, gas production from the wound, and the lack of normal tissue inflammatory healing. Accompanying signs include fever and respiratory difficulty, and on occasion, the patient presents in a delirious or confused state. If necrotizing fasciitis is left untreated, septic shock, renal failure, limb loss, or death could occur. Early treatment is surgical debridement, and it is a surgical emergency because it is often a limb- or life-saving procedure. Antibiotic therapy is considered, as is hyperbaric oxygen therapy (Edlich 2015). The incidence of necrotizing fasciitis is on the rise, due largely to the rising number of patients with chronic issues that affect their immune systems, such as those with diabetes, cancer, HIV, alcoholism, and vascular insufficiency. The average age of patients with this condition is ages 38 to 44 (Edlich 2015).

Group B Streptococcal Infections

Group B β-hemolytic streptococci (GBS) cause infections, endocarditis, septic arthritis, postpartum sepsis, pneumonia, meningitis, osteomyelitis, and soft-tissue infections (Woods 2015). These infections are uncommon in adults; however, they are also opportunistic and occur in patients with lowered resistance (Woods 2015). Group B β-hemolytic streptococci are indigenous to the upper respiratory, gastrointestinal, and female genitourinary tracts. In the elderly, GBS is strongly linked to congestive heart failure.

Group D Streptococcal Infections

Group D streptococcal infections includes two distinct bacteria: enterococcal and nonenterococcal species. These streptococci are commonly found in the gastrointestinal system (e.g., *Streptococcus bovis*), but they can also cause bacterial endocarditis, urinary tract infection, abdominal sepsis, cellulitis, and wound infections (Sinave 2015).

Signs and Symptoms

Because streptococci can attack almost any system, the signs and symptoms are not unique to this group of infections but to the body system affected. For example, pneumonia will have signs and symptoms unique to that infection, as will cellulitis; both are vastly different in presentation, yet both are caused by a streptococcal infection. The most common streptococcal presentation is pharyngeal infection from group A; strep throat presents with a bright red pharynx, fever, sore throat, lymphadenopathy, and tonsillar exudates (see chapter 13).

Referral and Diagnostic Tests

Patients exhibiting any signs of infection must be referred to a physician. Patients may present with symptoms or signs remote from the origin of the infection, as is the case in nonsuppurative infections. Laboratory blood tests showing a WBC count of 12,000 to 20,000/μL with 75% to 90% neutrophils indicate a streptococcal infection. See table 3.3 for normal CBC values. Tissue or blood culture can determine the specific cause of the infection (e.g., GAS, GBS), which in turn can dictate treatment (Sinave 2015; Khan 2015). Depending on the infection, urine or CSF may be tested (Woods 2015). A CBC sample cultured overnight and evaluated by microscopic examination provides confirmation, whereas the absence of streptococcal bacteria indicates other pathology.

Treatment and Return to Participation

The best medicinal treatment for streptococcal infections depends on the exact group and target tissue of the infectious agent. Patients must complete the course of their medication for complete effectiveness. Depending on the disease, isolation may be required (for example, scarlet fever), and to prevent all types of streptococci from spreading, any materials soiled with residue from the infection or infected person are handled as infectious waste.

The prognosis for return to activity after a confirmed streptococcal infection depends on the severity and duration of the symptoms, the tissues involved, how quickly it was diagnosed and treated, and the progression of the disease. Certain streptococcal infections, such as impetigo, require absence from participation until the skin has completely healed (see chapter 16) (National Athletic Trainers' Association 2005; 2007; Beaschler 2015; Parsons 2014).

Prevention of streptococcal infections includes proper sanitation, personal hygiene, and isolation of contagious persons until the period of communicability has passed.

Staphylococcal Infections

Staphylococcus aureus, the main culprit of staphylococcal infections, is found on up to 80% of healthy adults intermittently and up to 30% are permanent carriers, or colonized. Most commonly, the bacteria are found in the nares, but they can also be found in the throat, axilla, and rectum (Herchline 2015). Staphylococcal organisms are grape-like clusters of gram-positive bacteria that cause a tremendous number of infections in nearly every human body system. Table 15.5 compares staphylococcal infections, their normal environments, and the ailments most often caused. Immunocompromised patients, especially those with influenza, chronic pulmonary disorders, chronic skin conditions, diabetes mellitus, and surgical incisions, are prone to staphylococcal infections. Trans-mission is commonly through hand-to-hand contact during patient care and also by airborne transmission. In athletics, the biggest culprits are those associated with seemingly benign skin wounds and postsurgical infections.

Certain types of staphylococcal infections are caused by ingestion of infected or undercooked food. Toxic shock syndrome, previously described, is another preventable condition that results from a staphylococcal or GAS infection. Although rare, 30% to 79% of all cases are fatal (Venkataraman 2015).

An emerging problem with staphylococcal infections is the impediment to treatment with antibiotics, specifically methicillin-resistant *Staphylococcus aureus* (MRSA). The two most discussed MRSA infections are HA-MRSA (health care–associated MRSA) and CA-MRSA (community-associated MRSA). In the active population, it is CA-MRSA that is typically the culprit in staphylococcal infections. The first report of a CA-MRSA infection in athletes was in 1993, and such reports have steadily risen since then (Perloff 2014; Lindenmayer et al. 1998). At present, the low estimate is that 75,000 people are treated annually for MRSA (Centers for Disease Control and Prevention 2014a). CA-MRSA is quite treatable if recognized in its early stages and diagnosed, and with prophylactic treatment, its postsurgical infection rate is falling (Keller 2014; Schweizer et al. 2014).

Signs and Symptoms

Most CA-MRSA infections begin in a manner similar to other streptococcal infections, as a small lesion similar to a pimple, a mosquito bite, a recent injury or abrasion, or a wound from surgery. The wound quickly enlarges and becomes inflamed and quite painful. Athletes may run a low-grade fever that progresses to higher temperatures as the body fights the infection. The seemingly small infection is painful beyond expectation for the type of

TABLE 15.5   **Comparison of Staphylococcal Infections**

Bacterium	Normal location	Diseases or illnesses caused
Staphylococcus aureus	Skin, mucous membranes (nose, mouth); produces golden-yellow pigment	Boils, carbuncles, internal abscesses; toxins cause food poisoning, toxic shock syndrome
Staphylococcus aureus—methicillin resistant (MRSA)	Same as above	Same as above; resistant to many penicillin drugs
Staphylococcus aureus—vancomycin resistant	Becomes serious in nosocomial infections	Same as above; resistant to many vancomycin drugs
Staphylococcus epidermidis	Skin	None
Staphylococcus hominis	Frequently recovered in skin	Causes no known diseases
Staphylococcus saprophyticus	Anal area, genitals, nose, mouth	Urinary tract infection

pain a similar wound would cause. As the infection increases, so does the size of the area infected. It is not unusual for breakouts to occur among teammates (Rogers 2008; Perloff 2014).

Referral and Diagnostic Tests

A patient who presents with a wound that shows signs of infection, such as heat, swelling, and redness, and that is accompanied by pain is referred to a physician. Wounds that rapidly deteriorate or become enlarged are suspect. Unaware that they are fighting a serious condition, patients often try to drain the infection themselves and delay seeking treatment. Any athlete with a postoperative wound needs to be especially diligent in cleaning and inspecting the wound and must immediately report any increase in pain, swelling, or fever (Harris 2011).

Treatment and Return to Participation

If an infection is detected and the patient is referred early enough in the infection's development, a physician may be able to incise and drain (I&D) it and prevent further problems. The release of infectious materials coupled with an antibiotic and proper hygiene may be enough to prevent MRSA.

If the athlete is a staphylococcal carrier or has a history of resistance to penicillin treatment, other medications may be needed to eradicate the infection. The current antibiotic therapy for outpatient treatment is trimethoprim

 RED FLAGS FOR CA-MRSA

Systemic treatment and hospitalization for CA-MRSA may be required if two of the following signs are present (Perloff 2014):

- Temperature above 38 °C (100.4 °F) or below 36 °C (96.8 °F)
- Tachypnea above 24 breaths/min
- Tachycardia above 90 beats/min
- WBC count either above 12,000 cells/μL or below 400 cells/μL

with sulfamethoxazole (TMP-SMZ). Other effective medications are clindamycin, doxycycline, or linezolid (Perloff 2014; Baorto 2015). Hospitalization may be required for the athlete with high fever and pain unmanageable with outpatient medications.

An athlete confirmed to have MRSA cannot engage in contact athletic activity until proven infection free. Communal areas, including the weight rooms and athletic training clinics, need to be sanitized after every patient use (Rogers 2008; National Athletic Trainers' Association 2005; Parsons 2014; Beaschler 2015).

Prevention

Soap and water go a long way in the initial cleaning and disinfecting of wounds. The soap Hibiclens (Mölnlycke Health Care, Gothenburg, Sweden) is often prescribed

Vehicles for Transmission of CA-MRSA in the Athletic Setting

- Towels
- Water bottles
- Hydrocollator pad covers
- Velcro wraps
- Weights (handheld and bars)
- Tubs of balms
- Tape-cutting devices
- Bell and diaphragm of a stethoscope
- Ultrasound applicator head
- Rehabilitation equipment
- Freezable gel packs
- Paraffin baths
- Ice scoop (if left in the ice machine)
- Applicator pads for electrical stimulation modalities
- Cryotherapy devices (such as Gameready)

CA-MSRA = community-acquired methicillin-resistant *Staphylococcus aureus*.

for daily use by infected patients. Athletes must clean abrasions or turf burns as soon as possible after they occur and follow-up with hot water and soap in a shower; finally, the wounds are covered with a sterile dressing. Daily cleaning and inspection of wounds will indicate if an athlete may be slower to heal or prone to infection. To prevent further colonization in one who is a carrier, an antibiotic is prescribed for 5 to 7 d. A study involving over 38,000 surgical patients has demonstrated that rates of postoperative infection can be lessened dramatically by a presurgical preventive approach. Patients were screened for *S. aureus* via a nasal or buccal (mouth) swab at least a week before surgery. Those who tested positive as carriers for *S. aureus* were given intranasal mupirocin and asked to bathe with chlorhexidine for each of the five days before surgery. Those who were not identified as carriers bathed in chlorhexidine the night before surgery and were given a dose of cefazolin (Keller 2014; Schweizer et al. 2014).

Sexually Transmitted Diseases and Infections

Sexually transmitted diseases (STDs) and infections (STIs) are a group of infectious diseases that are transmitted through body secretions from an infected partner. There are documented rare occasions in which an STI may be contracted in a nonsexual fashion, such as through occupational hazard (e.g., needle sticks) or dental care (e.g., an infected health care provider); and fetuses can acquire an STI through the maternal placenta before or during birth.

The presentation and detection of STIs differ for each sex and are covered in detail in chapter 10.

Encephalitis

Encephalitis, literally translated, means "inflammation of the brain." In general, encephalitis is caused by a viral infection, but it can also be a sequela of immunizations or vaccines. The same organisms responsible for aseptic meningitis are also responsible for encephalitis, although their relative frequencies differ.

Encephalitis takes two forms: primary and secondary with complications from a viral infection. Primary encephalitis is caused by a direct viral invasion of the brain and spinal cord. The virus can be sporadic or epidemic. Sporadic infection arises from herpes simplex, varicella-zoster, measles, mumps, and other viruses (Porter and Kaplan 2011; Howes 2015). Epidemic encephalitis is typically caused by mosquito-borne arboviruses, with the exception of the Zika virus. **Arboviruses** are a large group of viruses recovered largely from bats,

rodents, and arthropods (e.g., insects and crustaceans). Disease is typically transmitted by blood-feeding insects such as mosquitoes and ticks. These arboviruses are also known as distinct disorders: eastern and western equine encephalitis, both named after the horses that are also attacked by the virus; St. Louis and La Crosse viruses, which are named for the areas of the United States where they were first discovered; and West Nile virus. Zika virus, also an arbovirus caused by a mosquito, does not cause encephalitis, and it is covered after this section.

Secondary encephalitis is typically a complication of a viral infection in another part of the body that then enters the brain. All forms of encephalitis have a similar presentation that may begin as a minor illness with headache and fever but then develop more serious symptoms. Whereas primary encephalitis is more serious, the secondary form is more common. People often do not seek medical care because of the milder nature of secondary encephalitis; therefore, physicians see more cases of primary encephalitis (Howes 2015).

Although encephalitis is rare, it is the most common mosquito-borne disease in the United States. The mortality rate varies with the source of the virus. Insect-borne sources might cause low morbidity one year but severe mortality the next.

Birds are the conduit that spread the virus to mosquitoes through their food chain. A newly infected bird carries high levels of the virus in its bloodstream before developing immunity. Mosquitoes who feed on these birds become lifelong carriers of the disease. Carrier mosquitoes then easily pass the infection on to more birds, which in turn spread it to more mosquitoes.

Although most mosquitoes would choose birds over mammals for their primary food source, they do attack humans and other warm-blooded creatures. The risk is highest during the warm months when birds and mosquitoes reproduce. The ease of modern travel has also contributed to a slight rise in some vector-borne diseases. Travelers can bring back infected mosquitoes from their trips to their homes. Because many athletes practice in the late afternoon and early evening during the warmer months, their activity coincides with the highest mosquito activity, so their risk is highest (Anderson 2004).

CLINICAL TIPS

Vector Transmission of Disease

Organisms that transmit disease from one animal host to another are called **vectors**. For example, mosquitoes are vectors for the transmission of encephalitis from small creatures, usually birds and rodents, to humans.

In addition, mosquitoes congregate in bodies of water however small. This would make puddles of water from a hydration station or a discarded water bottle a haven for these pests.

Eastern equine encephalitis is the most serious viral encephalitis found in North America, primarily in the eastern United States. It affects horses, as its name suggests, and humans. Western equine encephalitis also affects horses and humans and is prevalent in the central and western plains. It is a serious variety of encephalitis but is not fatal as often as the eastern variety. Both are rare in the United States (Howes 2015). Of the 100 cases of eastern equine encephalitis in 2014 in the United States, all were hospitalized and 25 died (Lindsey et al. 2015).

The St. Louis variety was first discovered in the Midwest and is responsible for approximately 67 neuroinvasive cases since 2004 (Centers for Disease Control and Prevention 2016a). La Crosse encephalitis is one of the few mosquito-borne viruses common in hardwood forests and is primarily found in the upper Midwest. It is transmitted to mosquitoes via chipmunks and squirrels rather than birds. However, it is the West Nile virus, with activity in all 50 states, that attracts the most media attention. The *Culex, Aedes,* and *Anopheles* mosquitoes are the primary culprits for West Nile virus, which was first reported in Africa, Europe, and Asia and reached the United States in 1999 (Centers for Disease Control and Prevention 2016a; Salinas 2015).

The West Nile virus has been transmitted through blood transfusions, through donated organs, by breastfeeding, and during pregnancy from mother to fetus. First reported in New York, West Nile virus is now found coast to coast. It has been found in birds, horses, dogs, squirrels, and bats, as well as humans (Salinas 2015). Prevention strategies have proven effective. In 2003, 264 fatalities resulted from more than 9,862 cases, whereas in 2014, 97 deaths resulted from 2,204 cases (Lindsey et al. 2015). In the same year, there were three reported deaths due to La Crosse encephalitis, and none due to St. Louis encephalitis.

Although symptoms of West Nile encephalitis are generally mild, the disease can become severe, especially in older people and those with weakened immune systems (Salinas 2015).

Signs and Symptoms

Signs and symptoms of encephalitis caused by a mosquito generally appear within 5 to 15 d of being bitten by an infected mosquito, and they have a presentation unique to the virus. For example, St. Louis encephalitis patients have dysuria and pyuria, whereas those suffering from West Nile encephalitis suffer from extreme lethargy (Howes 2015). In general, signs and symptoms of encephalitis include sudden fever, headache, vomiting, photophobia, stiff neck and back, confusion, drowsiness, clumsiness, unsteady gait, and irritability. Infection due to a virus (e.g., varicella-zoster virus, Epstein-Barr virus, measles, and mumps) includes a rash, lymphadenopathy, parotid enlargement, and hepatosplenomegaly (Howes 2015). Symptoms that require emergency treatment include loss of consciousness, seizure, poor responsiveness, muscle weakness, memory loss, sudden and severe dementia, impaired judgment, coma, and paralysis (Ferri 2016).

Differential diagnoses for encephalitis include bacterial meningitis, brain abscess, parasitic diseases, metastatic tumors, and collagen diseases.

Referral and Diagnostic Tests

Encephalitis is potentially serious and life-threatening. Early referral to a physician or hospital emergency department may be necessary. The cardinal symptoms for immediate referral include severe headache, stiff neck, photophobia, and mental disturbances (Salinas 2015). Because the origin of encephalitis can be autoimmune, bacterial, fungal, or vector-borne, a thorough history is paramount. History of travel, immunizations, close proximity with infectious people, and outdoor activity can all provide critical information to distinguish the variety of encephalitis.

The keystone diagnostic test is CSF examination and analysis. Neuroimaging studies, magnetic resonance imaging (MRI), computed tomography (CT) scan, both with and without contrast, and often an electroencephalogram (EEG) may be performed as well. Both the MRI and CT imaging may show edema or increased signal, indicating vector-borne virus (Harris et al. 2012; Howes 2015). An EEG is a graphic record of the electrical activity of the brain. Electrodes are placed on the patient's scalp to measure electrical waves, frequencies, and amplitudes. These tests help identify or exclude alternative diagnoses. They also determine whether the disease process is focal or diffuse.

Treatment and Return to Participation

Viruses are not responsive to antibiotics. Antiviral agents (such as acyclovir, which is used only in the early stages for the herpes simplex virus) are geared toward symptom management and maintenance of body systems. This will include adequate nutrition, ventilation, and hydration. Control of seizures and cerebral edema, along with prevention of secondary infection, may be necessary (Howes 2015).

The overall prognosis for recovery is good, depending on the infecting agent and the speed with which treatment is begun. Some cases are mild, and the patient experiences a full recovery. In severe cases, however, permanent impairment or death is possible within 48 h despite early treatment. The acute phase of the infection may last 1 to 2 wk. Resolution of fever and neurological symptoms may be sudden or gradual. Neurological symptoms may require many months of treatment before full recovery, and rehabilitation with speech therapy is often required.

Prevention and Public Health Implications

All cases of encephalitis caused by an arbovirus should be reported to the local public health authority. Each state authority is allowed to determine whether to report these diseases immediately, within 1 working day, or within 1 wk (Centers for Disease Control and Prevention 2016a).

Prevention of many forms of secondary encephalitis caused by a viral infection in another part of the body, such as mumps, chicken pox, rubeola, or rubella, is best achieved through immunization.

Public health measures that control mosquitoes can reduce the incidence of many types of viral encephalitis. Effective local mosquito control includes the use of appropriate pesticides and cleanup of containers with standing water that may offer breeding sites (Anderson 2004). Common containers that may hold enough water to breed mosquitoes include discarded cups and water bottles, football sleds, flowerpots, tire swings, and birdbaths. Individual prevention measures include wearing a hat, wearing long pants with pant legs stuffed into socks, and liberal use of an insect repellent that contains *N,N*-diethyl-*m*-toluamide (DEET) on the face, neck, ears, and arms.

Zika Virus

The Zika virus (ZIKV) is another arbovirus but not one that causes encephalitis. It is related to yellow fever, dengue, West Nile, and St. Louis encephalitis viruses (Hayes 2009). The consequences of ZIKV include loss of pregnancy and the birth defect microcephaly (Telxeira et al. 2016; Cauchemez et al. 2016; Scheler-Faccini et al. 2016). Microcephaly is caused by defective brain development, resulting in an unusually small head. There are other environmental and genetic causes for microcephaly, such as exposure to drugs or radiation, fetal alcohol syndrome, and some infections. Rubella, herpes virus, and syphilis are known genetic causes for microcephaly, and prior to November 2015, ZIKV was not considered a culprit (Telxeira et al. 2016). Mothers infected in the first trimester of pregnancy seem to be at highest risk for delivering babies with microcephaly (Cauchemez et al. 2016).

The *Aedes* mosquito has been identified as the carrier of the Zika virus, and it has two varieties: *Aedes aegypti* and *Aedes albopictus* (Centers for Disease Control and Prevention 2016h; Hayes 2009). The former is an African native, but it is found globally in tropical and subtropical areas. The latter is originally from Asia, and it is most known for being transported internationally in used tires. Both are found in the United States, although *Aedes albopictus* has a broader inhabitance, as it has been located in the entire southern and eastern United States from Texas to New England (Centers for Disease Control and Prevention 2016h).

Zika is named after an area in the Ugandan forest in Africa where it was first discovered in 1947 (Hayes 2009). The first human transmission was in 1952, but it was not until February 2016 that it was truly recognized as a public health emergency by WHO (Centers for Disease Control and Prevention 2016j). Once infected, humans can spread the virus. Zika has been found in blood, breast milk, and semen of infected people, and it can spread by maternal–fetus transmission as well as laboratory exposure (Hennessey, Fischer, and Staples 2016; Dupont-Rouzeyrol et al. 2016). A high correlation between ZIKV and Guillain-Barré syndrome has been observed. There are no known vaccines for ZIKV and no known cure (Centers for Disease Control and Prevention 2016b; 2016j; Dupont-Rouzeyrol et al. 2016; Hennessey, Fischer, and Staples 2016).

Signs and Symptoms

Unfortunately, many are unaware they have the Zika virus. It is believed that signs include a fine maculopapular diffuse rash, fever, and conjunctivitis. Symptoms can include joint or muscle pain and a headache (Centers for Disease Control and Prevention 2016j; Hayes 2009). Symptoms emerge within 2 wk of infection. The virus remains in the blood of infected people for about a week, and in the semen longer (Centers for Disease Control and Prevention 2016b). One case demonstrated ZIKV was present in semen over 2 mo after the onset of symptoms (Reuters Health Information 2016). Symptoms are mild and last less than a week. It is postulated that once infected, the person is immune from subsequent Zika virus infection (Centers for Disease Control and Prevention 2016j). Differential diagnoses for ZIKV include group A streptococcal infections, malaria, rubella, measles, and dengue (Hennessey, Fischer, and Staples 2016).

Referral and Diagnostic Tests

People with symptoms of ZIKV and a history of travel to countries with high ZIKV infection or a history of outdoor activity in areas known to have *Aedes* mosquitoes and reported infections should be referred to a physician for evaluation. Although there is no commercially available test for ZIKV, assessment is done to rule out other conditions (Hennessey, Fischer, and Staples 2016). Laboratory examination includes serological testing. Specifically, testing using RT-PCR or ELISA, depending on the time of onset of symptoms, is most reliable (Navalkele 2016). ZIKV has been found in urine more than 10 d following symptoms (Navalkele 2016). Fetal ultrasonography and amniocentesis may be used in pregnant women with symptoms, although there is no reliable research supporting amniocentesis.

Treatment and Return to Participation

Because up to 80% of patients with ZIKV are unaware they are infected, the return to participation may be unaffected (Centers for Disease Control and Prevention 2016j). For those with symptoms, appropriate fluid replacement is recommended, as is acetaminophen for pain and fever control. NSAIDs are not recommended because of the association of hemorrhagic consequences with similar conditions, such as dengue fever (Navalkele 2016).

Prevention and Public Health Implications

Prevention of the Zika virus begins with eliminating anything that may attract mosquitoes in general. Insect repellent should be the top layer, over clothing and over sunscreen. In addition to the measures previously discussed for encephalitis prevention, public education is paramount. Use air conditioning or screened windows when indoors (Hennessey, Fischer, and Staples 2016). Keep vegetation trimmed and grasses cut; cover, dump, or treat any vessel that can hold water to eliminate larva infestation (Centers for Disease Control and Prevention 2016h).

In 2016, the CDC issued a HAN (Health Alert Network) alerting the public to the possible routes of Zika virus transmission, including unprotected sexual relations (Centers for Disease Control and Prevention 2016b). Men with pregnant partners should use barrier protection to ensure that Zika virus is not transmitted. Women who are pregnant or anticipating a pregnancy should use extra caution, especially when determining travel to areas that host the *Aedes* mosquitoes (Hennessey, Fischer, and Staples 2016). ZIKV is a notifiable disease in the United States.

Viral Meningitis

Viral or aseptic **meningitis** is the most common form of meningitis, an inflammation of the meninges and CSF surrounding the brain and spinal cord (see figure 11.2 for an illustration of these structures).

Even though viral meningitis is a benign, self-limiting illness, it is associated with 26,000 to 42,000 hospital-

izations each year in the United States (Ferri 2016). It is generally less severe than bacterial meningitis and is rarely fatal in adults with normal immune systems. Care focuses on management of the symptoms, which typically last 7 to 10 d before complete recovery.

Many different viruses cause meningitis, including **enterovirus**, arboviruses, the mumps, varicella-zoster, influenza viruses, and herpes simplex virus. Arboviruses such as West Nile can also cause viral meningitis (Centers for Disease Control and Prevention 2016f; Hasbun 2016). The most common causative agent is enterovirus. Enteroviruses are a group of RNA viruses that can cause diseases in humans; they are typically found in respiratory secretions and stools of infected people. Other causes of infection can be bacteria, parasites, and drug use.

The organisms that cause viral meningitis are contagious. An enterovirus is most commonly spread through direct contact with respiratory secretions, such as the saliva, sputum, or nasal mucus of an infected person. The typical pathway for infection occurs by shaking hands with an afflicted person or by touching something that the person has handled before rubbing the nose, mouth, or eyes. Kissing an infected person on the mouth can also spread the disease (Wan 2015).

In temperate climates, most cases are seen in the summer and early fall. The incubation period for an enterovirus is generally between 3 and 7 d from the time of infection until symptoms develop. An infected person can spread the virus to someone else during a period of about 3 d after infection until approximately 10 d after symptoms develop.

Viral meningitis has been transmitted among athletes. In 2014, eight football players and two siblings of the athletes sought treatment at an emergency department. All were diagnosed with viral meningitis, and all survived (Croker et al. 2015). In 1989, 25% of students and staff at a high school suffered an outbreak of an enterovirus-like illness. Twenty-one percent of them were diagnosed with viral meningitis, and of them, the highest rates of infection were among members of the football team (Alexander et al. 1993). Another high school group traveling to Mexico became ill after swimming in the ocean. Twenty-one of the twenty-five-member group contracted meningitis, most likely due to improper sewage dumping into the sea (Begier et al. 2008). These three examples are a few among many reports of groups of active people contracting meningitis. They highlight the importance of proper hygiene and early recognition of an infectious condition.

Signs and Symptoms

Signs and symptoms of acute viral meningitis are common to all pathogens. Often the disease is accompanied or preceded by a nonspecific malaise or upper respiratory infection. Viral meningitis is similar in presentation to meningococcal infections because it appears with a sudden high fever, headache, and cervical rigidity. Nausea, vomiting, and diarrhea are found in more than 50% of patients (Wan 2015).

Other conditions to rule out include bacterial meningitis, migraine, Lyme disease, varicella zoster, and SLE (Ferri 2016).

Referral and Diagnostic Tests

The three indicators that occur abruptly and develop rapidly are severe headache, high fever, and stiff neck; these indicators should alert the health care provider to the need for immediate referral to a physician or hospital emergency department. Applying stress on the spinal cord through Brudzinski's sign (figure 15.8) or Kernig's sign can exacerbate pain in the meninges, but it is not as definitive an indicator of the disease as is a stiff neck (Porter and Kaplan 2011). These two signs are often described with many varieties in positioning, but the chief result is an elongated neural tube along the spine, resulting in pain.

In the early stages it is impossible to separate viral meningitis from acute bacterial or meningococcal meningitis without laboratory studies. It is necessary to examine the CSF to distinguish between the two infections as well as to rule out differential diagnoses. CSF is obtained through a spinal tap, which is also known as a lumbar puncture (see chapter 3). With viral meningitis, the spinal fluid on gross inspection is usually clear to the naked eye; no organisms are seen on microscopic examination, and they cannot be cultured. The glucose content also is normal (Wan 2015; Hasbun 2016).

RED FLAGS FOR MENINGITIS

Warning signs of meningitis that warrant immediate referral include the following:

- Severe headache
- High fever
- Stiff neck

Treatment and Return to Participation

Once a diagnosis of viral meningitis is made, treatment is supportive. It consists of symptom management with bed rest, increased fluids, analgesics, and medications to prevent or relieve nausea and vomiting. Antibiotics are not helpful with a viral disease.

Prevention and Public Health Implications

Although aseptic or viral meningitis is the most common type of meningitis, the Centers for Disease Control and Prevention (CDC, Atlanta, GA) in 1999 dropped it from the list of illnesses that need to be reported to the agency. It is still reportable to some state public health agencies. The time period within which to report a case or suspected case of aseptic meningitis varies from state to state but is usually within 1 wk. The National Enterovirus Surveillance System (NESS) is in place to gather information about enterovirus detection and outbreaks from state public health agencies and private laboratories as well as treating physicians.

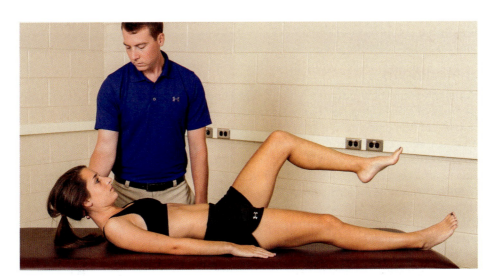

FIGURE 15.8 Brudzinski's sign involves passive neck flexion, thereby elongating the spinal cord. A positive sign is increasing localized pain, radiating in the lower extremity, or voluntarily flexing the hip or knee to alleviate spinal cord pressure; either action can indicate meningeal or nerve root irritation.

The most effective way to prevent enteroviral disease is adherence to good hygiene practices that include frequent and thorough hand washing and avoidance of shared utensils and drinking containers. In institutional settings, washing objects and surfaces with a dilute bleach solution (as described in chapter 1) can be an effective way to destroy the virus. Other preventive methods encompass the mosquito prevention techniques mentioned earlier.

Acute Bacterial Meningitis

Unlike viral meningitis, acute bacterial meningitis is a potentially life-threatening infection of the meninges and the CSF. Four types of bacteria account for more than 80% of all cases: *Streptococcus pneumoniae* (the most common cause of bacterial meningitis in adults), group B streptococci, staphylococci, and *Neisseria meningitidis* (a meningococcus) (Porter and Kaplan 2011). Incidences of pneumonia and meningococcal meningitis are decreasing due to increased use of vaccinations targeted to prevent them.

The health care provider needs to fully appreciate the severity of meningitis; if left untreated, it is fatal in 50% of the cases (World Health Organization 2015). The disease is expressed most commonly either as meningococcal meningitis, an inflammation of the membranes surrounding the brain and spinal cord, or as meningococcemia, a serious infection of the blood. Meningococcemia blood infections are caused by gram-negative *Neisseria meningitidis* but do not present with associated meningitis (Porter and Kaplan 2011). Most cases occur during the winter and spring (Centers for Disease Control and Prevention 2016g).

RED FLAGS FOR BACTERIAL MENINGITIS

- Headache increasing in severity is the first symptom, typically frontal or retroorbital
- Rapid onset of symptoms
- Fever up to 40 °C (104 °F)
- Nausea and vomiting, especially in the early stages
- Confusion
- Drowsiness, progressive lethargy
- Convulsions or seizures more common in children, especially with influenzal meningitis; rare in adults
- Cervical rigidity
- Positive Brudzinski's sign
- Positive Kernig's sign
- Skin rash, especially near the armpits or on the hands or feet
- Rapid progression of small petechiae under the skin
- Malaise
- Irritability
- Photophobia
- Muscle aches

Meningococcal meningitis can result in permanent brain damage, hearing loss, learning disability, limb amputation, kidney failure, or death. Meningococcal

CONDITION HIGHLIGHT

Bacterial Meningitis

Acute bacterial meningitis is a potentially life-threatening illness that develops quickly. Because it is prevalent in areas of close living, such as military barracks and college dorms, many colleges require the vaccine prior to admission to the university. The bacterium is carried in respiratory and pharyngeal tissues and spread by air and mouth contact either with an infected person or with something the infected person ate or drank from (e.g., shared utensils, cups, beverages). The condition begins as a harmless headache, accompanied by a stiff neck, rash, and eventually, a high fever. Because the meninges are involved, the patient can experience concussion-like symptoms including confusion, drowsiness, personality changes, and irritability. People with these signs and symptoms should be referred to a health care provider for immediate follow-up because bacterial meningitis can progress quickly, leading to limb amputation, coma, or death. Diagnosis is made via cerebrospinal fluid (CSF) examination through a lumbar spinal tap, and most health care providers will treat these symptoms as bacterial meningitis until a different diagnosis is confirmed. Treatment involves hospitalization and antibiotics. Bacterial meningitis is a health risk to the public and is a reportable disease.

disease is spread by the exchange of respiratory and throat secretions through such activities as coughing or kissing. Sometimes, however, bacteria have spread to other people who have had close or prolonged contact with a patient with meningitis caused by *N. meningitidis* (World Health Organization 2015). People in the same household, such as college students living in dormitories, or anyone in direct contact with a patient's oral secretions from coughing, sneezing, kissing, or oral contact with shared items, such as cigarettes, hookah mouthpieces, or drinking glasses, would be considered at increased risk of acquiring the infection. People who qualify as close contacts of a person with meningitis caused by *N. meningitidis* should receive prophylactic antibiotics to prevent them from getting the disease. *N. meningitidis* has been found in the nasopharyngeal passages of about 10% of uninfected adults (Gondim 2015). While these people carry the bacteria in their noses and throats without signs of illness, they can spread the disease to others.

Signs and Symptoms

As stated earlier, meningitis strikes suddenly; therefore, early diagnosis and treatment are especially important. All forms of acute meningitis, bacterial or viral, have common symptoms that may also be mistaken for the flu. This disease has also been erroneously dismissed as torticollis because of its proclivity for stiff neck (Gondim 2015). Patients complain of a respiratory illness or sore throat, followed by fever, headache, and a stiff neck (Ferri 2016). Other symptoms can include confusion, irritability, delirium, and coma (Hasbun 2016). In children, projective vomiting and seizures may be present. Symptoms can develop over several hours or a few days, but only 44% of adults with bacterial meningitis presented with

the classic diagnostic trio of headache, fever, and neck stiffness (Hasbun 2016). Another anecdotal observation is not to dismiss headache and stiff neck complaints from athletes the first few days in a sport requiring a helmet as the helmet adjustment period can often lead to headaches. Be certain to ask history questions germane to other signs or symptoms of meningitis.

A diagnosis of bacterial meningitis is not difficult to make with a careful review of the patient's clinical history and a physical examination that notes the sudden onset of severe headache accompanied by high fever and lethargy or confusion.

Referral and Diagnostic Tests

Bacterial meningitis is a medical emergency. A satisfactory outcome depends on the speed with which treatment is begun. As with viral meningitis, the three indicators that occur abruptly and rapidly are severe headache, high fever, and stiff neck, but they are not always present. Because Kernig's and Brudzinski's signs are positive in approximately 50% of patients with meningococcal disease, the practitioner should consider using them as clinical noninvasive tests (Porter and Kaplan 2011; Gondim 2015).

Diagnosis is based on clinical history, physical examination, and specific diagnostic tests. The definitive diagnosis of bacterial spinal meningitis is made by examination of CSF (table 15.6) obtained through a lumbar puncture (see chapter 3); opening pressure of the CSF will be elevated (>180 mm H_2O). On visual inspection the CSF appears cloudy or purulent. Further evaluation of the CSF includes culture, protein, glucose, and white blood cell count (Hasbun 2016). Other key laboratory tests include blood cultures, chest radiograph, and electrolyte

TABLE 15.6 Cerebrospinal Fluid Values and Indicators

Parameter	Normal value	Notes
Pressure	50–80 mm (H_2O)	High: Acute bacterial meningitis, cerebral hemorrhage, perhaps Lyme disease
Appearance	Clear	Cloudy: Infection, meningococcal meningitis Red: Cerebral hemorrhage, obstruction Orange: High protein, old bleeding
Protein	20–45 mg/dl	High: Tumors, trauma, infection, inflammation, acute bacterial meningitis, Guillain-Barré syndrome
Glucose	40–70 mg/dl	Low: Acute bacterial meningitis, hypoglycemia, infection, cancer High: Hyperglycemia
Leukocytes	Up to 5 cells/μL	500–10,000: Acute bacterial meningitis 0–500: Lyme disease 0–100: Guillain-Barré syndrome Presence of red blood cells (RBCs): Cerebral hemorrhage

Based on Porter and Kaplan 2011; Ferri 2016; Hasbun 2016

and glucose measurement. CT or MRI brain scanning may also be desirable.

Treatment and Return to Participation

Bacterial meningitis can be treated effectively with a number of antibiotics. Treatment is two-pronged. First, because of the severity and emergent nature of the disease, antimicrobial treatment is started before the results of the CSF cultures are known. Once the specific pathogen is identified, specific intravenous drug therapy is begun. Second, other associated complications, such as hearing loss, brain swelling, shock, convulsions, and dehydration, must be addressed with appropriate supportive treatment and drug therapy (Gondim 2015; Ewald and McKeag 2008).

The prognosis for bacterial meningitis depends on several factors, including the type of infecting organism and the speed with which medical treatment is initiated. Untreated bacterial meningitis can be fatal. The mortality rate for uncomplicated meningococcal meningitis and *H. influenzae* meningitis is about 5%. Meningococcal infections in the United States still cause about 500 deaths a year (Hasbun 2016). In general, early and effective treatment leads to recovery with no residual symptoms. Late or inadequate treatment may result in permanent damage. Common sequelae include memory impairment, decreased intellectual function, hearing loss, dizziness, seizures, and gait disturbances (Gondim 2015).

Return to participation will depend on the complete resolution of symptoms and medical clearance from the treating physician or medical team.

Prevention and Public Health Implications

Anyone exposed to meningococcal meningitis who has face-to-face contact (family member, housemate, teammate) should begin **prophylaxis**. Appropriate medications range from Rifampin to ciprofloxacin. Rifampin is targeted to children and tends to turn body fluids orange. A better choice for athletes is ciprofloxacin, a one-dose pill that assures compliance (Porter and Kaplan 2011).

At the national level, meningococcal meningitis is a reportable disease. State and local public health agencies also have their own guidelines for reportable diseases. Universities typically have guidelines for proper reporting procedures. Notification to local, state, and national agencies is usually done through the hospital or treating physician. Meningococcal infections require immediate reporting to the public health department (Centers for Disease Control and Prevention 2016g).

There are currently six vaccines available to prevent meningococcal conditions, and each covers specific subgroups of the infection (Centers for Disease Control and Prevention 2016g). The patient's age, health status, and risk evaluation all matter in determining which vaccine is most appropriate. The vaccine is 85% to 100% effective in preventing disease in older children and adults. The CDC, the American College Health Association (ACHA), and the American Academy of Pediatrics (AAP) recommend that parents and college students, particularly freshmen who plan to live in dormitories, learn about meningococcal disease and the potential benefits of vaccination. Other college undergraduates wishing to reduce their risk may also choose to be vaccinated. The CDC has issued updated vaccination criteria for meningococcal meningitis. The Advisory Committee on Immunization Practices (ACIP) recommends vaccination with the quadrivalent meningococcal conjugate vaccine (MCV4) for all persons ages 11 to 18, and for persons ages 2 to 55 if they are at increased risk for meningococcal disease (Centers for Disease Control and Prevention 2016c).

Summary

Infectious diseases commonly attack every system in the human body, but most are largely preventable. People who take advantage of immunizations and follow universal precautions will protect themselves from most common infectious diseases. The athletic trainer must consider infectious diseases when working with an athlete who has fever, unexplained fatigue, or a skin abrasion that does not heal in order to ensure that the athlete gets the best care possible and to protect other athletes who may have been exposed to an infectious agent.

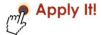 **Apply It!** The case study for this chapter looks at a 16-year-old soccer athlete diagnosed with bacterial meningitis. Read the scenario and answer the questions at www.HumanKinetics.com/MedicalConditionsInTheAthlete.

16

Dermatological Conditions

Dermatological conditions in athletes are common and are a major reason that many athletes miss practice or competition. In a national survey of U.S. high school athletes from 2009 to 2014, nearly 500 dermatological conditions were reported. Wrestling accounted for 73.6% of the infections, with football following at 18%. Nearly 70% of the infections were bacterial (including staphylococcal, streptococcal, and impetigo), and 28.4% were fungal (tinea) (Ashack et al. 2016). Although most dermatological conditions originate with skin-to-skin contact and resultant transmission, some may involve respiratory or airborne transmission. Others may result from allergic reactions, cancer, or insect bites. The five main types of dermatological conditions are general, bacterial, viral, fungal, and parasitic. This chapter reviews pertinent anatomy and discusses signs and symptoms, referral and diagnostic tests, and treatment and criteria for return to participation for simple dermatological conditions.

Overview of Anatomy and Physiology

The skin, or integument, is the largest organ of the body and can be divided into three layers: the **epidermis**, the dermis, and the subcutaneous tissue or hypodermis (figure 16.1). The epidermis is composed of up to five layers from deep to superficial: stratum basale, stratum spinosum, stratum granulosum, stratum lucidum (found only in the soles of the feet and palms of the hands), and stratum corneum.

Each layer of the epidermis, except for the stratum basale, is composed of dead cells. The epidermis is the body's primary protective shield; it constantly forms new cells and sloughs off old ones, and it produces a protective pigment known as melanin. The dermis, which is composed of a papillary layer and a reticular layer, contains a variety of vascular and sensory structures; hair follicles;

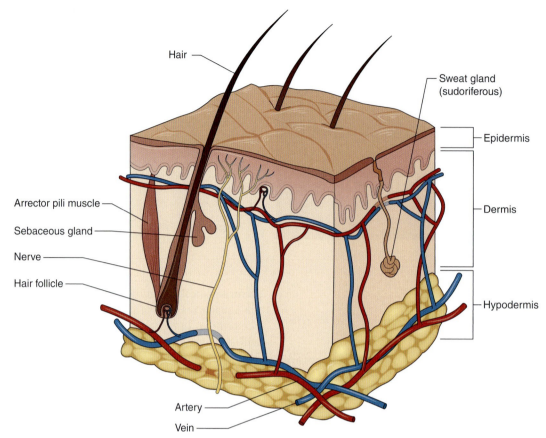

FIGURE 16.1 Anatomy of the skin.

sebaceous, sudoriferous, or sweat glands; and nails. Finally, the hypodermis is made up of connective tissue, which binds the dermis to the deeper structures, and adipose tissue, which provides insulation and cushioning. Together the epidermis, the dermis, and the hypodermis make up the integumentary system.

The integumentary system serves as the interface between the body and the external environment. It is a dynamic system that serves as a barrier against invading organisms and outside influences such as ultraviolet radiation, toxic chemicals, thermal changes, and penetrating forces. At the same time, it allows people to sense and to adapt to the environment in terms of thermoregulation; fluid loss; proprioception and kinesthesis; force dissipation; cutaneous absorption of gases, ultraviolet light, and toxins; and synthesis of vitamin D. Finally, the skin plays an important role in human communication by helping people to convey emotions through changes in skin color and texture as well as through facial expression.

Nails are made up largely of keratin and are found on the dorsal surfaces of all fingers and toes. The nail is a hard, clear surface that presents a pink color from the underlying highly vascular epithelial cell layer (figure 16.2). The lunula lies at the proximal end of all nails. It is a moon-shaped, white opaque layer that protects the nail matrix, which in turn produces new keratinized cells. The nail fold surrounds the lateral and proximal nail

and hooks onto the nail bed. It is in this area that certain bacterial conditions arise.

Evaluation of the Skin

The goal of a skin examination by the health care provider is to identify, or attempt to identify, unknown skin lesions in order to determine the need for referral, need for treatment, or activity status (i.e., to allow participation or to withhold from participation), and to prevent transmission among athletes. New or previously undiagnosed lesions must be diagnosed and treated or, at minimum, carefully watched for changes. A history and a visual inspection can be very revealing; exactly how revealing depends on the patient's history, the quality of the visual inspection, and the patient's willingness to be truthful in either reporting or trying to hide a skin lesion. The athletic trainer should be suspicious of an athlete-patient wearing a wrap or a bandage that the athletic trainer did not apply. When asking the patient to disrobe for a skin inspection, all tape, wraps, and bandages should be removed. Wrestlers have been known to self-abrade (e.g., using sandpaper) or to apply caustic chemicals (e.g., bleach) to skin lesions in an attempt to hide or remove the infection.

When working with athletes such as wrestlers whose sports put them in close skin-to-skin contact, skin examination should be performed often enough to detect

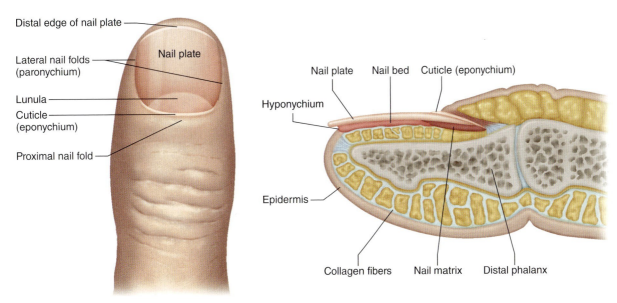

FIGURE 16.2   Anatomy of the nail.

newly forming and potentially contagious lesions early enough to initiate treatment and to prevent transmission to others. Weekly skin examinations are considered the norm; however, when the possibility of an active outbreak exists they should be performed often enough to detect new lesions immediately, thereby shortening the course of the outbreak among team or family members. For athletes, specific league rules may require that full-body skin examinations be performed at specified intervals; however, compliance with league rules should be viewed by the athletic trainer only as the minimal standard, especially when more frequent inspections are warranted.

A skin inspection should be conducted in a well-lit room that provides a private, respectful environment. For full-body examination, males should be wearing only shorts, while females should be wearing shorts and a sports bra or swimsuit top. Whenever possible, a health care provider of the same gender should be conducting the examination. Begin the examination with a history by asking the patient if he or she has any skin problems to report, and if they have felt ill or has nausea, fever, body aches, or fatigue. These symptoms may be especially indicative of viral or bacterial infections. The visual inspection is conducted with the patient standing erect, feet shoulder width apart, arms abducted to 90°, and palms forward with hands open. Avoid touching the patient whenever possible; however, this may be unavoidable when examining specific body parts, especially the scalp. If contact is necessary, athletic trainers should wear gloves and should change them and disinfect their hands between patients in order to avoid cross-contamination. Begin a systematic inspection of the patient, including all aspects of the upper and lower extremities and the torso, including the axilla, the neck, the face, and the scalp. The scalp is especially important because hair may conceal active infections. Patients should be able to adjust their

necks and move their hair to facilitate the inspection, but the athletic trainer may have to physically part the hair in order to visualize the scalp.

The athletic trainer should look for any abnormalities and should note specifically any lesion's pattern, color, and location:

- *Pattern:* Does the lesion appear scratched, raised, depressed, in groups or clusters, and is it bullous, moist, dry or crusted, or draining fluid?
- *Color:* What is the color of the lesion, the surrounding tissue, and the fluid or crust, and is the color uniform with well-defined borders and symmetry?
- *Location:* Is the lesion above or below the hairline on the scalp, on or near the genitals or mouth?

The athletic trainer is usually the first clinician to evaluate a dermatological lesion on an athlete. A **lesion** is synonymous with abnormal tissue. The key is to look for tissue abnormal to the surrounding area. That being said, a freckle is also one form of a lesion. Lesions are typically in the very early stages of development and can be difficult to differentiate without microscopic or laboratory testing. Because these types of diagnostic procedures are beyond the scope of many health care providers, the athletic trainer must use sound clinical judgment when determining the appropriate course of action for athletes with dermatological conditions.

When referral to a medical doctor for evaluation and treatment is necessary, the health care provider must understand the patient's signs and symptoms and be able to effectively describe findings to the physician using dermatographical nomenclature. The terminology used to describe the appearance of a skin lesion or condition is very specific (figure 16.3). The athletic trainer must

Primary lesions: Caused by a condition or a disease

Nonpalpable

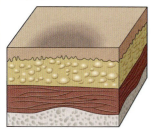

Type: Macule
Description: A flat area on the skin that is usually lighter or darker in color than the surrounding skin
Examples: Freckles, petechiae, vitiligo, café au lait spots

Palpable and solid

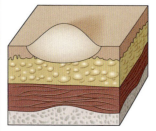

Type: Papule
Description: A small bump, palpable and circumscribed, and less than 5 mm in diameter; may be pigmented, erythematous, or flesh-toned
Examples: Elevated nevus (mole), prickly heat, psoriasis, melanoma

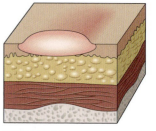

Type: Wheal
Description: A temporary elevation of the skin that itches, with a smooth surface, and is light pink to pale red in color; caused by acute inflammatory reaction in the skin; may appear, disappear, or change form abruptly within minutes or hours
Examples: Urticaria, anaphylaxis

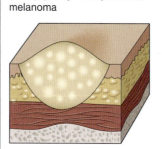

Type: Tumor
Description: A swelling or enlargement, any mass lesion; may be either malignant or benign
Examples: Lipoma, inflammatory reaction

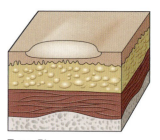

Type: Plaque
Description: A flat, raised patch on the skin or other tissue
Examples: Psoriasis, dental plaque

Palpable and fluid-filled

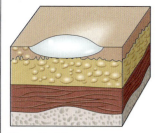

Type: Vesicle
Description: A small blister (up to 5 mm in diameter); filled with clear fluid
Examples: Herpes simplex (early stages), common blister

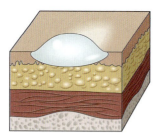

Type: Bulla
Description: A thin-walled, fluid-filled blister larger than 5 mm
Example: Impetigo

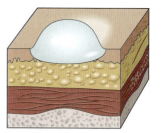

Type: Pustule
Description: An elevated, well-circumscribed lesion filled with white blood cells (WBCs) or bacteria
Examples: Acne vulgaris, herpes simplex, herpes zoster

> continued

FIGURE 16.3 Common skin lesions.

Secondary lesions: Caused by external forces

Damaged or diminished skin surface

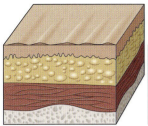

Type: Excoriation
Description: An abrasion of the outer layers of the skin due to scratching, rubbing, chemical irritant, burns, or trauma
Examples: Abrasion, scratched skin

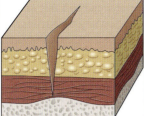

Type: Fissure
Description: A cleft, groove, or split through all epidermal layers of skin
Example: Athlete's foot

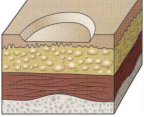

Type: Erosion
Description: Loss of epidermis that does not extend into dermis
Example: Ruptured chickenpox vesicle

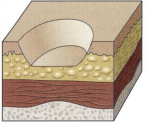

Type: Ulcer
Description: Loss of skin through the epidermis or mucous membranes; begins with inflammation and leads to necrosis and sloughing of damaged and dead tissue; healing results in scar formation; not unique to skin
Examples: Stasis ulcer, herpes simples

Augmented or increased skin surface

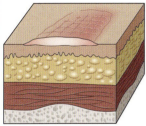

Type: Crust
Description: Dried plasma, serous exudates, blood, or debris on the surface of damaged or absent outer skin layers; fluid is often honey colored
Examples: Impetigo, eczema, seborrhea

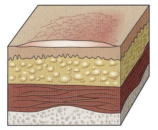

Type: Scale
Description: Flakes or plates on the skin; may vary in size, thickness, and consistency
Examples: Psoriasis scale (compact and thick), pityriasis rosea scale (thin and small)

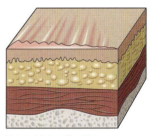

Type: Lichenification
Description: Epidermal thickening and roughening of the skin with increased visibility of skin surface furrows
Example: Chronic atopic dermatitis

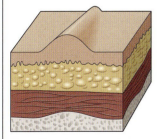

Type: Scar
Description: A permanent fibrotic change of tissue that forms to replace lost epidermal and dermal tissue
Examples: Surgical scar, acne scar

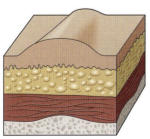

Type: Keloid
Description: An exaggerated response to tissue insult resulting in obvious, permanent, and raised scar tissue
Examples: Postsurgical scar, postacne scar

FIGURE 16.3 *> continued*

have the knowledge and resources necessary to make these distinctions. It is much easier and more efficient to describe the lesion as a *fissure* rather than as a "linear loss of epidermis and dermis with sharp, defined borders." The clinician must also understand that these terms are important to the description and are not a specific diagnosis.

Dermatitis, for example, is an inflammation of the skin or dermal layers and can be the result of a variety of dermatological conditions with various causes. The term *dermatitis* merely indicates a general inflammation of the skin, whereas **contact dermatitis** indicates an inflammation of the skin caused by direct contact with a specific allergen, and **actinic dermatitis** indicates inflammation of the skin from exposure to sunlight or another irritating light source.

Another way to describe dermatological conditions is by referencing the area of skin affected. Most physicians use millimeters (mm) to describe the width or breadth of a condition, but centimeters (cm) are used for larger surface areas. As a point of reference, 1 in. is equal to 25.40 mm or 2.54 cm (figure 16.4).

Urticaria

Urticaria is a group of distinct skin conditions characterized by itchy, wheal-and-flare skin reactions, commonly known as *hives*. Urticaria is a common skin pathology that is often seen in athletes. When histamine is released from mast cells, it produces a characteristic triple response: vasodilation causing local erythema, erythematous flare beyond the local erythema, and leakage of fluid causing local tissue edema (figure 16.5). Urticaria can occur with or without **angioedema** (subcutaneous or submucosal acute swelling), but up to 50% of patients present with both conditions (Wong 2015). Most cases are acute and can last up to a few weeks. The causes of urticaria are wide-ranging and include allergies to foods such as shellfish, nuts, and eggs; food additives such as salicylates, dyes, and sulfites; drugs such as penicillin, aspirin, and sulfonamides; bacterial, viral, and fungal infections; and allergens such as pollens, mold, and animal dander. Internal disease; physical stimuli such as dermatographism, exercise, cholinergic agents, cold, and sun; skin diseases; hormones that occur during pregnancy; and genetic predisposition can also trigger urticaria. The underlying cause of acute urticaria cannot be determined in about 50% of cases (Wong 2015). A more rare variety of the condition is chronic urticaria, which arises from chronic infection, intolerance to food additives, or autoreactivity. A typical hive is an intensely itchy erythematous or white edematous area. A discussion of general urticaria and specific conditions follows.

Signs and Symptoms

General urticaria may develop at any age and is extremely common. The characteristic appearance described previously is fairly easy to diagnose, and most cases are self-limiting, lasting from a few hours to a few weeks. The lesions are usually very itchy, or **pruritic**, but the intensity may vary. Also, the size may range from small, 2 mm lesions, to very large areas. They last 20 min to 3 h and can disappear and reappear in other areas (Wong 2015). This pattern repeats itself up to 48 h.

Referral and Diagnostic Tests

Referral to a physician is appropriate if symptoms persist for an extended period and if they are interfering with

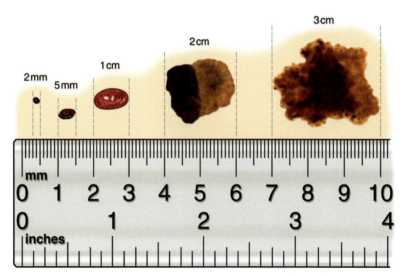

FIGURE 16.4 Comparison of size of lesion.

© Katie Walsh Flanagan

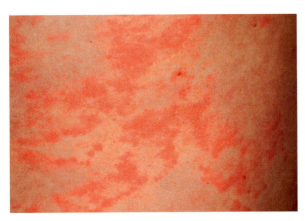

FIGURE 16.5 Urticaria, seen here in various stages of formation, is a local erythemic reaction to exercise, temperature changes, drugs, or allergies.

The Division of Dermatology at Brody School of Medicine, East Carolina University

daily activities. Immediate referral to a medical facility is necessary if an athlete shows signs or symptoms of **anaphylactic shock**. Diagnostic testing to determine the exact cause of urticaria can be highly expensive and endless, commonly with no resolution.

Treatment and Return to Participation

The most effective treatment for urticaria is to determine and eliminate the cause, but this is often extremely difficult. Most athletes will need an oral nonsedating antihistamine, such as loratadine (Claritin) or fexofenadine

RED FLAGS FOR ANAPHYLACTIC SHOCK

General urticaria may also indicate anaphylactic shock. Any athlete with the following signs or symptoms should be referred to a medical facility immediately:

- Facial edema
- Swollen tongue
- Respiratory distress
- Stridor
- Difficulty talking
- Difficulty swallowing
- Hoarseness
- Hypotension
- Syncope or near syncope

(Allegra), because the sedating antihistamines may impair performance. Another popular antihistamine commonly used for urticaria is cetirizine (Zyrtec), but it has mild sedative properties, although not as severe as the sedating antihistamines. If the aforementioned antihistamines are unsuccessful, the use of glucocorticoids (steroids) has been effective (Wong 2015). In emergencies, in which the athlete's airway is compromised, the use of epinephrine (EpiPen) injection prescribed for that athlete may be warranted (see chapter 4). Most cases resolve spontaneously and have a good prognosis. The athlete may return to participation if stable and comfortable. The best prevention for most urticarial conditions is to determine and eliminate the cause or allergen if possible.

Dermatographism

Dermatographism is one form of urticaria induced by rubbing or stroking the skin or by rubbing of skin with clothing. The exact cause is unknown, but recent infections or medications appear to be the most common cause. The hives develop within 1 to 3 min of stroking the skin and resolve in 30 to 60 min. The patients affected will go through periods of reactivity during their lifetimes, but dermatographism is more common in younger patients (Laube 2014).

Signs and Symptoms

Dermatographism presents with blanching and associated linear edema and erythema (figure 16.6). It can occur on any part of the body because it does not matter if the skin is covered by clothing or equipment. However, the friction caused by clothing or equipment may induce a dermatographical reaction.

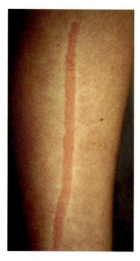

FIGURE 16.6 Drawing on the skin provided this reaction in a patient with dermatographism.

The Division of Dermatology at Brody School of Medicine, East Carolina University

Referral and Diagnostic Tests

If a patient presents with signs of dermatographism, referral may be warranted when the reaction is either severe or prolonged. The common test for this condition is to use a tongue blade to draw a line on the area to see the response. Any raised or discolored reaction is considered positive for dermatographism. No other diagnostic tests are needed.

Treatment and Return to Participation

Treatment ranges from conservative use of topical agents to the use of oral antihistamines as described for general urticaria. As with urticaria, it is not an infectious or contagious condition. The prognosis is excellent for dermatographism, and sport participation is not restricted. If the allergen is associated with the uniform or equipment needed to participate, it would be wise to alter the allergen within safety rules to prevent recurrence. Another means of preventing dermatographism is to wear a barrier between the allergen and the skin.

Cholinergic Urticaria

Cholinergic urticaria is caused by a physical stimulus. It was once thought to be triggered by heat, but the irritant is actually sweat (Schwartz 2015). It usually develops in younger patients between the ages of 10 and 30 and typically resolves within 30 to 90 min. Ninety-six percent of the people diagnosed with cholinergic urticaria are male (Schwartz 2015). This reaction consists of 1 mm to 4 mm hives with surrounding erythema that occur during or shortly after the patient experiences exposure to heat or overheating of the body during exercise or stress. Other inducers are hot food, hot water/bath/hot tub, sauna, emotional distress, and, of course, exercise (Schwartz 2015). This reaction typically occurs within 2 to 20 min of exposure but may be delayed for up to 1 h. Signs and symptoms are induced by the parasympathetic nervous system's release of acetylcholine and may last up to 3 h (WebMD 2015).

Signs and Symptoms

Symptoms of cholinergic urticaria include itching, burning, tingling, warmth, or irritation of the skin that appears following anything that would raise the core temperature or elicit sweating. It can occur anywhere on the body. Systemic symptoms of wheezing, angioedema, or hypotension may also occur. The patient will have a higher core temperature than is normal.

Referral and Diagnostic Tests

The athletic trainer refers the athlete with symptoms of cholinergic urticaria to a physician for definitive diagnosis, which is typically by history and clinical examination. The patient may also exercise in place or on a stationary bicycle for about 10 to 15 min while being observed for 1 h for the development of hives. This exercise will help to establish the diagnosis and is done only under the supervision of a physician at a medical facility.

Treatment and Return to Participation

Treatment consists of limiting strenuous exercise, stressful environments, and hot showers. Antihistamines may help before exercise, but most often a strong sedating antihistamine is needed. Rapid cooling upon the first signs or symptoms of cholinergic urticaria has also been effective in slowing the progress of the hives (Schwartz 2015). The athlete may also shower with hot water to induce a reaction, deplete the histamine stores, and begin a refractory period of about 24 h. Athletes known to be reactive should always exercise with someone else in case exercise anaphylaxis occurs.

Only a few cases of cholinergic urticaria spontaneously resolve because most of these patients will have persistent symptoms. Return to participation depends on the development of any additional symptoms, especially exercise-induced anaphylaxis.

Cold Urticaria

Cold urticaria is a reactive disorder that manifests as hives after exposure to cold. It is the most common form of physical urticaria (WebMD 2015). It can occur often in athletes because ice baths and ice therapy are a common treatment modality. There are two forms of cold urticaria: acquired and hereditary. The former occurs after exposure to cold, with hives rapidly appearing. Hereditary cold urticaria has a slower onset, with reactions appearing up to 24 to 48 h after exposure (WebMD 2015). Likewise, symptoms last longer, up to 48 h, with hereditary cold urticaria.

Signs and Symptoms

A patient will usually develop hives within 5 min of exposure to ice, cold water, or a sudden drop in air temperature. These lesions may last 1 to 2 h after removal of the stimulus. Systemic symptoms of generalized urticaria, angioedema, or anaphylaxis may also develop. Urticarial vasculitis, cholinergic urticaria, Raynaud's phenomenon, and dermatographism are all differential diagnoses for cold urticaria.

Referral and Diagnostic Tests

The athletic trainer refers any athlete with extreme reactions to cold to a physician for definitive diagnosis and evaluation for other systemic symptoms. Diagnosis is made in the physician's office by applying ice to the skin for 1 to 5 min or by exposing the forearm to cold water (0 °C to 8 °C; 32 °F to 46 °F) for 5 to 15 min and monitoring for hives (figure 16.7). This is recommended only under the supervision of a physician in a medical facility because systemic symptoms and anaphylaxis may develop.

Treatment and Return to Participation

Treatment consists of avoidance of sudden decreases in temperature and exposure to cold water or ice. The anti-

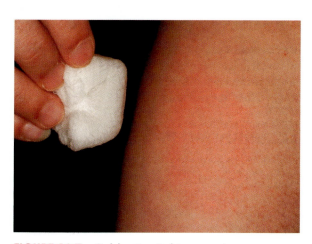

FIGURE 16.7   Cold urticaria hive reaction.

The Division of Dermatology at Brody School of Medicine, East Carolina University

histamine cyproheptadine and the tricyclic antidepressant doxepin have been shown to help suppress this reaction. Symptoms in most patients will resolve spontaneously. For those using cryotherapy to reduce the pain and inflammation of an injury, placing a barrier between the ice and the skin can help ameliorate symptoms of cold urticaria. Return to participation depends on the development of any other symptoms such as angioedema, general urticaria, or anaphylaxis. If the reaction is local, the athlete may return to participation if no other symptoms have developed within the next 1 to 2 h. If generalized symptoms develop, return to participation should be determined by a physician. Prevention of cold urticaria includes reducing exposure to ice, cold objects, and sudden decreases in temperature.

Solar Urticaria

Solar urticaria is a condition manifested by hives that occur within minutes of exposure to ultraviolet (UV) light and resolve within 1 to 3 h (Tajirian 2014).

Signs and Symptoms

The obvious sign of solar urticaria is the sudden onset of hives precipitated by exposure to UV light. Systemic reactions such as syncope have occurred but are rare. Syncope typically occurs in young adults and more commonly in females shortly after sun exposure.

Referral and Diagnostic Tests

The diagnosis of solar urticaria is based on the obvious hive or wheal formation and quick resolution. Further diagnostic testing includes phototesting and UV sleeve testing. UV sleeve testing exposes a section of skin to a given amount of UV light. The reaction determines whether the patient is reactive to that range of UV light. Polymorphous light eruption, sunburn, and photoallergic drug reaction are the differential diagnoses for solar urticaria.

Treatment and Return to Participation

Treatment consists of antihistamines, liberal use of sunscreen, hats, long-sleeved clothing, and graded exposure to UV light. Prognosis is unknown, but immediate return to play is reasonable if no systemic symptoms, such as angioedema, syncope, or anaphylaxis, have occurred (Tajirian 2014). A return to outdoor activity should include the use of appropriate sunscreens.

Prevention

Prevention of solar urticaria consists of decreasing the amount of sun-exposed skin; using sunscreens; and wearing long sleeves, pants, and hats when possible. Most sunscreen agents absorb the ultraviolet B (UVB) radiation (290 to 320 nm) responsible for the development of hives; however, sunscreens that contain avobenzone (also known as Parsol 1789) will absorb UVA I and UVA II wavelengths (340 to 400 nm and 320 to 340 nm, respectively), and sunscreens containing menthyl anthranilate and oxybenzone will absorb UVA II wavelengths (American Academy of Dermatology 2015a). All of these wavelengths are linked to hives and other skin injuries related to sun exposure (Tajirian 2014).

Epidermoid Cysts

Epidermoid cysts, also known as sebaceous, epidermal, or **keratinous cysts**, are very common from youth to middle age. These cysts may occur anywhere on the body, but the most common sites are the face, scalp, neck, and trunk (Fromm 2015). Because they are all of epidermoid tissue, this term is favored over sebaceous cyst, which indicates the cyst is only sebaceous in nature. Recall that the term *sebaceous* is related to sebum (oil in the skin), which is secreted near sweat (sudoriferous) glands. Epidermoid cysts have a thin wall filled with a white keratin material produced by the epithelium. One of the more common epidermal cysts is the pilonidal cyst that can form in the sacrococcygeal area of the lower back. Epidermoid cysts are slow growing, movable, and nontender (figure 16.8).

Signs and Symptoms

Cysts range in size from a few millimeters to several centimeters. They are usually soft, round, flesh-colored, mobile, and smooth and have some communication with the surface. Some originate from **comedones**, and these are usually found on the back. The cyst wall may rupture, and the keratin creates an inflammatory reaction within the dermis. They can become inflamed or infected; if they do, they become painful. Epidermoid cysts may reabsorb or recur. They do not itch or cause a localized increase in temperature. The differential diagnoses for **sebaceous cysts** include abscess, acne, boil, ganglion, and skin tumor.

Referral and Diagnostic Tests

The athletic trainer refers to a physician any athlete who has skin swelling contained within a specific area or one that does not diminish in size or is problematic because of its location. No specific diagnostic tests are needed, but referral is necessary so that the physician can incise and drain the cyst.

Treatment and Return to Participation

Asymptomatic cysts require no treatment. Symptomatic cysts may be treated by injecting them with triamcinolone or by the use of oral antibiotics (Fromm 2015). Should surgical intervention be required, a physician may incise and drain the cyst, although some require excision. The physician opens the cyst with a No. 11 blade, and the keratin material is expressed through the opening. A No. 1 curette is then used to remove the remaining excess material, and the wall is removed by either expressing the cyst edges or grasping the wall with small forceps. Infected cysts may require placement of a gauze drain after excision; the drain remains in place for 7 to 10 d. An oral antibiotic regimen may also be prescribed (Stevens et al. 2014).

Epidermoid cysts often recur. Sport participation is not restricted other than to prevent secondary infection.

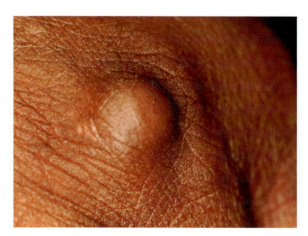

FIGURE 16.8 Sebaceous cyst.

The Division of Dermatology at Brody School of Medicine, East Carolina University

Dermatitis

The term *dermatitis* is used loosely. Dermatitis means inflammation of the skin, and the large variety of causes is beyond the scope of this chapter. This chapter discusses two conditions: eczema and psoriasis.

Eczema and Atopic Dermatitis

Eczema is often used synonymously with dermatitis and is the most common inflammatory skin disease. Whereas eczema itself often indicates vesicular dermatitis, some refer to it as atopic dermatitis (Bradby 2014). Atopic dermatitis (AD) is a dermatological reaction between environmental and genetic factors (Porter and Kaplan 2011). It is the most common inflammatory skin condition in children. There are both intrinsic and extrinsic causes of AD. Whereas the intrinsic form is not well understood, the extrinsic causes include allergic reactions to food and airborne allergens (e.g., mold, dander). AD has been thought to be an immunological disturbance resulting in immunoglobulin E (IgE) sensitization (Bradby 2014). IgE is responsible for the release and production of many inflammatory substances, and it can cause over- or underproduction of reactionary enzymes that manifest in AD and other inflammatory responses. AD has shown genetic tendencies (Bradby 2014; Porter and Kaplan 2011). AD affects an estimated 17% of the pediatric population in the United States (Bradby 2014). If left alone, most eczematous lesions will resolve, but patients are rarely able to avoid scratching.

Signs and Symptoms

Eczema consists of three stages: acute, subacute, and chronic. More often, the acute and subacute stages are seen in infants and young children, and the chronic presentation is found in adults. The acute stage consists of a red swollen plaque with small vesicles. These lesions are very itchy, appear within days after exposure, and last for days to weeks. The subacute stage consists of erythema and scales of various degrees, which may also itch. The chronic stage consists of thickened skin with increased skin markings and moderate to intense itching (Bradby 2014).

Differential diagnoses include contact irritants such as poison ivy, topical medicines including neomycin, fungal infections, nutritional deficiencies, **dyshidrosis**, scabies, and habitual scratching. Other conditions to consider are herpes simplex virus (HSV), psoriasis, systemic lupus erythematosus (SLE), or discoid lupus erythematosus.

Referral and Diagnostic Tests

Referral to a physician is warranted for an athlete exhibiting increasing or persistent symptoms consistent with eczema. Diagnostic tests may include microscopic examination with a **potassium hydroxide (KOH) preparation**. Patch testing may be needed to determine specific allergens. Patch testing involves covering the skin with various patches of allergens for 1 to 2 d to determine which ones cause an allergic response.

Treatment and Return to Participation

The most important treatment for eczema is removal from the allergen if possible. Because one of the consequences of AD is extremely dry skin, proper skin care is paramount. Patients must be counseled to bathe properly with mild (Dove) soap and to dry their skin and immediately apply emollient skin lotion (Bradby

2014). Topical steroids are appropriate for up to 2 wk following an acute onset. Antihistamines may be used to reduce itching, and antibiotics should be started if there are signs of infection. Systemic steroids may be needed to control the inflammation, but their use is controversial (Bradby 2014).

The prognosis of eczema depends on the severity of the reaction. Unless the reaction is severe or a significant infection has developed, the athlete may return to play without restriction.

Psoriasis

Psoriasis is a genetic, chronic, and recurring disorder that usually begins during childhood. It is a scaling, papular infection similar to eczema but without the epithelial eruptions, wet areas, and crusts. It is a hyperproliferation of *keratinocytes*, which form the tough outer protective layer of skin. Psoriasis affects an estimated 3% of the worldwide population (Meffert 2016). It is more common in Caucasians, and the average age of onset is age 28. It is believed to be associated with the immune system, and it can be triggered by trauma, infections, or certain medications (Porter and Kaplan 2011). Psoriasis has a gradual onset and usually has chronic remission and recurrence rates that vary in frequency and duration, but permanent remissions are rare. There are many forms of psoriasis that affect the nails, joints (psoriatic arthritis), and eyes. The most common form is plaque psoriasis, simply called *psoriasis.*

Approximately 5% to 30% of patients with psoriasis also experience psoriatic arthritis (Meffert 2016; Hammadi 2016). The exacerbation–remission cycle common to the skin disorder may coincide with the arthritic component. Most often, the distal interphalangeal joints of the fingers and toes are affected. Compared to rheumatoid arthritis (RA), psoriatic arthritis tends to enter remission more often and more rapidly than RA, and it lacks the typical joint nodules associated with RA. The patient with psoriatic arthritis may progress to chronic, disabling arthritis, so complaints of joint pain in the psoriatic person must not be overlooked (Hammadi 2016).

Signs and Symptoms

The distinctive lesion of psoriasis is a silvery white plaque with surrounding erythema with distinct borders (figure 16.9). The lesions usually begin as small, red, scaly papules that coalesce into round or oval plaques except in the skin folds, where they appear as deep red, macerated plaques. These lesions are most common on the extensor surfaces, such as the elbows and knees, but they are also very common on the scalp, fingernails, toenails, gluteal clefts, and previous sites of trauma. Psoriasis can also present with pain and itching at the site.

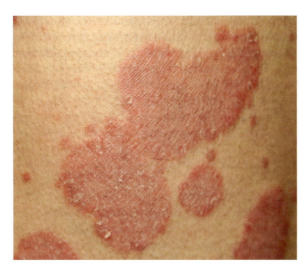

FIGURE 16.9 Psoriasis is characterized by scaly erythematous patches with silvery scales on the top.
The Division of Dermatology at Brody School of Medicine, East Carolina University

Forms of psoriasis may develop other than the general chronic plaque type just described. Another common form is scalp psoriasis. The scalp, which may be the only site affected, has a thick, erythematous, silvery scale in multiple areas. This lesion may extend onto the forehead. Psoriasis of the nails is another type and is demonstrated by pitting of the nails.

Streptococcal infections; pityriasis rosea; systemic lupus erythematosus (SLE); seborrheic dermatitis; rheumatoid arthritis; squamous cell carcinoma; secondary syphilis; candidiasis; drug eruptions generally caused by β-blockers, gold, or methyldopa; and pancreatic tumor are all differential diagnoses for psoriasis.

Referral and Diagnostic Tests

Any person suspected of having psoriasis is referred to a physician for medical evaluation and initiation of treatment. The clearly defined, dry, silvery scales are quite distinguishable and unique to psoriasis. Although diagnosis is rarely difficult, testing includes a complete blood count (CBC), including ESR (erythrocyte sedimentation rate), and a *Streptococcus* screening. Testing for rheumatoid factor is indicated if psoriatic arthritis is suspected. On occasion, biopsy of the lesion may be necessary to confirm the diagnosis and rule out other disorders (Meffert 2016).

Treatment and Return to Participation

Treatment for psoriasis is complicated and involves many options, from systemic to topical medications, stress reduction, phototherapy, and changing climate (Hennessey, Fischer, and Staples 2016). The American Academy of Dermatology (ADD) put forth treatment recommendations that therapy be tailored for each patient. Pharmaceutical treatment includes the use of methotrexate for as long as tolerated and cyclosporine intermittently (Menter et al. 2011). Topical steroids such as calcipotriol (Dovonex), anthralin ointment, and targeted UV light are first-line treatment options. Exposure to sun, sea bathing, and combination therapy with vitamin D have been successfully prescribed. Lubricating creams, including hydrogenated vegetable oil, white petrolatum, and crude coal tar, combined with exposure to UV light (280 to 320 nm), have been effective (Porter and Kaplan 2011). The prescription of oral steroids is contraindicated because of their side effects, which include severe exacerbations of psoriasis.

The prognosis for psoriasis is determined by the extent of the disease and whether the arthritic component is present. Traditionally, more severe attacks coincide with an earlier onset of the disease. Return to activity depends on whether arthritis is involved and the degree of debilitation. Most likely the patient will have no restrictions, but close follow-up is recommended to prevent flare-ups.

Environmentally Induced Dermatological Conditions

Skin Cancer

The inclusion of skin cancer in this chapter is not intended to provide definitive diagnosis but to encourage athletic trainers to recognize suspicious lesions and make timely referrals for treatment. Two types of skin cancer are discussed: nonmelanoma and melanoma. Each has subcategories based on the tissue invaded.

Nonmelanoma Skin Cancers

Nonmelanoma skin cancer (NMSC) is the most common skin cancer in humans worldwide. NMSC can be classified into two categories, basal cell carcinoma or squamous cell carcinoma, depending on which type of cell is affected. Both arise from keratinocytes. Basal cell carcinomas (BCCs) comprise 80% of NMSCs, whereas squamous cell carcinomas (SCCs) comprise only 20% (American Cancer Society 2016b). Together, about 5.4 million new cases of BCCs and SCCs are diagnosed each year in the United States. Due to the rising incidence of this largely preventable form of cancer, the National Collegiate Athletic Association (NCAA) issued a sports medicine guideline in 2012 that addresses safety from exposure to the sun (Wysong et al. 2012; Parsons 2014).

CONDITION HIGHLIGHT

Predisposition for Melanoma

- *Moles:* A mole is a benign skin tumor. Certain types of moles increase a person's chance of getting melanoma. People with many moles and those who have some large moles have an increased risk for melanoma.

- *Fair skin:* People with fair skin, freckling, light hair, or blue eyes have a higher risk of melanoma, but anyone can get melanoma.

- *Family history:* About 10% of people with melanoma have a close relative (e.g., mother, father, brother, sister, child) with the disease. A strong family history of breast and ovarian cancer could mean that certain gene changes or mutations are present. Men with this gene change have a higher risk of melanoma.

- *Immune suppression:* People such as transplant patients who have been treated with medicines that suppress the immune system have an increased risk of developing melanoma.

- *Ultraviolet radiation:* Too much exposure to UV radiation is a risk factor for melanoma. The main source of such radiation is sunlight. Tanning lamps and booths are other sources.

- *Age:* About one-half of melanomas occur in people over age 50, but younger people are also susceptible.

- *Gender:* Men have a higher rate of melanoma than women.

- *Xeroderma pigmentosum (XP):* XP is a rare, inherited condition. People with XP are less able to repair damage caused by sunlight and are at greater risk of melanoma.

- *Past history of melanoma:* A person who has already had melanoma has a higher risk of getting another melanoma.

Adapted from the American Cancer Society 2016c.

Whereas BCCs rarely metastasize and are infrequently fatal, SCCs, if left untreated, may lead to significant mortality. Actinic keratoses are considered to be precursors to SCC and are the most frequently treated lesions in humans. Actinic keratoses (AKs) are typically characterized as being "precancers" or premalignant because of the presence of atypical keratinocytes confined to the epidermis. They are rough patches of skin that appear on sun-exposed surfaces. An estimated 58 million Americans have AKs (American Cancer Society 2016b). Left untreated, up to 10% of AKs develop into SCC. Treatments of AKs include topical creams, photodynamic therapy, chemical peel, and laser surgery.

An estimated 5.4 million new cases of NMSC are diagnosed each year in the United States (American Cancer Society 2016b). The number of skin cancer cases in the United States has surpassed the number of cases of all other cancers combined. Approximately one in five Americans will develop skin cancer during their lifetime—more than 95% of which will be NMSC.

The most significant risk factor for developing NMSC appears to be a fair complexion, blonde or red hair, and light eyes (American Cancer Society 2016b). Other risk factors include environmental exposures: chronic or intermittent sun exposure, tanning bed use, radiation therapy, and smoking. The impact of exposure to the sun cannot be overstated. In a consensus report, the European Academy of Dermatology and Venereology found the occupational risk of developing BCC was 43% higher for outdoor workers than for their counterparts working indoors. SCC carried double the risk to the outdoor workers (John et al. 2016). In addition, a history of immunosuppression, scars, ulcers, or burns will also increase the chances of developing NMSC. Unlike melanoma, there is no genetic

CLINICAL TIPS

Skin Terms

Recall that the squamous cells comprise the middle layers of the epidermis; they continuously shed to give way to new cells. Deeper than that is the basal cell layer of epidermis that lies closest to the dermis (then the adipose layer). Basal cells also move up and change over time, becoming squamous cells. The basal layer produces melanocytes that give skin its pigment. Melanoma occurs when the melanocytes become cancerous.

predisposition to nonmelanoma skin cancer (Bader 2015).

Basal Cell Carcinoma

Basal cell carcinoma is the most common skin malignancy and occurs twice as often in males as in females. The incidence of BCC increases with age, and it is nearly 100-fold higher in those aged 55 to 79 than those 35 and younger (Bader 2015). It is the least likely cancer to metastasize to other areas.

There are many types of BCC. The most commonly occurring types are as follows:

- Nodular BCC
- Superficial BCC
- Pigmented BCC
- Morpheaform BCC

The first two are discussed next.

Nodular basal cell carcinoma is considered to be the classic and most common type, comprising 50% to 54% of all BCCs. It typically presents as a pearly, translucent pink papule with central telangiectasias on the head and neck regions, with a predilection for the nose (25% to 30%) (Bader 2015). A central ulceration with bleeding, crusting, and rolled borders may develop in this tumor, and it usually remains asymptomatic and rarely metastasizes. The nodular BCC may be mistaken for a benign nevus (plural, nevi) or an acneiform lesion.

Superficial basal cell carcinoma comprises 9% to 11% of all BCCs and usually is found in patients younger than those who have nodular basal cell carcinoma. This type presents as an asymptomatic, erythematous, scaly plaque that enlarges very slowly and typically occurs on the trunk or extremities (figure 16.10). Superficial BCC

may grow to be as large as 15 cm in diameter without ulceration or bleeding. It may be mistaken for psoriasis or a squamous cell carcinoma *in situ*.

Squamous Cell Carcinoma

The incidence of squamous cell carcinoma has risen over the last several decades at a rate of 3% to 10% per year, with more than 500,000 cases diagnosed yearly in the United States. SCC is associated with higher mortality in Caucasians, the elderly, and males (American Cancer Society 2016b). Classic invasive SCC is discussed next.

Classic Invasive Squamous Cell Carcinoma

Squamous cell carcinoma occurs on the mucous membranes as well as on sun-exposed skin. SCCs generally arise from AKs, which are considered premalignant precursors. Actinic keratosis presents as an erythematous crusted papule on sun-damaged skin. It is often recognized more easily by touch than by sight (figure 16.11). The presence of an AK indicates that skin has been sun-damaged and skin cancer may develop. The most common sites of occurrence include the head and neck, dorsal hands, lower lip, and genitalia. SCC commonly develops as a hyperkeratotic erythematous nodule or plaque on sun-damaged skin. Sites with a higher associated risk of metastases include the lip and ear as well as sites with scarring or inflammation.

Signs and Symptoms

Patients presenting with possible basal cell cancer must have a lesion with a pearly appearance. Often there is

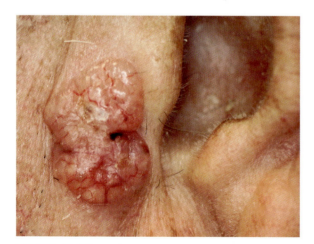

FIGURE 16.10   Nodular basal cell carcinoma.

The Division of Dermatology at Brody School of Medicine, East Carolina University

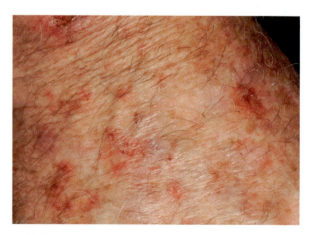

FIGURE 16.11   Actinic keratoses are often precursors of cancer. Because they are recurring rough patches of skin they are discovered more often by feel than by sight.

The Division of Dermatology at Brody School of Medicine, East Carolina University

a central depression or ulceration and perhaps crusting or bleeding from the lesion (Bader 2015). The skin texture feels rough over the lesion. There may be scaling or crusting (Monroe 2015). Lesions are different from surrounding skin, are slow growing, and occur on areas most often exposed to the sun (e.g., nose, lips, ears, hands, forearms).

Referral and Diagnostic Tests

Patients with lesions that are unusual are referred to a dermatologist. Suspicious lesions are biopsied and staged.

Treatment and Return to Participation

Although the standard treatment of NMSC is surgical excision, electrodesiccation and curettage, or cryosurgery are acceptable treatment options for appropriately selected tumors. Mohs micrographic surgery offers the highest cure rate for those that are high-risk (Brodland 2010). Mohs surgery is best for NMSCs that are recurrent, exhibit an aggressive histology, are larger than usual (>2 cm), or are located at sites that require tissue conservation. Mohs surgery is an office procedure in which the physician cuts around the tumor with a small scalpel, using local anesthesia, and evaluates the margins of the tumor. Other treatment modalities include radiation therapy, photodynamic therapy, laser ablation, topical chemotherapy (typically 5-fluorouracil or imiquimod), and systemic retinoid therapy.

Suspect but not confirmed lesions are often treated by a regimen of topical chemotherapy, followed by photodynamic therapy. The purpose of this treatment is to remove the most superficial layers of the skin, most likely taking with it the damaged, possibly precancerous aspects of it. The topical cream is applied to lesions and reacts to nontypical cells. During the time of treatment (typically 1 to 2 wk), patients are cautioned to remain out of the sun because the chemotherapy reacts to sunlight. Patients will report a gradual reddening of the skin, followed by possible open sores resembling fever blisters. The subsequent photodynamic therapy reacts to the topical cream, and although this treatment lasts only up to 30 min, the burn effect of the light continues for 24 to 48 h. During this time, the patient will report deepening reddening of the skin, tightness, and eventually peeling. It is imperative to avoid sunlight, even from windows, for the first several days after photodynamic therapy (Bader 2015; Monroe 2015). A biopsy may be performed after the chemotherapy or photodynamic care if lesions are still present or suspected.

Melanoma

Melanoma is a skin cancer arising from melanocytes. **Melanocytes** are found in the stratum basale (deepest layer of the epidermis), eye, inner ear, meninges, heart, and bone. They produce the pigmentation in skin, also known as **melanin**. Melanoma is not limited to the skin; it is also found in mucosa of the oral and genital cavities, nails, and the conjunctiva of the eye (Porter and Kaplan 2011). The risk of melanoma will surely grow with the increasing number of people exposed to UV light from either the sun or tanning booths (Simon 2015). The rate of malignant melanoma diagnoses has increased by an alarming 190% since the 1930s, and it has significantly increased among Caucasian women compared to men and over all racial groups of both genders (Centers for Disease Control and Prevention 2015). The American Cancer Society listed over 76,000 newly diagnosed cases of melanoma in the United States in 2016 and attributed to it over 10,000 deaths (American Cancer Society 2016a). It is 20 times more prevalent in Caucasians than in African-Americans and also in women aged 15 to 29, and the trunk is the most common site of melanoma (American Academy of Dermatology 2015b; 2016b). The most susceptible individuals have fair skin and blue eyes, sunburn easily, had multiple sunburns at an early age, and have a personal or family history of skin cancer (American Cancer Society 2016c). Because 40% to 50% of malignant melanomas arise from pigmented moles, people with moles or freckles should be especially cautious (Porter and Kaplan 2011).

Melanoma is recognized as a public health issue due to its recent rising incidence and overall mortality rate. Notably, melanoma kills young adults more often than most other cancers (American Cancer Society 2016a). Significant attempts have been made to increase public awareness through public sun protection campaigns for the past 25 yr (Simon 2015).

There are four recognized major types of primary cutaneous melanoma:

- Superficial spreading melanoma
- Nodular melanoma
- Lentigo maligna melanoma
- Acral lentiginous melanoma

The two most common, superficial spreading melanoma and nodular melanoma, are discussed here.

- *Superficial spreading melanoma (SSM)* is the most common type of melanoma, constituting 70% of all melanomas (Ferri 2016). The median age of occurrence is in the fifth decade, and it appears most frequently on the trunk in males and on the legs in females. Most notably, SSM has no preference for sun-damaged skin. SSM can arise anew or from an existing mole. It originates as an asymptomatic brown to black macule (see figure 16.3) with irregular or notched borders and color variegation such as red, blue, and white. Bleeding, itching, and ulceration may also be noted.

• *Nodular melanoma (NM)* is the second most common type of melanoma in fair-skinned people and develops most often during the sixth decade of life. It comprises 15% to 20% of all melanomas and occurs twice as often in males as in females (Ferri 2016). NM may develop at any sun-exposed body site, but it has a predilection for the head, neck, and trunk. It appears as a bluish-black or reddish-pink nodule that has been rapidly enlarging for months. Ulceration and bleeding may ensue. NMs are often misdiagnosed as blood blisters. NM exhibits vertical growth *de novo* and lacks the typical initial horizontal growth phase demonstrated by the other types of melanoma. Therefore, nodular melanoma tends to grow thicker, invade deeper, and associate with a poorer prognosis at the time of diagnosis.

It is important to recognize the risk factors for the development of melanoma. Unlike NMSC, risk factors for melanoma are both genetic and environmental. Genetic factors include fair skin, red hair color, a tendency to burn, and a family history of melanoma or atypical (dysplastic) moles or nevi. Environmental factors include intense intermittent sun exposure, sunburn, and geographic residence proximal to the equator. Other risk factors include having more than 50 atypical or large moles, being immunosuppressed, having a history of sunburns or skin cancer, and using tanning beds (American Academy of Dermatology 2016b; Simon 2015; John et al. 2016).

Although ocular (eye) melanoma is rare, comprising only 5% of all melanomas, patients with **dysplastic nevi** have a higher risk of ocular nevi. Dysplastic nevi are atypical moles that look different from other, more common forms of mole.

It is known that people who burn easily typically have fair skin, blonde or red hair, and blue eyes, and therefore have a higher risk of developing cutaneous (skin) mela-noma. However, it is currently not established whether there is any link between ultraviolet radiation exposure and the development of ocular melanoma (Richtig et al. 2004).

Signs and Symptoms

Patients presenting with atypical lesions must have a thorough medical history, focusing on the genetic and environmental risk factors such as a personal or family history of melanoma or atypical moles, fair skin type, a large number of moles, childhood history of sunburns, immunosuppression, and genetic syndromes with skin cancer predisposition. A detailed history about a suspicious lesion should be obtained regarding whether it was present at birth; any changes in appearance; symptoms such as itching, bleeding, burning, or pain; and any other systemic symptoms such as weight loss, fatigue, cough, or headache.

A complete total body skin examination should be performed to rule out any suspicious lesions. Both the American Academy of Dermatology and the American Cancer Society use the ABCDE mnemonic as a guide to better recognize suspicious pigmented lesions (American Academy of Dermatology 2015b). The ABCDE mnemonic is outlined in table 16.1.

Differential diagnoses for melanoma include basal cell carcinoma, squamous cell carcinoma, sebaceous carcinoma, dysplastic nevi, vascular lesions, and blue nevus (Tan 2016).

Referral and Diagnostic Tests

A mole or lesion should have clear, definitive borders. If it does not, or if it falls into any of the ABCDE categories, the lesion is suspect, and the patient needs to be evalu-

TABLE 16.1 **The ABCDEs of Melanoma**

Abbreviation	Descriptor	Parameters
A	Asymmetry	A melanoma lesion cannot be "folded in half"; in other words, the lesion does not have equal right and left sections or top and bottom sections.
B	Border	Benign lesions have a distinct border that can easily be traced, whereas malignant lesions may have borders that can fade off and be difficult to trace.
C	Color	Benign lesions have a uniform tan, brown, or black color, whereas malignant lesions may have variegated or multiple (i.e., red, white, and blue) color patterns. In addition, a sudden darkening in color or spreading into normal skin suggests a malignant lesion.
D	Diameter	Benign lesions usually have a diameter of less than 6 mm, whereas malignant lesions usually have a diameter greater than 6 mm (the size of a pencil eraser when diagnosed), but they can be smaller.
E	Evolving	A mole or lesion looks different from the surrounding area or is changing in shape, color, or size.

ated by a physician. The athletic trainer should refer to a physician any athletes with changes in shape, border, or size of a mole or lesion or the development of ulceration or bleeding, all of which are suggestive of melanoma. It is paramount to convey to patients with risk factors and an unusual lesion the urgent need to seek dermatological care because the prognosis for a patient with melanoma depends on the stage of the disease when it is diagnosed.

Diagnosis is typically based on a biopsy that is performed on a suspicious pigmented lesion. The preferred procedure is an excisional biopsy, where the lesion and the 1 to 3 mm margins are completely excised (Tan 2016). The lesion and its border are then evaluated under a microscope via histopathological examination. The pathologist can then clearly identify the types of cells in the lesion. Because the degree of atypia and the depth of invasion may not be uniform in a pigmented lesion, an excisional biopsy decreases the risk of sampling error by allowing the pathologist to examine the entire lesion (American Academy of Dermatology 2016a). Another type of biopsy is an incisional biopsy, also termed a punch biopsy, where only one part of the lesion is inspected microscopically.

Malignant melanomas are staged at the time of biopsy. An accurate staging system that groups patients at similar risk for disease progression and natural history is a necessary tool for the selection of optimal treatments. The staging of melanoma involves determining the tumor thickness and any involvement of the lymph nodes or organs. The system most commonly used to stage cancers is the TNM staging system (Tan 2015). It is described in chapter 3 and was created by both the American Joint Committee on Cancer and the International Union Against Cancer.

The local, regional, or distant extent of the melanoma strongly correlates with survival. In general, the prognosis for a patient with localized melanoma and no nodal or systemic metastases is favorable. There is a delineation between the stage I patients with low-risk melanoma with a depth less than 1 mm and the stage II patients with higher risk melanoma with a depth greater than 2 mm. Depth is an indicator of how deep melanoma cells have penetrated into the skin, and the TNM system and clinical (anatomical) and pathological staging are used to determine the patient's prognosis (American Academy of Dermatology 2016a). Stages I and II include localized melanoma with estimated five-year survival rates of 90% to 95% and 45% to 78%, respectively (Tan 2015). Involvement of regional lymph nodes (stage III) decreases the survival rate to 24% to 63%, and the presence of distant metastases (stage IV) correlates with only a 7% to 19% survival rate. Other prognostic indicators include gender, age, and anatomic site (American Academy of Dermatology 2016a; Tan 2015).

Patients diagnosed with malignant melanoma will undergo further testing to include chest radiography, MRI, CT scans, and PET scans to determine the extent of the cancer (Tan 2016).

Treatment and Return to Participation

Although benign moles, freckles, and age spots may provoke suspicion, it is wise to refer any questionable lesion to a medical doctor for inspection and likely a biopsy. If caught early, surgically removed melanoma has a high cure rate, but once it metastasizes to the lymph nodes, the five-year survival rate drops considerably. If organ involvement has occurred through this spread, the survival rate drops again (Tan 2015). Excision includes removing at least 1 cm lateral to the tumor. Large surgical areas may require skin grafts or loss of underlying tissue that could result in deformity of the area involved.

The "gold standard" for treatment of stage I and II primary melanoma is wide local excision with the appropriate margins determined by the depth of the tumor. The purpose of the wide excisional margins is to ensure complete removal of any migratory melanoma cells and to prevent local recurrence. Management options for stage III regional metastatic melanoma include sentinel lymph node biopsy, elective lymph node dissection, and adjuvant therapy by chemotherapy (typically interferon α-2b). Interferon α-2b is an anticancer and antiviral drug administered to high-risk patients and to those with melanoma stage IIb/III as adjuvant therapy after an initial treatment (two rounds) of dacarbazine (DTIC) chemotherapy. The most common toxic side effects of interferon α-2b are influenza-like symptoms and mood alterations. Current treatment options for stage IV include chemotherapy, radiation therapy, immunotherapy, biochemotherapy, and molecularly targeted therapy (Tan 2015; 2016).

Prognosis for the athlete with melanoma depends on the thickness of the tumor involved. Patients with tumors less than 1 mm have up to a 95% five-year survival rate, whereas patients with tumors greater than 4 mm thick have an approximately 45% survival rate for the same period (Tan 2015; American Cancer Society 2016c). The more tissue involved, the longer an athlete will need to recover.

Prognosis and return to participation also relate to the tumor's growth in other areas or tissues. An athlete with a melanoma contained within one mole will have a return-to-participation rate that is based on the sutures and the location of surgery as well as any additional treatment such as chemotherapy. Melanoma involving organs or the lymphatic system most likely will require cessation or at least a great reduction of activity until the cancer is fully under control.

Prevention

Because of the numerous data linking sun exposure to melanoma and other skin cancers, sun protection is imperative. "Sun-bathing" and the use of tanning beds are discouraged. Sun damage is cumulative, and 80% of the damage occurs before the age of 18 (American Cancer Society 2016c). In 2015, the FDA proposed new safety rules for indoor tanning bed use. These restrictions included banning tanning bed usage for anyone under age 18 and requiring all users to sign a safety statement acknowledging the health risks of using tanning beds (Simon 2015). It should be noted that both Australia and Brazil have banned indoor tanning, and 11 European countries forbid those under 18 from using them.

Sun avoidance during peak midday hours may be impractical for certain people, especially those whose occupations keep them outdoors and athletes who practice and participate outside. The public has been slow to embrace the use of sun-protective clothing. Clothing itself is not a prohibitive barrier, as it has been found that clothing typically yields a sun protection factor (SPF) of 5. Clothing with higher SPF values is available. Other protection from the sun includes hats with wide brims that can increase coverage to the face, neck, and portions of the shoulders. Long-sleeved shirts and pants aid in protection, as does wearing gloves when possible during gardening, golf, cycling, and other outdoor activities.

People can be genetically predisposed to melanoma. Overexposure to UV light, even for brief periods, can cause a twofold increase in the incidence of melanoma, so protection from the sun is paramount (Centers for Disease Control and Prevention 2015; American Academy of Dermatology 2016b). The liberal use of sunscreens with an SPF rating of at least 30 and those effective against UVA and UVB can greatly reduce exposure. Darker skinned athletes are not immune to melanoma and should be encouraged to follow these precautions as well. Ideal sunscreens for sport activities are those that are also waterproof and sweatproof. Furthermore, sunscreens need to be applied liberally to the sun-exposed skin to provide even coverage. They need to be applied at least 20 to 30 min before sun exposure and should be reapplied every 1 h or after water exposure (American Academy of Dermatology 2016b; American Cancer Society 2016c). In 2012, the NCAA added a new sports medicine guideline (2S) that addressed sun protection. It states that environmental factors such as latitude, altitude, minimal clouds, and reflective surfaces (water, snow, ice) can increase UV radiation exposure (Parsons 2014). It also states that more than 250,000 student-athletes practice outdoors, and UV rays can damage unprotected skin in as little as 15 min. The guideline offers protective measures that include avoiding the sun between 10 a.m.

CLINICAL TIPS

Proper Sunscreen Application

- Apply sunscreen at least 20 to 30 min before exposure.
- Use a sunscreen with a high sun protection factor (SPF), as well as one that has water-proof capabilities.
- Apply liberally to all exposed areas, including ears, back of the neck, and the posterior aspect of the legs.
- Reapply often (at least every hour) and after drying off from water activities.
- Realize that the sun does not need to be shining for one to be dangerously exposed to UVA or UVB light, so make using sunscreen a daily habit.
- Use sunscreen even when in the shade; sunlight reflected off water can also damage the skin.

UVA = ultraviolet A; UVB = ultraviolet B.

and 4 p.m., wearing sun-protective clothing, and using a broad-spectrum sunscreen with an SPF of 30 or higher when outdoors (Parsons 2014). The National Federation of State High School Associations (NFHS) has yet to publish a position on sun exposure, but prudent athletic trainers would align with the NCAA statement for the safety of athletes.

Sunglasses with UVA or UVB protection help protect the eyes not only from direct sun but also from reflected sunlight. To further protect the eyes from sun-induced damage, choose sunglasses that also wrap around the eyes to prevent light from entering the sides that can be reflected into the eyes. Polycarbonate lenses are recommended for children and athletes because they are the most shatter-resistant. Refer to chapter 12 for more information about sun protection for the eyes.

Ultimately, public health campaigns educate people about the importance of being proactive in performing regular skin self-examinations. Through monthly screenings using the ABCDE criteria, one may be able to detect subtle changes in a skin lesion much earlier than at the time of the annual skin examination. Early detection of melanoma yields the greatest chance of a cure. Benign lesions usually appear early in life, and malignant lesions typically arise from preexisting moles or appear spontaneously later in life. If suspicious lesions are recognized during evaluation or during normal daily interactions with athletes, referral to a physician is in order. Annual screening examinations by a board-certified dermatologist are critical for those who have genetic risk factors. It is recommended that everyone have an annual screening beginning at age 40, regardless of risk factors.

Frostbite

Prolonged outdoor cold exposure during sport or recreational activities may lead to frostbite or hypothermia. Hypothermia is a systemic presentation with minimal dermatologic features and is not discussed. Frostbite is caused by vasoconstriction in response to cold, resulting in freezing tissues of the affected body part. Frostbite occurs most commonly on exposed skin, especially on the ears, nose, cheeks, and wrists (Castellani et al. 2006). Cold injuries are most prevalent at –25 °C to –35 °C (–13 °F to –31 °F). Although the temperature and wind chill factors do not affect the severity of a cold injury, a significant risk factor is a prior cold injury. Intrinsic risk factors for frostbite include fatigue, circulatory impairment, malnutrition, and prior history of cold injury. Extrinsic and environmental risk factors include inadequate or constrictive clothing, wind chill, high altitude, and prolonged exposure to cold or moisture (Cappaert et al. 2008; Mechem 2016; Castellani et al. 2006; Castellani and Young 2012). Exposure to environmental cold affects younger athletes more severely than college- and middle-aged people. Athletes with lean body mass and those over age 50 are also at increased risk for hypothermia-related issues (Cappaert et al. 2008; Castellani and Young 2012).

Signs and Symptoms

Because of the body's protective vasoconstrictive mechanism in the cold environment, the core temperature of the trunk is maintained at the expense of the extremities, nose, and ears. Frostbite can occur while in contact with cold surfaces and fluids as well as cold equipment (Cappaert et al. 2008; Castellani et al. 2006; Castellani and Young 2012). Because the condition begins at superficial skin levels and progresses to deeper tissues, damage worsens as the exposure continues. This condition is a localized response to a cold environment and is different from hypothermia, which is a systemic reaction to cold whereby the core temperature drops. Frostbite is divided into four stages, which are detected only on rewarming.

- *First-degree frostbite (frost nip):* First-degree frostbite exhibits erythema, swelling, cutaneous numbness, and fleeting pain. Localized mild edema is not uncommon. The patient is expected to make a full recovery with only mild residual superficial skin peeling (Mechem 2016).

- *Second-degree frostbite:* Second-degree frostbite causes marked redness, swelling, and blister formation. It is a full-thickness skin freezing; the outer skin is hard but resilient with pressure to the underlying areas (Mechem 2016). Although it may heal, the patient may be left with long-term sensory neuropathy and cold sensitivity.

- *Third-degree frostbite:* Third-degree frostbite causes subdermal freezing with destruction of the skin, with the formation of hemorrhagic blisters and hard, waxy skin. This patient will have deep burning pain on rewarming, which can last up to 5 wk (Mechem 2016).

- *Fourth-degree frostbite:* Fourth-degree frostbite results in loss of the entire body part with full-thickness destruction of the skin, muscle, tendon, and bone. Severe injury to this degree usually requires amputation. Visual signs and symptoms include edema, redness, or mottled gray or white skin and accompanying numbness, tingling, or burning. Limited range of motion and cold, hard skin are also signs of fourth-degree frostbite (Cappaert et al. 2008; Mechem 2015).

Referral and Diagnostic Tests

Frostbite injuries are usually easily recognizable because of the clinical history and presentation. Determining the degree of a cold injury may be more challenging; however, radiological evaluation such as magnetic resonance imaging (MRI), radiography, and bone scan may help determine the extent of a cold injury.

Treatment and Return to Participation

The key goals in treating frostbite are removal from cold exposure, rewarming the tissues, and restoring circulation. Rewarming should be achieved slowly at room temperature or by placement next to another person's skin. In an emergency, when transportation to a medical facility is imminent, wrap the tissue in dry towels or blankets to ward off further exposure to cold (Mechem 2015). If using water to rewarm, use circulating water temperatures not exceeding 37 °C to 39 °C (98. 6 °F to 102.2 °F) (Cappaert et al. 2008; Mechem 2016). Warming is continued for 15 to 30 min or until tissue is thawed. It is not advisable to apply dry heat to the frozen extremity or to rub it. It is important to complete core body rewarming and to completely rehydrate the patient before attempting limb rewarming in order to avoid sudden shock and hypotension. The affected tissue should not be allowed to refreeze once the rewarming has begun, as necrosis could result (Cappaert et al. 2008; Castellani et al. 2006; Castellani and Young 2012; Mechem 2016).

Standard therapy consists of local wound care of the frostbitten area. Superficial blisters may be gently debrided to avoid further contact with the inflammatory mediators in the blister fluid. A tetanus prophylaxis should be administered. Other therapies include administration of topical aloe vera, which inhibits the inflammation in superficial frostbite. Thrombolytic therapies including heparin are useful, as are anti-inflammatory agents such as aspirin and pentoxifylline.

Prevention

Active people who participate at high elevations or in winter-like conditions need to prepare for the weather by wearing equipment designed for the conditions. High-quality hiking boots and appropriate gloves are two of the critical items needed for adverse conditions. Athletes who participate in colder weather should wear layers of clothing with wicking layers against the body, a middle layer that offers insulation, and a wind and water barrier as the outermost layer. Because wind can greatly affect colder temperatures, a windbreaker is one of the most critical pieces of protective gear. Other ways to prevent frostbite include maintaining proper nutrition and hydration status and avoiding standing still for long periods of time (Cappaert et al. 2008; Parsons 2014; Castellani and Young 2012). Alcohol, nicotine, and certain drugs affect a person's ability to adapt to colder environments and should be avoided.

Bacterial Conditions

Bacterial skin disorders include impetigo, abscesses, folliculitis, furuncles or boils, carbuncles, and paronychia or onychia. Healthy skin has many different bacterial and fungal organisms that are usually held in check and do not cause infection. However, if the bacteria, often *Staphylococcus aureus* or *Streptococcus pyogenes,* are introduced into a break in the skin, they may begin to

secrete toxins or interfere with cellular function, thereby producing symptoms.

S. aureus and *S. pyogenes* are responsible for most bacterial dermatological conditions. Bacterial and viral conditions may coexist within the same infection and complicate the diagnosis and treatment. It is important to note that one is not immune to a particular bacterial infection after recovery. Given the right conditions, infection is possible again.

The NCAA and the NFHS provide oversight over collegiate and scholastic sports, respectively. Both the NCAA and NFHS have singled out the bacterial infections of impetigo, folliculitis, furuncles, carbuncles (including methicillin-resistant *Staphylococcus aureus* [MRSA]), and staphylococcal diseases for particular restrictions (Parsons 2014; National Federation of State High School Associations 2013). In wrestling, time lost due to skin conditions accounted for 17% of time lost in the sport (Agel et al. 2007). Although the rules are meant especially for wrestlers, they apply to all athletes. Protecting others from infection is paramount, as is protecting the health and welfare of the infected athlete. These guidelines will be reiterated for each transmittable skin infection discussed in this chapter.

Impetigo

Impetigo is a highly contagious skin disorder caused by either *S. aureus* or *S. pyogenes* bacteria, with *S. aureus* accounting for the majority of the infections. It is one of the most common bacterial infections in children and occurs most often in warm temperatures and humid areas (Lewis 2015). Impetigo usually occurs in areas of previous skin disease or injury, such as sites of eczema, insect bite, varicella, or abrasion. Earlier damage to the skin by abrasion opens a pathway for invading bacteria, leading to impetigo. It is transmitted by skin-to-skin

NCAA and NFHS Participation Regulations for Wrestlers With Bacterial Infections

The following regulations apply to participation with the bacterial conditions of impetigo, folliculitis, furuncles, carbuncles, and staphylococcal diseases, including CA-MRSA:

- Completion of at least 72 h of antibiotic therapy.
- No new lesions for 48 h.*
- No moist, draining, or exudative lesions.
- If lesions are questionable, a Gram stain is required if available.
- Active lesions may not be covered to participate.

*NCAA regulation only (not NFHS)

Adapted from Parsons 2014; National Federation of State High School Associations 2013.

contact, with combative sports having a higher incidence of transmission than other activities (Ashack et al. 2016). Each year, it prevents a large number of athletes from participating. Impetigo is a self-limiting disease that typically heals within 2 to 3 wk without scarring (Lewis 2015). It is readily transmitted with skin-to-skin contact, as evidenced by a 2014 high school outbreak from a wrestling meet that hosted 24 schools. Of the 47 athletes who were subsequently infected, 47% contracted impetigo. The original contagion was an athlete who was allowed to illegally participate with uncovered lesions (Williams et al. 2015).

Signs and Symptoms

Athletes with impetigo generally are afebrile, but they may have localized **lymphadenopathy**. The two types of impetigo are nonbullous and bullous. The nonbullous form (about 70% of cases) typically appears as a yellow or honey-colored, crusted lesion on an erythematous base (figure 16.12). Bullous impetigo first presents with moist, red skin that resembles a burn and progresses to flaccid small to large vesicles that appear filled with clear or yellow fluid (Lewis 2015). Both bullous and nonbullous forms present lesions that may be small and pea-shaped or large and blister-like in appearance, or they may appear as ribbon-like strands.

Lesions of impetigo eventually erupt, leaving purulent discharge to dry on the skin. They are painless yet pruritic, which exacerbates and spreads the infection to other areas. The face, arms, legs, and trunk are the most common sites for impetigo. Differential diagnoses for impetigo include HSV, varicella-zoster virus (VZV), insect bites, and tinea infections (Lewis 2015).

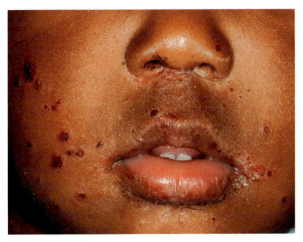

FIGURE 16.12 Nonbullous impetigo presents with a honey-yellow crust covering the lesion.

The Division of Dermatology at Brody School of Medicine, East Carolina University

Referral and Diagnostic Tests

The athletic trainer who suspects an athlete may have impetigo should remove the athlete from activity immediately to prevent the spread of the infection to others and make a referral to a physician (Zinder et al. 2010). Diagnosis is mostly by clinical examination and history, but a culture may be obtained if the diagnosis is unclear (Lewis 2015). In this case, the patient is treated for both impetigo and herpes simplex until the cultures return.

Treatment and Return to Participation

Treatment for a small area of impetigo consists of a topical antibiotic such as mupirocin (Bactroban) applied three times daily for 10 d or until the lesion has cleared. Larger areas of impetigo are generally treated with oral antibiotics that cover both *S. aureus* and *S. pyogenes,* such as penicillin, erythromycin, cephalexin (Keflex), and dicloxacillin (Lewis 2015).

The athlete washes the area with soap and water three times daily, removes the crusts before application of a topical antibiotic, and is not allowed to participate in contact activity until the lesions have completely cleared.

The athlete may return to play on complete resolution of the crusted, infected, exposed areas. In wrestling, the NCAA and NFHS have very specific regulations (see the sidebar "NCAA and NFHS Participation Regulations for Wrestlers with Bacterial Infections").

Prevention

Proper hygiene is paramount. The National Athletic Trainers' Association (NATA) and NCAA are clear and consistent about preventing skin infections, and the key aspects of their message are presented in the sidebar "Prevention Strategies for Infectious Dermatological Conditions in Athletes." When impetigo recurs multiple times, family members or close contacts may need to produce samples for nasopharyngeal culture because 30% to 40% may be asymptomatic carriers of the causative bacteria *(S. aureus).* A carrier who tests positive will need to apply mupirocin ointment to the nasal passages twice daily for 5 d (Lewis 2015). Equipment that may have come in contact with athletes who have lesions must be sanitized daily to prevent the spread of infection or recurrence. Equipment, in this case, includes all mats, towels, protective gear, water bottles, clothing, and uniforms (Zinder et al. 2010).

Folliculitis

Folliculitis is another common bacterial skin infection. There are two types of bacteria that cause folliculitis: *S.*

Prevention Strategies for Infectious Dermatological Conditions in Athletes

The National Athletic Trainers' Association and the National Collegiate Athletic Association have provided the following prevention strategies:

- Organizational support must be adequate to limit the spread of infectious agents.
- A clean environment must be maintained in the athletic training facility, locker rooms, and all athletic venues.
  - Clean and disinfect gym bags or travel bags and all protective gear on a regular basis.
  - Inspect playing fields for animal droppings that could cause bacterial infections of cuts or abrasions.
  - Sanitize athletic lockers between seasons.
  - Weight room equipment, including benches, handles, and bars, should be sanitized daily.
- Health care practitioners and athletes should follow good hand hygiene practices.
- Athletes must be encouraged to follow good overall hygiene practices.
- Athletes must be discouraged from sharing the following:
  - Towels
  - Athletic gear
  - Water bottles
  - Disposable razors
  - Hair clippers
- Athletes with open wounds, scrapes, or scratches must avoid whirlpools and common tubs.
- Athletes are encouraged to report all abrasions, cuts, and skin lesions and to seek attention from an athletic trainer for proper cleaning, treatment, and dressing.

Adapted from S.M. Zinder et al., 2010, "National Athletic Trainers' position statement: Skin diseases." *Journal of Athletic Training* 45(4):411-428. This work is licensed under a Creative Commons Attribution 3.0 License.

---

aureus and *Pseudomonas aeruginosa*; the latter is often associated with infections acquired in hot tubs.

Folliculitis is an inflammatory reaction in the hair follicles and most often occurs on the face, chest, axilla, buttocks, groin, and legs. The most common cause is shaving with a razor blade. When a razor blade nicks the skin, the opening allows bacteria to be introduced into the tissue (figure 16.13). Folliculitis may also be caused by friction from helmets, equipment padding, or straps.

The other common bacterial cause of folliculitis is *Pseudomonas,* which is commonly referred to as hot tub folliculitis (figure 16.14). This type usually appears 2 to 3 d after exposure to water contaminated with *P. aeruginosa.* The most common conduits are poorly maintained hot tubs, pools, baths, water slides, and contaminated waters. There does not appear to be any skin-to-skin transmission with *P. aeruginosa.*

Signs and Symptoms

Clinical presentation of folliculitis demonstrates small, tender, red papules or bumps in the hair follicles, with a

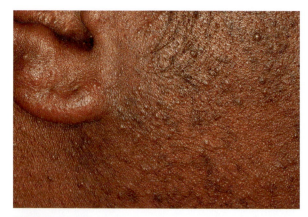

FIGURE 16.13   Folliculitis in a beard, characterized by superficial infection of hair follicles.

The Division of Dermatology at Brody School of Medicine, East Carolina University

hair shaft within the papule. These lesions tend to occur in multiples and are often pruritic (Zinder et al. 2010). The typical presentation of itchy red papules around

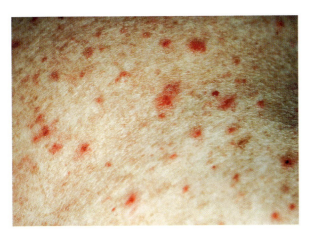

FIGURE 16.14 *Pseudomonas* folliculitis reaction resulting from exposure in a hot tub; the rash appears in areas covered by a swimsuit.

DermPics / Science Source

hair follicles occurs in many areas of the body but most commonly under areas covered by the swimming suit.

Differential diagnoses for folliculitis include *Pityrosporum* folliculitis, dermatophytic folliculitis, gram-negative folliculitis, HSV, acne, pityriasis rosea, molluscum contagiosum, and syphilis.

Referral and Diagnostic Tests

The clinician refers patients who have persistent symptoms despite conservative treatment or those with an unusual presentation. Physician diagnosis is made on the basis of clinical examination, but a Gram stain and culture may be obtained if the results of the examination are nonspecific or if the symptoms persist.

Treatment and Return to Participation

Treatment for folliculitis includes topical or oral antibiotics that provide coverage for both *S. aureus* and *S. pyogenes*. Warm saline compresses and a topical antimicrobial ointment such as bacitracin may also benefit the patient (Porter and Kaplan 2011). The athlete should follow the hygiene protocols outlined in the "Prevention Strategies for Infectious Dermatological Conditions in Athletes" sidebar. In cases of recurrent folliculitis, the patient may benefit from a nasal culture for *S. aureus* (National Athletic Trainers' Association 2005). Sometimes antibiotic treatment is required. Treatment of *Pseudomonas* is not needed because this type of folliculitis usually resolves spontaneously in 7 to 10 d as long as there is no additional exposure. The patient may return to participation immediately and without restrictions.

An athlete may return to participation when the lesions of folliculitis begin to heal. In wrestling, the NCAA and NFHS recommend that the athlete not return until there have been no new lesions for the last 48 h and the athlete has been taking antibiotics for the last 72 h. As with impetigo, nonactive lesions must be covered with durable, nonporous bandaging for participation (National Athletic Trainers' Association 2007; National Federation of State High School Associations 2013; National Federation of State High School Associations 2015a; Parsons 2014). The amount of time it takes for these lesions to heal may depend on their location; some areas, such as the beard, take much longer to heal, especially if the athlete wears headgear with a chin strap that may irritate the condition. The athlete with *Pseudomonas* may participate without restriction.

Abscesses, Furuncles, and Carbuncles

Furunculosis is similar to folliculitis but occurs when lesions are deeper in the hair follicle cavity and contain pus. These lesions are also bacterial skin infections, and they are caused by *S. aureus* and include abscesses, furuncles, and carbuncles, which is a conglomeration of multiple furuncles. An **abscess** is a collection of pus that arises in a variety of locations. A **furuncle**, or boil, is a walled-off abscess containing pus that usually develops in a preexisting site of folliculitis. Boils commonly occur at sites of trauma or friction, such as the beltline, waistline, axilla, groin, thighs, and buttocks; they are more common after puberty (Zinder et al. 2010).

A **carbuncle** is a collection of several coalescing furuncles. Carbuncles are common among wrestlers and readily transmitted by skin-to-skin contact. Methicillin-resistant *S. aureus* (MRSA) has become especially problematic in athletics when athletes are allowed to participate as long as they are receiving medical treatment. In response to MRSA, the NFHS, NATA, and others established policies on the condition (Perloff 2014; Rogers 2008; National Federation of State High School Associations 2015; National Athletic Trainers' Association 2005). Resistant strains cause the athlete to sustain the effects of the infection for a longer period of time, allow more opportunity to spread the disease, and may result in severe systemic illness. (For a more detailed discussion of MRSA, please see chapter 15.)

Signs and Symptoms

The lesion usually begins with a tender, deep, firm, erythematous papule that enlarges and becomes painful and fluctuant over a period of days (figure 16.15). The abscess remains deep, reabsorbs, or drains through the skin. Elevated temperatures and malaise are not uncommon.

Differential diagnoses include folliculitis, sebaceous cyst, skin cancer, severe HSV infection, **hidradenitis**

MRSA

Methicillin-resistant *Staphylococcus aureus* (MRSA) was first observed in 1961. At the time, it was presumed to be associated only with nosocomial infections. However, in the decades that followed, MRSA has spread outside the hospital environment to pervade community settings. In particular, community-acquired MRSA (CA-MRSA) has become a persistent and growing medical problem among the young and healthy population, including athletes. CA-MRSA epidemics have even been reported in entire communities. Because of its ubiquitous presence, it is important to recognize and treat CA-MRSA early to prevent its spread within the community, especially in young athletes participating in contact sport.

Preventing MRSA involves following good hygiene practices in sport that are outlined in the sidebar "Prevention Strategies for Infectious Dermatological Conditions in Athletes." For more on CA-MRSA, see chapter 15.

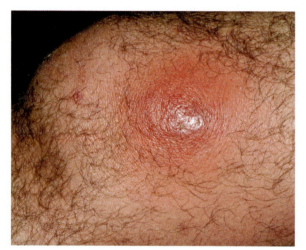

FIGURE 16.15 A furuncle, or boil, is an enlarged swollen purulent mass.

SPL / Science Source

 RED FLAGS FOR CONTAGION ALERT

Moist compresses or heat packs used on infectious skin disorders *must* be disinfected before use on another patient!

Treatment and Return to Participation

Treatment of furuncles consists of warm, moist compresses applied often throughout the day. If this fails, a physician incises and evacuates the abscess. Antibiotics are usually not effective once the abscess has developed, although they are still often prescribed.

A patient who often develops furuncles may need topical antibiotic ointment for the nasal passages to eradicate a carrier state, as happens with impetigo. Return to sport with protection is allowed when the infection begins to heal. In wrestling, however, the NCAA and NFHS recommend that an athlete not return until there have been no new lesions for the last 48 h, among other criteria listed in the sidebar "NCAA and NFHS Participation Regulations for Wrestlers With Bacterial Infections." As with the other bacterial infections, active lesions should not be covered to allow for participation (Parsons 2014; National Federation of State High School Associations 2013).

Prevention

Preventive measures include treating the athlete and close contact members for *S. aureus* carrier states and recurrent infections. Other prevention techniques mentioned with folliculitis and impetigo will also help to retard the spread of furuncles.

suppurativa if located in the axilla or groin, and **pilonidal cyst** if the furuncle is located in the gluteal cleft.

Referral and Diagnostic Tests

The clinician refers to a physician any patient who presents with an elevated temperature, malaise, vomiting, and persistence of furuncles after conservative treatment. Diagnostic tests include a Gram stain for gram-positive cocci and a culture to determine the organism involved, but a culture is usually reserved for persistent infections that do not respond to treatment. A blood culture with antibiotic sensitivities may be obtained with symptoms of a systemic infection, such as fever and malaise (Zinder et al. 2010).

Acne

Acne is a common problem among adolescents, but very little information exists about acne and sport participation. Acne is a condition of the pilosebaceous unit and most commonly occurs where the concentration of sebaceous or sweat glands is the greatest, such as on the face, neck, chest, and back (figure 16.16). The condition is common in both males and females.

Signs and Symptoms

Acne consists of inflammatory and noninflammatory lesions. Inflammatory lesions are composed of erythematous papules, pustules, or deep cysts; noninflammatory lesions are made up of open and closed comedones. Open comedones are commonly referred to as *blackheads,* and closed comedones are commonly referred to as *whiteheads.*

The bacterium involved is *Propionibacterium acnes* and not *S. aureus* or *S. pyogenes.* The follicular shaft becomes plugged, and the proliferation of *P. acnes* secondarily increases keratin formation. This is known as a *noninflammatory reaction,* but when white blood cells are attracted to these lesions, the acne becomes inflammatory. Symptoms range from a few open or closed comedones on the face or another area to multiple comedones, pustules, and deep, large, painful cysts.

The differential diagnoses for acne include bacterial folliculitis, *Pityrosporum* folliculitis, pseudofolliculitis, perioral dermatitis, human papillomavirus (HPV), HSV infections, and contact dermatitis.

Referral and Diagnostic Tests

Many people with simple episodic acne do not need referral. Typical over-the-counter treatments, such as antimicrobial soaps and washes, often contain benzoyl peroxide or retinoids focused on drying the skin, and they can be a great first-line treatment. These should be tried prior to referral if possible. Patients with acne are referred to a dermatologist if they have chronic or widespread acne. If personal hygiene is not the culprit, pharmaceutical intervention can help ameliorate most forms of acne (Rao 2015).

Treatment and Return to Participation

Depending on the type, acne responds well to a variety of agents. Noninflammatory acne responds well to topical adapalene (Differin), tretinoin (Retin-A, Avita), azelaic acid (Azelex, Finevin), and tazarotene (Tazorac). Benzoyl peroxide is an antibacterial agent but also works well for noninflammatory acne. Inflammatory acne responds well to topical benzoyl peroxide either alone or in combination with an antibiotic as well as topical and oral antibiotics. For resistant or severe cystic acne, isotretinoin (Accutane) is used, but it has a significant number of side effects. Oral antibiotics or hormonal therapy are usually prescribed, but steroid injection and chemical peels have also been used in some cases (Rao 2015).

The athletic trainer and physician counsel athletes during acne treatment about the side effects of some acne medications; these medications may cause sensitivity to sunlight and, as a result, may increase the likelihood of sunburn.

Acne is not considered contagious or a limitation to activity, so athletes are allowed to participate without restrictions.

Paronychia or Onychia

Paronychia is an infection that affects the proximal or lateral nail fold that separates the skin from the nail, and **onychia** is an infection of the nail matrix. The infection may occur after manipulation, other infection, or trauma. The organism usually involved is *S. aureus,* but it can also be a fungal infection if the athlete is immunocompromised. Other, more obscure causes include prolonged water exposure, herpes simplex, or candidal vaginitis (Porter and Kaplan 2011).

Signs and Symptoms

A paronychia is a bright red swelling of the folds of tissue surrounding a nail, which may show an accumulation of purulent material (figure 16.17). In contrast, an onychia is an infection of the nail bed. Differential diagnoses for paronychia include bacterial infections, fungal infections, *Pseudomonas,* and trauma.

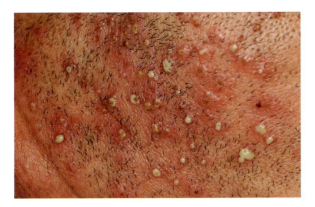

FIGURE 16.16 Acne is typical among athletes.
The Division of Dermatology at Brody School of Medicine, East Carolina University

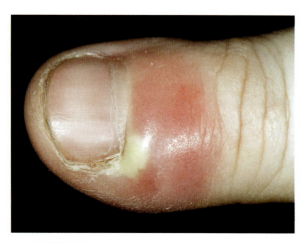

FIGURE 16.17   Paronychia infection of a thumb.

Dr P. Marazzi / Science Source

Referral and Diagnostic Tests

Athletes with infected nail beds are referred when conservative care is ineffective. Referral is also indicated for immunocompromised patients or those with persistent or worsening symptoms. If the patient is immunocompetent, no further diagnostic testing is needed unless the symptoms persist, and then a Gram stain, KOH preparation, and culture of the fluid are obtained.

Treatment and Return to Participation

Conservative treatment consists of warm to hot soaks and acetaminophen (Tylenol) for mild pain. If the infection is large, especially painful, or disabling, a small incision into the corresponding location will relieve the pressure by draining the infection. Sometimes antibiotics are needed if incision and drainage are inadequate. Prevention of paronychial or onychial infections consists of good nail and skin hygiene and limited manipulation with careful nail cutting. Keeping fingers and toes clean and dry will retard these infections (Ferri 2016).

Participation is not restricted with a paronychial infection, and the prognosis after treatment is good. If the area was drained, the athletic trainer should follow basic wound care protocol to prevent further infection.

Viral Conditions

Viral infections are some of the most difficult and challenging problems in athletes, especially wrestlers. The viruses presented in this section include herpes simplex virus (HSV), varicella-zoster virus (VZV), molluscum contagiosum, and human papillomavirus (HPV).

Herpes Simplex

HSV is addressed in chapter 10. It is an extremely contagious viral infection and presents as cold sores or fever blisters, genital herpes, and **herpes gladiatorum**. There are more than 80 types of HSV, but the most common types are HSV-1, which typically occurs above the waist, and HSV-2, which typically occurs below the waist. Both types, however, can be found in both areas, and typing may only be significant for predicting future outbreaks and responses to treatment.

It is estimated that by age 30, 50% of people in higher socioeconomic regions and 80% of those in lower socioeconomic areas test positive for HSV-1 (Salvaggio 2015). Not everyone develops symptoms once infected, and each person experiences a different rate of recurrence. HSV enters the skin through a site of previous injury, such as a cut or abrasion, or damage, such as eczema, and follows the nerve root to the dorsal root ganglion in the spinal cord. One may not develop symptoms or a rash during the primary infection. Subsequent infections of HSV can be triggered by stress, sunburn, or even menstrual cycles (Salvaggio 2015).

At various times, HSV will follow the nerves back to the skin and produce symptoms along the dermatomal distribution. HSV is never eradicated, but symptoms present in varying degrees. Approximately 70% of genital herpes is transmitted by asymptomatic shedding of the virus in people who report never having had the infection (Salvaggio 2015).

When HSV occurs on the face and trunk, it is commonly known as herpes gladiatorum. The NFHS has established a position statement on this condition and has created a document that physicians can use in clearing high school wrestlers after infection (National Federation of State High School Associations 2013; 2015). Estimates indicate that 2.6% of high school wrestlers and 7.6% of collegiate wrestlers have been infected with HSV, and approximately 20% to 40% of NCAA Division I wrestlers have been infected (Landry and Chang 2004). These numbers probably underestimate the problem because some lesions remain unrecognized. The infection typically spreads by direct skin-to-skin contact with an infected person. Outbreaks are usually found on the head and trunk but are not limited to these areas.

Complications of HSV are numerous and include chronic recurrences, skin lesions, possible scarring, eye or corneal scarring, and blindness. **Herpes keratoconjunctivitis** is a highly infectious condition of the cornea of the eye that may lead to corneal damage, scarring, or even blindness (Landry and Chang 2004). HSV keratoconjunctivitis is the leading infectious cause of blindness in the United States. The infection may occur either by direct contact or by reactivation of HSV through the ophthalmic branch of the trigeminal nerve.

So-called fever blisters or cold sores are also caused by HSV, and people with active lesions can transmit the virus to otherwise healthy body areas (figure 16.18). Also known as *herpes labialis,* cold sores can be exacerbated by UV light from the sun, which is why wearing a lip balm with sunblock is one good preventive idea.

Signs and Symptoms

Typical symptoms for the primary HSV infection mimic the flu and include fever, sore throat, lymphadenopathy, malaise, and vesicles on an erythematous base. Recurrent HSV infection symptoms include grouped vesicles of the same shape and age on an erythematous base. On occasion, tingling or pain precedes the outbreak (Salvaggio 2015).

Outbreaks may present in many ways, however, and they do not always present as the typical vesicles on an erythematous base. In the early stages, they are often easily confused with ringworm, impetigo, acne, and eczema. Sometimes wrestlers break open the vesicles, cover the rash with makeup, sandpaper the rash, or even use bleach to alter the rash in order to continue to wrestle (Landry and Chang 2004; Landry, Chang, and Mees 2004). Obviously, diagnosis is then even more difficult and the infection can spread more easily to others.

Differential diagnoses for HSV include bacterial infections such as impetigo, acne, and various types of folliculitis; viral varicella-zoster; and fungal tinea infections.

Referral and Diagnostic Tests

The clinical diagnosis in many cases of HSV is made on the basis of symptoms and exposure. The most definitive method of diagnosis is to unroof an intact moist vesicle and culture the base for HSV. This method may take 48 h to yield results, so once a diagnosis is suspected, the ath-

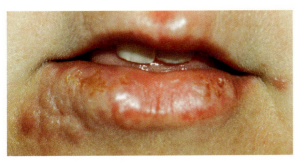

FIGURE 16.18 Herpes simplex, also called a *cold sore,* presents as tight vesicles that develop into pustules and ulcers.

Biophoto Associates / Science Source

lete should be kept out of contact with other athletes (Cyr 2004; Salvaggio 2015). Another test, polymerase chain reaction (PCR), is accurate and fast and can also detect asymptomatic shedding. The direct fluorescent antigen test yields results in 2 to 3 h and, as with culturing, takes samples scraped from the ulcer base (Salvaggio 2015). Withholding an athlete from contact activity before a culture is taken and medications are started is absolutely necessary to prevent the spread of the disease.

Treatment and Return to Participation

Oral antiviral medications include acyclovir (Zovirax), valacyclovir (Valtrex), and famciclovir (Famvir). Doses differ depending on whether the condition is a primary or recurrent outbreak. For wrestlers, prophylactic medications should be continued after the outbreak for the remainder of the wrestling season. Prophylactic doses are acyclovir, 400 mg two times daily; valacyclovir, 1000 mg daily; and famciclovir, 250 mg daily (Salvaggio 2015). The athlete must shower with antibacterial soap and launder all towels and uniforms daily. Although drug reactions with antiviral medications are rare, dehydration is a possible concern in wrestlers or in someone who has poor renal function, and it can lead to severe kidney problems (Cyr 2004). Athletes taking antiviral medications are encouraged to increase fluid intake for the duration of the medical course.

Current NCAA recommendations require that the athlete be withheld from contact sports until the athlete is asymptomatic (Parsons 2014). The NFHS also has recommendations for HSV but separates them into cold sores and herpes gladiatorum. Primary outbreaks have a longer time requirement for oral antiviral medications (10 to 14 d compared to 5 d required by the NCAA), but the NFHS is less restrictive in the case of new lesions: The NFHS requires 48 h with no new lesions, whereas the NCAA mandates 72 h (Parsons 2014; National Federation of State High School Associations 2013).

Varicella-Zoster

VZV, otherwise known as *chicken pox* (for the initial infection with the varicella virus) and *shingles* (for reactivations with the herpes zoster virus), is another common viral infection.

As presented in chapter 15, chicken pox is a common childhood disease with some cases presenting in adolescence or adulthood. This infection is very contagious and is spread by respiratory droplets or direct skin-to-skin contact. Patients are contagious from about 2 d before the onset of the rash until all lesions have crusted over (Anderson 2015).

NCAA Participation Regulations for Wrestlers With Viral Infections

Primary HSV Infection

- Free of systemic symptoms such as fever and malaise.
- No new lesions or blisters within the past 72 h.
- No moist or exudative lesions, and all existing lesions must be dry with a firm, adherent crust.
- Completion of at least 120 h (5 d) of an appropriate systemic antiviral therapy.
- Active lesions *may not* be covered to allow for participation.

Secondary (Recurrent) HSV Infection

- No moist or exudative lesions, and all existing lesions must be dry with a firm, adherent crust.
- Completion of at least 120 h (5 d) of an appropriate systemic antiviral therapy.
- Active lesions *may not* be covered to allow for participation.

Herpes Zoster (Shingles)

- All existing lesions must be dry with a firm, adherent crust.
- There must be no evidence of a secondary bacterial infection.

Molluscum Contagiosum*

- All lesions must be removed (frozen or curetted) before participation.
- Isolated or small clusters of lesions may be covered with a gas-permeable membrane and stretch tape that cannot be dislodged to allow for participation.

Verrucae (Warts)*

- Verrucae plana or vulgaris must be adequately covered for participation.
- Athletes with multiple facial verrucae digitata that cannot be adequately covered with a mask or curetted away may not participate.
- Solitary or scattered lesions may be curetted for participation but may not be seeping.

*The NFHS does not consider these to be very contagious and requires no treatment or restrictions for high school athletes.

Adapted from Parsons 2014; National Federation of State High School Associations 2013.

Herpes zoster, or shingles, is a reactivation of VZV involving the skin along its dermatomal distribution. It occurs at all ages but increases in frequency with advancing age. Reactivation may result from advancing age, immunosuppression, lymphoma, stress, and radiation therapy (Janniger 2016). Shingles most commonly is the result of reactivation from a previous VZV infection, not from direct contact with someone with shingles.

Signs and Symptoms of Varicella

Symptoms of chicken pox are presented in chapter 15 and include low-grade fever, headache, and malaise before the rash begins; the patient will develop a papular or vesicular rash. The rash evolves in size and scope as it begins on the trunk, spreading to the extremities and face. Intense itching is often secondary to the rash.

Differential diagnoses for varicella include herpes simplex, bullous impetigo, various types of folliculitis, and contact dermatitis.

Signs and Symptoms of Herpes Zoster

Typical symptoms of shingles include pain, tingling, burning, or itching before the onset of the rash along a single dermatome, and they may present along more than one dermatome or may cross the midline. The most common complication is postherpetic neuralgia (PHN), which may require strong analgesic medications to control the pain (Janniger 2016; Landry and Chang 2004).

Differential diagnoses for herpes zoster include migraine, acute dermatitis, spinal nerve compression, renal calculi, HSV infection, contact dermatitis, bullous impetigo, and conjunctivitis (Janniger 2016).

Treatment and Return to Participation

Patients diagnosed with varicella are typically prescribed the antiviral medication acyclovir, 800 mg four times per day for 5 d initially, to help prevent complications from varicella. Pediatric doses may vary depending on the age and weight of the patient. These medications are used to help reduce the viral shedding, pain, and frequency of PHN. Symptomatic treatment also includes lotions and antihistamines to reduce itching. Sometimes prednisone is prescribed to reduce the chance of PHN. Narcotic analgesics are also used to help with pain control.

Prevention

The best prevention for chicken pox is the varicella vaccine at 12 mo. Limited exposure at a young age to known cases will prevent the athlete from contracting the condition later in life when the disease presents more dramatically.

Molluscum Contagiosum

Molluscum contagiosum is a viral infection commonly found in children and in sexually active adults. It most commonly appears on the face, trunk, arms, legs, and genital areas. Palms and soles are usually not involved. It is easily spread via direct contact, such as children sharing a bath or athletes sharing equipment (Bhatia 2015). The disease is self-limited and typically resolves spontaneously after several months. It is caused by a virus in the *Poxviridae* family and is more common in swimmers, wrestlers, and gymnasts (Cyr 2004).

Signs and Symptoms

Molluscum contagiosum presents as a small, skin-colored, sometimes erythematous, smooth, dome-shaped papule with a central punctum (figure 16.19). It is very contagious and is spread by **autoinoculation** and direct skin-to-skin contact. The lesions usually spontaneously resolve in 6 to 12 mo. Differential diagnoses include HPV, sebaceous hyperplasia, and squamous cell or basal cell carcinoma (Bhatia 2015).

Treatment and Return to Participation

Conservative treatment of molluscum contagiosum is effective for most patients, but wrestlers and those in other contact sports may require aggressive therapy sooner.

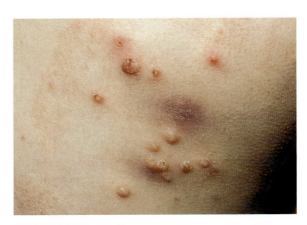

FIGURE 16.19 Molluscum contagiosum.

Dr. P. Marazzi / Science Source

Lesions may be treated by freezing each one with liquid nitrogen or by curetting with a comedone extractor or small needle, although slight scarring is possible with these two procedures. After these treatments, the lesions are no longer contagious.

If the lesions are solitary or grouped, they can be covered with a gas-permeable membrane such as OpSite (Smith & Nephew Healthcare, Hull, UK), Tegaderm (3M, St. Paul, MN), or Bioclusive (Johnson & Johnson, New Brunswick, NJ) followed by prewrap and stretch tape so that participation can be allowed. If the lesions are too numerous or cannot be covered, then all lesions must be curetted or frozen before return is allowed.

Human Papillomavirus

HPV, or warts, are most common in children and young adults but may occur at any age. More than 65 types of HPV have been identified and can be seen any place on the skin. Some warts may spontaneously resolve in less than 2 yr, but others last a lifetime. Warts are spread by skin-to-skin contact and usually occur at sites of trauma, abrasion, or eczema, most commonly on the hands and feet.

Signs and Symptoms

The diagnostic feature of warts is their distortion or obscuring of the normal skin lines. Warts present as small, smooth, skin-colored papules that may progress to a rough surface, a flat-topped surface, or a deep, callus-like lesion (figure 16.20). Some warts have small black dots, which represent thrombosed capillaries. These dots are often considered a diagnostic sign of warts.

Differential diagnoses include molluscum contagiosum, seborrheic keratosis, actinic keratosis, squamous cell and basal cell carcinoma, corns, and calluses.

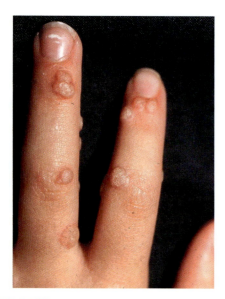

FIGURE 16.20 Warts, also called verrucae, can appear anywhere on the skin.

The Division of Dermatology at Brody School of Medicine, East Carolina University

Referral and Diagnostic Tests

No specific tests are needed unless the diagnosis is atypical. In rare cases, a biopsy may aid in the diagnosis. Referral is indicated when conservative treatment has failed or when symptoms interfere with daily activities.

Treatment and Return to Participation

The many treatments for warts include salicylic acid, liquid nitrogen, and podophyllin. Blunt dissection and laser treatment are reserved for resistant cases. Imiquimod (Aldara) has been approved for genital and perianal warts, and research shows it may have some merit in treating common warts (Gearhart 2015).

Prognosis is generally good because most lesions do eventually resolve spontaneously. Return to participation for an athlete recovering from warts is unlimited. In collegiate wrestling, however, competitors with multiple facial digitate warts will be disqualified if the warts cannot be covered with a mask. Wrestlers with multiple flat warts and common warts should cover them adequately before competition (Parsons 2014). The National Federation of State High School Associations places no restrictions on wrestling with warts or molluscum contagiosum (National Federation of State High School Associations 2013). Athletic trainers should check regional or state guidelines to be certain they are following local safety policies. Acid or freezing treatment of warts may result in a blood-tinged blister that eventually resolves into a scab. While the blister is present, it should be covered during participation. The best prevention for HPV is good skin hygiene that will help prevent transmission through damaged skin areas. There is currently a vaccine series for men and women that prevents certain strains of HPV that can cause cervical cancer (Arends, Wyllie, and Bird 1990; Daley et al. 2010).

Fungal Conditions

Fungal infections are extremely common in athletes, especially wrestlers. Fungal infections are often found on the skin, hair, and nails, with the most common infection sites being the scalp, face, extremities, trunk, groin, and feet. **Dermatophytes** are superficial fungal infections of the skin, and they are the most common infectious agents among humans (Kao 2015).

The dermatophytes discussed here are surface, or topical, fungal conditions and include tinea corporis, tinea cruris, tinea unguium, tinea pedis, tinea capitis, tinea barbae, and tinea versicolor. Tinea infections are named according to the affected body area. All are true fungal infections except for tinea versicolor, which is categorized as a yeast disorder. Table 16.2 lists the common tinea infections, their location on the body, and typical treatment. As a group, these conditions tend to be transmitted person to person or animal to person. Most respond well to topical antifungal ointments, but newer systemic oral medications have proven to be effective alternatives to their topical counterparts (Ferri 2016).

Fungal infections are usually diagnosed on the basis of appearance alone, but each can be distinguished by microscopic examination with a KOH stain. Athletes who have recently used a topical over-the-counter antifungal medication may present with a false-negative KOH stain (Winokur and Dexter 2004). In general, medical treatment is continued for at least 2 wk after resolution of the lesions (Porter and Kaplan 2011).

Preventive measures for all fungal infections include keeping wet materials away from the body; fully drying clothing, towels, and uniforms before using them; and allowing light and air exposure to the skin as practical. Additional measures include good personal hygiene outlined in the sidebar "Prevention Strategies for Infectious Dermatological Conditions in Athletes," including not sharing clothing, towels, or personal items such as grooming accessories, and wearing foot protection when using common shower facilities. Showering with hot water and soap and washing hair with shampoo immediately after practices or athletic events will help prevent fungal and skin diseases in general (Landry, Chang, and Mees 2004; Levy 2004; Zinder et al. 2010; National Athletic Trainers' Association 2007).

TABLE 16.2 **Comparison of the Tinea Fungi**

Name	Body part affected	Signs and symptoms	Treatment
Tinea corporis	Ringworm on the body	Scaling, deep erythema; well-defined margins; pruritic	Topical antifungal agents; difficult or recurrent cases may need griseofulvin or oral terbinafine
Tinea pedis	Athlete's foot	Within the interdigital web spaces; maceration, pruritic	Topical cream-based anti-fungals such as Tinactin (tolnaftate) or Lamisil (terbinafine) are often used; oral antifungals may be necessary in difficult cases
Tinea unguium	Nails of the hands or feet	Nail thickening; multiple nails involved; hyperkera-tosis	Griseofulvin, terbinafine, itraconazole (topical anti-fungal agents not effective)
Tinea capitis	Scalp	Scaly, patchy alopecia; pruritic	Oral antifungal agents; antibiotics if necessary; oral steroids to prevent scarring, hair loss
Tinea cruris	Jock itch, primarily in the groin	Scaly, erythematous rash; pruritic	Same as tinea corporis
Tinea barbae	Beard or base of neck	Inflammatory folliculitis on face; often scars	Oral terbinafine

Unless specifically addressed in the categories that follow, unexposed tinea infections have no restrictions, and the athlete can participate as tolerated. All active lesions and capitis infections have specific constraints in collegiate wrestling, and the NCAA has given express permission to the examining physician or certified athletic trainer to determine the participation of athletes with tinea on an individual basis, whereas the NFHS has allowed the participation of athletes with warts that can be covered (Parsons 2014; National Federation of State High School Associations 2013). Athletes with tinea infections require 72 h of medication before returning to high school participation. When no longer contagious, these athletes should cover lesions with bio-occlusive dressings (National Federation of State High School Associations 2013).

Tinea Corporis

Tinea corporis, otherwise known as *ringworm*, is caused by the *Trichophyton, Microsporum,* and *Epidermophyton* species. The organism most commonly identified is *T. tonsurans*, which accounts for 47% of tinea corporis cases (Lesher 2015).

Tinea corporis is common in wrestling and is spread mostly by skin-to-skin contact. Wrestlers develop mat burns, abrasions, and scrapes during competition that pro-vide easy entry for fungal infection. Fungus also develops best in dark, damp, humid conditions. Sites inside shoes or in damp clothing that has not been properly laundered and is hung in a dark, enclosed locker are particularly favorable (Landry, Chang, and Mees 2004).

Signs and Symptoms

The lesions of tinea corporis are erythematous, scaly areas of varying size and may have a clear area in the center (figure 16.21). The active areas of infection are at the border, and the central clearing develops as the fungus digests cells as it moves away from the center. Tinea corporis may be itchy or asymptomatic. It is important to also check the feet of someone with tinea because this may be the original source.

The differential diagnoses for tinea corporis include contact dermatitis, psoriasis, atopic dermatitis, seborrheic dermatitis, pityriasis alba, pityriasis rosea, pityriasis versicolor, subacute lupus erythematosus, and erythema migrans (Lesher 2015).

Referral and Diagnostic Tests

Diagnosis is made by clinical and microscopic examination. The lesion is scraped onto a slide and examined with KOH staining under a microscope. Multiple hyphae (the branches of the fungus cell) are seen on active lesions.

NCAA and NFHS Participation Regulations for Wrestlers With Tinea Infections

- At least 72 h of oral or topical therapy for skin lesion must be completed.
- The NCAA Skin Evaluation and Participation Status form shall be used to document the duration of therapy.*
- Status of lesion treatment can be judged by KOH preparation or review of documented therapy.*
- On-site medical personnel will disqualify wrestlers with extensive, multiple lesions following assessment.*
- For scalp lesions, at least 2 wk of systemic antifungal therapy must be completed.
- If active lesions are closely clustered and can be "adequately covered," a wrestler may participate.*
- If active lesions cannot be adequately covered, the athlete may not participate.
- Final disposition of the student-athlete participation status may be decided on an individual basis by the on-site physician or certified athletic trainer.*

*NCAA regulation only (not NFHS).

Adapted from Parsons 2014; National Federation of State High School Associations 2013

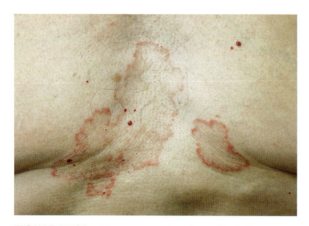

FIGURE 16.21 Tinea corporis, also called *ringworm*, presents with a red, scaly border.

The Division of Dermatology at Brody School of Medicine, East Carolina University

Athletes with extensive skin involvement, persistence of symptoms despite treatment, and any lesions that are questionable should be referred to a physician.

Treatment and Return to Participation

Treatment employs topical or oral antifungal medications. The most commonly used medications are the topical antifungal creams. Typical treatment with topical antifungal medication for noninflammatory tinea corporis includes twice-daily treatment for 1 to 4 wk, depending on the type of cream. Each antifungal is different and is individually dose-adjusted. On occasion, the lesions are too extensive for topical treatment, and oral medications such as terbinafine, itraconazole, and fluconazole are used. Doses of these medications must typically be taken for up to 4 wk to be fully effective (Lesher 2015).

In addition, athletes should shower and clean the affected area daily. Clothing needs to be laundered after each practice or competition; sweaty clothes or towels should not be left in a closed locker.

The prognosis for tinea corporis is good if the athlete uses the treatment as directed. If infection recurs, then the fungus is resistant to the medication used, the treatment was not administered properly, or another source of infection exists that has not been detected. Athletes, especially wrestlers, may return to activity after 3 d of topical antifungal treatment for tinea corporis. Small local lesions are treated by washing with an antifungal shampoo (selenium sulfide or ketoconazole), applying a fungicidal cream (terbinafine or naftifine), covering with a semipermeable membrane (e.g., OpSite or Bioclusive), and wrapping with a prewrap followed by flexible tape. This process is repeated after each practice or match to allow the lesion to air dry.

Prevention

Many isolated cultures from the lesions are the same species as those cultured from the scalp. Therefore, it may be beneficial to have athletes, especially wrestlers, shampoo with an antifungal shampoo such as Head & Shoulders (Procter & Gamble, Cincinnati, OH) or Nizoral (Johnson & Johnson), both of which are active against

T. tonsurans. Mats need to be cleaned daily and allowed to dry before storing.

Many wrestlers use wipe-on foams such as Kenshield or KS Skin Protection (Kennedy Industries, Horsham, PA) before practice and competition to provide a barrier against fungal and bacterial infections. Limited research has been done to evaluate their effectiveness; they have not yet been shown to be beneficial. They may, in fact, have an adverse impact by giving athletes a false sense of security and encouraging less strict adherence to hygiene (Cyr 2004).

Tinea Cruris

Tinea cruris, or *jock itch,* is another common fungal infection. This infection usually occurs in the warm summer months. Although it is more common in men, women may also experience this fungal infection. It affects the inner thigh, perineum, and perianal regions, with the scrotum, penis, and vagina typically not affected (Porter and Kaplan 2011). Most often, the culprit is tight-fitting clothing and humid conditions. Members of the military, athletes, and prison inmates have an increased risk of contracting tinea cruris because their clothing may be tight fitting and they may not be able to completely dry it out before re-wearing it. Bathing suits that have not completely dried out can also can cause tinea cruris (Wiederkehr 2015).

Signs and Symptoms

Signs and symptoms of jock itch are similar to those for other fungal infections. It presents with a well-demarcated, scaly, erythematous rash that tends to be pruritic (Wiederkehr 2015). As previously noted, it is localized to the groin area. Athletes who complain of symptoms from tinea cruris are referred to a physician if conservative over-the-counter treatment fails.

The differential diagnoses for tinea cruris include heat rash, candidiasis, erythrasma dermatitis from clothing or soap, or skin abrasion from clothing. If the lesions appear with a beefy red color and involvement of the scrotum, most likely the condition is candidiasis and not tinea cruris.

Treatment and Return to Participation

Antifungal agents are the treatment of choice for tinea cruris. Treatment includes completely drying off after showering and applying antifungal ointment. Loose-fitting clothing will promote healing, as will maintaining proper hygiene. Changing clothes often and laundering them in hot water also help to break the cycle (Wiederkehr 2015; Landry, Chang, and Mees 2004). All areas of the body with an active tinea infection must be treated simultaneously to prevent recurrence (Wiederkehr 2015). Antifungal powders and sprays may help to prevent tinea cruris; however, creams are more effective treatments.

Tinea Unguium

Tinea unguium is also known as *ringworm of the nails.* It can occur in both the fingernails and toenails but is more common in the fingernails (Porter and Kaplan 2011).

Signs and Symptoms

The most telling signs of tinea unguium are thickening and a lusterless, opaque coloring of the nail. As the condition progresses, the nail plate separates from the nail bed, and the nail itself may be destroyed. Athletes who present with thickened, yellowish nails are referred to a physician for medication to treat the fungus causing the problem. The differential diagnosis for tinea unguium is injury to the nail.

Treatment and Return to Participation

Treatment of this condition is especially tedious and lengthy. Topical antifungal treatment is typically ineffective. Instead, oral systemic medication taken twice daily is required for up to 4 mo. Unlike antibiotics, this medication does not need to be taken until all signs of the fungus are gone. The systemic drugs bind to the nail plate and continue to work after oral administration is complete (Porter and Kaplan 2011).

As with many of the tinea infections, participation is not restricted for athletes with tinea unguium. Certain conditions, however, make athletes more prone to tinea unguium. This includes wearing hand protection that covers their nails (e.g., soccer goalkeepers, hockey players). The dark, moist environment is an excellent place for this fungus to flourish. Equipment, especially equipment used in the summer or during twice-daily practices, is not always allowed to completely dry before reuse.

Prevention

Using open-finger gloves, such as those used in cycling and weightlifting, is one way to reduce the risk of infection, but this is not possible in some sports. Athletes would be wise to avoid the warm, moist, dark conditions that encourage tinea infections, such as keeping fingers and toes clean and dry; removing socks, shoes, and hand wear immediately after practice; allowing hand wear to completely dry before wearing again; and always wearing clean, dry socks.

Tinea Pedis

Tinea pedis, also known as *athlete's foot*, is the most common dermatophyte infection because shoes promote dark and moist conditions.

Signs and Symptoms

The most common sites for tinea pedis are between the toes and on the lateral areas of the feet and soles. The affected area between the toes is usually macerated and scaly (figure 16.22). The foot may also demonstrate the classic ringworm pattern of tinea corporis. The lateral edges and soles usually have dry, scaly, erythematous areas, and these lesions are usually, but not always, itchy. It is not uncommon for cracks or fissures to develop in the macerated skin (Robbins 2015). Diagnostic tests include scraping the scales for a microscopic evaluation with a KOH preparation. The athlete is referred to a physician if symptoms persist despite treatment.

Differential diagnoses for tinea pedis include impetigo, erythrasma, pitted keratolysis, *P. aeruginosa* infection, psoriasis, allergic dermatitis, cutaneous candidiasis, dyshidrosis, and contact dermatitis (Robbins 2015).

Treatment and Return to Participation

Treatment consists of topical antifungal creams, first with application twice daily for 2 to 4 wk. If the infection does not respond, another antifungal drug family is tried.

Athletes can help prevent tinea pedis fungal infections by wearing wicking socks, by wearing sandals, or by frequently removing their shoes to allow their feet to dry. Wearing sandals in public showering facilities will also help prevent transmission of the fungus.

Participation is not limited unless the athlete lets the condition go too far and develops secondary lymphangitis, cellulitis, or osteomyelitis. These dangerous sequelae must be managed before a full return to participation (Robbins 2015).

Tinea Capitis

Tinea capitis, or *scalp ringworm*, occurs commonly in children and is spread by pets or other infected people. In addition to the scalp, tinea capitis can be found in the eyebrows and eyelashes. It has several varieties with slight differences in presentation.

In general, the infection starts in the scalp and moves into the hair shaft. Black dots on the scalp where the follicle has broken or small semibald patches surrounded by lusterless hairs may be present (Kao 2015). Often, there is a raised inflammatory response to the fungus resembling an abscess that quickly heals. The fungus may be limited to a small area in the hair, or it may persist, affecting the entire scalp.

Signs and Symptoms

The tinea capitis infection may be either inflammatory or noninflammatory. Most commonly, identifiable areas of hair loss, scales, and broken hair shafts are seen in the scalp (figure 16.23). Sometimes the infection causes an exaggerated inflammatory response and produces one or more inflamed, boggy, tender areas on the scalp called **kerions**. Because of this, the patient may present with low-grade but persistent inflammation (Porter and Kaplan 2011). The hair shafts are usually destroyed, and scarring is common after the kerion resolves.

The differential diagnoses for tinea capitis include **alopecia areata**, psoriasis, atopic dermatitis, and seborrheic dermatitis.

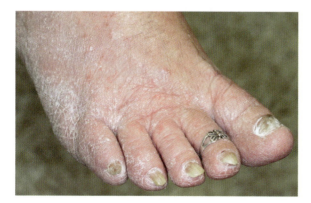

FIGURE 16.22 Tinea pedis starts in the moist areas between toes and is shown here spreading to the top of the foot.

The Division of Dermatology at Brody School of Medicine, East Carolina University

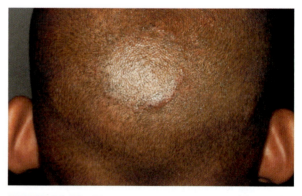

FIGURE 16.23 Tinea capitis is ringworm of the scalp, and it can lead to hair loss.

The Division of Dermatology at Brody School of Medicine, East Carolina University

Referral and Diagnostic Tests

Athletes who experience patchy hair loss, who have been exposed to tinea capitis, or who have signs of tinea capitis are referred for medical treatment. Diagnosis is determined by clinical and microscopic examination. Hairs easily removed are examined with a KOH stain under a microscope. Multiple spores are seen either inside or outside infected hair shafts. A **Wood's lamp**, which provides ultraviolet light, demonstrates fluorescence in the case of some fungal infections, but it is not useful in identifying *T. tonsurans* (tinea corporis).

Treatment and Return to Participation

Topical antifungal medications are not as effective with tinea capitis, and oral antifungal medications are often needed. Griseofulvin is the most common medication used in the treatment of tinea capitis. Treatment is continued until 2 wk after KOH preparations are negative. Prednisone and systemic antibiotics may also be used to treat tinea capitis.

The NCAA and NFHS have specific regulations about unrestricted return to activity (see the sidebar "NCAA and NFHS Participation Regulations for Wrestlers With Tinea Infections" (Parsons 2014; National Federation of State High School Associations 2013). Return-to-sport participation is up to the discretion of the treating physician and may be less of an issue in noncontact sports or sports with helmets.

Because tinea capitis is easily transmitted on inanimate objects, all combs, brushes, hats, and other headgear worn by the athlete must be cleaned. Spores of tinea are shed into the air around infected persons and their clothing, so preventive measures must include laundering bed linens, towels, and clothing. Roommates or family members of affected athletes should also be examined for tinea capitis (National Federation of State High School Associations 2015; Landry and Chang 2004; Landry, Chang, and Mees 2004).

Tinea Versicolor

Tinea versicolor is a common yeast infection seen in adolescents and young adults. This infection is not contagious and is common in high-humidity environments and sometimes in areas that feature prolonged use of topical corticosteroids. Tinea versicolor is marked by areas of hyper- or hypopigmentation. It may go unnoticed for months to years, and it usually produces very few symptoms, if any (Ferri 2016).

This yeast is part of the normal skin flora, but it can produce an infection that is found mostly on the trunk, arms, neck, abdomen, and sometimes the groin. It is more common on the face and forehead in children but not in adults.

Signs and Symptoms

Versicolor starts as multiple, small, round, scaly macules that enlarge radially. They may present as white, brown, or pink areas of the skin that increase, and they may or may not cause itching (figure 16.24). These areas typically will not tan when exposed to the sun or ultraviolet light (Burkhart 2016).

The differential diagnoses for versicolor include vitiligo, postinflammatory hypopigmentation, pityriasis alba, pityriasis rosea, nummular eczema, guttate psoriasis, seborrheic dermatitis, and tinea corporis.

Referral and Diagnostic Tests

Patients who have patchy areas that do not tan, who have varying pigmentation, or who do not respond to conservative treatment are referred to a physician. Scraping the scales onto a slide and examining them microscopically confirm the diagnosis. Microscopic examination with KOH staining reveals a "spaghetti and meatballs" appearance. Wood's light may demonstrate a pale yellow, white, or even a blue-green fluorescence pattern (Burkhart 2016).

Treatment and Return to Participation

Versicolor is treated in many ways. The most common treatment is with a selenium sulfide 2.5% lotion (Selsun Blue shampoo; Chattem, Chattanooga, TN), which is applied for 10 min and then washed off. Alternatively,

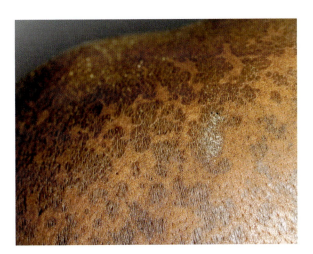

FIGURE 16.24 Tinea versicolor is often first noted as an area that does not tan.

The Division of Dermatology at Brody School of Medicine, East Carolina University

the shampoo may be applied at bedtime to all body areas except the scrotum and washed off in the morning. The typical course of treatment is 7 d (Burkhart 2016).

Another treatment is ketoconazole cream or shampoo (Nizoral) applied once daily for 2 wk. For resistant cases, both cream and oral antifungal medication may be prescribed.

Prevention

Prevention of reinfection includes ketoconazole or selenium sulfide treatments once weekly or every other week. Using a salicylic acid, sulfur, or pyrithione zinc bar may also be helpful.

Parasitic Conditions and Bites

Parasitic infestations and insect bites are common causes of skin inflammation and infection. A wide range of insects can cause skin eruptions. The most common infections caused by parasites are pediculosis and scabies. **Pediculosis**, an infection caused by lice, occurs in three forms: head lice, body lice, and pubic lice. Lice feed on human blood after injecting their victim with saliva. In many, lice cause severe pruritus due to an allergic reaction to the parasite's saliva (Guenther 2016). **Scabies** is caused by the mite *Sarcoptes scabiei*. Both are spread by person-to-person or person-to-object transmission. These parasites do not hop or fly; they move by crawling.

Head Lice

It is estimated that 6 to 12 million people are infested annually with head lice, also known as *Pediculus humanus capitis* (Centers for Disease Control and Prevention 2013). The presence of head lice is not an indicator of a person's hygiene or environment. They occur most frequently in children ages 3 to 11, and they are less common among African-Americans than in other races (Centers for Disease Control and Prevention 2013). A single female louse lays three to six eggs (nits) per day that are glued to the base of hair shafts. The eggs hatch after 8 to 9 d. The hatched nymphs begin at 1 mm in length; they reach maturity in 9 to 12 d and can begin laying eggs (Guenther 2016). When mature, these tiny insects are about 1/10 to 1/8 in. long and live on the human scalp while feeding on human blood. The lice themselves are hard to see, but the nits can be seen at the hairline behind the ears or on the base of the scalp (figure 16.25). Both forms of lice are transmitted by contact with a person who is already infested, through sharing personal items such as combs, towels, hats, helmets, or other clothing as well as bedding, carpet, couches, stuffed animals, or pillows (Guenther 2016). Lice cannot survive without a human

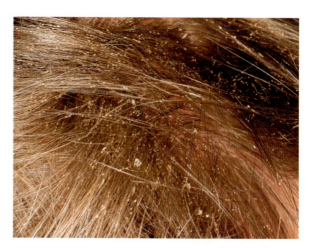

FIGURE 16.25 Pediculosis humanus capitis.
The Division of Dermatology at Brody School of Medicine, East Carolina University

host for longer than 48 h (Centers for Disease Control and Prevention 2013).

Signs and Symptoms

Clinical presentation consists of intense itching of the scalp and the sighting of nits. The itching may not start until several weeks after infestation.

Referral and Diagnostic Tests

An athlete who shows signs of lice is referred to a physician for confirmation of infestation. Nits that are attached more than 1/4 in. from the scalp are already hatched or dead, but the presence of dead nits may not be an indicator of a current infestation with head lice (Guenther 2016). It is critical to continue to inspect for crawling nits, as they can be seen with the naked eye.

Treatment and Return to Participation

Treatment consists of the application of topical medications, including Nix, RID, malathion (Ovide), and lindane (Kwell). Nix (Insight Pharmaceuticals, Langhorne, PA) and RID (Bayer HealthCare, Morristown, NJ) are the initial treatments of choice because lindane has been associated with neurological toxicity in some cases. The lice are usually killed with one treatment, but a second treatment may be needed 7 to 10 d later. After the first treatment, a nit comb is used to remove the eggs. Any nits found more than 1/2 in. along the hair shaft are old and dead; nits less than 1/4 in. along the hair shaft 1 wk after treatment may be new and may necessitate retreatment. The person needs to be checked for lice every 2 or 3 d for 2 wk. Do not use a cream rinse, conditioner, or combination shampoo and conditioner before using medication as it will negate the effects of the treatment. The hair should not be rewashed for 1 to 2 d after treatment (Guenther 2016; Centers for Disease Control and Prevention 2013).

It is also imperative to wash all bedding and recently worn clothing in hot water at a temperature greater than 54 °C (130 °F) and to dry them on a hot cycle for at least 20 minutes. Nonwashable clothing is dry-cleaned. Items that cannot be washed or dry-cleaned, such as helmets, headgear, and shoes, can be placed in a double plastic bag for 2 wk. Vacuuming the floor and furniture completes the extermination procedure. On occasion, fumigation or chemical dusting may be required of the living space (Guenther 2016).

Athletes can resume normal activity levels when all lice and nits are confirmed gone. However, the NCAA recommends that athletes be treated with pediculicide and reexamined for complete extermination of lice before return to sport. Avoiding exposure to infected people and their personal items is the best preemptive tool against lice infestation.

Body Lice

Body lice, or *Pediculus humanus corporis*, unlike head lice, do not live on the human body but in clothing. The nits are found in the seams of clothing and the bedding of infested humans or in body hair. The lice only leave clothing to feed on humans, typically at night (Guenther 2016). Also, unlike head lice, female body lice lay 15 to 20 eggs per day in clothing or bedding, and the mature louse lives up to 30 d. Infestation usually occurs when poor hygiene and crowded environments necessitate frequent close contact with others. Homeless people without regular access to bathing facilities or clean clothes are particularly vulnerable. People who bathe regularly are seldom infested.

The usual clinical presentation is itching and a rash, usually around the waist, groin, and thighs. Body lice are treated by changing clothes regularly, bathing regularly, washing all clothing in hot water at a temperature above 54 °C (130 °F), drying it in a hot dryer for at least 20 min, and using RID or Nix shampoo applied to the body (Ferri 2016). Compared to other types of lice, body lice are more likely to require fumigation to eradicate.

Pubic Lice

Pubic lice, or *Pthirus pubis*, commonly referred to as *crabs,* are usually found in the genital area but may also be seen on the legs, axilla, mustache, beard, eyebrows, and eyelashes. These lice are usually spread through sexual contact rather than through contact with infested towels, clothing, or bedding. They typically live 2 wk, and females lay one or two eggs a day. Pubic lice can migrate from the pubis, crawling up to 10 cm per day (Guenther 2016).

Clinical presentation is usually intense itching in the genital area. The lice and nits are much easier to identify than head or body lice. Treatment for crabs is with RID, Nix, or lindane shampoo, followed by removal of nits with fingernails or nit combs. Clothing is washed in hot water at a temperature greater than 54 °C (130 °F), dried in a hot dryer for at least 20 min, and changed regularly; sexual partners need to be informed and treated as well and sexual activity avoided until appropriate treatment has successfully eradicated the infestation.

Scabies

The other common parasite associated with skin infection is the mite *S. scabiei,* which causes scabies. Worldwide, approximately 300 million cases of scabies are reported annually (Barry 2015). Mites burrow under the upper layer of the skin and lay their eggs, which cause a pimple-like lesion and intense itching. Spread is usually the result of direct contact, sexual contact, or sharing of infested clothes or bedding. It is common in overcrowded areas such as prisons, nursing homes, and other close-quarters living arrangements. These mites can survive away from the host for 48 to 72 h and therefore can be more challenging to eradicate than lice (Ferri 2016).

NCAA Participation Regulations for Wrestlers With Parasitic Conditions

The following regulations apply to participation with the parasitic conditions of pediculosis (lice) and scabies:

- Pediculosis must be treated with pediculicide and must show no infestation on reexamination.
- Scabies must have a negative scabies prep at the time of competition.

Adapted from Parsons 2014.

Signs and Symptoms

Intense itching that interferes with sleep is commonly associated with scabies. The wrists, fingers, and ankles are the most obvious sites, but the itching may occur anywhere on the body, with the head and neck usually spared. The patient develops small red bumps that may be arranged in a linear fashion after itching (figure 16.26).

Differential diagnoses for scabies include drug reactions, folliculitis, insect bites, lice, urticaria, and dermatographism (Barry 2015).

Referral and Diagnostic Tests

Diagnosis is usually made through clinical examination; however, finding a mite is extremely difficult and requires scraping the skin for a sample that is then examined under a microscope for a live mite. Sometimes a Burrow ink test is used for diagnosis. This test involves rubbing a washable felt marker across a suspected site, followed by removal of the ink with alcohol. The presence of scabies is confirmed when the ink penetrates the upper layer of the burrow, leaving a mark (Barry 2015). A diagnosis may also be confirmed microscopically via the presence of mite eggs or fecal matter (scybala).

Treatment and Return to Participation

Medications used to treat scabies (scabicides) are available only with a physician's prescription. Treatment is with 5% permethrin cream (Elimite) applied to the body from the neck down and washed off in 8 to 14 h, or 1% lindane per 1 oz of lotion, or 30 g of cream applied from the neck down and washed off after 8 h. Ivermectin taken

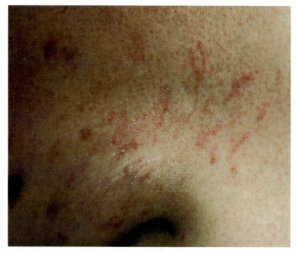

FIGURE 16.26 A pruritic infestation of scabies.

The Division of Dermatology at Brody School of Medicine, East Carolina University

orally is an alternative treatment (Centers for Disease Control and Prevention 2010; Barry 2015). The patient will likely need an antihistamine because itching may last for at least 2 wk after treatment begins. As with lice, all bedding and recently worn clothing need to be laundered in hot water above 54 °C (130 °F) and dried on a hot cycle for at least 20 min; nonwashable clothing needs to be dry-cleaned. Items that cannot be washed or dry-cleaned, such as helmets, headgear, and shoes, can be placed in a double plastic bag for 2 wk (Centers for Disease Control and Prevention 2010). In addition, all floors and furniture must be vacuumed. The infected person needs to review close and sexual contacts within the past 30 d and notify those people for treatment as necessary (Barry 2015).

The NCAA wrestling rules stipulate that athletes who have had scabies must present a negative preparation for scabies before being allowed to resume participation (see the sidebar "NCAA Participation Regulations for Wrestlers With Parasitic Conditions") (Parsons 2014).

Insect Bites

Dermatological reaction to insect bites is extremely common. In the United States, 1 to 2 million people are severely allergic to insect venom. These bites also can lead to anaphylaxis, which causes 90 to 100 deaths in the United States each year (U.S. National Library of Medicine 2016). These data may be underrepresented, as many deaths are attributed to heart attacks or heat stroke. Exposure to insects becomes a possibility for physically active people during outdoor practice and events.

In addition to mosquitoes, covered in chapter 15, chiggers, ticks, wasps, bees, ants, and spiders can produce particularly bothersome reactions. Bites and stings can cause direct irritation from the insect's body parts or secretions, immediate or delayed-hypersensitivity responses, or specific effects from venoms, or they can serve as vectors for secondary invaders (U.S. Food and Drug Administration 2015). Common reactions may be localized or spread across a larger part of the body and may include redness, pain, and swelling that may last as long as 10 d. Individuals with a prior history of allergic reaction to specific insect bites or stings can be extremely vulnerable and often carry an EpiPen (an epinephrine injection) when participating in outdoor activities (U.S. National Library of Medicine 2016).

The brown recluse spider has received wide attention because of the possible dramatic reaction associated with its bites. Dermonecrotic arachnidism, described in the next section, is a condition that can result when this type of spider deposits venom within a host (Arnold 2016). The brown recluse, also called the *fiddleback spider*, is very small at about 1.5 cm long and has a characteristic dark, violin-shaped marking on its dorsum with the broad base of the marking or "violin" located near the head and the narrow stem pointing toward the abdomen. The brown recluse spider is most prevalent in the southern half of the United States and prefers dark, quiet spaces under porches, woodpiles, and rocks or inside closets, barns, picture frames, and basements. It has also been found in dormitories, and it bites when a person is putting on clothing or rummaging through other materials where the spider resides (National Institute for Occupational Safety and Health 2015).

Signs and Symptoms

Insect bites can range from a nuisance to an emergency. Chigger bites can cause extreme discomfort for days and possibly lead to secondary lesions with bacterial infection as a result of scratching. Wasp and bee stings can be extremely dangerous when the person stung has an allergic reaction, which may quickly progress to anaphylaxis in sensitive individuals; therefore, first aid kits should be equipped with EpiPens for emergencies. Symptoms resulting from tick bites, which can result in Rocky Mountain spotted fever or Lyme disease, do not develop immediately, often making diagnosis a challenge.

A brown recluse spider bite can produce a dramatic and prolonged reaction called **dermonecrotic arachnidism**. The initial bite produces a bee sting-like pain and often only mild erythema and swelling, but these bites can create a severe reaction and may become necrotic within 6 h. In some cases, the wound begins to ache and becomes pruritic over the first 8 h, and subsequently a rapid blue-gray macular halo develops around the bite that represents local hemolysis. The area may become oblong or irregular and result in a sudden increase in pain. The macule then widens and sinks below the level of intact skin and may advance to necrosis, affecting the underlying muscle and broad areas of skin or even an entire extremity (Arnold 2016). In such cases, when the dead tissue sloughs, a large ulcer persists, resulting in significant scarring and prolonged healing. Systemically, patients with severe reactions often experience fever, chills, nausea, vomiting, myalgias, and weakness. These reactions are rare and generally limited to children (National Institute for Occupational Safety and Health 2015).

Referral and Diagnostic Tests

A patient who presents with a history of a bite with associated local severe reaction, fever, or systemic manifestations is referred to a physician immediately.

Treatment and Return to Participation

Insect bites usually are treated conservatively with ice and elevation of the affected extremity. Strenuous exercise, heat, and surgery are avoided (U.S. National Library of Medicine 2016). Topical antibiotic ointment may be applied under a sterile dressing to retard infection. Antibiotics for *S. aureus* or *S. pyogenes* may be initiated, and a tetanus booster should be administered by a physician if the term of the vaccine has lapsed. Serious bites become evident in the first 24 to 48 h; in this event, the athlete is

---

🚩 RED FLAGS FOR INSECT BITES

- Take the bites of any venomous insect seriously because the secretions, venom, and insect body parts can provoke dramatic or life-threatening reactions in sensitive individuals.

- Be aware of the insect varieties common to the geographical location.

- Recognize and refer athletes with signs and symptoms of anaphylaxis: agitation, chills, facial edema, swollen tongue, wheezing, difficulty breathing, flushing, generalized urticaria, hoarseness or difficulty talking, palpitations, near-syncopal or syncopal episodes, profuse sweating, palpitations, cardiovascular collapse.

- Have epinephrine on hand for emergency use in the event of a severe reaction.

CLINICAL TIPS

Proper Application of Insect Repellant

- Only use insect repellant approved by the Environmental Protection Agency (EPA).

- Do not use insect repellant on babies or pets.

- Repellant used on older children should have less than 10% DEET.

- Do not apply insect repellent to children's hands or faces.

- Spray repellant on clothing or skin but not on the face.

- Read the label to determine effectiveness time as well as specific insect(s) the product deters.

- Completely wash hands with soap and water after application.

U.S Food and Drug Administration 2015.

referred for medical treatment immediately (U.S. Food and Drug Administration 2015).

Prevention

Prevention of most insect bites involves avoiding the insects' habitat, including shrubs and wooded and bushy areas. Use chemical repellants properly by applying them over clothing. Use structural barriers, such as window screens, netting, and protective clothing, to prevent contact with insects (U.S. Food and Drug Administration 2015). When putting on shoes, socks, and other apparel that have been left unattended outdoors, athletes must thoroughly shake them out. Exercise caution during storms and floods that may drive insects from their normal habitats.

Summary

This chapter introduces athletic trainers, educators, and students to the pathology of common skin conditions. Signs, symptoms, diagnostic tests, treatments, and suggestions for appropriate times to seek referral for dermatological disorders are discussed. A dermatological condition can be prevented from becoming more severe through early identification and referral for diagnosis and treatment. This chapter also presents the NCAA and NFHS guidelines for determining when wrestlers with various skin conditions may be allowed to participate. These regulations may differ or may vary from school district guidelines, amateur sport organization regulations, or the rules of other governing entities. Become familiar with the rules for specific areas of athletic interest and must remain abreast of changes as they occur.

Because these recommendations may be revised as research is conducted and made public, health care practitioners should continue to seek out new information as it becomes available. A prudent athletic trainer continues to educate athletes about their personal responsibility for skin care, hygiene, and prevention with regard to transmission of infectious skin disorders.

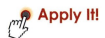 **Apply It!** The case study for this chapter looks at a high school wrestling athlete complaining of an inflamed neck. Read the scenario and answer the questions at www.HumanKinetics.com/MedicalConditionsInTheAthlete.

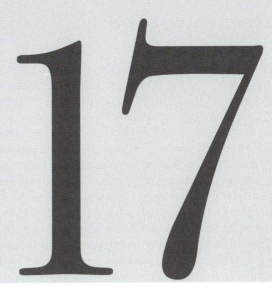

Psychological and Substance Use Disorders

Layne A. Prest

OBJECTIVES

At the completion of this chapter the reader should be able to do the following:

- Recognize emotional and behavioral signs of common substance use disorders and psychological problems, including mood, anxiety, eating, and attention deficit hyperactivity disorders.

- Intervene appropriately with the affected athlete through discussion, supportive confrontation, education, and referral.

- Be aware of and establish collaborative relationships with qualified physical and mental health professionals in the recognition and treatment process.

- Identify a variety of educational and supportive resources (printed, Web based, and organizational materials) that are available to both professionals and patients affected by these disorders.

The 21st century is supposed to be the era of healthier people, and of course, athletes are by definition among the healthiest. Therein lies the main dilemma when assessing and intervening in potential mental health concerns of athletes. Many people, perhaps athletes more than the average person, have been conditioned to minimize or even deny physical health problems, and they are even more inclined to do so with mental health issues. Being sick or disabled physically is one thing; being weak mentally or emotionally is quite another! Professionals working with athletes are becoming more and more likely to have been educated about mental health issues or to know of someone who has struggled with emotional or behavioral problems. We can hope that more open discussion about these disorders will increase the likelihood of early detection and appropriate intervention (Neal et al. 2013). This chapter is designed to teach you about the signs, symptoms, and prognoses of the most common mental health disorders. It is not intended to teach you how to counsel athletes—this is beyond the scope of practice—but rather to know when to refer them. To that end, this chapter outlines the mental health problems most commonly experienced by athletes, suggests red flags for early detection, and describes strategies for intervention.

According to the World Health Organization (WHO), mental and behavioral health conditions account for 4 of the 10 leading causes of disability worldwide, and they affect a quarter of the world's population at some time in their lives (World Health Organization 2001). These four leading causes of disability are depression, anxiety disorders, suicide, and alcohol use. Other serious disorders include schizophrenia, bipolar disorder, dementia, obsessive–compulsive disorder, posttraumatic stress disorder, and panic disorder. Problems with attention and concentration, disordered eating, personality issues, and other forms of substance abuse also contribute greatly to the disease burden throughout the world (Murray and Lopez 1996). Some of these difficulties, chiefly depression, anxiety, and substance abuse problems, are ubiquitous in the United States. The others, including attention deficit hyperactivity disorder (ADHD), personality disorders, and disordered eating, are not as common. All can impair athletic performance and overall life adjustment. These conditions also can be difficult to treat, especially if allowed to escalate. Therefore, athletic trainers working with physically active people must be able to identify these potentially serious problems as early as possible. Following a description of typical physical and emotional symptoms, diagnostic criteria, and potential red flags, suggestions are made for initial intervention, referral, and treatment. The diagnostic criteria are taken from the *Diagnostic and Statistical Manual of Mental Disorders,* 5th edition (DSM-V) (American Psychiatric Association 2013).

Understanding the Role of Mental Health Professionals

At the outset, a full and comprehensive treatment plan must be developed in the context of the athlete's relationship with a trusted, licensed professional operating within the scope of professional practice. The athletic trainer, who may be among the first to detect a problem, can be instrumental in getting the athlete needed help. Athletic trainers need to be familiar with the mental health professionals to whom they may refer someone for professional services. A reasonable place to start is with the patient's primary care physician.

The U.S. federal government identifies five disciplines as competent to provide mental health services: (1) psychiatry, (2) psychology, (3) marriage, couple, and family therapy, (4) social work, and (5) psychiatric nursing (table 17.1). Other professionals who provide mental health services include professional counselors and clergy members. Licensure and certification for most of these professionals are becoming standardized within

each discipline, and boundaries are delineated between disciplines. A fair amount of overlap remains, however, and providers in any of these categories can potentially help with the clinical problems this chapter addresses. Referrals may be guided somewhat by the discipline of the professional but more importantly by the person's clinical specialty.

The training of psychiatrists and psychiatric nurse practitioners enables them to assess the patient from a medical point of view and to prescribe medicine to address the underlying physiological or chemical components of the problem. They may also provide supportive counseling, psychoeducation, or assistance in problem solving. If a major mental disorder is suspected and medical intervention is needed, a referral to one of these professionals would be appropriate.

The various types of psychologists—clinical, educational, and counseling—have different but overlapping training, experience, and areas of expertise. They can be trained at either the master's or doctoral level. Typically, psychologists are the professionals to contact if psychological or educational testing is needed. Psychologists also provide psychotherapy services.

Marriage, couple, and family therapists (MCFTs), especially medical family therapists, assess problems from the biopsychosocial point of view. Consequently their clinical approach considers various aspects of the person's life. MCFTs work with typical mental health issues, such as depression, anxiety, eating disorders, and ADHD, but they will often do so by including part or all of the family and in collaboration with a primary care provider.

Social workers usually specialize in addressing macroissues, such as housing, income, or food deficiencies and insurance needs, or micro-issues, such as psychotherapy. Social work as a discipline also takes a holistic perspective on the client. A number of social workers also provide psychotherapy services similar to those of other mental health providers.

Mental health professionals (MHPs) increasingly are being called on to demonstrate the effectiveness of their

TABLE 17.1 **Disciplines Providing Mental Health Services**

Discipline	Typical credentials	Approach
Psychiatry	MD, DO	Medical approach, including medication
Psychology	MS, PhD, PsyD, EdD	Psychological testing and psychotherapy; individual psychotherapy
Marriage, couple, and family therapy	MA, MS, PhD	Biopsychosocial assessment; family systems therapy
Social work	MSW	Holistic approach; social services
Psychiatric nursing	RN, APRN	Medical approach, including medication

work with clients. As a result, more attention is being focused on the development of evidence-based protocols. Therapy typically begins with an intake session during which the professional gathers background information (e.g., family of origin details), a description of the problem and previous attempts to address it, and the client's goals. A contract governing the frequency and duration of sessions is negotiated, and parameters of confidentiality are discussed. If MHPs wish to contact other professionals, including the athletic trainer or family members working with the client, they will obtain a signed consent for release of information.

Overview of Mental Health Issues in the Athlete

Everyone has symptoms of some type of mental health issue at some time in life when one or several stressors overwhelm the person's ability to self-regulate or repair. The symptoms are usually, and arbitrarily, labeled either physical or mental. This artificial dichotomy usually does not align with the affected person's reality. Rarely is an athlete with a strained hamstring not also worried about the injury or distressed by the pain. Similarly, the most common initial warning signs of depression are the physical symptoms of tension, restlessness, and disturbed sleep, energy, and appetite. This is because we have overlapping systems of mind, body, spirit, and relationships, each integrally connected to the others. When the homeostasis of one or more systems is disrupted, people instinctively try to correct the problem regardless of its origin. In the mental health domain, signs of distress are emotional, mental, behavioral, and physical.

Framework for Understanding Mental Health

In almost all situations, a variety of overlapping factors contribute to symptom development. The **biopsychosocial–spiritual model (BPSS)** is a framework for understanding the person's responses in a given situation and the development of symptoms. Symptom etiology may be conceptualized as a pie. Figure 17.1 shows how these various factors overlap and contribute to well-being. In a given person, the various pieces of the BPSS pie may be larger or smaller at any one time. The relative sizes of the pieces greatly influence the person's symptoms and ability to adapt.

For example, two runners may have identical injuries, but the impact of the injury and the course of rehabilitation in these two athletes will usually differ. The amount of pain they have, as well as the length of time until they are ready to compete again, will be influenced not only by the difference in respective levels of physical condi-

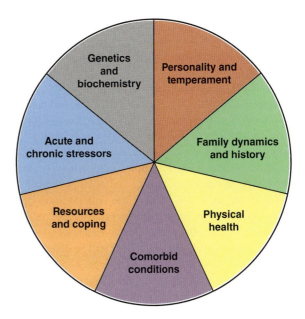

FIGURE 17.1 The biopsychosocial–spiritual model is a framework for understanding a person's responses in a given situation and the development of symptoms.

tioning and injury history but also by other physical and emotional conditions such as pain tolerance, attitude, perception of the problem, and its implications for life. The situation may also be affected by personality and temperament issues, variable resources for coping, and so on. Another example involves two wrestlers who seem to be equally competitive, but wrestler A, in a struggle to make or maintain weight, develops more obviously disordered eating patterns than wrestler B. Perhaps wrestler A has a family history of obesity and is genetically predisposed toward weight gain more than the other; temperamentally, wrestler A may tend to think more negatively about life challenges, become somewhat self-defeating in the face of adversity, and find emotional comfort in food and the process of eating. Often a variety of factors will help to explain the development of clinically significant problems.

This interplay of variables is the same for athletes as it is for others who are physically active, regardless of whether the symptoms of an injury or condition are physical or emotional. Whereas one athlete may become depressed, another's symptoms may include anxiety or outbursts of anger and physical aggression. Sometimes one piece of the BPSS pie is so big that it seems to account for virtually the whole reason that someone is symptomatic (e.g., the chemical disequilibrium that comes with bipolar disorder). For this reason, it is a good practice to regularly consider the possibility that an organic cause may be the culprit and refer the person for a medical evaluation.

The treatments that have proven effective for the problems discussed in this chapter are based on the same BPSS approach as the assessment and diagnosis. Different strategies can be useful, depending on the biopsychosocial–spiritual components that are implicated in the assessment process. Practitioners often recommend treatment plans based on their assessment and experience, and then these are negotiated with the patient or family members according to personal preferences. The treatment may be offered on either an inpatient or, more commonly, an outpatient basis.

Treatment may also involve the collaboration of a variety of treatment professionals. For example, eating disorder treatment often involves a physician, a registered dietitian, and a psychotherapist. This will be determined based on the severity of symptoms, the difficulty the athlete has in making changes, the amount of support the athlete has, and other resources that affect care, including financial concerns or insurance benefits. The important first step in treatment is accurate assessment followed by clear and well-timed communication and education with the athlete and family. The athletic trainer can play a valuable role here because people are much more likely to engage in treatment or some type of change process if they become convinced that there is a problem, they know what it is, and they know that something can be done about it. This is because most people will want to know what is going on with themselves, how they "got it," and what they can do to "get rid of it" or at least cope more effectively. Additional treatment recommendations specific to various clinical problems are listed in subsequent sections.

Implications for Participation in Athletics

Early identification and treatment are very helpful in preventing problems from worsening, but sometimes the stigma still associated with mental health conditions prevents people from recognizing these problems in themselves or others. In those cases, functioning in one or more areas of life can be affected, sometimes severely. Restricting participation in a sport, if necessary, will depend on the assessment of the athlete's level of functioning by the athlete, the coach, and the athletic trainer. Initially, while the medication dosage is being adjusted, the athlete could experience adverse effects that could affect participation or performance, such as nausea, headache, sedation, disturbed balance, or overstimulation. The National Collegiate Athletic Association (NCAA) has no restrictions on the medications typically used to treat these conditions except for pemoline, a medication prescribed to treat ADHD (National Collegiate Athletic Association 2015).

The last general point to be made is that some people experiencing psychological or substance use disorders may consider suicide or become homicidal. Most health care professionals or other professionals are required by law or by a professional code of ethics to report to the authorities if a patient is a danger to self or others. Athletic trainers, too, may encounter an athlete with depression, panic disorder, or substance abuse who is considering suicide or harming someone else. The athletic trainer must seek immediate consultation if in doubt about the need to report. An assessment of whether one is suicidal or homicidal includes determining whether the person has a specific plan, the means to carry it out, the intention to carry it out, and how lethal the plan is. Those with a personal or family history of this type of ideation or action or whose judgment is impaired, perhaps through the use of substances, are more at risk to follow through.

Role of Stress in Psychological and Substance Use Disorders

A related topic for the health care professional to consider is the role of stress in the life of an athlete. Determining how much stress an athlete is experiencing, and how well he or she is coping, is an important part of assessing the overall level of functioning. First of all, what is stress? Stress is alternately considered bad, normal, healthy in moderation, or an inescapable fact of life. In fact, all of these are true. Stress is the word we use for the impact our physical, emotional, psychological, and social experiences have on us. Athletes, like all human beings, experience stress just by living life, and because of the demands that training places on them, athletes have additional stress with which to contend. But stress is a two-sided coin. We need the stimulation, challenge, and motivation that come from being stressed. Because we are stressed, we strive to meet basic survival needs for ourselves and our loved ones. Being stressed is what helps us to push toward a goal and rise to the occasion in competitions. But too much stress can be debilitating. Ineffective stress management contributes to the psychological and substance use disorders described in this chapter. When overloaded with demands, athletes can begin to decompensate, becoming less effective and ultimately failing in their pursuits. The discussion of stress for the last several decades has focused on both sides of the coin. Research and clinical experiences suggest that we should strive for a balance between rest and activity, pushing for improvement and adjusting to limitations, and between a goal-directed orientation and being in the experience. Athletic trainers should help the athletes with whom they work to pause and reflect on the amount of stress they are under and whether the effects are helpful and motivational or undermining and disabling.

There are a variety of tools for measuring stress—some adapted for specific populations. One that has been used in studying athletes in a variety of sports is the COPE inventory (full and brief versions; the latter is included here). By having an athlete complete this inventory, the athletic trainer can get a clearer sense about the athlete's coping strategies and the degree to which she or he is coping successfully and constructively.

Anxiety Disorders

Anxiety is one of the most common human experiences despite some cross-cultural differences (Asnaan et al. 2010). For example, most people have experienced a momentary sensation of "butterflies" in the stomach. In fact, the ability to respond with anxiety is considered normal and even desirable, and anxiety is what helps us "get our game face on." However, given the right set of factors—physiology, central nervous system sensitivity, perceptual filters, belief system, coping, and support system—people may respond to one or more acute or chronic stressors by developing anxiety serious enough to be considered a disorder. This is a case of too much of a good or necessary thing. The individual is wracked with very serious and debilitating apprehension, excessive and ongoing worry, overwhelming fears, panic attacks, or compulsive behaviors. Slightly more than 18% of the American population experiences one of the more debilitating forms of anxiety and has been diagnosed with an anxiety disorder (Anxiety Disorders Association of America 2016; Asnaan et al. 2010). Another study indicates that 31.9% of adolescents suffer from serious anxiety (Merikangas, He, and Burstein 2010).

Red flags for problems with anxiety include outbursts of irritability or anger, substance abuse, changes in athletic performance, or other behaviors that are uncharacteristic for the athlete. Anxiety symptoms include both somatic–behavioral and emotional–cognitive disturbances (Anxiety Disorders Association of America 2016; Merikangas, He, and Burstein 2010). The presence of some or all of these symptoms may signal an anxiety problem or even an anxiety disorder:

- Difficulty getting to sleep
- Shortness of breath
- Dizziness, lightheadedness
- Sweating
- Feeling of choking
- Impairment of performance
- Feelings of unreality
- Worry, nervousness
- Appetite disturbance
- Paresthesias
- Chills or hot flashes
- Gastritis, nausea
- Psychomotor agitation
- Irritability
- Fear of losing control
- Feelings of going crazy or dying

People can be screened for anxiety disorders using a variety of standardized measures, such as the Generalized Anxiety Disorder-7 (GAD-7) (Spitzer et al. 2006).

Generalized Anxiety Disorder

Generalized anxiety disorder (GAD) is a condition in which the person is worried or nervous about many or most things in life. The person may complain on a regular basis of one or more of the anxiety symptoms listed previously. Criteria for diagnosing generalized anxiety are

- excessive daily anxiety or worry for 6 mo;
- difficulty controlling the worry;
- three or more anxiety symptoms; and
- impairment in social, academic or occupational, or relational functioning because of the anxiety.

It has been estimated that 6.8 million people, or 3.1% of the U.S. population, have this disorder in a 12 mo period of time. Women are twice as likely as men to report generalized anxiety (Anxiety Disorders Association of America 2016). Adolescents and young adults into their 20s are prone to develop anxiety as well (Merikangas, He, and Burstein 2010). Consistent with the BPSS model described previously, the causes of GAD and other anxiety problems are varied. Fortunately, a number of effective treatment approaches and self-help measures are available (Antony and Hood 2012; Gorman 2002).

Panic Attacks

Among the 6 million people (2.7% of the U.S. population) who experience panic attacks, some say that these episodes seem to come out of nowhere when, in fact, they are probably in response to an accumulation of stressors. At other times, the attacks may be stimulated by an identifiable, acutely stressful event (Antony and Hood 2012). Symptoms that seem to be cardiovascular, such as chest pain or shortness of breath, are especially striking during these episodes. The attacks can be so overwhelming and can produce such fear and intense anxiety that the affected person may begin avoiding stressful situations and other stimuli perceived as triggers (Antony and Hood 2012). As a result, the panic attacks may become **panic disorder** accompanied by agoraphobia, avoiding open

Brief COPE Inventory

These items deal with ways you've been coping with the stress in your life. There are many ways to try to deal with problems. These items ask what you've been doing to cope with this one. Obviously, different people deal with things in different ways, but I'm interested in how you've tried to deal with it. Each item says something about a particular way of coping. I want to know to what extent you've been doing what the item says. How much or how frequently. Don't answer on the basis of whether it seems to be working or not—just whether or not you're doing it. Use these response choices. Try to rate each item separately in your mind from the others. Make your answers as true FOR YOU as you can.

1 = I haven't been doing this at all.
2 = I've been doing this a little bit.
3 = I've been doing this a medium amount.
4 = I've been doing this a lot.

_____ I've been turning to work or other activities to take my mind off things.
_____ I've been concentrating my efforts on doing something about the situation I'm in.
_____ I've been saying to myself "this isn't real."
_____ I've been using alcohol or other drugs to make myself feel better.
_____ I've been getting emotional support from others.
_____ I've been giving up trying to deal with it.
_____ I've been taking action to try to make the situation better.
_____ I've been refusing to believe that it has happened.
_____ I've been saying things to let my unpleasant feelings escape.
_____ I've been getting help and advice from other people.
_____ I've been using alcohol or other drugs to help me get through it.
_____ I've been trying to see it in a different light, to make it seem more positive.
_____ I've been criticizing myself.
_____ I've been trying to come up with a strategy about what to do.
_____ I've been getting comfort and understanding from someone.
_____ I've been giving up the attempt to cope.
_____ I've been looking for something good in what is happening.
_____ I've been making jokes about it.
_____ I've been doing something to think about it less, such as going to movies, watching TV, reading, daydreaming, sleeping, or shopping.
_____ I've been accepting the reality of the fact that it has happened.
_____ I've been expressing my negative feelings.
_____ I've been trying to find comfort in my religion or spiritual beliefs.
_____ I've been trying to get advice or help from other people about what to do.
_____ I've been learning to live with it.
_____ I've been thinking hard about what steps to take.
_____ I've been blaming myself for things that happened.
_____ I've been praying or meditating.
_____ I've been making fun of the situation.

With kind permission from Springer Science + Business Media; *International Journal of Behavioral Medicine*, "You want to measure coping but your protocol's too long: Consider the Brief COPE," Vol. 4, 1997, pgs. 92-100, C.S. Carver.

spaces or public places. Panic disorder can be so severe and distressing that some victims might consider suicide as the only way out; in fact, up to 20% of those affected consider this step. Women experience panic attacks at twice the rate of men (Gorman 2002).

Posttraumatic Stress Reactions

Similar to the intense responses involved in panic attacks are varying degrees of posttraumatic stress reactions (e.g., **acute stress disorder [ASD]**, **posttraumatic stress disorder [PTSD]**) experienced by approximately 7.7 million Americans (Asnaan et al. 2010; Merikangas, He, and Burstein 2010). These reactions are in response to exposure to life-threatening events or other situations outside the normal range of human experience (e.g., war, serious physical or sexual assault, motor vehicle accident). ASD and PTSD result because the survivors have witnessed or experienced events that include serious injury, life-threatening trauma, or death. Examples of situations that have caused some of those involved to develop PTSD are the 9/11 attacks, the Iraqi and Afghani wars, and the various domestic terrorism-related assaults and killings that have occurred in the last decade. People can be so overwhelmed by the event or series of events that they will go to great lengths to avoid similar situations, as well as the thoughts or feelings associated with the original experience, because their responses involved intense fear, helplessness, or horror.

Fairly often, people will replay or reexperience the traumatic event in the form of recurrent or intrusive and distressing recollections, images, thoughts, perceptions, dreams, illusions, or hallucinations. They often have strong physiological reactions to these experiences, and therefore they try to avoid stimuli and to numb their responses. This leads them to avoid thoughts, feelings, conversations, activities, places, and people they associate with the traumatic event. At times, this process of compartmentalization can be so severe that it leads to an inability to recall important aspects of the event, marked **anhedonia**, detachment or estrangement, restricted range of affect, and a sense of a foreshortened future. Without intervention to help survivors deal with what they have experienced, PTSD can develop and cause many physical, emotional, and social difficulties for years to come (American Psychiatric Association 2013).

Obsessive–Compulsive Disorder

Approximately 19 million people, or 8.7% of the U.S. population, displays characteristics of anxiety in a more circumscribed manner by developing phobias to specific triggers or fears about specific issues. These include abnormal anxiety about being in social situations, fear of public speaking, fear of flying, or preoccupations with

CLINICAL TIPS

Diagnostic Criteria for Obsessive–Compulsive Disorder

- Obsessions or recurrent and persistent thoughts, impulses, or images that are not simply about life problems
- Attempts to suppress or neutralize such thoughts with other thoughts or actions while recognizing they are a product of the person's own mind
- Compulsive thoughts or actions engaged in accordance to rigid rules even though they may not be rationally connected to the intrusive thoughts

germs or disease (American Psychiatric Association 2013; Anxiety Disorders Association of America 2016). These manifestations of anxiety can be manageable if the person can avoid the stimuli without compromising normal activities, but otherwise they can be quite disruptive. Some aspects of anxiety can be useful. For example, attention to detail and the ability to be thorough can be valuable in environments such as athletic competition, where excellent performance is rewarded. However, taken or driven to the extreme, these impulses can be debilitating.

Obsessive–compulsive disorder (OCD) is a condition that affects approximately 2.2 million people in the United States and is equally common among men and women. The basis for OCD is persistent thoughts, impulses, or images about exaggerated or imaginary circumstances. The thoughts the person has are experienced as intrusive or inappropriate to the situation. Compulsive or repetitive behaviors are paired with the obsessions, with the goal of eliminating, reducing, or ignoring the resultant anxiety. As with the obsessions, the person often recognizes that the compulsive behaviors are, to some degree, excessive or unreasonable, especially if they impede the person's performance, routine, or social activities. The most common obsessive thoughts are those concerning contamination, doubts, loss of order, horrible trauma, and sexuality. Table 17.2 summarizes common compulsive behaviors.

Treatment of Anxiety Disorders

Treatment plans for anxiety disorders are often recommended by the practitioner on the basis of assessment and experience, and then negotiated with the individual or family members according to personal preferences. The treatment plan for anxiety can include one or all of

TABLE 17.2 **Common Compulsive Thoughts and Behaviors Associated With Obsessive–Compulsive Disorder**

Worrisome thoughts	Compensatory behaviors
Contamination or infection	Washing of hands Excessive cleaning
Doubts	Requesting or demanding assurance
Loss of order	Ritualized behaviors Certain order to getting dressed
Personal safety	Making sure doors are locked Checking to make sure appliances are turned off (e.g., stove and coffee maker)
Sexuality	Religious or psychological correction Self-flagellation Defense

a group of evidence-based interventions (Anxiety and Depression Association of America 2015).

When there is a strong family history of anxiety problems, there is probably a biological or physiological predisposition that can be managed with medications. One class of **psychotropic medications** often used includes those that act on the serotonin system. These include selective serotonin reuptake inhibitors such as fluoxetine (Prozac), paroxetine (Paxil), and escitalopram (Lexapro). When anxiety coexists with depression, medications that affect dopamine or norepinephrine, as well as serotonin, can be useful. These include venlafaxine (Effexor) and mirtazapine (Remeron). **Benzodiazepines** have been used for many years to treat anxiety and are fairly well known. These medications include clonazepam (Klonopin), diazepam (Valium), lorazepam (Ativan), and alprazolam (Xanax).

The antianxiety drugs are prescribed according to their rate of onset, effects, and adverse effect profiles. Medication can be used from the outset or added after treatment begins. It is usually recommended that the person stay on the medication for 9 to 12 mo or until symptoms are fully resolved. The dosage may need to be adjusted, or a different type or class of medication altogether may be needed. In the case of first or second episodes of anxiety, medication can be discontinued after the person has developed healthy coping strategies. If the anxiety recurs, then the person may need to take the medication for the duration.

Other important steps to take to reduce anxiety on a physical level are to get regular exercise and regulate sleep. Exercise, especially aerobic exercise, has been shown to significantly reduce levels of anxiety. This may be a moot point for those who are already physically active, but, at times, people will stop exercising if they are distressed enough. For the injured athlete, maintaining aerobic conditioning during rehabilitation is important for mental as well as physical well-being. Most people

should be encouraged to slowly reestablish healthy patterns of physical activity. Similarly, good sleep hygiene addresses the basic human need for restful sleep, which in turn supports well-being and stable functioning:

- Establish regular times for going to bed and awakening.
- Minimize distractions and noises.
- Avoid stimulating activity or substances before bedtime (e.g., exercise, caffeine).

Negative patterns of thought or behavior can exacerbate anxiety. Therefore, cognitive–behavioral psychotherapy is used to help people recognize automatic thoughts and reflexive behaviors and replace them with more constructive ones. On a related note, minimizing stress and distinguishing controllable from uncontrollable events are important to addressing anxiety problems. Stress management strategies include breathing exercises, progressive muscle relaxation, guided imagery, meditation, and prayer. Problem-solving and conflict resolution skills can be learned. Developing social support systems is also helpful.

Generalized anxiety disorder (GAD), obsessive–compulsive disorder (OCD), and panic attacks are often treated through a combination of medication and support techniques. These include stress management, conflict resolution, problem solving, supportive relationships with others, exercise, and good sleep hygiene. In addition, psychotherapy emphasizing cognitive–behavioral and interpersonal therapy is important. Acute or posttraumatic stress disorders often benefit from group therapy because this process helps to normalize the sense of unreality or disconnection that victims of trauma often experience. People with phobias do not usually respond to the use of medication; instead, a process of systematic desensitization helps to lessen or even eliminate their phobic responses (Roy-Byrne et al. 2002).

Mood Disorders

Transient feelings of sadness or depressed mood are normal in response to life's ups and downs. At the other end of the spectrum, however, depression can be so severe that people experience psychotic symptoms. Like anxiety, depression can appear as changes in physical, mental, emotional, relational, or spiritual well-being. Depression can be mild, moderate, or severe, and it can be situational or global. The incidence of depression is highest in middle aged people. According to the World Health Organization, it accounts for the heaviest burden of disability among mental and emotional disorders, and it is among the most devastating of all health problems (second only to heart disease) (Hedden, Kennet, and Lipari 2014).

Depression can affect people at any time of life. Up to 2.5% of children, 8.3% of adolescents, 5.8% of adult men, and 9.5% of adult women are affected each year (Baron et al. 2013). Athletes tend to be less vulnerable to depression due to their goal-directed activities, internalized locus of control, and generally stronger health status, but they remain vulnerable to depressive experiences (Baron et al. 2013). In addition, comorbidity between anxiety and mood disorders is high (Levine, Cole, and Chengpappa 2001). Some people become depressed in response to situational stressors (e.g., a change in performance or playing status, a move, illness in a family member) or developmental stressors (e.g., the transition from high school to college, birth of a baby in the family). In most cases, depression will come and go within a limited time.

Persistent symptoms, however, may be a sign of a more serious problem. For those people who develop more serious forms of depression and are not adequately

RED FLAGS FOR DEPRESSION

- Depressed mood
- Diminished interest in usual activities
- Irritability or anger
- Diminished performance
- Substance abuse
- Social withdrawal or isolation
- Preoccupation with escape or death

treated, 35% will relapse within 2 yr and 60% will relapse within 12 yr (Hedden, Kennet, and Lipari 2014; World Health Organization 2011). As with the other conditions discussed in this chapter, the development, progression, and recovery or relapse of depression are affected by many things, which again reflect the pieces of the BPSS pie (Hedden, Kennet, and Lipari 2014; Levine, Cole, and Chengpappa 2001). In more serious forms of depression, the person demonstrates both depressed mood and diminished interest in daily activities.

Typical physical symptoms include both somatic–behavioral and emotional–cognitive disturbances. The athlete may experience changes in sleeping patterns, such as waking very early and being unable to return to a restful sleep or wanting to sleep all the time. Other symptoms include either a loss of appetite or eating more than usual, a loss of energy, and concentration difficulties (American Psychiatric Association 2013).

A depressed athlete is also very likely to complain of various somatic pains or irregularities, such as muscle aches, bowel problems, or headaches. A depressed person is often sad, can become self-critical, and feels out of control, despair, and hopeless, even to the point of being suicidal (American Psychiatric Association 2013; Hedden, Kennet, and Lipari 2014).

The minor form of a mood disorder is called an *adjustment disorder*. The DSM-V guidelines, although somewhat arbitrary, suggest that an adjustment disorder is two to four symptoms with onset within 3 mo and resolution within 6 mo of termination of the stressor. If the symptoms are more severe in number or quality, an even more significant problem may have developed. This more serious form, major depressive episode, involves a greater number and more severe depressive symptoms for at least 2 wk (American Psychiatric Association 2013). Criteria for a major depressive episode are listed.

At least 2 wk of the following:

- Lack of interest in usual activities
- Depressed mood

CLINICAL TIPS

Stressors That Sometimes Lead to Depression in Athletes

Situational Stressors

- Not meeting performance expectations of self or others
- Change in playing status, coaches, teams, partners
- Death or serious illness in a family member
- Relationship breakup

Developmental Stressors

- Major life transitions (e.g., move, change of schools)
- Birth of a baby in the family

Plus four or more of the following:

- Appetite change along with weight gain or loss
- Insomnia or hypersomnia
- Psychomotor agitation or retardation
- Fatigue
- Worthlessness or guilt
- Difficulty concentrating or indecisiveness
- Recurrent thoughts of death or suicide

Mood disorders such as major depressive episode can be assessed according to the diagnostic criteria listed, but the busy practitioner or athletic trainer who is not an expert in this area can use one or more screening instruments to measure the level of impairment. One example is the **Zung Self-Rating Depression Scale** (Zung 1965). The National Institute for Mental Health (NIMH) publishes another scale called the *Center for Epidemiological Studies Depression Scale* (CES-D). The CES-D is free to use and is available at the National Institute of Mental Health website (Hedden, Kennet, and Lipari 2014). The only depression screening tool specifically developed for use with athletes is the Baron Depression Screener for Athletes (BDSA). While its validity and reliability have not been studied, it holds promise because its items pertain to the athlete's experience (Baron et al. 2013).

Even depressed people can have periods from days to weeks or even months during which they do not feel so bad and can rally to perform well. Some people have cyclical fluctuations in mood, energy, and appetite. Not surprisingly, one mood disorder is termed **cyclothymia**. In this case, the athlete may perform well in practice or competitions for several days or weeks but then inexplicably hit a slump. Another form of fluctuating depression, **seasonal affective disorder (SAD)**, is tied to exposure to changing amounts of sunlight. The prevailing theory is that sunlight, by way of the optic nerve, stimulates the brain to produce melatonin, which is a chemical related to serotonin. The hormone serotonin helps to regulate mood, appetite, activity level, and the wake–sleep cycle. When there is relatively less exposure to sunlight, less of this chemical is being produced, which in turn leads to depression (American Psychiatric Association 2013; Asnaan et al. 2010). These cycles are often tied to the changing of the seasons. Therefore, the changes in mood, energy, and performance may take place over longer periods.

The most debilitating mood disorder, manic–depressive illness or **bipolar disorder**, is associated with significant fluctuations of symptoms. In this condition, people may experience periods of depression (hypodepression), mania (hypomania), or both. Mania and hypomania are on a continuum with a normal sense of well-being and the depression previously described.

Mania is characterized by extremes of energy, euphoria, irritability, frustration, and rapid or grandiose thinking, speaking, and acting. In more moderated circumstances, people can be very productive and creative, but in extreme situations, they can be driven to put themselves and others at risk because of impulsivity, poor judgment, and lack of focus and concentration. Mania is also characterized by thrill seeking, such as risky sexual behavior, substance use, impulsive travel, or buying sprees.

Treatment of depression is actually fairly similar to the treatment of anxiety problems because the biopsychosocial–spiritual issues underlying these disorders overlap. Therefore, the interventions are those mentioned previously: medication, psychotherapy, sleep hygiene, exercise, skill building, stress management, and social–spiritual support.

Research has shown that in cases of adjustment disorders and even mild or moderate depression, medication is usually not needed (Larzelere, James, and Arcuri 2015; Manbar, Allen, and Morris 2002; Wang and Patten 2002). People tend to heal with time, reassurance, supportive relationships with others, exercise, good sleep hygiene, and sometimes a short course of psychotherapy, either cognitive–behavioral or interpersonal therapy. When the depression is more serious, research-based practice indicates that psychotherapy and medication can both be helpful (Wang and Patten 2002). Whereas medication is more effective in the short term, therapy tends to be more helpful over longer periods. Severe depression requires aggressive treatment with both medication and psychotherapy. The other strategies are helpful additions to the treatment plan in both moderate and severe depression (Larzelere, James, and Arcuri 2015).

Eating Disorders

It is estimated that 5 million Americans are affected by eating disorders each year, but many more experience disordered eating (Smink, van Hoeken, and Hoek 2012). Perhaps this is because Americans have a love-hate relationship with food and their bodies. We are surrounded by cheap, high-calorie foods that contain generous amounts of fat and sugar. A growing focus on fitness and healthy lifestyles is paired incongruously with record levels of obesity and related health problems, such as diabetes, coronary artery disease, and stroke (Zung 1965). The resulting disordered patterns of eating often have their onset in childhood and early adolescence (Smink, van Hoeken, and Hoek 2012). This is a time when the person is becoming increasingly aware of him- or herself and attuned to peer group messages about acceptability, attraction, and competence.

Even though athletes are usually more physically active and fit than the average person, the demands of

RED FLAGS FOR EATING DISORDERS

- Frequent comments about feeling fat or overweight
- Fluctuations or other changes in weight
- Secretive, peculiar, or ritualized eating habits
- Avoidance of social situations involving food
- Mood changes
- A history of weight problems
- Excessive training regimen
- Gastrointestinal problems
- Dizziness
- Dental or oral problems
- Ability to recall specific details about food portions
- Wearing baggy clothing

performance, such as maintaining a certain body weight or proportions, can strongly affect the athletes' approach to food. Wrestlers, gymnasts, dancers, and swimmers are especially prone to developing problems with food and weight. One recent estimate is that up to one-third of female athletes display disordered eating patterns (Bratland-Sanda and Sundgot-Borgen 2013; Mitan 2002).

Like the other issues discussed in this chapter, disordered eating can be viewed on a spectrum of severity. People with these problems often do not fit into clear-cut categories.

Anorexia Nervosa

Anorexia nervosa is a potentially life-threatening condition with long-term mortality rates approaching 20% (Bratland-Sanda and Sundgot-Borgen 2013; Mitan 2002).

CLINICAL TIPS

Criteria for Anorexia Nervosa

- Refusal to maintain weight at a minimum of 85% of expected
- Intense fear of gaining weight or being fat
- Disturbed perception of body weight or body image
- Absence of at least three consecutive menstrual cycles

Anorexia develops when the person restricts or otherwise compensates for eating to the point that the person drops below 85% of ideal body weight (American Psychiatric Association 2013). An important point for athletic trainers to consider is that overtraining is a common compensatory behavior.

Anorexia is a relatively rare condition, with about 5 to 10 new cases per 100,000 persons each year and a prevalence of 0.5%. The vast majority of cases of anorexia are found in females, but approximately 10% to 15% of cases occur in males (Martinsen and Sundgot-Borgen 2013; Raevuori, Keski-Rahkonen, and Hoek 2014). It occurs more often in industrialized than in nonindustrialized societies. The two subtypes of anorexics are the restricting type and the binge eating–purging type. Individual patients' behaviors may vary from time to time (Smink, van Hoeken, and Hoek 2012).

The possible physical sequelae include gastrointestinal problems (stomachache, diarrhea, constipation, heartburn), amenorrhea or other menstrual irregularities, dehydration, electrolyte imbalance, bradycardia, hypotension, decreased muscle mass and body fat, musculoskeletal injuries, lowered core body temperature, development of **lanugo** hair on the body, and fatigue and weakness (Bratland-Sanda and Sundgot-Borgen 2013; Smink, van Hoeken, and Hoek 2012). Emotionally and mentally, people develop a distorted body image, emotional lability, cognitive rigidity, perfectionist attitudes, social isolation, an intense fear of becoming fat, and eventual impairment of mental functions (American Psychiatric Association 2013).

Bulimia

Bulimia is another type of eating disorder that affects athletes and is more common than anorexia. Even though the athlete is often at or slightly above normal weight, bulimia can also be life-threatening. It is characterized by binge eating followed by an inappropriate compensatory act designed to prevent weight gain and, perhaps more importantly, to combat the person's sense of being out of control (American Psychiatric Association 2013; Smink, van Hoeken, and Hoek 2012). These compensatory acts include restricting food (dieting or fasting), vomiting, laxative or diuretic use, and exercise. A stereotypical binge involves eating large amounts in secret in a short period of time. In fact, people may or may not be especially secretive, and the amount of food constituting a binge is a matter of perception. People with bulimia who believe they have eaten too much may see even one too many cookies or slices of pizza as a binge. In response, they engage in one or more compensatory behaviors.

The results of this behavior include fluid and electrolyte imbalance, gastrointestinal difficulties, inflammation of the esophagus and parotid glands, dental conditions, visual disturbances, muscle weakness, and menstrual irregularities. Vomiting, laxatives, or diuretics usually are what cause the problems. From psychological and behavioral points of view, people with bulimia often exhibit excessive concern about body weight and shape, irritability, social withdrawal, depression, and impulsive behavior (American Psychiatric Association 2013; Smink, van Hoeken, and Hoek 2012).

Binge Eating Disorder

A third category, recently added to the DSM-V, is **binge eating disorder** (American Psychiatric Association 2013). Considered to be the most common eating disorder, it is characterized by eating in binges that result in emotional or physical discomfort similar to bulimia but without the obvious compensatory behaviors mentioned previously (Smink, van Hoeken, and Hoek 2012).

Treatment of Eating Disorders

Eating disorders of all types require a thorough assessment and multidisciplinary treatment. This treatment can be done on an outpatient basis, but for more serious problems that create life-threatening electrolyte imbalances or starvation, inpatient stabilization may be needed. The most effective treatment teams include medical, nutritional, and mental health practitioners. The antianxiety and depression medications described previously are used to treat underlying or comorbid conditions. These medications are especially useful in treating the dysphoria associated with low self-esteem and disturbed identity, the anxiety that comes with changed eating behaviors (e.g., eating but not purging, fear of gaining weight), and the obsessive–compulsive nature of the disorder (Martinsen

and Sundgot-Borgen 2013; Raevuori, Keski-Rahkonen, and Hoek 2014).

Group therapy, or more generally milieu therapy, can help the patient to confront unrealistic expectations, maladaptive behaviors, and distorted thinking. Nutritionists work with eating-disordered patients to help them gain a more realistic understanding of the body's physiology and nutritional needs and to establish expectations about diet and exercise. Individual and family therapy is especially helpful with children and adolescents, and it addresses dysfunctional social, cultural, and family dynamics within which eating behaviors are often embedded (Raevuori, Keski-Rahkonen, and Hoek 2014).

Substance Use and Dependence

As with eating and weight issues, the social messages around drug and alcohol use seem to conflict and to exacerbate the problems. On one hand, alcohol use in the United States is legal and normative for those over the ages of 18 to 21, depending on state laws. On the other hand, millions of dollars are spent on alcohol and drug awareness programs for school children to combat the problems associated with their use. Peer pressure among younger adolescents often encourages alcohol use. The use of mind- or mood-altering substances takes many forms, including use, misuse, abuse, and dependence (American Psychiatric Association 2013; Hedden, Kennet, and Lipari 2014).

It can be difficult to draw the line among appropriate use, misuse, abuse, and dependence, but from a health care professional's point of view, the lines might be defined by the impact the use is having on the athlete's health and well-being, including athletic performance.

Drug or alcohol use involves using the substance without meaningful impairment. Substance misuse includes occasional use of an illegal substance or use of a legal substance to excess, resulting in impairment of one's ability to function. Substance abuse is a maladaptive pattern of substance use occurring within a 12 mo period that causes impairment in social or occupational functioning. A substance abuser will continue this pattern of use despite its ongoing or increasingly negative consequences. Substance dependence or addiction is a maladaptive pattern of substance abuse occurring within a 12 mo period that leads to significant impairment or distress and is characterized by either tolerance—the need for markedly increased amounts of the substance or markedly diminished effects from continued use of the same amounts—or withdrawal, even if withdrawal does not happen because the patient uses a substance to relieve or avoid withdrawal symptoms (American Psychiatric Association 2013).

CONDITION HIGHLIGHT

Alcohol Abuse

Depression gets a lot of press. Anxiety is the most common disorder afflicting average Americans, including athletes, but the behavior that is associated with more risk taking and results in the most injuries and fatalities is the abuse of alcohol. The top three contributors to morbidity and mortality among people aged 16 to 24 are homicide, accidents, and suicide, all three of which are more likely to occur when people overuse alcohol. Athletes are more likely to be victims of physical or sexual assault when alcohol and other drugs are being consumed. Alcohol is often used by athletes who are suffering from mood and anxiety disorders to self-medicate, exacerbating the underlying mental health condition. Therefore, athletic trainers must be careful not to normalize the consumption of alcohol or to ignore the impact that it can have on the well-being and performance of their athletes.

Alcohol, illegal street drugs (e.g., cocaine, methamphetamine, ecstasy), and other substances (e.g., inhalants such as glue, gasoline, propellants) can be used for their intoxicating effects. The highest rates of inhalant use are found among children aged 8 to 12 (Hedden, Kennet, and Lipari 2014). The highest rates of illicit drug use, at 36%, are found in 16- to 20-year-olds, with alcohol and marijuana being the most commonly used drugs. In a 2010 study, binge drinking prevalence (28.2%) and intensity (9.3 drinks) were reported to be highest among persons aged 18 to 24 (Centers for Disease Control and Prevention 2012).

Alcohol is the third leading cause of preventable mortality, contributing to 100,000 deaths each year (National Institute on Drug Abuse [NIDA] 2016). Increasingly, prescription drugs are being obtained by deception or theft and used or distributed to others, including in schools and universities. An estimated 20% of people in the United States (including 15% of high school seniors) have used prescription drugs for nonmedical reasons (National Institutes of Health [NIH] 2015). The types of drugs most often misused and abused include narcotic painkillers (e.g., oxycodone, hydrocodone), sedatives and tranquilizers (e.g., Xanax, Valium, Ambien), and stimulants (e.g., Ritalin, Provigil) (National Institute on Drug Abuse (NIDA) 2016). Over-the-counter drugs, such as no-sleep or diet aids (for stimulative effects) and cough syrups (containing dextromethorphan and used for sedative effects), can also be misused, abused, or become part of a person's dependency (National Institutes of Health [NIH] 2015). Although misuse of these drugs accounts for a rather small fraction of the problem, athletic trainers need to be aware of it (Hedden, Kennet, and Lipari 2014).

The misuse of substances can be found in families of all socioeconomic, racial, and ethnic backgrounds, and it negatively affects the lives of family members at many levels because of the potential relational, social, and legal difficulties. Paradoxically, substance abusers are often enabled by family members who may cover for such compulsive or addictive behavior patterns. The impact of substance abuse on the user and the family depends on the type of drug, length of use, amount being used, and any comorbid conditions. In cases where athletes are having training- or performance-related difficulties, the athletic trainer should consider substance abuse as a potential contributor. A simple set of screening questions is represented by the mnemonic CAGE:

C: Have you ever tried to cut down on your (substance) use?

A: Have you ever felt angry or annoyed when someone asks or confronts you about your substance use?

G: Have you ever felt guilty about your substance use?

E: Have you ever used an eye-opener (used your substance of choice first thing in the morning to get going)?

Denial is often a complicating factor when working with these people and their families. Often they will not want to acknowledge or discuss substance abuse problems. Because of the possibility of denial, the athletic trainer must be alert for simple clues such as performance problems, absenteeism, marital discord, or vehicular and everyday accidents. It also helps if the athletic trainer can provide a safe, nonjudgmental environment within which athletes can share personal struggles. Successful intervention is based on the person's desire to stop, willingness to find alternative coping strategies, and, when indicated, effective detoxification, treatment of dual diagnoses, or relapse prevention through individual or family treatment or participation with groups such as Alcoholics or Narcotics Anonymous.

Substance abuse is associated with many possible comorbid conditions that either contribute to or result from the substance abuse itself (Hedden, Kennet, and Lipari 2014). Comorbid conditions associated with substance abuse include the following:

- Mood and anxiety disorders
- Marital or family dysfunction
- Partner or child abuse
- Physical injury to self
- Engaging in dangerous behaviors
- Driving while intoxicated
- Falls (especially in older adults, elderly)
- Overdosing
- Physical complaints
- Gastrointestinal problems
- Malnutrition
- Numbness
- Weakness and fatigue
- Hypertension

Many people with comorbid problems self-medicate with alcohol or other drugs to correct or compensate for the difficulty with mood, anxiety, or concentration.

The first step in substance abuse intervention is usually assessment by a qualified professional such as a certified drug and alcohol abuse counselor, mental health practitioner, or physician trained in addictions. If the person is determined to be dependent on alcohol or other drugs, inpatient or outpatient detoxification may be necessary. This person needs to be educated and even confronted about the effects of the substance abuse. Treatment options include a referral to a 12-step group (e.g., Alcoholics Anonymous, Narcotics Anonymous), an alternative treatment method (e.g., Rational Recovery [RR], Moderation Management), outpatient individual or group psychotherapy, or inpatient treatment and aftercare follow-up. The RR is an alternative to the 12-step model and is based on a perspective of substance use as a pattern of problematic behavior and thinking but not a lifelong addictive disease. RR is not a group-based approach; rather, the organization provides information and training on their alternative to AA.

Relapse is a normal part of the change process with most lifestyle, behavioral, or addiction problems. This is obviously the case with substance abuse. In addition to education and referral, the athletic trainer can play an important role in offering ongoing support for the person to stay with the behavior change and recovery process.

Attention Deficit Hyperactivity Disorder

Attention deficit hyperactivity disorder (ADHD) is a neurobehavioral condition that impairs a person's ability to sustain attention or to control activity and impulses in at least two settings, such as home and school or work (American Psychiatric Association 2013). As with the other conditions discussed in this chapter, ADHD can be mild, moderate, or severe in its impact on one's ability to function. It is often first detected in childhood, especially when children enter school; however, adult ADHD is increasingly becoming a focus of clinical concern. An estimated 4% to 12% of children are affected by ADHD; it appears to affect boys more than girls by a ratio of 3:1. Girls are more likely to manifest the inattentive type, and boys generally display the hyperactive or combined type (Giedd 2003). Differences in socialization may account for some of this discrepancy.

ADHD among adults is gaining more attention because of its long-term consequences if unrecognized and untreated (Committee on Quality Improvement: Subcommittee on Attention-Deficit/Hyperactivity Disorder 2011). Initially, the athlete with ADHD is much less likely than the student with ADHD to come to the attention of teachers or other concerned adults. This is because the athlete may just seem to have more energy than peers, but eventually coaches and even teammates may become irritated or frustrated with the athlete's inability to sit still, listen to directions, or follow through on plans.

ADHD is seen in several forms: primarily hyperactive, primarily inattentive, or mixed (American Psychiatric Association 2013). People with primarily hyperactive ADHD can be very easy to detect because they are "wound up like a top." Those with primarily inattentive disorder may be more difficult to detect because they fade into the academic woodwork. Most people with ADHD have elements of hyperactivity, impulsivity, and inattention. Typical symptoms of hyperactivity, impulsivity, and inattention are as follows:

Hyperactivity and Impulsivity

- Difficulty unwinding
- Restless, fidgety, or always "on the go"
- Talking excessively or interrupting
- Difficulty remaining still when required (e.g., waiting turns)
- Difficulty engaging in quiet activities
- Irritability
- Impulsive behavior (e.g., clowning around, unnecessarily touching others)

Inattention

- Difficulty paying attention, especially to details
- Problems concentrating on instructions
- Failure to follow directions
- Difficulty following through to a goal
- Making careless mistakes
- Distractibility
- Memory problems (e.g., appointments, deadlines)

In general, people with ADHD do not perform academically as well as they should according to their standardized test scores. If ADHD is suspected in an athlete, questions about classroom performance and standardized tests can be helpful. It is also useful to understand the diagnostic criteria for ADHD.

There is high comorbidity among ADHD, substance abuse, mood and anxiety disorders, and other mental health and behavioral problems (Giedd 2003). In fact, people with untreated ADHD are almost twice as likely as those who are treated with medication to develop substance abuse problems (Giedd 2003). Many professionals believe that people with ADHD who also use or abuse substances are, at least in part, self-medicating the underlying problem. Therefore, treatment needs to address the medical, behavioral, family, and psychoeducational needs of the patient with respect to ADHD and these comorbid conditions.

The clinical practice guidelines of the American Academy of Pediatrics recommend that assessment begin with an interview, a medical checkup, and administration of checklists (Committee on Quality Improvement: Subcommittee on Attention-Deficit/Hyperactivity Disorder 2011). To be diagnosed with attention deficit hyperactivity disorder, a person must, for at least 6 mo, experience inattention, including the following:

- Problems attending to details or making careless mistakes
- Difficulty sustaining attention
- Appearance of not listening
- Difficulty with follow-through on tasks or instructions
- Difficulty with organization
- Avoidance or dislike of tasks requiring sustained mental effort
- Problems losing things
- Distraction occurs easily
- Forgetfulness

From a medical standpoint, first-line ADHD treatment includes the use of stimulant medication, such as methylphenidate in its various forms. Some alpha-2a blockers typically used for blood pressure control (e.g., guanfacine, intuniv) have an endorsement from the FDA for use alone or in combination with stimulant medications. Older tricyclic antidepressants such as imipramine, newer dopaminergic agents such as bupropion (Wellbutrin), or drugs that block norepinephrine reuptake such as atomoxetine (Strattera) are also being used. Bupropion is indicated for the treatment of ADHD in adults, and atomoxetine is useful for people with comorbid ADHD and depression because of its norepinephrine effects.

Other treatment options for attention deficit hyperactivity disorder are as follows:

Mild

- Educate patient and family about the disorder.
- Develop adaptive strategies that increase organizational skills and concentration.

Moderate–Severe

- Add medication.
- Use individual therapy to problem solve.
- Add family therapy.
- Reinforce adaptive strategies.
- Address problematic interpersonal dynamics.

Children, adolescents, and adults with ADHD all benefit from education about the nature of the disorder. Those with ADHD also benefit from coaching to reinforce coping strategies that address the problematic behavior and thought processes, such as eliminating distraction, setting short-term goals, and seeking frequent feedback on performance. Family sessions can help others develop realistic expectations for the person and can open up communication about what may have been a very painful and disruptive set of behaviors. Similar communication with teachers, coaches, or work supervisors can be valuable as well (Committee on Quality Improvement: Subcommittee on Attention-Deficit/Hyperactivity Disorder 2011).

Stages of Readiness

The concerned athletic trainer will routinely screen troubled athletes for one or more of the problems described in this chapter. The athletic trainer who finds a problem that needs to be addressed will be able to educate the athlete about the problem and to discuss options. The screening process should include an assessment of the athlete's readiness to recognize that a problem exists and a desire to do something about it. Prochaska and DiClemente developed a useful framework for this step. It involves assessing the athlete's readiness for change (Prochaska et al. 2013; Prochaska and DiClemente 1983). People in need of change can be in one of five different stages of the change process:

1. *Precontemplation stage:* The athlete has not considered that there might be a problem with substance use, eating habits, or mood. This person needs to be educated and encouraged to consider the presence of a problem.

2. *Contemplation stage:* The athlete has begun to think about the problem and has wondered whether it is time to change, that is, to stop using the substance or to seek medical treatment. This

should be encouraged, and an athletic trainer can help the athlete to look honestly at the impact of the condition on performance, satisfaction, or general life circumstances.

3. *Preparation stage:* Once the athlete has decided to change or seek help, there needs to be a plan. The athletic trainer can help by brainstorming possible components of an effective plan for change.

4. *Action stage:* The athlete has begun making behavioral, situational, or attitudinal changes, including seeking professional help. Referrals from the athletic trainer can be very important now.

5. *Follow-up or relapse prevention stage:* This involves continued implementation or changes to the plan despite possible setbacks. The athletic trainer can use contacts with the athlete on the field or in the office to support the athlete's decision to address the problem, to support progress, or to confront relapse.

It will not be a productive use of time or relationship capital for the athletic trainer to try to get the athlete to do something she or he is not ready to do. You cannot persuade athletes to develop a plan of action or even take steps to correct a problem when they are still in denial about it. You will be more effective by first assessing and asking good questions, providing support, and offering educational input. When the athlete moves from precontemplation to contemplation and preparation, then it is time for the athlete and the athletic trainer to partner in developing a plan.

What to Do in a Crisis

Even during the best of times, athletes can become overwhelmed by feelings, psychological tensions, or interpersonal conflicts. An acute stressor (lost a match, breakup of a relationship, conflict with teammates or coach) can precipitate strong emotional responses. There may be preexisting problems with depression or anxiety, or the reaction may seem to come out of the blue. In these situations, the athletic trainer may be called on to help defuse the crisis and arrange for acute follow-up care. This is especially important when the AT can identify certain factors that indicate the likelihood of heightened risk for the athlete or others (Parsons 2014):

- Inconsolable emotion (e.g., sobbing, rage)
- Drastic change in typical behavior
- Use of alcohol or drugs
- Suicidal or homicidal ideation, threats, or plans
- History of suicidal or homicidal ideation

The most important goal is to help the person to deescalate and see through the emotion to a more hopeful or less distressing future. The following are some strategies for doing so:

- Engagement with the athlete should be by someone who is skilled *and* likely to be trusted.

- Speak in a calm, soothing tone without being patronizing. (Avoid statements such as "I know how you feel..." unless it is clear that you have the life experience to prove that you do.)

- Ask open-ended questions to encourage the person to talk and allow sufficient time to talk things out (e.g., "I can see you are upset. I'd like to help if I can. Can you tell me what's going on?").

- Reassure the athlete that, unless there is a legal exception, revealing the source of the crisis won't be held against him or her.

- Help the person to verbalize feelings and validate them (e.g., "You look really mad. Could it be that you are feeling guilty about how you did today? Are you afraid the team is mad at you?" [If there is an affirmative response] "That makes a lot of sense. I can see why you might feel that way.").

- Then move on to help the athlete begin to rationalize and think things through. (e.g., "Have you ever been through something like this before? What happened then? Did you feel the same way? How did you get past it that time? What do you think you need now? Is there something you think would help?")

At times, even the most highly trained mental health practitioner may not be able to help someone calm down and begin to cope effectively. In these circumstances, other steps need to be taken:

- When possible, ensure that the person is not in immediate jeopardy or a threat to others (e.g., remove objects or weapons with which the person might cause injury, prevent the person from driving).

- Call 911.

- Take the person to the nearest emergency department.

It is important to involve a psychiatrist or psychologist as part of the sports medicine team. The ability to recognize when an athlete may be in trouble and to refer that athlete for professional help before the situation escalates to a dangerous level may help to defuse a difficult situation.

Summary

The certified athletic trainer attends to the athlete as a whole person and not just to the athlete's physical health and performance. This is because performance, physical health, mental health, behaviors, and life situation affect each other. This chapter highlights the most common mental health conditions of athletes that athletic trainers need to recognize. On the basis of this chapter and continuing education, athletic trainers should be able to identify emotional and behavioral signs of common mental health issues, including anxiety, mood, eating, substance use, and attention deficit hyperactivity disorders.

Informed athletic trainers will be equipped to intervene with affected athletes through discussion, supportive confrontation, education, and referral. This involves knowing when and to whom to refer for qualified professional services. This chapter also mentions educational and supportive resources, such as organizational procedures, printed materials, and Web-based resources, that are available to both professionals and patients affected by these disorders.

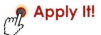 **Apply It!**   The case study for this chapter looks at a high school basketball player exhibiting atypical behaviors. Read the scenario and answer the questions at www.HumanKinetics.com/MedicalConditionsInTheAthlete.

18

Working With Special Populations

Monique Mokha

OBJECTIVES

At the completion of this chapter the reader should be able to do the following:

- Discuss aspects of the general medical history as needed when assessing persons with selected disabilities.
- Recognize the importance of the preparticipation physical examination in identifying baseline norms in the athlete with a disability.
- Identify typical symptoms and clinical signs of pathological conditions seen in athletes with selected disabilities.
- Apply typical treatment and prevention measures for pathological conditions seen in persons with selected disabilities.
- Explain how common medical conditions can have devastating consequences to a person with a disability.
- Communicate effectively with athletes with selected disabilities.

Participation in organized sports and recreation by athletes with disabilities has increased significantly, with more than 3 million participating in the United States alone. This has created a deeper field of competition, requiring athletes to train and compete at higher levels to attain success. Athletes in wheelchairs have broken the four-minute mile and have completed marathons in less than 90 min. Alan Oliveira has run the 100 m on two prosthetic legs in 10.77 s. In January 2015, the Eastern College Athletic Association became the first NCAA-sanctioned conference to adopt an inclusive strategy to provide new athletic opportunities for student-athletes with a variety of disabilities at the collegiate level. War also has had an effect on participation by persons with disabilities. A combined 38 active-duty service members and veterans represented the United States at the 2012 London and 2014 Sochi Paralympic Games (U.S. Paralympics 2016).

In the United States, special education programs make school attendance possible for more than 6.4 million children with disabilities (National Center for Education Statistics 2016). Adapted physical education provides opportunities to participate in sports and recreation through training in physical conditioning, noncompetitive and competitive sports, outdoor physical activities, and health centers. Quality sports medicine care in special populations is as important as it is in the able-bodied population.

Although risks of injury and illness are inherent in all physical activity, and injury rates for athletes with disabilities are within the same range as for athletes without disabilities (Webborn, Willick, and Reeser 2006), athletes with disabilities pose some unique challenges. Ferrara and Buckley (1996) developed the first disability register for athletes with disabilities and found that musculoskeletal injuries accounted for 79.7% of reported injuries. General medical problems (that is, illness or disability related) accounted for 20.3% of those athletes who were unable to participate. Athletic trainers working with world-class athletes will note that Paralympians file more therapeutic use exemptions with the governing bodies than do their Olympic counterparts; this is due to the more complex nature of their medical conditions.

Person-first terminology should be used to refer to athletes with disabilities. Person-first terminology recognizes the individual before the disability (DePauw and Gavron 2005). For example, the health care provider identifies the athlete as a person with spina bifida or an athlete with a visual impairment, rather than a disabled or blind athlete. Using appropriate terminology reflects an overall philosophy of the person being first and the disability being second. It also supports a social model of disability in which the focus is on changing attitudes, facilities, structures, and policies to promote participation rather than the medical model of disability, in which the focus is on the limitations, abnormalities, and impairments of the athlete. The social model is preferred by persons with disabilities.

This chapter focuses on issues related to the general medical concerns for the athlete with a disability. The disabilities covered are traumatic tetraplegia and paraplegia, spina bifida, poliomyelitis, cerebral palsy, amputations, sensory disabilities, and intellectual disabilities.

Preparticipation Examination for Athletes With Disabilities

Athletes must complete a thorough preparticipation physical examination (PPE) so that baseline norms can be established. The general approach of the PPE for athletes with disabilities is similar to that for athletes without disabilities (see figure 1.2). However, often the focus is on the primary condition or disability, and the athletic trainer and other members of the sports medicine team may overlook medical issues beyond the primary disability. This is known as **diagnostic overshadowing** (Boyajian-O'Neil et al. 2004; Patel and Greydanus 2010). Patel and Greydanus (2010) stress the importance of a detailed history and suggest that the PPE be completed by a sports medicine team that is involved in the athlete's long-term care that is familiar with the athlete's baseline functioning. It is also suggested that the mass or station method of conducting PPEs be avoided with these athletes. The decreased mobility of some athletes also makes this method impractical. Specific recommendations include talking at eye level with athletes in wheelchairs, asking the athlete what movement patterns are possible and which parts of the body have normal sensation, and being aware of skin conditions and pressure sores.

Athletes with histories of seizures have two and a half times more injuries than those with no seizure history (Ramirez et al. 2009). This further necessitates a careful PPE during which the clinician obtains information such as seizure history and documentation of antiseizure medication, including type, dose, frequency of use, and performance-related side effects.

Many athletes with spinal cord disabilities have constant or residual pain from their disabilities, and they may not be able to distinguish the pain of a sport injury from the pain of their disability. Having a baseline appreciation for the athlete's condition will help with the assessment process should a general medical condition arise later. Another part of the examination includes ensuring proper fit and adequacy of any prostheses, orthoses, sports wheelchairs, or other assistive devices (Hawkeswood et al. 2014). Stump care in athletes with amputations and bowel and bladder habits in athletes with spinal cord injury, will also be in the athletic trainer's purview of questioning during the PPE. It may be necessary to have a parent or guardian present to help in obtaining an accurate history from an athlete with an intellectual disability. Athletic trainers should seek assistance from professionals with expertise in the specific area of disability. Other points to consider during the PPE for an athlete with a disability including the following:

- Inspect all braces, orthoses, wheelchairs, and other assistive devices.
- Make sure braces are clean and free of rough areas.
- Ensure a proper fit of all braces for the athlete.
- Obtain a resting blood pressure in at least two positions: supine and sitting or standing.
- Inquire about bladder and bowel habits.
- Ask about his or her management plan.
- Determine the method of voiding and evacuating (e.g., catheter, bag).
- Inquire about autonomic dysreflexia and the offending agent.
- Inquire about a history of heat-related illnesses.
- Inquire about experiences with stimuli that cause spasms.
- Note the history and frequency of urinary tract or bladder infections.
- Note the history of spina bifida.
- Note the presence of a cerebral shunt.
- Note the history of latex allergy.
- Note the history of poliomyelitis.
- Note the history of seizures and the management plan (medications, last seizure, type of seizure).

- Note the history of visual impairment (age at onset, cause, protective lenses).

To identify medical problems, collect baseline data and identify training goals. Jacob and Hutzler (1998) developed the Sports-Medical Assessment Protocol (SMAP), which is a tool for the evaluation of athletes with neurological disabilities. The SMAP includes a clinical interview, cardiopulmonary testing, and physical and functional assessments. Concerning participation guidelines, the American Academy of Orthopaedic Surgeons developed a sport participation possibility chart designed to provide initial guidance for the athlete and sports medicine team about which sports are appropriate. Factors in matching athletes to sports include psychological maturity, adaptive and protective equipment, modification of the sport, the athletes' and parents' understanding of the risks of injury, current health condition, and level of competition and position played (Patel and Greydanus 2010). Boyajian-O'Neill and colleagues (2004) suggest the following questions could be asked of athletes with particular disabilities during the PPE:

- Does the athlete have a history of seizures, hearing loss, or vision loss? Are the seizures controlled? These are common abnormalities seen in Special Olympic athletes. Uncontrolled seizures often require a consultation with a neurologist and a delay in clearing the athlete for sport participation.

- Does the athlete have a history of cardiopulmonary disease? Congenital cardiac disorders, including heart murmurs, ventricular septal defects, and endocardial cushion defects, are more common in people with Down syndrome.

- Does the athlete have a history of renal disease or unilateral kidney? Various renal anomalies, such as hypoplasia, dysplasia, and obstruction, are more common in people with Down syndrome.

- Does the athlete have a history of atlantoaxial instability? Spontaneous or traumatic subluxation of the cervical spine is a potential risk in athletes with Down syndrome.

- Has the athlete had heatstroke or heat exhaustion? Thermoregulation in athletes with spinal cord injuries is impaired because of skeletal muscular paralysis and loss of autonomic nervous system control. Medications used for pain and bladder dysfunction can interfere with the normal sweat response.

- Has the athlete had any fractures or dislocations? Ligamentous laxity and joint hypermobility are prominent features in athletes with Down syndrome.

- What prosthetic devices or special equipment does the athlete use during sport participation? Health care providers need to be aware of an athlete's need for adaptive equipment and regulations concerning its use in different sports.

- Does the athlete use an indwelling urinary catheter or require intermittent catheterization of the bladder? Athletes with spinal cord injuries or other neurologic disorders often have bladder dysfunction or neurogenic bladders.

- Does the athlete have a history of pressure sores or ulcers? Athletes who use wheelchairs are prone to pressure ulcers at the sacrum and ischial tuberosities, and athletes who use prostheses are prone to pressure ulcers at prosthesis sites.

- At what levels of competition has the athlete previously participated?

- What is the athlete's level of independence for mobility and self-care?

- What medications is the athlete taking?

- Is the athlete on a special diet?

- Does the athlete have a history of autonomic dysreflexia? This is an acute, potentially life-threatening syndrome of excessive, uncontrolled sympathetic output that can occur in athletes with spinal cord injuries at or above the sixth thoracic spinal cord level.

Overview of Anatomy and Physiology

The anatomy and physiology pertinent to traumatic spinal cord injury are also pertinent to spina bifida, poliomyelitis, and cerebral palsy. Chapters 11 through 13 discuss the anatomy and physiology related to intellectual and sensory disabilities and amputation. Recall from chapter 11 that the spinal cord is a cylindrical mass of nerve tissue that consists of 31 pairs of spinal nerves and extends from the medulla to the first or second lumbar vertebra (figure 18.1*a*). It is protected by the vertebral column, which consists of 7 cervical, 12 thoracic, 5 lumbar, 5 fused sacral, and 4 or more fused coccygeal vertebrae (figure 18.1*b*). The lumbar and sacral roots of the spinal cord fan out like a horse's tail at L1–L2, giving rise to the term **cauda equina**.

Nerve impulses are conducted by the spinal cord and nerves between the brain and other parts of the body, and trauma to the spine can severely affect these intricate processes. In addition, the nervous system has other, nonmotor functions. The autonomic nervous system consists of the sympathetic and parasympathetic systems. The sympathetic system controls increases in heart rate, blood

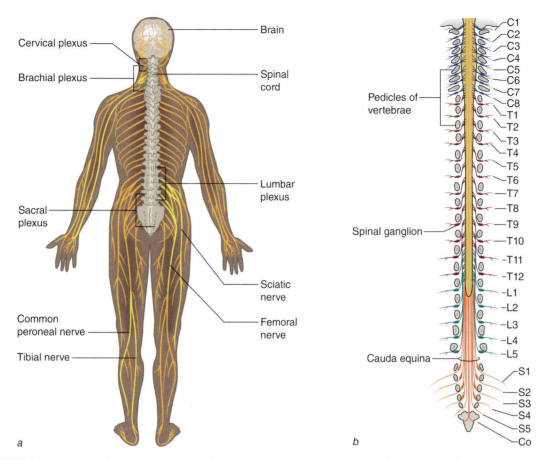

Cervical plexus

Brachial plexus

Brain

Spinal cord

Pedicles of vertebrae

C1
C2
C3
C4
C5
C6
C7
C8
T1
T2

Lumbar plexus

Sacral plexus

Spinal ganglion

Common peroneal nerve

Tibial nerve

Sciatic nerve

Femoral nerve

Cauda equina

T3
T4
T5
T6
T7
T8
T9
T10
T11
T12
L1
L2
L3
L4
L5
S1
S2
S3
S4
S5
Co

a

b

FIGURE 18.1   The spinal cord has 31 pairs of nerves that interpret sensory and motor stimuli and allow movement to occur. The level of a lesion to the cord is associated with the type of disability, typically sensory and motor, and will affect all areas distal to the lesion.

pressure, and temperature, whereas the parasympathetic system controls decreases in heart rate, blood pressure, and temperature.

Pathological Conditions

Spinal cord disability results from some form of injury or disease to the vertebrae or the nerves of the spinal column. Usually some degree of paralysis accompanies the disability. The degree of the paralysis is a function of the location of the injury on the spinal column and the number of neural fibers that are destroyed by the injury. The level of function for an athlete with a spinal cord disability depends on the level of the lesion. The lower the level of the lesion on the spinal cord, the greater the athlete's functional ability. Table 18.1 provides a summary of the relationship between level of lesion and functional ability. Note that athletes with lesions above S2 will experience bowel and bladder concerns. It is appropriate for the clinician to discreetly ask the athlete how bowel and bladder issues are controlled.

The pathological conditions associated with spinal cord injury (SCI), whether tetraplegia or paraplegia, spina bifida, or poliomyelitis, are often seen in cerebral palsy as well. Sequelae unique to specific conditions are discussed here.

Pathological conditions associated with amputations, sensory disabilities, and intellectual disabilities are also covered in this chapter.

Traumatic Tetraplegia and Paraplegia

The extent of an SCI is generally described by means of a five-point grading system. The American Spinal Injury Association (ASIA) advocates an impairment scale according to which an athlete will be classified as ASIA A (complete), ASIA B (incomplete with sensation only), ASIA C (incomplete with nonfunctional motor ability), ASIA D (incomplete with motor function), and ASIA E (normal motor and sensory function). A full explanation of this impairment scale can be found in figure 18.2. An

TABLE 18.1   **Level of Spinal Cord Lesion Related to Functional Ability**

Level of lesion	Functional abilities
C4	Use of neck and diaphragm Needs total assistance for transfers Limited respiratory endurance Controls electronic wheelchair by mouth-operated joystick
C7	Ability to extend elbow and flex and extend fingers Uses wheelchair independently Transfers to some extent independently Weak grasp
T1–T9	Ability to use upper extremities Little or no use of lower extremities Lower-level injury: some control of upper back, abdominal, and rib muscles; may ambulate with braces
T10–T12	Complete control of upper back, abdominal, and rib muscles Ambulates mainly with use of long leg braces or crutches Uses wheelchair for convenience; wheelchair sport possible
L1–L3	Hip joint flexibility and ability to flex hip Ambulates independently with short leg braces, cane, or crutches
S1	Ability to flex knees and lift feet Ambulates without crutches but may need ankle braces or orthopedic shoes

athlete with complete **tetraplegia** (formerly called quadriplegia) has a lesion above T1 that involves the cervical spine and affects all four limbs, has no trunk control or sitting balance, and usually uses a high-backed sports wheelchair. The athlete will also be strapped in for safety. An athlete with complete **paraplegia** has a lesion below T1 that affects the lower extremities, has full use of the upper extremities, and may or may not have trunk control and sitting balance. A training apparatus is available to encourage correct movement.

Athletes with incomplete spinal lesions will have varied and unpredictable responses to many neurological tests. For example, a wheelchair basketball player with a T10 incomplete lesion may respond within normal limits to dermatome testing below T10.

Athletes with SCI have higher resting heart rates and lower blood pressures than their able-bodied counterparts. The higher heart rate is due primarily to the smaller venous return from the nonworking muscles in the lower extremities. To maintain cardiac output when stroke volume is reduced, the heart compensates by increasing its rate. In turn, the blood pressure lowers to accommodate a decreased perfusion need in the nonworking limbs. Clinicians know that the baseline blood pressure for adults with tetraplegia may be as low as 90/60 mmHg and that peak heart rates for persons with tetraplegia typically do not exceed 130 beats/min. As part of the PPE, blood pressure should be obtained in two of three positions: supine and sitting or standing, as applicable

(Dec, Sparrow, and McKeag 2000). A change of less than 10 mmHg between positions is acceptable. Resting pulse is checked, as tachycardia (heart rate >120 beats/min) may be the only sign of pneumonia or pulmonary embolus in an athlete with a high-level SCI.

Autonomic Dysreflexia

Autonomic dysreflexia (AD), also known as hyperreflexia, is a clinical phenomenon unique to people with SCI above the major sympathetic nervous system outflow tract. It is a potentially life-threatening complication from SCI particular to those with lesions above T6, although attacks are possible in athletes with lesions to T10. With AD, the athlete's blood pressure rises to dangerous levels (systolic blood pressure can reach 300 mmHg [Karlsson 1999]) and, if not treated, can lead to stroke or death. In a clinical context, it is defined as a sudden rise in systolic blood pressure of more than 20 mmHg above baseline (Gee, West, and Krassioukov 2015). Herein lays the importance of obtaining a baseline blood pressure because athletes with cervical SCI will have a lower resting blood pressure than those with lower SCI, and they may present with a relatively "normal" blood pressure while experiencing AD.

AD is an imbalanced reflex sympathetic discharge that occurs when there is a painful, irritating, or even strong stimulus below the level of injury, such as an insect bite, bone fracture, or distended bowel or bladder. Other

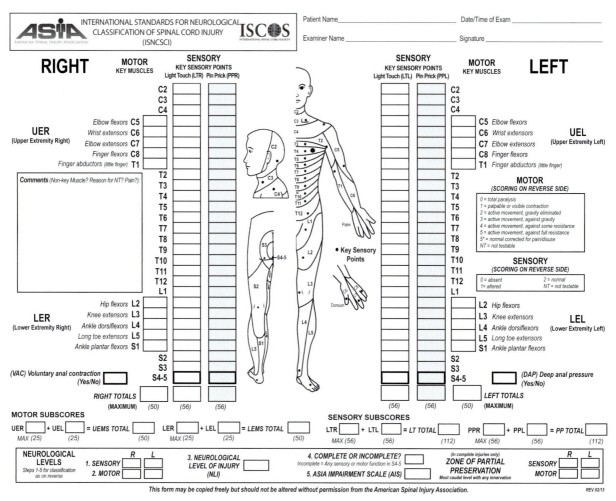

FIGURE 18.2 American Spinal Injury Association's standard neurological classification of spinal cord injury.

Reprinted from American Spinal Injury Association, 2014, *Standard neurological classification of spinal cord injury.* © The Academy of Spinal Cord Injury Professionals, Inc. 2014. Available: https://www.ncbi.nlm.nih.gov/pmc/articles/PMC4066420/figure/F2/.

physiological causes of AD include a urinary tract infection, epididymitis or scrotal compression, menstruation, gastritis or gastric ulcers, bowel impaction, or appendicitis. External causes of AD can include constricted clothing, uniform, shoes, equipment, contact with sharp objects, blisters, sunburn, or ingrown toenails. Finally, the environment can play a role in AD, as temperature fluctuations can trigger it. Intact peripheral sensory nerves transmit impulses that stimulate sympathetic neurons in the spinal cord below the level of the lesion. The inhibitory outflow above the SCI is increased, but it cannot pass below the SCI. The large sympathetic outflow causes the release of various neurotransmitters, such as norepinephrine and dopamine, causing systemic vasoconstriction and a sudden rise in blood pressure. Vasomotor brainstem reflexes try to lower blood pressure by increasing parasympathetic stimulation to the heart through stimulation of the vagus nerve, resulting in bradycardia. Because the

parasympathetic system's messages cannot pass through the SCI, the blood pressure remains elevated. The most common cause of AD is impairment in the urinary system (bladder distension or UTI). Everyday training and rehabilitation sessions can provoke AD.

Signs and Symptoms

AD is characterized by sudden-onset high blood pressure and slowed heart rate, profuse sweating above the lesion level, piloerection (goose bumps), flushing of the skin above the lesion level, headache, and nasal congestion (Gee, West, and Krassioukov 2015). It is possible for signs or symptoms to be absent despite the elevated blood pressure. It is critical to take a blood pressure reading when AD is suspected. Special attention is paid to any blood pressure reading more than 20 mmHg to 40 mmHg above the reference range for systole. To detect

> continued

Muscle Function Grading

0 = total paralysis

1 = palpable or visible contraction

2 = active movement, full range of motion (ROM) with gravity eliminated

3 = active movement, full ROM against gravity

4 = active movement, full ROM against gravity and moderate resistance in a muscle specific position

5 = (normal) active movement, full ROM against gravity and full resistance in a functional muscle position expected from an otherwise unimpaired person

5* = (normal) active movement, full ROM against gravity and sufficient resistance to be considered normal if identified inhibiting factors (i.e. pain, disuse) were not present

NT = not testable (i.e. due to immobilization, severe pain such that the patient cannot be graded, amputation of limb, or contracture of > 50% of the normal range of motion)

Sensory Grading

0 = Absent

1 = Altered, either decreased/impaired sensation or hypersensitivity

2 = Normal

NT = Not testable

Non Key Muscle Functions (optional)

May be used to assign a motor level to differentiate AIS B vs C

Movement	Root level
Shoulder: Flexion, extension, abduction, adduction, internal and external rotation **Elbow:** Supination	C5
Elbow: Pronation **Wrist:** Flexion	C6
Finger: Flexion at proximal joint, extension. **Thumb:** Flexion, extension and abduction in plane of thumb	C7
Finger: Flexion at MCP joint **Thumb:** Opposition, adduction and abduction perpendicular to palm	C8
Finger: Abduction of the index finger	T1
Hip: Adduction	L2
Hip: External rotation	L3
Hip: Extension, abduction, internal rotation **Knee:** Flexion **Ankle:** Inversion and eversion **Toe:** MP and IP extension	L4
Hallux and Toe: DIP and PIP flexion and abduction	L5
Hallux: Adduction	S1

ASIA Impairment Scale (AIS)

A = Complete. No sensory or motor function is preserved in the sacral segments S4-5.

B = Sensory Incomplete. Sensory but not motor function is preserved below the neurological level and includes the sacral segments S4-5 (light touch or pin prick at S4-5 or deep anal pressure) AND no motor function is preserved more than three levels below the motor level on either side of the body.

C = Motor Incomplete. Motor function is preserved below the neurological level**, and more than half of key muscle functions below the neurological level of injury (NLI) have a muscle grade less than 3 (Grades 0-2).

D = Motor Incomplete. Motor function is preserved below the neurological level**, and <u>at least half</u> (half or more) of key muscle functions below the NLI have a muscle grade ≥ 3.

E = Normal. If sensation and motor function as tested with the ISNCSCI are graded as normal in all segments, and the patient had prior deficits, then the AIS grade is E. Someone without an initial SCI does not receive an AIS grade.

** For an individual to receive a grade of C or D, i.e. motor incomplete status, they must have either (1) voluntary anal sphincter contraction or (2) sacral sensory sparing <u>with</u> sparing of motor function more than three levels below the motor level for that side of the body. The International Standards at this time allows even non-key muscle function more than 3 levels below the motor level to be used in determining motor incomplete status (AIS B versus C).

NOTE: When assessing the extent of motor sparing below the level for distinguishing between AIS B and C, the **motor level** on each side is used; whereas to differentiate between AIS C and D (based on proportion of key muscle functions with strength grade 3 or greater) the **neurological level of injury** is used.

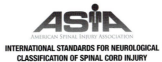

AMERICAN SPINAL INJURY ASSOCIATION

INTERNATIONAL STANDARDS FOR NEUROLOGICAL CLASSIFICATION OF SPINAL CORD INJURY

ISCOS
INTERNATIONAL SPINAL CORD SOCIETY

Steps in Classification

The following order is recommended for determining the classification of individuals with SCI.

1. Determine sensory levels for right and left sides.
The sensory level is the most caudal, intact dermatome for both pin prick and light touch sensation.

2. Determine motor levels for right and left sides.
Defined by the lowest key muscle function that has a grade of at least 3 (on supine testing), providing the key muscle functions represented by segments above that level are judged to be intact (graded as a 5).
Note: in regions where there is no myotome to test, the motor level is presumed to be the same as the sensory level, if testable motor function above that level is also normal.

3. Determine the neurological level of injury (NLI)
This refers to the most caudal segment of the cord with intact sensation and antigravity (3 or more) muscle function strength, provided that there is normal (intact) sensory and motor function rostrally respectively.
The NLI is the most cephalad of the sensory and motor levels determined in steps 1 and 2.

4. Determine whether the injury is Complete or Incomplete.
(i.e. absence or presence of sacral sparing)
If voluntary anal contraction = **No** *AND all S4-5 sensory scores =* **0** *AND deep anal pressure =* **No**, *then injury is* **Complete**.
Otherwise, injury is **Incomplete**.

5. Determine ASIA Impairment Scale (AIS) Grade:

Is injury **Complete?** If YES, AIS=A and can record ZPP (lowest dermatome or myotome on each side with some preservation)

NO ↓

Is injury Motor **Complete?** If YES, AIS=B

NO ↓ (No=voluntary anal contraction OR motor function more than three levels below the motor level on a given side, if the patient has sensory incomplete classification)

Are <u>at least half</u> (half or more) of the key muscles below the <u>neurological</u> level of injury graded 3 or better?

NO ↓   YES ↓

AIS=C   AIS=D

If sensation and motor function is normal in all segments, AIS=E
Note: AIS E is used in follow-up testing when an individual with a documented SCI has recovered normal function. If at initial testing no deficits are found, the individual is neurologically intact; the ASIA Impairment Scale does not apply.

FIGURE 18.2   *> continued*

RED FLAGS FOR AUTONOMIC DYSREFLEXIA

Immediately examine an athlete who presents with the following signs or symptoms of autonomic dysreflexia, and treat by removing the offending stimulus:

- Sudden onset of elevated blood pressure
- Accompanying lowered heart rate
- Profuse sweating above the level of impairment
- Piloerection
- Flushing of the skin above the level of impairment
- Headache
- Nasal congestion

this, the athletic trainer must know the athlete's normal blood pressure. Because impacted bowels and distended bladders can lead to AD, the clinician should also inquire about bowel and bladder habits.

Treatment and Return to Participation

The response to AD must be quick and thorough. First and foremost, the offending stimulus must be removed. The athlete should be in a sitting position because sitting leads to pooling of blood in the lower extremities and may aid in reducing blood pressure. Clothing is loosened, as is protective equipment. A thorough inspection should begin with the urinary system. Indwelling catheters are checked along the entire length of the system for constrictions, obstructions, or kinks. Health care providers must be familiar with the mechanism of these catheters because they are common to many athletes with SCI. The bladder should be drained; fecal matter is evacuated. If neither bladder nor colon is full, the clinician checks for other causes such as sunburn, pressure sores, ingrown toenails, and insect bites. A physician may administer sublingual nifedipine (a drug used to lower arterial blood pressure in emergent situations) to reduce the blood pressure while the causes of AD are being sought. Caution is recommended when using antihypertensives with older adults or those with coronary artery disease. Most athletes susceptible to AD, those with lesions above T6, will typically have had extensive education on the hazards of AD from an SCI therapist; however, the athletic trainer should never assume that the athlete is fully aware of the causes or the signs and symptoms.

It is essential that the underlying causal agent be found and removed. If symptoms do not seem to resolve immediately or if the cause of the AD has not been identified, emergency medical services should be summoned. Return to play should be based on a physician's clearance. The athlete's symptoms and blood pressure are monitored for at least 2 h after resolution of the episode to ensure that AD does not reoccur.

Prevention

Prevention is the key with AD. Because most episodes result from forgetfulness or carelessness about urine needs (Sherrill 2004), athletes should inspect catheters and void the bladder before activity. Athletes must be asked what type of bowel and bladder management program they maintain. They should avoid the risk of sunburn by using sunscreen, wearing hats or visors, seeking shade during nonactivity, and covering susceptible areas. Careful inspection after training or competition by the athlete and the athletic trainer for contributors such as blisters, sunburn, pressure sores, and constricting clothing or equipment will aid in preventing episodes of AD. To date, no specific relationship has been documented between AD and age. Because more males sustain SCI, AD is primarily a male phenomenon.

Boosting

Boosting is a dangerous technique used by some athletes with SCI to gain an advantage over an opponent or to improve race times. It is the intentional induction of AD for the purpose of enhancing performance through increased blood circulation. Athletes with SCI can induce AD by holding their urine or clamping their catheters before an event, sitting on a sharp object, sitting for a prolonged period of time, strapping their legs very tightly, or aggressively pinching or striking themselves. Self-induced lower leg fractures have also been reported (Patel and Greydanus 2010).

Improvements of approximately 10% in track and swimming times have been reported in athletes with disabilities who used this tactic (Bhambhani 2002). This would be equivalent to reducing the able-bodied 26-mile marathon record by 12 min! However, this practice is, at the very least, unethical and must be prevented at all costs. The International Paralympic Committee (IPC) bans boosting as a method of doping and sees it as a safety risk. The athletic trainer must know that this is an extremely risky behavior and must strongly discourage it. Athletes may think they are only receiving a catecholamine response and heart rate reserve that could normally be attained if uninjured. However, the significant rise in blood pressure that occurs with AD cannot be controlled by the body's autonomic nervous system. Other factors, such as inadequate hydration, fatigue, thermal stress, illness, or anxiety, can add to the AD and push the athlete to the point of autonomic shutdown, which can lead to death.

Athletes who have boosted will typically present at the starting line with profuse sweating, goose flesh, and significant leg spasms. These athletes should be immediately suspected. The athlete's blood pressure is monitored, and those with elevated measures (the IPC uses 180 mmHg systole as a cut point) are given 10 min to bring it down; if a diagnosis of AD, whether intentional or not, is confirmed, the competitor is withdrawn from the event. Athletes anecdotally report that boosting is obvious when watching competitors at the starting line (Shepherd 2003). A study by Bhambhani et al. (2010) reported that 66% of respondents surveyed at the 2008 Paralympic Games had experienced AD, and 16.7% had intentionally boosted.

Thermoregulation Concerns

Evaporative cooling is the most effective heat loss mechanism for the body, providing more than 80% of heat loss in the able-bodied athlete. Those with spinal cord injury cannot depend on the autonomic nervous system to lower their core temperature by regulating blood flow. In addition, sweating is often impaired below the level of the spinal cord lesion, requiring the athlete's body to rely on less surface area for evaporative cooling (Griggs, Price, and Goosey-Tolfrey 2015). Therefore, athletes with SCI are at greater risk of heat illness than their able-bodied counterparts, and the athletic trainer must keep careful watch over athletes during high-energy sports that raise their core temperature. Athletes with tetraplegia and those with lesions above T6 are especially vulnerable to heat illness because they cannot increase heart rate to sustain cardiac output when blood must flow to both the muscle and the skin (Griggs, Price, and Goosey-Tolfrey 2015).

Likewise, in cold conditions these athletes may lack normal warming mechanisms, such as piloerection, shivering, and circulatory shunting. A lack of working muscle mass below the level of lesion contributes to temperature regulation problems. Even temperatures around 10 °C (50 °F) may pose problems for an athlete with a cervical or high thoracic lesion. Impaired or absent sensation intensifies the risk of **hypothermia** because these athletes may be unaware of the loss of body heat. Athletes with spinal cord injury are particularly susceptible to cold. The athlete, athletic trainer, coaches, and other team members need to be sensitive to not only the environmental conditions but also inadequate clothing, prolonged levels of inactivity during competition, improper warm-up, and dehydration.

Signs and Symptoms

Recognizing the early warning signs and symptoms of dehydration is crucial in preventing severe complications from heat stress. Signs and symptoms include thirst, irritability, fatigue, headache, weakness, dizziness, decreased performance, erratic wheelchair propulsion, flushed skin, head or neck heat sensations, vomiting or nausea, and general discomfort. In able-bodied athletes chills and muscle cramps are common; such signs may not be present in athletes with SCI if piloerection is impaired. Cramping of the gastrocnemius and abdominal muscles is common, but these muscles are often nonworking in athletes with SCI.

Dehydration can also occur in hyperthermal situations during cold weather or when hypothermia also exists. Dehydration causes reduced blood volume, resulting in less fluid available to cool or warm tissues. Low temperatures accentuated by wind and dampness can pose a major threat to any athlete but especially to the athlete with a spinal cord injury, who may lack the normative mechanisms for warming.

Referral and Diagnostic Tests

Thermoregulatory problems are often incorrectly attributed to fatigue, illness, hypoglycemic reactions, concussion, or head injury (Prentice 2014). To determine

---

CONDITION HIGHLIGHT

Hyperthermia

Hyperthermia occurs when an athlete's body temperature rises and remains above the normal 37 °C (98.6 °F due to the body's failure to thermoregulate. Athletic trainers need to alert all athletes to the factors that can contribute to temperature-related illnesses. Health care providers must also be able to recognize conditions that put athletes at risk for hyperthermia and understand that these factors may occur in combination to create a risky environment for the athlete. These factors contribute to heat-related illness:

- Hot, humid conditions
- Recent illness
- Inability to sweat
- Lack of acclimation to temperature
- High-intensity workout
- Dehydration
- Dark-colored clothing
- Use of medications or dietary supplements
- Lack of fitness
- Excessive motivation
- Behavior risks (e.g., lack of sleep, alcohol intake)
- Amount and type of clothing or equipment causing impaired evaporation

The most severe form of hyperthermia is **heatstroke**, a life-threatening emergency characterized in the able-bodied population by a core temperature over 40.5 °C (105 °F) (Casa et al. 2015); a rapid increase in pulse is present as well (160–180 beats/min). The chief symptom of heatstroke is central nervous system dysfunction. Other symptoms are similar to those associated with concussions, namely confusion, agitation, inappropriate behavior or language, apathy, vacillating emotions, stupor, and coma or death if untreated.

hyperthermia, the clinician feels a distressed athlete for hot skin. Because the person with SCI has a diminished ability to regulate blood flow beneath the lesion, rectal temperatures may not provide accurate readings of core temperature in athletes with spinal cord injuries (Armstrong et al. 1995). In addition, when the thermoregulatory system is impaired, typical signs such as shivering might not be observable. It is critical that the health care provider be able to review a thorough medication and nutritional supplement history for the athlete that includes prescriptions and over-the-counter products. Sympathomimetics and anticholinergics affect thermoregulation, as do diuretics and excessive caffeine (Patel and Greydanus 2010). Emergency referral is warranted if the athlete is not responding to treatment or if heatstroke is suspected.

Treatment and Return to Participation

Treating thermoregulatory problems in the athlete with a spinal cord disability is similar to treatment for the able-bodied athlete. For hyperthermia, the athlete is moved to a shaded or cooled area, clothing is loosened, equipment removed, oral fluids are administered, and cooling is accomplished with cold water. Intravenous fluids are administered if the athlete is not coherent. If heatstroke is suspected, emergency measures to reduce the athlete's temperature (e.g., sponge application of cool water, fanning body with a towel) are performed first; then the athlete must be transported to an advanced emergency care facility (Casa et al. 2015). Although immersion in an ice bath has been recommended for able-bodied athletes, this treatment should be used with caution for an athlete with a spinal cord injury, especially one with a complete, high level of lesion because the thermoregulatory system is impaired. Cooling may occur too rapidly. To date, research in this area for athletes with SCI is incomplete. Therefore, indications and contraindications should be discussed with the physician who is most familiar with the athlete.

Treating hypothermia involves administering warm fluids, transporting the athlete to a warm environment, removing wet clothing immediately, and replacing them with warm, dry clothing. The use of heating pads or hot water bottles on paralyzed areas should be avoided because using heat on areas without sensation is contraindicated.

The National Athletic Trainers' Association established an Inter-Association Task Force that created a statement on exertional heat illness containing return-to-activity guidelines for able-bodied athletes (Casa et al. 2015). In general, these guidelines include clearance by a physician and a gradual and monitored return to activity, and they may be used for the athlete with SCI.

Prevention

Heat-related illnesses are entirely preventable. The availability of proper hydration and rehydration techniques, appropriate adaptation to environmental conditions, wearing appropriate clothing, and screening for a prior history of heat-related illnesses can prevent hyperthermia. Wheelchair athletes should attach a water bottle for drinking and a spray bottle for surface cooling to the wheelchair. A tented area adjacent to the competition for ready access to shade should be provided. The medications that athletes are taking should be monitored. Some prescriptions, over-the-counter, and recreational drugs, as well as nutritional supplements, can adversely affect heat production and heat loss. The risk of heat illness in able-bodied athletes is much greater for those who consume these drugs. It stands to reason that some medications could influence similar mechanisms in athletes with SCI. Certain medications may also predispose the athletes to temperature regulation problems in the cold.

Preventing hypothermia includes encouraging the athlete to drink plenty of fluids, warm up properly, wear adequate layers of clothing, change wet clothing immediately after exercise, and wear a hat. Athletic trainers should screen participants for a past history of hypothermia.

Special Concerns in the Adolescent and Mature Athlete

As with the able-bodied athletic population, athletic trainers should closely monitor youth or master's level athletes for thermoregulatory issues (Casa et al. 2015). Children tend to absorb more heat from their surroundings, have a lower sweating capacity, and produce more metabolic heat per mass unit than adults. Therefore, exercise time and intensity are reduced when environmental conditions are extreme. In addition, athletic trainers should make sure that children have 10 to 14 d of acclimatization. Older adults may have decreased fitness levels, decreased lean body mass, and chronic diseases, and they may use prescription medications, all of which may affect the athlete's reaction to the environment. The athletic trainer should check for fitness, acclimatization, and frequent intake of fluids, as well as should consult with the athlete's physician about medications.

Skin Breakdown and Pressure Sores

The inability of athletes with complete SCI to feel sensations makes them susceptible to skin breakdown. Wrinkled socks, poorly fitted shoes, or orthoses can create blisters that become infected. Inattention to personal hygiene may also cause skin breakdown (Sherrill 2004). Circulatory problems related to paralysis increase the risk of infection and slow healing. Pressure sores, or decubitus ulcers, result in a loss of training and competition time and could lead to bed rest, hospitalization, or, in extreme cases, such as that of the late actor Christopher Reeve, death. Skin over bony prominences is at the greatest risk (e.g., sacrum, buttocks, and ankles). Athletes with pressure sores should not be allowed to compete.

Sports wheelchairs are designed so that the athlete's knees are at a higher level than the buttocks, which is a position that leads to increased pressure over the sacrum and ischial tuberosities. This is due to the weight of the body that creates shear and compressive forces when combined with the moisture created by competitive activity. Impaired circulation is exacerbated by friction with the chair and perspiration. Wheelchair athletes, such as tennis and basketball players, who may train without shirts or in perspiration-soaked shirts, can develop skin breakdown on their upper backs from contact with the backs of their chairs.

Signs and Symptoms

Skin appearance will vary with the severity of the breakdown (figure 18.3). A stage I sore is red or discolored, but the skin is not broken. The discoloration or redness does not disappear within 30 min of pressure being removed from the site. In a stage II sore, there is partial-thickness skin loss; the epidermis or top layer is broken, creating a shallow, open sore, but drainage may or may not be present. In a stage III sore, the break in the skin has extended deep through the dermis or second layer into the

subcutaneous and fat tissue creating a full-thickness tear, and drainage is present. Stage IV is more severe in that the breakage extends into the muscle tissue and possibly down to the bone, and extensive tissue necrosis and drainage are present. Signs and symptoms that indicate further complication of a pressure sore include fever, black areas around the sore, greenish drainage, and an odor.

Referral and Diagnostic Tests

Sores are typically overlooked because an athletic trainer or other health care provider may not inspect for them, or they are dismissed as abrasions or contusions from equipment. The athletic trainer and the athlete should thoroughly inspect the skin over at-risk body parts. Young athletes need special reminders to make this inspection a habit. When a pressure sore is discovered, the offending pressure needs to be removed (e.g., the athlete transfers from the wheelchair to a treatment table or the athlete stops lying or sitting on that particular skin area). If the discoloration or redness does not disappear within 30 min, the location and color should be noted, along with any drainage, in the athlete's medical file. If there is drainage, the health care provider inspects, monitors, and notes the color and odor and refers the athlete to a physician.

Treatment and Return to Participation

Keeping pressure off the sore is the first and foremost treatment. If this is not possible during athletic activity and the sore is not severe enough to warrant the athlete's

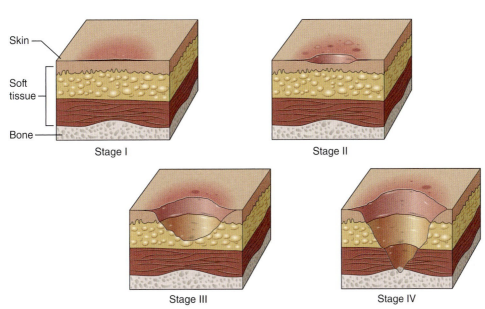

FIGURE 18.3 Staging of pressure sores.

restriction from activity, the athlete must relieve pressure from the area when not participating in athletics. These sores must be cleaned and treated as potential infections. Appropriate hygiene and sanitation must be maintained and medicated dressing applied if necessary. Treatment for pressure sores is stage-dependent:

Stage I

- Remove pressure
- Practice proper hygiene (avoid vigorous scrubbing; pat dry)
- Evaluate diet for nutritional deficits
- Evaluate mattress, wheelchair cushions, transfer techniques
- Apply Tegaderm (3M, St. Paul, MN) or similar dressing to prevent friction
- Refer if sore persists 3 to 5 d

Stage II

- Complete stage I plan
- Cleanse with saline and pat dry
- Apply dressing such as Tegaderm or DuoDERM (ConvaTec, Skillman, NJ)
- Refer if sign of infection

Stage III

- Complete stage I and II plans except for dressing
- Use pressure-relieving mattress (physician can authorize)
- Apply advanced wound care for cleansing, debriding, and packing; most likely will need referral
- Administer oral or topical antibiotics
- Refer if sign of infection

Stage IV

- Consult with physician immediately
- Undergo surgery, as is often required

Only when a pressure sore is completely healed will the area be able to receive pressure. The epidermis should not be broken and there should not be any redness or discoloration. One recommendation for determining whether a sore is completely healed is to gradually allow pressure to be accepted by the area again. For example, 15 min of pressure could be allowed, followed by 15 min of waiting for the redness to subside. If the discoloration does not subside, the area is not ready to accept pressure. If the redness does subside, the procedure can be repeated in 1 h. After three successful and consecutive 30 min trials, the area is usually ready to accept pressure. Athletes with pressure sores should not be allowed to compete.

Prevention

Prevention of pressure sores and skin breakdown includes regular inspection of the skin, the use of seat cushions in the everyday wheelchair, changing position often, proper transferring mechanics to avoid shear, good hygiene, adequate nutrition, and keeping the skin dry. Athletes should promptly towel dry to remove perspiration after heavy exercise, swimming, and bathing or showering.

Children especially need to be reminded of the preventive measures that can be taken to avoid skin breakdown, such as proper hygiene, adequate nutrition, and routine visual inspections (Patel 2004). Because the skin of older adults who are physically active will be more inclined to break down, it is paramount that preventive measures be stressed with this group of participants as well.

Spasms

Spasms can occur in athletes with spinal cord lesions above L1. Spasms are caused by excessive reflex activity below the lesion level and appear as the sudden, involuntary jerk of a body part. In an able-bodied person, the brain coordinates reflex activity, but in spinal paralysis impulse, transmission is impaired. A spasm in a muscle group can be strong enough to launch an athlete out of a wheelchair. Spasms are frustrating for the athlete but have been considered good for circulation, especially for those who use wheelchairs (Sherrill 2004). Most people in wheelchairs experience spasms, although ambulatory people with incomplete SCI can get them, too.

The stimuli that provoke spasms differ from one person to another. Three main stimuli are responsible: (1) sensory input, generally from touching hot or cold items, (2) pathology, such as bladder infections or skin breakdowns, and (3) menstrual period. Spasms are not inherently negative, and they may not be preventable because they are associated with the reflex activity in spinal cord lesions above L1. However, because bladder infections may contribute to the intensity and frequency of spasms, avoiding such infections is critical.

Signs and Symptoms

A spasm may vary in its duration and intensity but is most often a sudden, rapid, involuntary jerking of the paralyzed limb. The strength, frequency, and duration of the spasms should be noted and compared with the athlete's norm; this information will vary from athlete to athlete. Spasms can be confused with seizure disorders or spasticity.

Referral and Diagnostic Tests

Clinicians must obtain a history of spasms during the PPE in order to have comparison data. During the general medical assessment, questions about stimuli that can cause spasms are also noted. Again, having a record of the athlete's baseline when problems arise is the reason why a complete history is essential. For example, an athlete who reports severe or more frequent spasms might be asked about a possible bladder infection. The athlete is referred to a physician for a complete urinalysis when bladder infection is suspected. The athlete is always referred to a physician if conservative measures do not alleviate the spasms and improve the condition.

Treatment and Return to Participation

Typically, no treatment is necessary for spasms, especially once the cause is addressed. However, when spasms are too severe, treatments such as stretching, drug therapy (e.g., baclofen, dantrolene, diazepam [Valium]), nerve blocks, and surgery are options.

Athletes usually do not need to be restricted from activity because of spasms. If the spasms are excessive for the athlete, then the underlying cause must be addressed. Otherwise, spasms usually pose no medical threat to participation.

Bladder Dysfunction

Athletes with SCI have a neurogenic bladder, meaning that the bladder does not always empty properly or completely. This can lead to infections, kidney stones, and obstructions.

The health care provider must ask the athlete about his or her bladder management plan. Ideally, this is done during the PPE. Perhaps the athlete uses an indwelling catheter to drain the bladder. Athletes who use indwelling catheters usually have frequent, if not constant, bacteria in their urine (Hill et al. 2013). Bacteria in the bladder can spread to the kidneys and bloodstream to cause further illness and even death. Athletes who use intermittent catheterization, such as self-catheterization only when the urge to urinate is sensed, are also at risk for bladder infections, although to a lesser degree than those who use indwelling catheters. The clinician should be aware if timely access to appropriate facilities is a problem. These factors, as well as inadequate hydration, lead to an increased risk for urinary tract infections among athletes with SCI.

Athletes with SCI also have problems with constipation and stool retention that require that they regularly follow a bowel regimen.

Signs and Symptoms

The athlete with a spinal cord injury will not sense symptoms of pain and burning as an able-bodied athlete does. Other signs and symptoms include bacteria in the

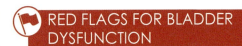

RED FLAGS FOR BLADDER DYSFUNCTION

Identify and immediately treat athletes with spinal cord injury who have bladder dysfunction because this condition can lead to autonomic dysreflexia (AD); AD, when untreated, can cause death because of the combination of high blood pressure and lowered heart rate.

urine, discolored urine, and fever. As stated previously, a bladder problem is the most common cause of autonomic dysreflexia, which can cause death. Kidney infection; kidney stones; bladder infection; urinary tract infection; contusion to ureter, bladder, or urethra; urethritis; and cystitis are the differential diagnoses for bladder dysfunction.

Referral and Diagnostic Tests

A proper assessment includes in-depth questions about the bowel and bladder routine (e.g., type, frequency, hygiene), an inspection of the catheter, urinalysis, body temperature assessment, and hydration history. The athletic trainer should be aware that, while on road trips, athletes have often been known to withhold hydration; therefore, avoiding the perceived hassle of bladder voiding, but arriving at the competition in a less than hydrated condition. Chapter 3 provides a description of how to take a dipstick reading for an on-site evaluation for many properties of the urine; table 3.2 lists the normal values for urine.

Treatment and Return to Participation

Antibiotics are the typical treatment for bladder infections. Athletes refrain from training and competition for at least 8 h after initiating antibiotic treatment, in addition to being free from fever for at least 24 h.

Prevention

Athletes need to drink at least 2 L of water a day in order to regularly flush the bladder. They should be advised to use sterile voiding techniques in order to avoid contamination during catheterization and urinary drainage. In addition, the athletic trainer creates and promotes an environment in which athletes do not feel self-conscious about taking care of their bowel and bladder needs.

Children need education and encouragement about independent care of bowel and bladder habits. Different routines (e.g., new environment, school), accidents, and odor may cause embarrassment in the young athlete (Patel 2004). The young athlete may also be too preoccupied with the sporting activity to adhere to a prescribed routine.

This adds to the risk of infection, as well as embarrassment should an accident occur.

Spina Bifida

Spina bifida is a congenital spinal cord disability in which the neural tube fails to close completely during the first 4 to 6 wk of fetal development. Subsequently, the posterior arch of one or more vertebrae does not develop properly, leaving an opening in the spinal column. It occurs most often in the low back and is more prevalent in females than in males. It causes muscular weakness or paralysis below the deficit. From least to most severe, the types of spina bifida are (1) occulta, (2) meningocele, and (3) meningomyelocele. Spina bifida occulta is given its name because the defect is hidden under the skin (*occult* meaning hidden or secret). This mild form of spina bifida does not cause paralysis or muscle weakness. However, it is associated with low back pain in adults. In some people with spina bifida occulta, a birthmark, dimple, or a tuft of hair will mark the occulta. Usually diagnosis is obtained incidentally by radiographs for other problems.

Meningocele is characterized by the protruding of the meninges, the spinal cord covering, through a vertebral cleft into a sac, resulting in weakness in the lower extremities (figure 18.4).

The most common type of spina bifida is meningomyelocele, also termed *myelomeningocele* (figure 18.5). In this condition, the spinal cord and nerve roots exit through

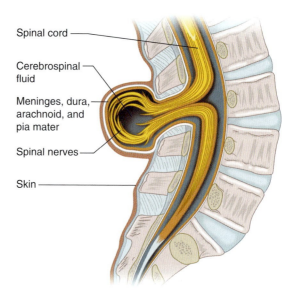

FIGURE 18.5 Meningomyelocele, or myelomeningocele, is a form of spina bifida that is apparent at birth. The herniation contains cerebrospinal fluid and a portion of the spinal cord.

a vertebral cleft and fill a tumorous sac, causing a significant deficit below the lesion. The latter two conditions require surgical correction for spinal cord fluid leakage into the sac. Spina bifida is nonprogressive; the defect at the spine will not become worse with time.

Athletes with spina bifida experience many problems common to all forms of spinal paralysis, including bladder and bowel dysfunction, spasms, and skin lesions. However, problems are greater for children (Sherrill 2004). Without sensation to the lower extremities, children with meningomyelocele might not notice and report skin lesions until serious infection occurs. This is due to children's proclivity to play with abandon, disregarding seemingly mild contusions and abrasions. Children are also more likely to be wearing splints and braces than adults. The health care provider needs to be diligent in the visual inspection of areas covered by assistive devices. Proper fitting of assistive devices must be ensured to avoid skin problems.

In addition, people with spina bifida often have a heightened **gag reflex**, which is related to the vagus nerve (Umphred et al. 2013). The exaggerated gag reflex may make swallowing pills, having the throat examined, or having a complete cranial nerve assessment more difficult for these athletes.

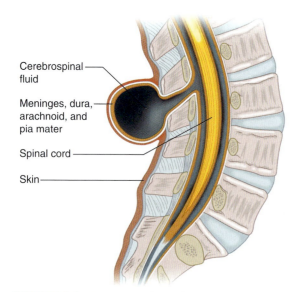

FIGURE 18.4 Meningocele is a form of spina bifida in which the meninges herniate through an incomplete closure in the spinal column, forming a sac that protrudes from the skin. The resulting cyst is filled with cerebrospinal fluid but no neural tissue.

Cerebral Shunts

The athlete with spina bifida may have an implanted cerebral shunt to control cerebrospinal fluid that backs up into the ventricles of the brain. The shunt relieves

hydrocephalus, that is, the buildup of cerebrospinal fluid in the ventricles. One end of a tube, which has a one-way valve for outflow of fluid, is inserted into the ventricles; the other end is threaded just under the skin down to the abdomen, where fluid is then reabsorbed by blood vessels in the membranes surrounding internal organs (Umphred et al. 2013). Athletic trainers should be sure to inquire, during the PPE, about shunts. Shunts typically pose no restrictions on activity except avoidance of trauma to the head, such as the type experienced in soccer heading. Some athletes will wear an appropriate helmet or headgear for protection. A small scar may be noticed behind the ear of an athlete with spina bifida who has a shunt. The athlete with suspected shunt problems should be referred to a physician. Clinical features of shunt malfunction include headaches, thoracic pain, vomiting, drowsiness, and **papilloedema**. If this athlete sustains an impact sufficient to cause a laceration to the skin overlying the shunt, referral to a neurosurgeon should occur immediately (Patel and Greydanus 2010).

Latex Allergy

Athletes with spina bifida have a higher incidence of latex allergy. Latex products such as gloves, stretch bands or rubber tubing, adhesive bandages and tape, and rescue breathing masks should never come into contact with athletes with spina bifida. The clinician must have nonlatex substitutes available when working with athletes with spina bifida. It is wise to have substitutes on hand for the general athlete population because latex allergies can exist in any athlete. Although most reactions are mild, some people may have a life-threatening reaction to latex.

Treatment for severe reactions includes the use of a prescription epinephrine-injecting pen (EpiPen; see chapter 4). Because the best method is prevention, the use of nonlatex products on athletes known to have this allergy is crucial. An allergist can conduct testing to confirm the allergy.

Poliomyelitis

Poliomyelitis, or polio, is a form of paralysis caused by a viral infection that affects motor cells of the spinal cord. Sensation, as well as bowel and bladder control, is not affected in the athlete with polio. The severity and degree of paralysis depend on the number and location of the motor cells destroyed by the virus. Because of the widespread use of the Salk vaccine, developed in the 1950s, the occurrence of polio is rare in school-aged athletes. However, in countries such as Nigeria, India, and Pakistan, polio continues to cause paralysis.

Many people who have previously had polio have experienced a recurrence of many of the symptoms of polio years after the initial attack. These symptoms include new muscle and joint pain, muscle weakness at old and new sites, severe fatigue, muscle atrophy, and new respiratory problems (National Institute of Neurological Disorders and Stroke 2016). This combination of symptoms is known as **post-polio syndrome**. According to the National Institute of Health's National Institute of Neurological Disorders and Stroke, post-polio syndrome affects 25% to 40% of people who have previously had polio.

Polio is similar to SCI and spina bifida in that muscles are paralyzed. However, because the virus does not attack sensory nerve fibers, sensation is intact. The paralysis is often incomplete, which makes judging the level of lesion difficult (Sherrill 2004). Therefore, a complete assessment of functional abilities should be conducted during the PPE.

Other than the possible presence of post-polio syndrome, few general medical conditions are unique to these athletes. The overall general medical assessment process is facilitated in this group of athletes because they have sensation and can detect pain.

Cerebral Palsy

Cerebral palsy (CP) is a chronic neurological disorder caused by a lesion in the brain that affects movement and posture. CP occurs before, at, or soon after birth and is not hereditary or progressive. CP affects the ability to move and maintain balance and posture because of the damage to those areas of the brain that control muscle tone and spinal reflexes. The disorder varies from mild, evidenced by general clumsiness and a slight limp, to severe, in which the affected person is dominated by reflexes, unable to ambulate without a motorized chair, and nonverbal.

 RED FLAGS FOR LATEX ALLERGY

Note: Athletes with spina bifida may have a higher incidence of latex allergy. Signs and symptoms of latex allergy include the following:

- Sneezing or runny nose
- Itchy, red, watery eyes
- Coughing
- Rash or hives
- Shock
- Chest tightness and shortness of breath
- Change in voice or hoarseness
- Difficulty breathing

The United States Cerebral Palsy Athletic Association uses a classification system based on an athlete's functional ability. This system also includes athletes with other conditions characterized by nonprogressive brain lesions. Neurotrauma, such as stroke and traumatic brain injury, are included in the classification because many Paralympic sports use a functional classification system across disabilities rather than isolated competition within disabilities. The system is controversial but was designed to allow for the grouping of athletes with similar abilities to compete within specific categories.

Some individuals with CP may have associated conditions such as deafness, vision disturbances, impaired hand–eye coordination, intellectual disabilities, and seizures. Seizure conditions are common in athletes with disabilities. However, athletic trainers should know that exercise actually decreases the incidence of seizures, and athletes with CP should not be discouraged from participation on the basis of seizure history. These factors influence the risk of injury but not necessarily illness in the athlete with CP. Because the affliction can be complicated by other impairments, communication with the athlete with CP is critical.

CP is characterized by **spasticity**, **athetosis**, or ataxia. Athletes with CP may be further grouped according to how many limbs are affected and what functions they have. Athletes may present with decreased musculotendinous flexibility, decreased strength, and considerable muscle imbalance. Flexibility is the most important fitness goal in the athlete with CP.

Spastic Cerebral Palsy

Spastic CP, the most common type of CP, is characterized by hypertonic muscle tone during voluntary movement. Typically, the flexor muscles are stronger than the extensor muscles. Associated with spasticity is an exaggerated myotatic reflex. This reflex normally serves as a protective mechanism, but in athletes with an exaggerated myotatic reflex (a reflex reaction in response to stretching a muscle), mild stretching may evoke a heightened response varying from a mild recoil to a violent withdrawal of the limb. In some athletes, this reflex is so disruptive that they strap their limbs down. Athletes with CP should start stretching after a period of warming up. This stretching is slow and sustained to prevent activation of the myotatic reflex.

Athletes who are ambulatory may walk with a scissors gait, which is characterized by a pigeon-toed walk caused by extreme tightness of the hip flexors, adductors, and internal rotators. The knee flexors and ankle plantar flexors are also abnormally tight, causing the knees to be bent when walking and causing the athlete to walk on his or her toes. The health care provider needs to be aware that spasticity increases with stress and fatigue.

Communication Considerations: Athletes With Cerebral Palsy

- Be patient and allow the athlete enough time to communicate; speech may be very slow or difficult to understand.
- Position the athlete carefully during assessment because incorrect positioning on a treatment table can elicit abnormal reflexes that will interfere with movement.
- Use word boards or other visual aids related to the general medical condition.
- Avoid ballistic movements during assessment; move the athlete's body parts slowly to avoid increased muscle tone or abnormal reflexive responses.

Athetoid Cerebral Palsy

Athetoid cerebral palsy, the second most common type, is characterized by constant, purposeless, and unpredictable movement that is caused by fluctuating muscle tone. Fluctuating muscle tone occurs when muscles are **hypertonic** and are then periodically **hypotonic**. This causes characteristics of drooling, lack of head control, and troubles with speaking, eating, and writing. Most people with athetosis are tetraplegic; some use wheelchairs and others walk with an unsteady gait. Signs and symptoms of athetosis increase with stress and fatigue.

Ataxic Cerebral Palsy

Ataxic cerebral palsy, the least common type, can result from disorders to the spinal cord as well as the brain. It varies from mild to severe and occurs in approximately 10% of people who have CP. It is diagnosed only in persons who can walk unaided. Athletes with ataxia have balance and coordination disturbances. These athletes can usually maintain balance when his or her eyes are open but not when they are closed. Walking on uneven ground, managing stairs, and stepping over objects pose problems for athletes with CP.

Seizures

Seizure control is a common medical issue in athletes with CP. Seizures should be identified at the PPE and then carefully monitored on an ongoing basis. The sports medicine team should be especially familiar with the different options available for antiseizure medication, as well as the potential side effects. Side effects include impaired attention span, ataxia, nystagmus, strabismus, and cognitive impairment. Seizure medications are chosen for an individual on the basis of the type of seizure. Because no one drug controls all types of seizures, athletes with CP may be taking various medications, and some may require a combination of seizure medications to achieve good seizure control. Carbamazepine is often recommended for this athletic population with caution as it has been known to cause **hyponatremia** (Crutchfield 2014). Seizures during aerobic activity are rare, but that does not preclude the need for caution. Compliance with medication is extremely important. Therefore, medications are kept on the athlete's person so that doses are not missed. During competition that involves travel, athletic trainers need to prompt athletes to take medications at the correct times because travel often disrupts routines, making many athletes more likely to forget doses. Also, the health care provider should know when athletes have had their antiseizure medications adjusted. The athlete, physician, and athletic trainer work together to set up the most appropriate seizure control plan.

Pathological Reflexes

In infants, the involuntary, predictable muscle and postural tone shifts that occur are normal and considered important for development. However, reflexes that are not integrated at the developmentally appropriate times become pathological and affect the smoothness and coordination of movement. These reflexes can be elicited spontaneously or by an external stimulus.

Patients with CP often exhibit these pathological reflexes. During an assessment, the athletic trainer should be aware of what reflexes the athlete has not integrated so that the athlete can be positioned in a way that does not elicit those reflexes that may interfere with the examination. Although a comprehensive discussion of the more than 25 primitive reflexes that might be present in this population is beyond the scope of this chapter, there are some that should be mentioned. There are four problematic reflexes that can manifest in athletes with CP; these reflexes are considered troublesome because they are initiated by head movements.

• *TLR-prone (prone tonic labyrinthine reflex)* is a reflex that is characterized by increased flexor tone elicited by a change in the position of the head. When gravity pulls the head downward and the body responds by assuming a flexion posture, this is evidence of the TLR-prone reflex.

• *TLR-supine (supine tonic labyrinthine reflex)* is characterized by increased extensor tone in response to any change in head position. If the head is thrown backward and the body responds in an extension posture, this is evidence of the TLR-supine reflex.

• *ATNR (asymmetrical tonic neck reflex)*, which is also known as the fencing reflex because, when activated, the upper extremities assume the "en garde" position of fencers. Rotation or lateral flexion of the neck causes obligatory extension of the arm on the face side and simultaneous flexion on the nonface side. Taking a position in front of the athlete before addressing him or her (to avoid head turning) will reduce the chance of eliciting this reflex.

• *STNR (symmetrical tonic neck reflex)* is characterized by bilateral arm and leg responses to up and down head movements. Head flexion causes flexor tone of the upper body and extensor tone of the lower body; head extension elicits the opposite. Positioning at eye level with the athlete will help to reduce the chance of eliciting this reflex.

Health care providers need to remember that these reflexes are involuntary motions or postures, and although they are not painful, they can compromise certain body positions. Communication with the athlete can be enhanced by understanding the reflexes and working around the stimuli that elicit them.

Amputations

Congenital or acquired disorders may necessitate limb amputation. Common indications for amputation include a necrotic extremity associated with peripheral vascular diseases or diabetes; life-threatening emergency conditions related to cancer or infection; and congenital deformity or injuries to the brachial plexus, which cause the arm to be hypersensitive, such that it is sometimes deemed a "nuisance extremity" (Lai, Standish, and Standish 2000). War and terrorist attacks have had an impact on the emergence and development of disability sport as well. Young, physically active men and women who have been injured during armed conflicts still want a competitive or fitness outlet.

People who have had amputations can continue to participate in sporting events despite the loss of one or both of the upper or lower extremities. Track and field and swimming events are the most popular for athletes with amputations. Athletes with double amputations compete in wheelchair tennis or basketball events. In track and field, the rules for individual events are the same as for able-bodied competition. The athletes may use prostheses, but no other assistive device is allowed. Prosthesis use is optional in most events but is not permitted in the high jump. Balance may be adversely affected in athletes with amputations because of the changes in their center of gravity.

Sport governing bodies have rules that allow or disallow participation with prosthetic devices. At present in the United States, the National Federation of State High School Associations does not prohibit prostheses and leaves the decision to each state association. The National Collegiate Athletic Association has guidelines and standards regulating the use of artificial limbs in its *Sports Medicine Handbook* (Parsons 2014). Factors considered include the type of amputation and prosthesis, the potential harm to other players, and the question of an unfair advantage for the athlete because of the prosthetic device. Extremity prostheses can give an athlete full range of motion for competitive success in a variety of sports, including basketball and throwing sports.

Amputations are categorized by location (AE, above the elbow; AK, above the knee; BE, below the elbow; BK, below the knee) and number for identification in sport classifications:

A1: AK double
A2: AK single
A3: BK double
A4: BK single
A5: AE double
A6: AE single
A7: BE double
A8: BE single
A9: Combined lower and upper limbs

The primary medical problems seen in athletes who have had amputations are skin breakdown and **phantom leg pain**.

Skin Breakdown

The athlete with an amputation is generally aware of skin irritation or breakdown when it begins. Prevention includes ensuring that the prosthesis fits properly. An excessively loose or tight fit will increase stress at the junction. Prostheses can increase local skin pressure and contribute to abrasions, blisters, and rashes. Other skin disorders affecting an athlete with an amputation include contact dermatitis (e.g., from cleaning agents, ointments, lotions, perfumed powders), cysts, folliculitis, fungal infections, adherent scars, and eczema. Various materials, such as gels, silicone, soft materials, and foam padding, have been used between the skin and the socket to reduce the stress from vigorous athletic activity. It is necessary to clean and thoroughly dry the stump and to change any padding that has become moist from perspiration. Morning washes are not advised unless a stump sock is worn because the damp skin can swell inside the prosthetic socket. A fragrance-free soap or antiseptic cleaner should be used, and the skin should be dried thoroughly. The socket of the prosthetic should also be cleaned and dried often. Talcum powder and antiperspirant roll-ons are commonly used to control perspiration buildup in the socket. If skin breakdown is in an advanced state, the athlete may have to temporarily discontinue use of the prosthesis and reduce athletic participation; many times stump rest is the best prescription. An athlete participating in wheelchair sports does not have to discontinue play. For minor skin irritations, lotions, such as ALPS skin lotion (silicone based; Alps South, St. Petersburg, FL) or Derma Prevent (Otto Bock Healthcare, Minneapolis, MN), or a film-like OpSite (Smith & Nephew Healthcare, Hull, UK) can be used. If a minor abrasion is present, medicated lotions such as those with zinc oxide are helpful.

Younger athletes with amputations have special needs because appliances are small and require frequent adjustments to accommodate growth. However, skin breakdown is less frequent at younger ages.

An athletic trainer may be required to assist in or perform wrapping of the stump. Although therapists may have subtle differences in the way they wrap, the basic technique for providing edema control and support without restricting circulation is the same:

- Apply the bandage with the limb extended to prevent contractures.
- All turns of the bandage should be diagonal, versus circular, to promote circulation.
- Wrap the bandage less firmly in the distal to proximal direction on the stump. No skin should be showing except for the joint itself, which usually is not bandaged at all.
- Wrap right up to the crease of the buttocks and around the waist (similar to the common hip spica wrapping technique) of an athlete with an above-the-knee amputation.
- No pain should be associated with the wrapping.

Encourage athletes to wash their bandages by hand, and squeeze rather than wring out the water. Spread them out on a flat surface to dry; never put them in a dryer. Some athletes may use **shrinkers**, which are elastic compression "socks" that are pulled over the stump. They are not as effective as wraps in controlling edema, but they are easier to use. The shrinker should fit tightly but not be painful or restrict blood flow. Avoid allowing athletes to roll or fold down the top of the shrinker, as this compromises its effectiveness.

Abnormal Sensation and Phantom Pain Syndrome

Abnormal sensations can be felt from the amputated body part, ranging from mild to severe. These include feelings of size, position, movement, itchiness, heat, cold, and touch. In some people with amputations, the abnormal sensation is pain. This is known as phantom pain syndrome and is more common in adults than children. It can also range from mild to severe. For severe pain, antidepressants have been used to provide relief. In the nonathletic population, narcotics have also been prescribed. Any person using narcotics for phantom pain needs to consult with a physician before entering an exercise program (American College of Sports Medicine 2009).

Sensory Disabilities

Athletes with sensory disabilities make up a unique segment of the athletic population. The general treatment of illness and sport-related injuries in athletes with sensory disabilities is similar to treatment for other athletes. The only special concern regards communication (Lai et al. 2000). The medical team should be prepared to find alternative ways to deliver and obtain information. In each of the following sections, recommendations for communication will be presented. Sensory disability in this chapter refers to visual impairments and blindness, as well as deafness and hardness of hearing.

Visual Impairments and Blindness

Athletes with visual impairments have visual acuity that ranges from legal blindness with partial sight to total blindness. Athletes with visual impairments compete and excel in a variety of sports, such as track and field, wrestling, swimming, tandem cycling, power lifting, goal ball, judo, gymnastics, skiing, baseball, and golf. Participation may be facilitated by the use of assistive technology such as a joint optical reflective display (JORDY 2) system (Enhanced Vision, Huntington Beach, CA), sighted guides, step or stroke counting, a tether or guide wire, or a sound source, depending on the degree of visual impairment. Table 18.2 lists the classification system for sport competition used by the United States Association of Blind Athletes.

The cause of the athlete's blindness should be noted. Blindness can be caused by birth defects, including congenital cataracts and optic nerve disease. Excessive oxygen in incubation in babies born in the 1950s was a common cause but has decreased. Other causes include tumors, albinism, injuries, and infectious diseases. In older people, common causes of blindness are diabetes, macular degeneration, glaucoma, and cataracts.

During the PPE the useful vision of the athlete is determined. About 80% to 90% of people who are blind have some **residual vision** (American College of Sports Medicine 2009). Residual vision can be ascertained by questioning the athlete in detail about what he or she sees, in addition to conducting a visual acuity examination. The health care provider must also be sensitive to the fact that lighting in the clinic or athletic training clinic may affect the athlete's ability to see. The athletic trainer should determine at what age this athlete became visually impaired and if loss of sight was congenital or occurred later in life.

Overall, there are few special concerns in sports medicine regarding the athlete with visual impairment. First and foremost is the issue of communication. It is up to the athletic trainer to effectively communicate information to the athlete, especially because so much of the general assessment is gained through the preparticipation history. Thorough documentation will help the athletic trainer and coach provide a positive athletic experience and can be obtained through a variety of communication modes.

Some people who are blind often exhibit **blindisms**, that is, repetitive movements such as rocking, hand waving, finger flicking, or digging the fingers into the eyes. There is no inherent harm in displaying blindisms other than social stigma. Many parents, teachers, and coaches have worked with children who are blind to stop these movements in certain situations. Postural deviations, such as a forward head and slumping, may also be

TABLE 18.2 United States Association of Blind Athletes Visual Classification System for Sport Competition

Level	Characteristics
B1	From no light perception in either eye up to light perception, but inability to recognize the shape of a hand at any distance or in any direction
B2	From ability to recognize the shape of a hand up to visual acuity of 20/600* and a monocular visual field of less than 5 degrees in the best eye with the best practical eye correction
B3	From visual acuity above 20/600 and up to visual acuity of 20/200 and a monocular visual field of less than 20 degrees and more than 5 degrees in the best eye with the best practical eye correction
B4	From visual acuity above 20/200 and up to visual acuity of 20/70 and a monocular visual field greater than 20 degrees in the best eye with the best practical eye correction

*See chapter 12 for a discussion of visual acuity as expressed according to Snellen eye chart numbers.

Adapted, by permission, from U.S. Association of Blind Athletes, *U.S. Association of Blind Athletes (USABA) visual classification*. Available: http://usaba. org/index.php/membership/visual-classifications/

Communication Considerations: Athletes Who Are Visually Impaired

- Always start an interaction by stating your name; for example, "James, hi. It's Tamika, and I'm going to discuss your symptoms with you." Do not expect the athlete to recognize you by the sound of your voice.

- Ask the athlete if assistance is needed with mobility. Do not grab the athlete's arm; rather, offer an upper arm and allow the athlete to grasp it.

- Provide the athlete with verbal cues that indicate changes in surface, location of the examining table, doors to be opened in or out, steps up or down.

- Use tactile sense when performing an assessment; allow the athlete to follow the examiner's hands through the evaluation.

- Demonstrate a maneuver within the athlete's field of vision.

- Conduct assessment in a brightly lit area and use colored instruments or materials that contrast with the background (e.g., brightly colored stethoscopes and reflex hammers, colored tape around edges of furniture or doorways).

- Understand that athletes who have albinism and glaucoma can better distinguish solid-colored objects under nonglare lights and away from the glare from sunlight.

- Ask the athlete's preference when providing material that is usually in a written format, such as treatment instructions or medical staff contact information; ask what works best (e.g., large print, Braille, audio clips, computer software–based files).

- Keep the examination and treatment areas free of clutter and low-hanging objects.

prevalent, especially in those athletes who are congenitally blind and have never seen others sit, stand, and move. Most experienced adult athletes develop proper posture through cueing and physical activity. Some novice athletes with visual impairments may exhibit poor balance, fewer social skills, and low cardiovascular fitness.

Documentation of illness and other general medical conditions in athletes who are visually impaired is extremely limited. Musculoskeletal injury data show that these athletes have a high proportion of lower extremity injuries. Athletes with visual impairments expend more energy than matched sighted athletes and therefore are more likely to fatigue quickly. This could be an important consideration when determining return-to-play guidelines after illness.

Albinism

Albinism is characterized by a lack of pigment in the iris and throughout the body. The eyes of an athlete with albinism are sensitive to light. Therefore, this athlete may need to wear tinted glasses inside and outside to help reduce glare. Nystagmus may also be present and should be noted in the PPE. Because athletes with albinism are more susceptible to sunburn, the athlete who exercises outdoors, even in overcast or cool weather, should generously and repetitively use sunscreen. Hats or visors and long-sleeved shirts are also advised.

Glaucoma

Glaucoma is an increase in pressure in the globe of the eye, caused by inability of the intraocular fluid to properly drain. This excess pressure damages the optic nerve. Visual loss may be gradual, sudden, or present at birth. An athlete reporting that lights appear to have halos around them may be experiencing the early stages of glaucoma. Athletes with glaucoma must avoid isometric activities, swimming underwater, inverted body positions, excess fluid intake, the use of antihistamines, and other practices that could increase eye pressure (Winnick 2011). Athletes with glaucoma may also need to use moistening eyedrops.

Deafness and Hardness of Hearing

In the United States, people who are deaf do not consider themselves disabled but rather members of a subculture of American society. Person-first terminology, discussed at the beginning of this chapter, is not supported by these athletes. The preferred terminology is "Deaf," with an uppercase D. **Hearing loss** is a general term that describes people who are hard of hearing or Deaf. **Hardness of hearing** is defined as a condition that makes understanding speech difficult through use of the ears alone, with or without a hearing aid. The term previously used for hardness of hearing was "hearing impaired." Deafness is a condition in which a person is unable to understand speech through the use of the ears alone, with or without a hearing aid. Hearing loss can range from mild to profound and is classified as one of three types: conductive, sensorineural, and mixed.

Conductive hearing loss is mechanically caused; sound does not pass through the external and middle ear to reach the inner ear (analogous to a radio with the volume on low) (Winnick 2011). A buildup of impacted wax, injury, or infection in the external ear can cause conductive loss. Athletes with conductive hearing loss typically have intelligible speech and may wear hearing aids to increase the volume. See chapter 13 for other conditions related to temporary hearing loss.

Sensorineural hearing loss is more serious and involves the inner ear, where sensory receptors convert sound waves into neural impulses that are transmitted to the brain for translation. Most people who are born deaf have this type of loss (analogous to a radio that is not well tuned). Causes of this type of loss are generally idiopathic. Others identified include hereditary factors, meningitis, measles, scarlet fever, mumps, and encephalitis. The speech of athletes with sensorineural loss may be difficult to understand. Those with more loss will most likely use sign language to communicate. Balance problems sometimes accompany this type of loss.

The mixed type of hearing loss is a combination of conductive and sensorineural losses. It is more common in seniors and might not be seen as often in the athletic population as the other types of losses.

Communication is the primary concern in the care of Deaf athletes, and it needs to be addressed during the PPE. In addition to the standard preparticipation examination,

ask the following questions of athletes who are hard of hearing or Deaf:

- Has the hearing loss progressed? Has it worsened, stayed the same, improved with aids?
- At what age did the loss occur?
- What method of communication does the athlete prefer (e.g., sign language, speech reading)?
- Does the athlete use hearing aids or have cochlear implants?
- Does the athlete use earplugs during swimming and water activities?
- Does the athlete have a history of ear infections?
- Is the hearing loss related to or accompanied by balance problems or vertigo?

It is up to the practitioner to find alternative ways to communicate. One method of communication that is relatively easy for medical personnel to learn is American Sign Language (ASL). Although there are shortcuts to certain words and phrases, the simple alphabet can be articulated by hand signs; it is depicted in figure 18.6.

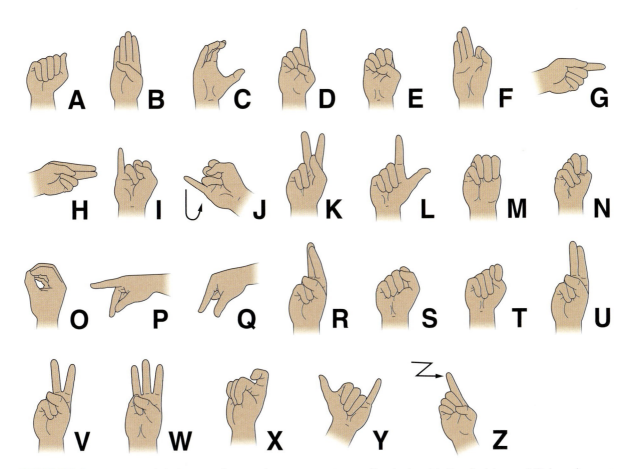

FIGURE 18.6   The ASL alphabet can be used to communicate effectively with Deaf athletes. ASL has shortcuts and abbreviations for words or phrases that facilitate communication, but this alphabet shows the basis for the language.

Hearing Aids and Implants

A variety of hearing aids exist for the Deaf. Hearing aids do not clarify or make speech sound clearer; they simply amplify sound. The four basic types of hearing aids are (1) on the chest or body, (2) behind the ear, (3) in the ear, and (4) on the eyeglasses.

Cochlear implants are recommended for those people for whom a hearing aid is not helpful. The implants are surgically placed in the inner ear and are activated by an external speech processor worn on a belt or in a pocket. A microphone is worn as a headpiece externally behind the ear. Sound is translated by the speech processor into distinctive electrical signals that travel up a thin cable to the headpiece and are transmitted across the skin via radio waves to the implanted electrodes in the cochlea. The auditory nerve is stimulated, and information is transmitted to the brain, where it is interpreted (figure 18.7). Some newer models do not have external wires. While cochlear implants are not promoted by the National Association for the Deaf, they are being increasingly implanted in children with sensorineural loss (Winnick 2011). The external apparatus should be removed during exercise to reduce the chance of electrostatic discharge (American College of Sports Medicine 2009). Athletes with cochlear implants must also stay away from plastic or rubber mats, balls, and equipment to avoid exposure to electrostatic discharge that can damage the electrodes.

Once communication barriers, type and care of hearing aids or implants, and any related conditions (e.g., balance problems, ear infections) have been addressed, the general medical assessment will not be any different from that for an athlete who is not Deaf or hard of hearing.

Intellectual Disabilities

Intellectual disabilities were formerly called mental retardation in the United States. In October 2010, President Barack Obama signed a bill called "Rosa's Law," which mandated that federal statutes would no longer use the terms *mental retardation* and *mentally retarded*. The law instead promotes the term *intellectual disability*. Intellectual disabilities are among the best known disabilities because of the visibility they receive from the Special Olympics. Athletes with intellectual disabilities compete in more than 30 individual and team sports, such as aquatics, basketball, gymnastics, figure skating, and alpine skiing. Special Olympics competition began in 1968 by Eunice Kennedy Shriver as a means for awareness, attitude change, and equal opportunity. It is the premier sport event for persons with intellectual disabilities.

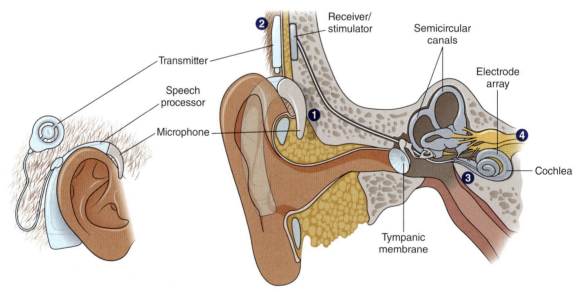

1 Sounds are picked up by and enter the system through a microphone.

2 The sound is transferred through the coil to the implant just under the skin to the receiver.

3 The implant sends a pattern of electrical pulses to the electrodes in the cochlea.

4 The auditory nerve (CN VIII) picks up the electrical pulses and sends them to the brain. The brain receives the signals and CN VIII interprets them as sound.

FIGURE 18.7   A cochlear implant can restore hearing through electronic assistive devices.

Communication Considerations: Deaf Athletes

- Speak directly to the athlete and not to a guest or interpreter who might be present.

- Maintain eye contact and face the athlete in order to facilitate speech or lip reading; even the best speech readers will understand only about 30% of what is said.

- Speak normally if the athlete uses a hearing aid.

- Use facial expressions, body language, gestures, and common signs such as thumbs up or down for "OK" and "not OK."

- Demonstrate any technique before performing it on an athlete.

- Use video, computer movie files, or other visual media as another form of demonstration.

- Use visual and tactile cues.

- Learn basic American Sign Language.

- Orient the athlete to all aspects of the facility, with special attention to exits and fire evacuation procedures.

- Do not pretend to understand the athlete if speech is unclear to you; instead, ask for repeats.

- Use instant messaging, e-mail, or other similar electronic methods to communicate.

- Use strobe fire alarms or other visual alerting devices in the facility so that the athlete has notification in the case of an emergency; point out these systems to the athlete.

- Avoid loud or constant music or background noise, even at low levels, it reduces hearing aid effectiveness and may even cause the athlete to develop headaches.

- Avoid "visual noise" such as extra physical or visual movements behind a person who is speaking.

The World Health Organization (WHO) defines intellectual disability as a "significantly reduced ability to understand new or complex information and to learn and apply new skills (impaired intelligence). This results in a reduced ability to cope independently (impaired social functioning), and begins before adulthood, with a lasting effect on development" (World Health Organization 2016). The International Classification of Diseases of the WHO subdivides intellectual disabilities into the following levels of severity according to the intelligence quotient (IQ) scale: mild (IQ, 50–55 to 70–75), moderate (IQ, 35–40 to 50–55), severe (IQ, 20–25 to 35–40), and profound (IQ, below 20–25). Note that the average IQ is 100 (World Health Organization 2016).

Athletic trainers will most likely be serving athletes who are in the category of mild intellectual disability. In general, these people will function academically between the third and sixth grades (Sherrill 2004). Terminology and directions used in the assessment of athletes with intellectual disabilities need to be clear and concise. Athletic trainers should provide ample time for athletes to familiarize themselves with the treatment or athletic training facility. Demonstrating the task first is best accompanied by simple, one-step instructions reinforced to the athlete verbally and continually. Athletes should be asked to repeat instructions to ensure that they understand.

Down syndrome is the most common chromosomal abnormality that causes intellectual disability. It is an autosomal chromosomal condition that results in a host of medical concerns in addition to those seen in other athletes with intellectual disabilities. Medical conditions associated with Down syndrome include atlantoaxial instability, balance deficits, obesity, poor hand–eye coordination, postural or orthopedic posture problems (e.g., kyphosis, club foot, lordosis), vision concerns (e.g., strabismus, nystagmus, cataracts) and cardiac issues (e.g., ventricular septal defect, atrioventricular canal defect, mitral valve prolapse).

People with intellectual disabilities vary so widely in abilities and medical issues that generalizations are difficult. Assessment during the PPE is the best method of determining normative values for each athlete. In addition to a thorough history and physical examination, echocardiograms may be indicated to screen for cardiac defects such as atrioventricular septal defects, ventricular septal defects, and atrial septal defects (Klenck and Gebke 2007). Maximal heart rates of persons with intellectual disabilities are 8% to 20% lower than expected. They exhibit maximal heart rates of 10 to 15 contractions/min below expected levels, and people with Down syndrome have even lower maximal heart rates (e.g., approximately 30–35 contractions/min below expected levels). In the general population, people with cognitive disorders have lower fitness levels than those without intellectual disabilities.

Associated Medical Concerns

Documented medical concerns that are associated with intellectual disabilities include seizures, pain insensitivity, and medication use. Seizures occur in approximately 20% of individuals with mild intellectual disabilities. The PPE should include inquiries about seizure control methods and medications. Approximately 25% of people with intellectual disabilities show signs of pain insensitivity or indifference that place them at serious medical risk (Orlander and Symons 2006). Reports have documented individuals with intellectual disabilities who have died from appendicitis and bowel obstruction that went undiagnosed because they did not report pain (Sherrill 2004). The health care provider needs to carefully check for signs of trauma and must not rely exclusively on what the athlete reports. Anticonvulsive, hypnotic, neuroleptic, and antidepressant medications are commonly used in this population. Hypothyroidism is common in persons with Down syndrome, and many of these athletes may be receiving thyroxine replacement therapy. Side effects of some of these hypothyroidism medications can cause angina until a stable dose has been determined (American College of Sports Medicine 2009). Vision problems are common in people with intellectual disabilities, necessitating a careful visual examination during the PPE.

Atlantoaxial Instability

Atlantoaxial instability is a term used to describe laxity of the ligaments and muscles that surround the first and second cervical vertebrae. Approximately 17% of persons with Down syndrome have atlantoaxial instability (Birrer 2004). The Special Olympics requires radiographic results to confirm the condition.

RED FLAGS FOR DETERMINING PAIN

Athletes who are intellectually disabled may have insensitivity or indifference to pain, or they may not be able to articulate the severity of pain they are experiencing. It is essential that the athletic trainer thoroughly evaluate for signs of trauma or illness if there is cause to believe something is wrong.

Full participation of the medical team in completing a thorough PPE that screens for the previously described health problems is paramount. An athlete with Down syndrome should have the presence of atlantoaxial instability ruled out before unrestricted participation in sport is approved. Without medical clearance on file, athletes with Down syndrome are restricted from participating in judo; equestrian sports; snowboarding; alpine skiing; squat lifting; gymnastics; butterfly stroke events, flip-turns, and diving in swimming; high jump; pentathlon events; soccer; and warm-up exercises that place pressure on the head and neck muscles (Birrer 2004). This restriction can be waived by an acknowledgment of risks signed by the adult athlete or his or her parent or guardian if the athlete is a minor and written certifications from two physicians, excluding the examining physician on record (Oberlander and Symons 2006).

Summary

Although athletes with disabilities do not have a higher incidence of general medical conditions than their able-bodied counterparts, they do present with some unique conditions that the athletic trainer must be prepared to recognize through assessment. Athletes with spinal cord injury are susceptible to autonomic dysreflexia, thermoregulatory problems, bowel and bladder complications, spasms, and skin breakdown. In addition, athletes with spina bifida may have latex allergies.

The athletic and medical teams need to be creative and committed when communicating with athletes who are sensory impaired, whether they are Deaf, hard of hearing, visually impaired, or blind. Knowing the common limitations associated with each disability can enable the athletic trainer to be prepared to provide quality care to these athletes.

Appreciating the critical importance of a thorough PPE enables the clinician to discover possible future problems and address them before they arise. The PPE is the most powerful tool team members have for managing the sports health care of the athlete with a disability. Each athlete presents with unique characteristics, and baseline measurements are imperative.

 Apply It! The case study for this chapter looks at a 27-year-old war veteran with paraplegia. Read the scenario and answer the questions at www.HumanKinetics.com/MedicalConditionsInTheAthlete.

GLOSSARY

abdominal aortic aneurysm (AAA)—Enlargement of the lower part of the aorta.

abscess—A cavity containing pus and surrounded by inflamed tissue, formed as a result of suppuration in a localized infection.

absorption—The process of getting drugs into the body through a variety of routes, including oral, rectal, vaginal, intravenous, intramuscular, inhalation, and topical application to the skin.

acne—A disease of the skin common where sebaceous glands are numerous.

actinic dermatitis—An inflammation of the skin from exposure to sunlight or another irritating light source.

acute pancreatitis—A sudden inflammation of the pancreas.

acute stress disorder (ASD)—Dissociative symptoms following a traumatic event; these symptoms are characterized by a decrease in emotional responsiveness, difficulty concentrating, and a feeling of detachment.

adenoids—Pharyngeal tonsils.

adenoma—A tumor of glandular epithelium, in which the cells of the tumor are arranged in a recognizable glandular structure.

administration—The direct application of a single dose of a drug.

adnexal—In relation to accessory organs.

adventitious breath sounds—Abnormal breath sounds superimposed over normal breath sounds: crackles, rhonchi, wheezes, pleural friction rubs.

afebrile—Without fever; pyretic.

afferent pupillary defect—When pupils react differently to light shown in one pupil at a time.

agonist—A drug that exerts its effect by attaching to cellular receptors in the body, causing stimulation of the receptor.

alopecia areata—A disease of unknown cause in which well-defined bald patches occur.

ambient temperature—The encompassing prevailing temperature.

amblyopia—A condition resulting from no apparent pathology in which vision is reduced or dimmed; also known as *lazy eye*.

amyloidosis—A disease in which a waxy, starch-like glycoprotein (amyloid) accumulates in tissues and organs, impairing their function.

anaphylactic shock—A severe, sometimes fatal systemic hypersensitivity reaction to a sensitizing substance, such as a drug, vaccine, food, serum, allergen extract, insect venom, or chemical.

anastomosis—A connection between two vessels, or a surgical connection between two vessels, ducts, or intestine.

anemia—A decreased number of red blood cells or a decreased hemoglobin concentration in the blood.

aneurysm—A sac filled with fluid or clotted blood that results from dilation of the wall and that can cause stenosis of the coronary artery.

angina—Pain or pressure in the chest.

angioedema—An acute, painless dermal, subcutaneous, or submucosal swelling of short duration. It involves the face, neck, lips, larynx, hands, feet, genitalia, or viscera.

angiotensin-converting enzyme (ACE) inhibitor—A protease inhibitor found in serum that promotes vasodilation by blocking the formation of angiotensin II and slowing the degradation of bradykinin and other kinins.

anhedonia—Inability to experience pleasure in acts that are typically pleasurable.

anisocoria—Unequal pupil sizes commonly associated with head trauma.

anorexia nervosa—Eating disorder that results in loss of weight, emaciation, intense fear of weight gain, and distorted body image; characterized by stringent diet restrictions, refusal to eat, or purging of ingested food.

antagonist—A drug that exerts its effect by binding to a cellular receptor but does not cause stimulation of the receptor.

antiemetic agent—A medication used to alleviate symptoms of nausea or vomiting.

antiphospholipid antibodies—Associated with immune-mediated illnesses, syphilis, and stroke; thought to result from a hypercoagulable disorder.

antipyretic—A medication to reduce fever, or an agent used to stop itching.

aortic dissection—Occurs when the innermost layer of the aorta tears, allowing inner and middle layers to separate due to blood flow into the area. If the blood-filled area ruptures through the outside aortic wall, it is usually fatal.

aortic stenosis—Narrowing or structure of the aortic valve.

AP view—Positioning depicted on a radiograph from front (anterior) to back (posterior), most commonly associated with the direction of an X-ray beam.

apical systolic murmur—A cardiac murmur occurring during systole that is heard over the apex of the heart.

aplastic anemia—A deficiency of all the formed elements of blood representing a failure to the cell-generating capacity of bone marrow.

apnea—Absence of spontaneous respiration.

appendicitis—Inflammation of the vermiform appendix.

arboviruses—A large group of viruses recovered largely from bats, rodents, and arthropods (e.g., insects and crustaceans).

arrhythmogenic right ventricular dysplasia (ARVD)—A rare cardiomyopathy in which fat or fibrous tissue replaces the normal muscle properties of the right ventricle.

arthrocentesis—Aspiration of a joint.

asepsis—Absence of infectious organisms.

aseptic technique—Technique to prevent transfer of microorganisms.

Asherman's syndrome—Adhesions or scars within the uterus.

ataxia—An abnormal condition characterized by impaired ability to coordinate movement.

athetosis—A condition in which involuntary, slow, irregular, twisting movements occur in the extremities, especially in the hands and fingers.

athlete's heart—An enlarged but otherwise normal heart of an athlete trained for endurance.

athletic amenorrhea—A condition where a woman does not have a period because of high exercise levels and low body fat percentage.

atrioventricular (AV) block—A disorder of cardiac impulse transmission that reflects prolonged, intermittent, or absent conduction of impulses between the atria and ventricles.

atropine—A drug used to dilate the pupils or relax muscles.

attention deficit hyperactivity disorder (ADHD)—Neurobehavioral condition that impairs the person's ability to maintain attention.

autoinoculation—The inoculation of a microorganism obtained by contact with a lesion on one's own body, producing a secondary infection.

autonomic dysreflexia (AD)—A potentially life-threatening condition characterized by the sudden onset of excessively high blood pressure in persons with lesions at or above the sixth thoracic nerve; also known as hyperreflexia.

bacterial vaginosis—A bacterial infection of the vagina.

bactericidal—Causing bacterial cell death.

bacteriostatic—Inhibiting further replication of bacteria but not causing cell death.

bacteriuria—Bacteria in the urine.

balanitis—Inflammation of the foreskin of the penis.

bell clapper deformity—Failure of the testes to be secured to the scrotum, leaving them free, much like a clapper within a bell.

benzodiazepine—A psychotropic medication used to alleviate anxiety.

bifid—Cleft, or split into two parts, or branches.

biguanides—A member of the class of oral antiperglycemic (a substance that prevents or counteracts high blood levels of glucose) agents that works by limiting glucose production and glucose absorption.

biliary colic—Painful contraction of the gallbladder that results from a gallstone that had obstructed the cystic duct.

binge eating disorder—Eating in binges that results in emotional or physical discomfort similar to bulimia but without the compensatory behaviors of bulimia.

biopsychosocial–spiritual model (BPSS)—Framework for understanding a person's response in a given situation.

bipolar disorder—Mental disorder marked by episodes of mania and depression.

bisferiens pulse—An arterial pulse that has two palpable peaks, the second of which is slightly weaker than the first.

bleb—Accumulation of fluid under the skin.

blepharospasm—Squeezing of the eyelid.

blindisms—Repetitive movements such as rocking, hand waving, finger flicking, or digging the fingers into the eyes.

boosting—The intentional induction of autonomic dysreflexia for the purpose of enhancing performance through increased blood circulation.

bradypnea—Abnormally low rate of breathing.

bronchial breath sound—A loud, high-pitched, and predominantly expiratory sound that represents air moving through large airways; normally heard only over the trachea in the anterior chest midline.

bronchophony—Increased intensity and clarity of vocal resonance due to increased density of lung tissue.

bronchovesicular breath sounds—Heard when air moves through medium-sized airways such as the main stem bronchi; can be heard both anteriorly and posteriorly, toward the center of the thorax. These sounds are of medium pitch and moderate intensity. Inspiratory and expiratory phases are approximately equal.

Brudzinski's sign—An involuntary flexion of the arm, hip, and knee when the neck is passively flexed. It occurs in patients with meningitis.

bruit—An abnormal blowing or swishing sound or murmur heard while auscultating a carotid artery, the aorta, an organ, or a gland, such as the liver or thyroid, and resulting from blood flowing through a narrow or partially occluded artery.

Buerger's disease—An occlusive vascular condition, usually of a leg or a foot, in which the small and medium-sized arteries become inflamed and form a clot.

bulbar conjunctiva—Conjunctiva overlying the sclera.

bulimia—Eating disorder characterized by repeated incidences of binge eating and self-induced vomiting, diarrhea, or excessive exercise.

bulla—Air- or fluid-filled sac in the chest.

candidiasis—An infection caused by a species of *candida* found most often in skin folds, the rectum, and nails. Oral candidiasis is also possible and is known as thrush.

carbuncle—A large site of staphylococcal infection containing purulent matter in deep, interconnecting subcutaneous pockets.

cardiac stress test—A graded test, typically on a stationary bicycle or treadmill, that challenges the heart activity.

cardioangiography—The process of producing a radiograph of the heart and its great vessels.

cataract—Clouding of the lens of the eye.

cauda equina—The terminal portion of the spinal cord and the spinal nerves below the first lumbar nerve.

cephalocaudal—In the case of an examination, covering all areas from head to toe.

cerebral palsy (CP)—A chronic neurological disorder caused by a lesion in the brain that affects movement and posture.

cerebrovascular accident (CVA)—Cerebral vascular hemorrhage in the brain resulting in ischemia of brain tissues normally perfused by the damaged vessels.

cerumen—The wax-like substance normally found in the external canal of the ear; earwax.

cheerleader's nodules—Laryngitis caused by excessive use of the voice.

chemoprophylaxis—Antimicrobial medication that prevents the spread of pathogens from one area of the body to another.

Cheyne-Stokes respiration—Breathing pattern characterized by periods of apnea.

choanae—The posterior openings in the nasal cavity that connect the nasal cavity with the nasopharynx, allowing the inhalation and expiration of air.

cholecystitis—Acute or chronic inflammation of the gallbladder.

cholelithiasis—Gallstones.

cholinergic—An agent that stimulates the elaboration of acetylcholine at the myoneural junction.

cholinergic urticaria—Skin condition, which results in hives, caused by sweat.

choriocapillaris—Vascular tissue between the retina and the sclera.

chronic fatigue syndrome (CFS)—A condition characterized by disabling fatigue accompanied by symptoms such as muscle pain, mulitjoint pain, and a headache.

claudication—Cramp-like pains in the calves caused by poor circulation of blood to the leg muscles.

clearance—The measure of the body's ability to eliminate a drug.

cold urticaria—Reactive disorder that manifests as hives after exposure to cold.

colonoscopy—A process of viewing into the colon of the digestive tract with a colonoscope.

comedones—A blackhead; the basic lesion of acne vulgaris, caused by an accumulation of keratin and sebum within the opening of a hair follicle.

commotio cordis—Damage to the heart, frequently fatal, resulting from a forceful nonpenetrating blow to the adjacent body surface.

comorbid—Two or more medical conditions that exist at the same time but that may be unrelated.

complete blood count (CBC)—A blood test looking at the major components of the blood under a microscope to determine if each component is within the usual range or value.

computed tomography (CT) scan—Computerized diagnostic imaging technique using electromagnetic radiation in a 360° motion around the patient to create an image of the body in cross-sectional slices for examination.

conductive hearing loss—A hearing loss caused by a mechanical deviation whereby sound does not pass through the external and middle ear to reach the inner ear.

congenital aortic valve stenosis (AS)—Narrowing or structure of the aortic valve present at birth.

congestive heart failure (CHF)—An abnormal condition that reflects impaired cardiac pumping and the inability to maintain the metabolic need of the body.

conjunctivitis—Inflammation of the vascular tissue covering the anterior sclera and the posterior surface of the eyelids; commonly caused by bacteria, allergies, or viral infection.

contact dermatitis—An inflammation of the skin caused by direct contact with a specific allergen.

contraindication—Situation in which a drug or treatment should be avoided.

contrast venography—The use of dye to detect the actions elicited in a vein.

cosmesis—The appearance of a patient or wound. Wound closure methods are intended to improve the cosmesis of the wound.

crackles—Adventitious sounds that occur as a result of disruption of airflow in the smaller airways, usually by fluid; also known as rales.

CREST syndrome—A syndrome consisting of *c*alcinosis cutis, *R*aynaud's phenomenon, *e*sophageal dysfunction, *s*clerodactyly, *t*elangiectasia, as well as scleroderma, carpal tunnel syndrome, and Buerger's disease.

cribriform plate—A perforated structure in the posterior portion of the ethmoid bone.

Crohn's disease—A chronic inflammatory bowel disease (IBD) characterized by inflammation of the gastrointestinal tract.

croup—Acute viral infection of the upper and lower respiratory tract.

cyclothymia—A form of season affective disorder where the athlete may perform well in practice or competitions for several days or weeks but then inexplicably hit a slump.

cystoscopy—The process of examining the lining of the bladder and the urethra.

deep vein thrombosis (DVT)—A disorder involving a thrombus (blood clot) in one of the deep veins of the body, most commonly the iliac or femoral vein.

dehiscence—Splitting open, separation of the layers of a surgical wound.

déjà vu—The sensation or illusion that one has encountered an experience or place before.

dermatitis—An inflammatory condition of the skin. Various cutaneous eruptions occur and may be unique to a particular allergen, disease, or infection. The condition may be chronic or acute; treatment is specific to the cause.

dermatographism—An urticaria due to physical allergy in which a pale, raised welt or wheal with a red flare on each side is elicited by stroking or scratching the skin with a dull instrument.

dermatophyte—Any of several fungi that cause parasitic skin disease in humans.

dermonecrotic arachnidism—Tissue destruction caused by spider venom.

diabetic ketoacidosis (DKA)—Diabetic coma; a life-threatening condition in uncontrolled diabetes mellitus.

diagnostic imaging—The use of radiographic, sonographic, nuclear, and other technologies to create visual representations for medical analysis and evaluation.

diagnostic overshadowing—The tendency for clinicians to attribute all signs and symptoms to the major condition (disability), leaving other coexisting conditions undiagnosed.

diagnostic testing—Process of using diagnostic imaging and procedures to identify a condition or disease.

dilutional pseudoanemia—"Anemia" due not to a low red blood cell count but to increased blood volume; not a true anemia.

diplopia—Condition in which the patient sees two of a single object; also known as *double vision*.

dispensing—The act of delivering a medication to an ultimate user pursuant to a medical order issued by a practitioner authorized to prescribe.

distribution—The process of getting drugs delivered throughout the tissues and fluids of the body.

dysautonomic cephalgia—A dysfunction in the autonomic system causing headaches in the back of the head.

dysdiadochokinesia—An inability to perform rapid alternating movements.

dyshidrosis—Any disorder of eccrine sweat glands.

dysmenorrhea—Abnormally painful or irregular menstruation.

dysmetria—Uncontrolled movements in a specific muscle group.

dyspareunia—Pain during sexual intercourse that is not normal.

dysphagia—Difficulty swallowing.

dysplastic nevi—An atypical mole or freckle.

dyspnea—Labored or difficult breathing.

egophony—Altered voice sound in a patient with pleural effusion.

electrocardiogram (ECG)—A graphic recording of the heart's electrical activity in the form of a PQRST wave.

electrocardiography—The process of having an electrocardiograph performed on a person.

electroencephalogram (EEG)—Electrodes placed on scalp that detect the electric potential produced by brain cells. The record of this test is the *gram* aspect of this test, whereas electroencephalography is the process of the recording.

electromyogram (EMG)—Process of applying electrodes to skeletal muscle to measure the electrical activity during muscle contraction.

electromyography—Record of the electrical activity in skeletal muscle.

elimination—Process of getting a drug out of the body.

encephalitis—An inflammatory condition of the brain, usually caused by an infection.

endocrine glands—Glands that secrete hormones directly into the bloodstream, allowing specific body functions to occur.

enophthalmos—Recession of the eyeball deeper into the orbit.

enterovirus—A group of RNA viruses that can cause diseases in humans, typically found in the respiratory secretions and stools of infected people.

epidermis—The superficial avascular layers of the skin made up of an outer dead, cornified part and a deeper living, cellular part.

epidermoid cysts—A painless, slow growing cyst that is noncancerous and arises from the upper layers of the skin.

erythema migrans—A skin lesion that begins as a small papule and spreads peripherally. It is sometimes associated with Lyme disease.

eustachian tube—A mucous membrane–lined tube that joins the nasopharynx and the middle ear cavity; opened during yawning, chewing, and swallowing to allow for equalization of air pressure.

exercise-induced laryngeal obstruction (EILO)—Wheezing and dyspnea caused by transient obstruction of the upper airways during exercise.

exophthalmos—An abnormal condition characterized by a marked protrusion of the eyeballs.

factor V Leiden anticoagulant gene mutation—A genetic mutation of factor V that causes venous thrombosis (blood clots).

fibromyalgia—A form of nonarticular rheumatism characterized by musculoskeletal pain, spasm and stiffness, fatigue, and sleep disturbances.

fluoroscopy—A diagnostic imaging device creating immediate radiographic imaging on a fluorescent screen for visual examination in real time.

folliculitis—Inflammation of the hair follicles.

fornices—The loose arching folds connecting the conjunctival membranes on the inside of the eyelid and those covering the eyeball.

furuncle—A localized suppurative staphylococcal skin infection originating in a gland or hair follicle and characterized by pain, redness, and swelling.

furunculosis—An acute skin disease characterized by boils or successive crops of boils that are caused by staphylococci or streptococci.

gag reflex—A reflex contraction of the muscles of the throat elicited by touching the soft palate or posterior pharynx.

gastritis—Diffuse inflammation of the lining of the stomach.

gastroenteritis—Inflammatory condition of the stomach and intestines that is usually caused by bacteria or a virus.

gastroesophageal reflux disease (GERD)—Condition in which stomach acid travels up through the lower esophageal sphincter into the esophagus or even into the back of the throat.

generalized anxiety disorder (GAD)—Disorder marked by worry over or nervousness about many or most things in life.

gingiva, gingivae—The gum tissue of the mouth that encircles the necks of the teeth.

gingivitis—An inflammation of the gingivae in which the margins close to the teeth are red, swollen, and bleeding.

glaucoma—Group of eye diseases characterized by increased intraocular pressure.

goiter—A visible swelling on the anterior neck due to an enlarged thyroid gland.

gonorrhea—A common sexually transmitted infection that affects the genitourinary system and often the rectum and pharynx.

Graves' disease—The common name for hyperthyroidism.

gustatory hallucinations—A false taste sensation of either food or beverage.

hairy leukoplakia—A white plaque visible on the surface of the tongue that is most often associated with severe immunodeficiency.

half-life—The length of time that it takes for blood or tissue levels of a drug to decrease by one-half.

hardness of hearing—A condition that makes understanding speech difficult through the use of the ears alone, with or without a hearing aid.

hearing loss—A general term that describes people who are hard of hearing or Deaf.

heatstroke—A life-threatening emergency characterized in the able-bodied population as having a core temperature over 40.5 °C (105 °F).

hemoglobin electrophoresis—A blood test used to differentiate different forms of hemoglobin.

hemoglobinuria—Abnormal presence in the urine of hemoglobin that is not attached to red blood cells.

hemolysis—The breakdown of red blood cells and the release of hemoglobin that occur normally at the end of the life span of a red blood cell.

hemolytic anemia—A disorder characterized by acute or chronic premature destruction of red blood cells.

hemoptysis—Productive cough of sputum that may contain blood.

hemothorax—Collection of the blood in the pleural cavity of the thorax.

hepatomegaly—An abnormal enlargement of the liver that is usually the sign of a disease.

hepatosplenomegaly—Enlargement of the spleen and liver.

herpes gladiatorum—Herpes simplex virus (HSV) found on the trunk that is typically transmitted via skin-to-skin contact, such as in the sport of wrestling.

herpes keratoconjunctivitis—A highly contagious form of herpes simplex that affects the cornea of the eye.

herpes zoster—An acute infection caused by reactivation of the latent varicella-zoster virus, which mainly affects adults.

hidradenitis suppurativa—An infection or inflammation of the sweat glands.

hirsutism—Excessive body hair in a masculine distribution pattern as a result of heredity, hormonal dysfunction, porphyria, or medication.

Hodgkin's lymphoma—A malignant condition of lymphoreticular origin; different from Non-Hodgkin's lymphoma because of the presence of Reed-Sternberg cells.

Holter monitor—Device worn over a period of time to capture prolonged electrocardiograph recordings.

homatropine—A drug used to dilate the pupils; less potent than atropine.

Horner's syndrome—A condition caused by damaged sympathetic trunk nerves.

hot spots—Locations on a nuclear diagnostic image that illuminate due to higher levels of detected radiation as a result of increased absorption of radionuclide.

hydrocephalus—The accumulation of cerebrospinal fluid in the ventricles of the brain.

hydronephrosis—Swelling of one kidney due to the failure of normal drainage of urine from the kidney to the bladder.

hydrophilicity—The degree to which a compound is soluble in water.

hyperalgesia—A heightened sensitivity to pain.

hyperandrogenism—A condition in which there are excessive levels of androgens in the body.

hyperemia—An increase in blood flow to a body part; characterized by reddening of the skin.

hyperinsulinemia—An excessive amount of insulin in the body.

hyperlipidemia—An excess of lipids, including glycolipids, lipoproteins, and phospholipids, in the plasma.

hyperopia—Farsightedness, in which a person can see objects in the distance clearly, but closer objects are out of focus.

hyperpnea—Rapid breathing with very large breaths; >24 breaths/min.

hyperthyroidism—An abnormal endocrine condition characterized by hyperactivity of any of the four parathyroid glands with excessive secretion of the parathyroid hormone (PTH).

hypertonic—Increased muscle tension whereby muscle tone is abnormally rigid and range of motion may be hampered.

hypertrophic cardiomyopathy (HCM)—An abnormal condition characterized by gross hypertrophy of a ventricle of the heart, but having a normal chamber size.

hyphema—Blood in the anterior chamber of the eye.

hypogonadism—Deficiency in the activity of the gonads; testes for males, ovaries for females.

hyponatremia—A condition where the level of sodium in the blood is drastically depleted, which can lead to coma and death. Overhydrating can cause this.

hypopnea—Shallow, slow breathing.

hypothermia—A potentially life-threatening emergency characterized in the able-bodied population as having a core body temperature under 35 °C (95 °F).

hypotonic—Diminished or flaccid muscle tone whereby muscle contraction speed is slow and strength is impaired.

immunosuppressed patient—A patient who has a condition that produces an inhibited ability to respond to antigenic stimuli.

impetigo—A streptococcal, staphylococcal, or combined infection of the skin beginning as focal erythema and progressing to pruritic vesicles, erosions, and honey-colored crusts.

in situ—The natural or original position or place.

indication—Condition for which a drug has been found to have a therapeutic effect.

infectious mononucleosis—Disease caused by the Epstein-Barr virus; associated with symptoms of fatigue, pharyngitis, fever, and lymphadenopathy; also known as the kissing disease.

inflammatory bowel disease (IBD)—A group of intestinal disorders that cause prolonged inflammation of the digestive tract.

international normalized ratio (INR)—A standardized measure of time it takes for blood to clot.

intravenous pyelogram (IVP)—A specific type of X-ray that shows images of the kidneys, the bladder, the ureters, and the urethra.

ipsilateral miosis—Ipsilateral pertains to the same side of the body, and miosis is a constricted pupil. Together this means only one pupil (of the eye) is constricted.

irritable bowel syndrome (IBS)—Disorder of gastrointestinal motility with abnormal cycles of muscle contraction and relaxation.

islets of Langerhans—Clusters of cells within the pancreas that produce insulin, glucagon, and pancreatic polypeptide. They are important regulators of carbohydrate metabolism.

jamais vu—A sensation of being a stranger to a previously known place or person.

Kaposi's sarcoma—A malignant condition beginning with dark papules on the feet or hard palate of the mouth that metastasizes to lymph nodes or other organs. It is associated with autoimmune or immunodeficiency conditions as well as with lymphomas.

Kawasaki's disease—Rare, inflammatory condition of unknown origin that usually occurs in young childhood.

keratinous cysts—An epithelial cyst containing keratin.

kerions—An inflamed, boggy granuloma that develops as an immune reaction to a superficial fungus infection, generally in association with tinea capitis of the scalp.

Kernig's signs—A diagnostic sign for meningitis that occurs when the patient cannot straighten the leg when it is fully flexed at the knee and hip.

Kiesselbach's plexus—An area of small, fragile arteries and veins located in the nasal septum; the root of most nosebleeds.

Korotkoff sounds—A series of sounds produced by distention of an artery by the blood pressure cuff; the level at which the sound disappears is the diastolic pressure, often referred to as the fifth or last Korotkoff sound.

Kussmaul breathing—Deep, rapid, sighing breaths characterized by diabetic ketoacidosis.

labial agglutination—When the labia majora stick together.

lactic acidosis—A disorder characterized by an accumulation of lactic acid in the blood, resulting in a lowered pH in muscle and serum.

lagophthalmos—Inability to close the eyelids completely, usually the result of a severe subconjunctival hemorrhage.

lanugo—Fine, downy hair covering the body.

laparoscopic—Surgical procedure in which a laparoscope is used to examine the abdominal cavity through one or two small incisions in the abdominal wall.

laparoscopy—A process of viewing within a body cavity with a laparoscope.

laryngitis—Inflammation of the larynx.

lateral view—Positioning on a radiograph taken from the outermost side, most commonly associated with the direction of an X-ray beam.

lesion—A wound, injury, or pathological change in body tissue. Any visible, local abnormality of the tissues of the skin, such as a wound, sore, rash, or boil. A lesion may be described as benign, cancerous, gross, occult, or primary.

leukemias—Uncontrolled proliferation of white blood cells in the bone marrow, which accumulate and replace normal blood cells in the marrow.

leukocytosis—An abnormal increase in the amount of circulating white blood cells.

leukopenia—An abnormal decrease in the number of white blood cells, fewer than 5,000 cells per cubic centimeter.

leukoplakia—White plaque found on the lateral borders of the tongue that may be folded or smooth in appearance; associated with severe immunodeficiency.

lipophilicity—The degree to which a compound is soluble in fat.

long QT syndrome (LQTS)—An inherited cardiac disorder characterized by prolongation of the QT interval.

lymphadenopathy—A condition where either a lymph node is diseased or a disease of the lymph nodes.

lymphocytosis—A proliferation of lymphocytes, as occurs in certain chronic diseases.

lymphoreticular system—A system composed of the primary lymphoid organs, such as bone marrow or the thymus, which serve to produce lymphocytes.

lymphosarcoma—Any of a heterogeneous group of malignant tumors involving lymphoid tissue.

maculopapular rash—A skin eruption characterized by distinctive macules or papules.

Marfan syndrome—An autosomal dominant, heritable disorder of connective tissue.

mastication—Chewing, tearing, or grinding food with teeth while it becomes mixed with saliva.

melanin—A black or dark brown pigment that occurs naturally in hair, skin, and the iris and choroid of the eye.

melanocyte—A body cell capable of producing melanin.

melanoma—Any group of malignant neoplasms that originate in the skin and are composed of melanocytes.

meningitis—Any infection or inflammation of the membranes covering the brain and spinal cord.

meningoencephalitis—An inflammation of both the brain and meninges, usually caused by a bacterial infection.

metabolism—In pharmacology, the process by which a drug is changed into one or more chemical entities.

metastasis—A process that occurs when cancerous cells establish a remote colony of cancerous cells from the original cancer.

metastatic—The process of tumor cells spreading from an initial disease site to another area of the body.

methicillin-resistant *Staphylococcus aureus* **(MRSA)**—An infection caused by a strain of staphylococcus (staph) bacteria that is resistant to many medications used to treat other staph infections.

microcytic anemias—Include iron deficiency, thalassemia, lead poisoning, sideroblastic anemia.

mitral regurgitation—A backflow of blood from the left ventricle into the left atrium in systole across a diseased mitral valve.

mittelschmerz—Abdominal pain mid-way through the menstrual cycle associated with the release of the ovum (ovulation).

molluscum contagiosum—A viral disease of the skin and mucous membranes caused by a poxvirus that involves nodules that are small, smooth, painless, and have a pink coloration. When the area is compressed, a milky fluid is produced.

mononucleosis (mono)—An abnormal amount of mononuclear leukocytes in the blood; represented by swollen glands and chronic fatigue.

MRI (magnetic resonance imaging) scan—Diagnostic imaging technique using radio-frequency pulses from a powerful magnetic field to produce high-resolution images of organs, soft-tissue structures, and bone.

Murphy's sign—Sudden cessation of inspiration during deep palpation over the liver when the patient takes a deep breath; may be a result of gallstones.

myocardial bridging—Strands of myocardial fibers lying over the coronary arteries. If long or deep enough, they may cause asystole, myocardial infarction, or necrosis of the affected tissue.

myocarditis—An inflammatory process of the cardiac myocytes.

myocytes—Muscle cells.

myopia—Nearsightedness, in which patients can see objects up close clearly, but objects in the distance are out of focus.

nares—The pair of openings in the front and back of the nasal cavity that allow air to pass to the pharynx.

nasopharynx—The uppermost portion of the three regions of the throat (pharynx), extending from the posterior nares to the level of the soft palate.

nebulizer—A machine that uses compressed air to cause aerosolization of a liquid drug, which is then inhaled through a mask or a mouthpiece.

necrotizing fasciitis—A rapid tissue death that results from a bacterial infection.

nerve conduction study (NCS)—An electrodiagnostic test that involves placing an electrical stimulator over a nerve and measuring the time required for an impulse to travel over a measured segment of the nerve. It is used to test the integrity of peripheral nerves.

nerve conduction velocity (NCV)—An electrodiagnostic test of the integrity of the peripheral nerves.

nongonococcal urethritis (NGU)—An infection of the urethra in males that is characterized by mild dysuria and penile discharge. The discharge may be white or clear, thin or thick.

nonspecific urethritis (NSU)—Inflammation of the urethra not caused by a specific organism. Symptoms are often related to sexual intercourse. Symptoms include urethral discharge in men and reddening of the urethra mucosa in women.

nonsuppurative—Pertaining to inflammation without forming pus.

nosocomial infection—Infection that is acquired at a hospital after the patient is admitted for hospital care for something other than the infection.

nuchal rigidity—A resistance to flexion in the neck, usually seen with patients suffering from meningitis.

nuclear stress test—A diagnostic test using a radioactive tracer to measure the blood flow to the heart at rest and in stress. It can illuminate areas of ischemic heart tissue.

obsessive–compulsive disorder (OCD)—Anxiety disorder characterized by persistent behaviors that markedly impair the person's functioning.

oligomenorrhea—Abnormally light menstruation or reduction in menstruation.

onychia—Inflammation of the nail bed.

oophoritis—The process of inflammation involving the ovaries.

open globe—Eyeball that has been ruptured after blunt trauma, allowing leakage of intraocular fluid or extrusion of intraocular tissue.

orbital emphysema—"Crunchy" sensation under the skin associated with an orbital fracture; results from air from the sinuses being trapped under the skin.

orchitis—Inflammation of one or both testes.

orthopnea—Shortness of breath while lying down.

orthostatic hypotension—Abnormally low blood pressure that occurs when an individual suddenly assumes the standing position.

orthostatic syncope—Brief lapse in consciousness while moving from a lying or sitting to a standing position.

otalgia—Pain in the ear.

otolaryngologist—A physician who specializes in the treatment and evaluation of the ears, nose, and throat.

otorrhea—Any discharge from the external ear.

oxygenation—In respiration, the exchange of gases in the alveolar–capillary beds.

PA view—Positioning depicted on a radiograph from back (posterior) to front (anterior), most commonly associated with the direction of an X-ray beam.

palliative therapy—Therapy designed to relieve the intensity of symptoms and support the patient; does not produce a cure.

palpebral conjunctiva—The part of the conjunctiva lining the eyelids.

palpitations—A pounding or racing of the heart.

panic disorder—Anxiety disorder marked by an acute period of intense fear or anxiety.

papilloedema—Swelling of the optic disk in the eye usually caused by pressure in the brain or intracranial pressure.

paraplegia—Impairment in motor or sensory function of the legs and possibly the trunk, caused by a lesion below the first thoracic nerve or a congenital condition affecting the neural elements of the spinal cord.

parenchyma—Functional tissue or cells of an organ.

paronychia—An infection of the fold of skin at the margin of a nail.

parotitis—Inflammation of the parotid salivary glands.

paroxysmal nocturnal dyspnea—Disorder characterized by sudden attacks of respiratory distress that awaken a person after a few hours of sleeping in a reclining position.

pectus deformity—A chest deformity normally resulting in convex or concave abnormalities.

pediculosis—An infestation with blood-sucking lice.

peptic ulcer disease (PUD)—Ulcer found in the stomach or duodenum.

periodontitis—An inflammation or infection of the supporting structures of the teeth.

peripheral arterial disease (PAD)—Also referred to as peripheral vascular disease, a condition caused primarily by atherosclerosis.

perirenal fat—Accumulation of fat outside of the peritoneal cavity surrounding the kidney.

person-first terminology—An example of disability etiquette that places the individual (e.g., athlete) before the descriptive phase (e.g., with a disability) thereby focusing on the person rather than the disability.

petechiae—Tiny purple or red spots appearing on the skin as a result of tiny hemorrhages within the dermal or submucosal layers.

phantom leg pain—Also known as *phantom limb pain*. Sensations, such as tingling, numbness, pain, heat, or cold, that are perceived by people with amputated limb(s).

pharmacodynamics—Study of the actions of a drug on the body, including mechanism of action and medicinal effect.

pharmacokinetics—Study of how the body acts on a drug, including the absorption, distribution, metabolism, and elimination of the drug.

photophobia—Pain occurring when light is shone into the eye.

photopsia—Sensation of flashes of light.

pilonidal cyst—A cyst that often develops in the sacral region of the skin.

pleural rubs—Sounds that occur outside the respiratory tree and result from friction between visceral and parietal pleura.

pleurisy—Inflammation of the lining of the lungs.

pneumothorax—Presence of air or gas in the pleural space, causing the lung to collapse.

polycystic ovarian disease—An endocrine disorder that can result in hirsutism, and a lack of ovulation, menstruation, and fertility.

polycythemia—An increase in red blood cell count and circulating red blood cell mass that may be primary or secondary to pulmonary disease, heart disease, or prolonged exposure to high altitudes.

polydipsia—A feeling of excessive thirst.

polymenorrhea—A condition in which the menstrual cycle is abnormally recurrent; more than one cycle per month.

polyphagia—A feeling of persistent hunger.

polyuria—A condition of increased urination.

positron emission tomography (PET) scan—Computerized radiographic technique that requires ingestion or injection of a biochemically radioactive substance that is used to measure metabolic activity in the desired body structure with color-coded images.

posterior vitreous detachment (PVD)—When the vitreous liquefies and peels away from the retina, resulting in "floaters" in the field of vision.

postphlebitic syndrome—A condition that occurs when valves of veins become damaged, allowing fluid to pool distally from the weakened valve.

post-polio syndrome—A neurological disorder characterized by new and progressive muscular weakness, pain, and fatigue that affects polio survivors years after recovery from the initial infection of the poliomyelitis virus.

posttraumatic stress disorder (PTSD)—Psychiatric disorder in response to a traumatic event, resulting in intense psychological distress.

potassium hydroxide (KOH) preparation—Using a surface scraping of the affected tissue, a KOH solution is added to the scraping and viewed under a microscope. The results determine if a skin condition is present or not.

preauricular lymphadenopathy—Small, tender lymph node located just in front of the tragus of the ear and commonly associated with conjunctivitis.

premature atrial contraction (PAC)—An atrial depolarization that occurs earlier than expected; an early P wave.

premature ventricular contraction (PVC)—A ventricular depolarization that occurs earlier than expected, portrayed as an early and wide QRS complex without a preceding related P wave.

presbycusis—Hearing loss due to aging.

presbyopia—Loss of flexibility of the crystalline lens inside the eye, resulting in an inability to focus on near objects.

prodromal—Pertaining to early symptoms that may mark the onset of a disease.

prophylaxis—Using preventative measures to avoid disease or illness.

proptosis—Downward or forward displacement of the eyeball as a result of swelling; also referred to as *exophthalmos*.

prostate-specific antigen (PSA)—A protein produced by the prostate that is abnormally high in patients with cancer or other disease involving the prostate.

prostatic calculi—Calcifications formed within the prostate.

prostatic tuberculosis—Tuberculosis of the prostate caused by bacteria.

prothrombin time (PT)—Test used to time clot formation; can detect defects in the ability of the blood to coagulate, which are usually caused by a deficiency of factor V, VII, or X (normal PT, 11–12.5 s).

pruritic—The symptom of itching, an uncomfortable sensation leading to the urge to scratch.

pruritus—A condition of itching.

psoriasis—A common chronic skin disorder characterized by circumscribed red patches covered by thick, dry, silvery adherent scales that are a result of excessive development of epithelial cells.

psychotropic medication—A medication that alters a person's psychic function or behavior.

ptosis—Drooping of upper eyelid.

pulmonary embolus—A blockage of the pulmonary artery by fat, air, tumor tissue, or a thrombus that usually arises from a peripheral vein (most frequently one of the deep veins of the legs).

purulent—Producing or containing pus.

pyelonephritis—A bacterial infection that causes inflammation to the kidney.

radiofrequency catheter ablation—Unmodulated high-frequency alternating current flow that is applied to the heart tissue to raise its temperature and injure cells for the purpose of destroying the ectopic foci and accessory pathways.

radionuclide bone scan—Noninvasive injection of a radioactive substance for visualization of a bone with an image produced by the emission of radioactive particles.

Raynaud's disease—Intermittent attacks of ischemia in the extremities of the body, especially the fingers, toes, ears, and nose, caused by exposure to cold or emotional stimuli.

Raynaud's phenomenon—Vasospasm of the arteries caused by an underlying issue.

Reed-Sternberg cells—Large, abnormal, multinucleated cells found in Hodgkin's disease.

renin–angiotensin system—The regulation of sodium balance, fluid volume, and blood pressure.

residual vision—The remaining vision the person has; what the individual can see.

retractions—Visible sinking in of the soft tissue of the chest.

Reye's syndrome—A combination of acute encephalopathy and fatty infiltration of the internal organs that may follow viral infections.

rhabdomyolysis—A potentially fatal syndrome caused by the breakdown of skeletal muscle fibers.

rhinitis—Inflammation of the mucous membranes of the nose, typically accompanied by swelling of the mucosa and nasal discharge.

rhinoplasty—A procedure in which the structure of the nose is altered by plastic surgery.

rhinorrhea—Thin, watery discharge from the nose or flowing of cerebrospinal fluid from the nose after injury to the head.

rhinovirus—Ribonucleic acid–based virus that causes acute respiratory illness.

rhonchus, rhonchi—Low-pitched, sonorous wheeze.

rubella—Another term for German measles, which is a viral disease that can cause a low fever, swollen glands, joint pain, and a fine red rash on the skin.

rubeola—Another term for measles, also called red measles, which is a virus that causes a skin rash.

salpingitis—The process of inflammation involving the fallopian tubes.

scabies—A contagious disease caused by *Sarcoptes scabiei*, the itch mite, characterized by intense itching of the skin and excoriation from scratching.

scleroderma—Chronic hardening and thickening of the skin caused by new collagen formation.

seasonal affective disorder (SAD)—Mood disorder characterized by lethargy and depression due to shorter exposure to daylight and longer exposure to darkness during the fall and winter.

sebaceous cysts—A misnomer for epidermoid, epidermal, or pilar cysts. Sebaceous cysts arise from the oil glands in the skin.

seminoma—A tumor on the testis.

sensorineural hearing loss—Hearing loss involving the inner ear, where sensory receptors convert sound waves into neural impulses that are transmitted to the brain for translation. Most people who are born deaf have this type of loss.

serology—Test that identifies specific antibodies in the blood.

shrinker—An elastic sock pulled over the stump of an amputated limb that is designed to control edema, promote healing, and assist in shaping the stump.

sickle cell anemia—A severe, chronic, hereditary disease that causes red blood cells to be misshapen (sickle-shaped), leading to blockages that cause damage to areas distal from the blockage.

sideroblastic anemia—A form of anemia in which the bone marrow does not produce healthy red blood cells but rather ringed sideroblasts (abnormal immature red blood cells) that cannot transform readily available iron sources into hemoglobin.

sinusitis—Acute or chronic inflammation of the sinus with or without purulent drainage.

Sjogren's syndrome—A disorder of the immune system marked by inefficient production of certain glands (e.g., salivary, lamictal) resulting in dryness.

slit-lamp—An instrument equipped with a high-intensity light source that can be focused to shine as a slit; used to examine structures at the front of the eye for any existing pathologies.

solar urticaria—Wheals caused by exposure to the sun.

spasticity—Motor disorder characterized by involuntary, sudden movement or muscle contraction, increased muscle tone, and exaggerated tendon jerks.

splenomegaly—An enlarged spleen.

Stevens-Johnson syndrome—Severe form of erythema multiforme caused by a dermatological reaction to antibiotics; characterized by malaise, headache, fever, and arthralgia.

stridor—High-pitched sound caused by obstruction in the larynx or trachea.

subconjunctival hemorrhage—Bright red blood appearing in a sector of the eye under the clear conjunctiva.

sulfonylureas—An oral antibiotic that increases insulin production in the pancreas.

suppurative—To form pus.

syncope—A brief lapse in consciousness caused by transient cerebral hypoxia (fainting).

syphilis—A sexually transmitted infection that has distinct stages that cover years; can affect almost any body organ.

T1—In the case of MRI scans, T1 is a technical term that allows certain structures to be lighter or darker on imaging. In terms of the vertebrae, T1 is the first thoracic vertebra.

T2—In the case of MRI scans, T2 provides more intensity (lightness) for fat, water, and fluid. In terms of the vertebrae, T2 is the second thoracic vertebra.

tachypnea—Rapid breathing; >24 breaths/min.

tactile fremitus—Palpable vibration generated from the larynx and transmitted through the bronchi and lungs to the chest wall.

tension pneumothorax—Air in the pleural space caused by a rupture through the chest wall.

tetraplegia—Impairment in motor or sensory function of all four extremities, usually caused by a lesion of the cervical spinal cord; also known as quadriplegia.

thalassemia—Production and hemolytic anemia characterized by microcytic, hypochromic red blood cells.

thoracentesis—Surgical procedure that perforates the chest wall or pleural space to aspirate fluid for diagnosis or treatment purposes.

thrombocytopenia—Any disorder of the blood coagulation mechanism caused by an abnormality or dysfunction of platelets.

thrombophlebitis—Inflammation of a vein accompanied by the formation of a clot.

thrush—White patches on the tongue caused by *Candida*; typically benign in children, but it can be caused by an immunodeficiency condition.

thyroid gland—A gland in the anterior throat that secretes hormones that regulate growth and metabolism.

tinea corporis—A superficial fungal infection of the non-hairy skin of the body, most prevalent in hot, humid climates and usually caused by species *Trichophyton* or *Microsporum*.

tinea versicolor—A fungal infection of the skin caused by *Malassezia furfur* and characterized by finely desquamating, pale tan patches on the upper trunk and upper arms that may itch and do not tan.

tinnitus—The sensation of ringing in the ears.

tonic–clonic seizure—Convulsive seizure that affects the entire brain.

torsades de pointes—An extremely rapid ventricular tachycardia determined by a changing QRS complex as seen on an electrocardiogram (ECG); may be self-limited or may progress to ventricular fibrillation.

traumatic iritis—Inflammation of the iris secondary to blunt trauma.

traumatic mydriasis—Condition in which one pupil is dilated; usually associated with traumatic iritis.

trephination—A technique where a burr hole is drilled into a hard surface such as a nail or a flat bone.

trichomoniasis—Infection of the vagina caused by *Trichomonas vaginalis*. Symptoms include itching, burning, frothy, light yellow discharge.

triphasic—Having three phases.

Turner's syndrome—An abnormality in females marked by the absence of one X chromosome.

tympanogram—A test providing graphic representation of the acoustic impedance and air pressure in the middle ear, as well as the mobility of the tympanic membrane.

ultrasound—Imaging technique projecting high-frequency sound waves into the body, producing a real-time image of internal structures from the reflective properties of sound waves.

urinalysis (UA)—A process of analyzing urine for certain attributes or components.

urticaria—A group of distinct skin conditions characterized by itchy, wheal-and-flare skin reactions, commonly known as hives.

uterine synechiae—Scars or adhesions on the uterus.

vector—An organism that carries and transmits a disease, usually from one species to another.

venous puncture—Poking a hole into a vein for the purpose of extracting blood, injecting a substance, or inserting an IV.

ventilation—In respiration, the process by which air moves through the respiratory tract.

ventilation–perfusion scan—A scan to determine if one or more areas of the lungs are getting air but not blood or blood but no air.

vesicular breath sounds—Normal sound of rustling or swishing that represents air moving into the smaller airways.

Wernicke's aphasia—A type of aphasia that involves impairment in the comprehension of written and spoken words.

Western blot—A blood test used to determine if specific antibodies are present.

wheezes—Adventitious breath sounds that represent airway obstruction by mucus, spasm, or even a foreign body.

whispered pectoriloquy—Whispered speech heard clearly through the stethoscope.

Wolff-Parkinson-White (WPW) syndrome—A disorder of atrioventricular conduction involving an accessory pathway. This syndrome is often identified by a characteristic delta wave seen on an ECG at the beginning of the QRS complex.

Wood's lamp—An illuminating device with a nickel oxide filter that holds back all light except for a few violet rays of the visible spectrum and ultraviolet wavelengths of about 365 nm.

X-ray—Electromagnetic radiation at a shorter wavelength than visible light, transmitted through the body to investigate the integrity of underlying structures, particularly bone.

Zung Self-Rating Depression Scale—A 20-item instrument for use with patients being evaluated for depression.

REFERENCES

Chapter 1

American Academy of Family Physicians, American Academy of Pediatrics, American College of Sports Medicine, American Orthopaedic Society for Sports Medicine, and American Osteopathic Academy of Sports Medicine. 2010. *Preparticipation Physical Evaluation*. 4th ed. Elk Grove Village, IL: American Academy of Pediatrics.

Beaschler, R. 2015. *Wrestling 2015–16 and 2016–17 Rules and Interpretations*. Edited by National Collegiate Athletic Association. Indianapolis, IN: National Collegiate Athletic Association.

Board of Certification. 2016. BOC Standards of Professional Practice. Last modified 2016. Accessed June 1, 2016. www.bocatc.org/resources/standards-of-professional-practice.

Centers for Medicare and Medicaid Services. 2015. ICD-10 basics. Accessed June 7, 2016. www.roadto10.org/icd-10-basics/.

Commission on Accreditation of Athletic Training Education. 2015. Standards for the accreditation of professional athletic training programs. Last modified December 4, 2015. http://caate.net/wp-content/uploads/2015/12/2012-Professional-Standards.pdf.

Fainaru-Wada, M. 2008. Autopsy reveals UCF's Plancher had gene trait tied to 10 similar deaths. In *College Football*. Available at www.ESPN.com.

Hetzner, A. 2009. Jury finds clinic not negligent in Arrowhead football injury. *Milwaukee Journal Sentinel*, September 22. Available at archive.jsonline.com/news/waukesha/6046992.html.

Kennedy v. Syracuse University. In No. 94-CV-269: U.S. Dist. 1995.

Kleinknecht v. Gettysburg College. In F. Supp. 2d: MD 1992.

Letchworth, B. 2009. Update: Schools respond to lawsuit. *The Daily Reflector*, December 4.

National Athletic Trainers' Association. 2013. NATA Code of Ethics. Last modified 2013. www.nata.org/membership/about-membership/member-resources/code-of-ethics.

National Federation of State High School Associations. 2015. General guidelines for sport hygiene, skin infections and communicable diseases. Last modified October 2015. www.nfhs.org/sports-resource-content/general-guidelines-for-sport-hygiene-skin-infections-and-communicable-disease/. Accessed March 27, 2016.

Parsons, J.T., ed. 2014. *2014–2015 NCAA Sports Medicine Handbook*. Indianapolis, IN: National Collegiate Athletic Association.

Price, J. 2005. O'Neal's family files lawsuit; death linked to meningitis. *Columbia Missourian*, August 24.

United States Department of Education. 2016. Family Educational Rights and Privacy Act. Accessed June 1, 2016. www2.ed.gov/policy/gen/guid/fpco/ferpa/index.htm.

United States Department of Health and Human Services. 2016. Health information privacy. Accessed June 1, 2016. www.hhs.gov/hipaa/.

United States Department of Labor. 2016a. Most frequently asked questions concerning the bloodborne pathogens standard. Accessed June 2, 2016. www.osha.gov/pls/oshaweb/owadisp.show_document?p_table=INTERPRETATIONS&p_id=21010&p_text_version=FALSE.

United States Department of Labor. 2016b. Occupational Safety & Health Administration. https://www.osha.gov.

United States Department of Labor. 2016c. Quick reference guide to bloodborne pathogen standard. Accessed June 2, 2016. www.osha.gov/SLTC/bloodbornepathogens/bloodborne_quickref.html.

United States Department of Labor. 2016d. Regulations standard 29 CFR, bloodborne pathogens. www.osha.gov/pls/oshaweb/owadisp.show_document?p_table=STANDARDS&p_id=10051.

United States Environmental Protection Agency. 2016. Selected EPA-registered disinfectants. Last modified March 14, 2016. Accessed June 2, 2016. www.epa.gov/pesticide-registration/selected-epa-registered-disinfectants.

Wong, G., and A. Apostolopoulou. 1999. Infection detection: HIV testing policies ought to be put in place before problems arise. *Athletic Business* 12:24–26.

Chapter 2

Armstrong, L, D.J. Casa, M. Millard-Stafford, D. Moran, S. Pyne, and W. Roberts. 2007. ACSM position stand: Exertional heat illness during training and competition. *Medicine and Science in Sports and Exercise* 39 (3): 556–72.

Ball, J., J. Dains, J. Flynn, B.S. Solomon, and R.W. Stewart. 2014. *Seidel's Guide to Physical Examination*. 8th ed. St. Louis: Mosby.

Bickley, L. 2012. *Bates' Guide to Physical Examination and History-Taking.* 11th ed. Philadelphia: Lippincott, Williams & Wilkins.

Binkley, H.M., J. Beckett, D.J. Casa, D.M. Kleiner, and P.E. Plummer. 2002. National Athletic Trainers' Association position statement: Exertional heat illnesses. *Journal of Athletic Training* 37 (3): 329–43.

Casa, D.J. 2011. *Preventing Sudden Death in Sport and Physical Activity.* Boston: Jones and Bartlett.

Casa, D.J., K.M. Guskiewicz, and S.L. Anderson. 2012. National Athletic Trainers' Association position statement: Preventing sudden death in sports. *Journal of Athletic Training* 47 (1): 96–118.

Ferri, F.F. 2016. *Ferri's Clinical Advisor 2016.* Philadelphia: Elsevier.

Jarvis, C. 2012. *Physical Examination & Health Assessment.* 6th ed. St. Louis: Elsevier/Saunders.

Longo, D., A. Fauci, D. Kasper, S. Hauser, J. Jameson, and J. Loscalzo. 2013. *Harrison's Manual of Medicine.* 18th ed. New York: McGraw-Hill.

Perry, A.G., P. Potter, and W.R. Ostendorf. 2014. *Clinical Nursing Skills & Techniques.* 8th ed. St. Louis: Mosby.

Potter, P., and A.G. Perry. 2011. *Basic Nursing: Essentials for Practice.* 7th ed. St. Louis: Mosby.

Rakel, R., and D. Rakel. 2011. *Textbook of Family Medicine.* Philadelphia: Elsevier/Saunders.

Spring, B. 2015. Exertional heat illness. In *Sports Medicine for the Emergency Physician*, edited by Ana Waterbrook, 390–407. Cambridge: Cambridge University Press.

Zimmerman, A.B., K.L. Lust, and M.A. Bullimore. 2011. Visual acuity and contrast sensitivity testing for sports vision. *Eye Contact Lens* 37 (3): 153–59.

Chapter 3

Akinpelu, D. 2015. Treadmill stress testing technique. *Medscape.* Last modified November 22, 2015. Accessed April 24, 2016. http://emedicine.medscape.com/article/1827089-technique.

emedicine. 2016. CT scan (CAT scan, computerized axial tomography). *emedicine health.* Accessed April 24, 2016. www.emedicinehealth.com/ct_scan/article_em.htm.

Johns Hopkins Medicine. 2016. Bone scan/Bone scintigraphy. www.hopkinsmedicine.org/healthlibrary/test_procedures/orthopaedic/bone_scan_92,p07663/.

Radiological Society of North America. 2015. Positron emission tomography. Last modified June 11, 2015. Accessed April 24, 2016. www.radiologyinfo.org/en/info.cfm?pg=pet.

Radiological Society of North America. 2016. Contrast materials. Last modified March 16, 2016. Accessed April 24, 2016. www.radiologyinfo.org/en/info.cfm?pg=safety-contrast.

WebMD. 2016. Magnetic resonance imaging (MRI). www.webmd.com/a-to-z-guides/magnetic-resonance-imaging-mri.

Chapter 4

Bavry, A.A., F. Thomas, M. Allison, K.C. Johnson, B.V. Howard, M. Hlatky, J.E. Manson, and M.C. Limacher. 2014. Nonsteroidal anti-inflammatory drugs and cardiovascular outcomes in women: Results from the Women's Health Initiative. *Circulation: Cardiovascular Quality and Outcomes* 7 (4): 603–10.

Brunton, L.L., B. Chabner, and B. Knollmann, eds. 2011. *Goodman & Gilman's The Pharmacological Basis of Therapeutics.* 12th ed. New York: McGraw-Hill.

Clinical Pharmacology Gold Standard. 2016. www.elsevier.com/solutions/drug-database. Elsevier, Inc.

Food and Drug Administration (FDA). 2016. Mission of the FDA. www.fda.org/AboutFDA/WhatWeDo/default.htm.

Hajart, A.F., F. Pecha, M. Hasty, S.M. Burfeind, and J. Greene. 2014. The financial impact of an athletic trainer working as a physician extender in orthopedic practice. *Journal of Medical Practice Management* 29 (4): 250–54.

Health Canada. 2016. Drugs and health products. Last modified January 18, 2016. Accessed April 8, 2016. http://hc-sc.gc.ca/dhp-mps/index-eng.php.

Kahanov, L., J. Roberts, and E.M. Wughalter. 2010. Adherence to drug-dispensation and drug-administration laws and guidelines in collegiate athletic training rooms: A 5-year review. *Journal of Athletic Training* 45 (3): 299–305.

Kanbayashi, Y., and H. Konishi. 2015. Predictive factors for NSAIDs-related gastrointestinal toxicity: Can COX-2 selective inhibitor prevent it? *Hepatogastroenterology* 62 (140): 787–89.

Lakshmanan, S., G.K. Gupta, P. Avci, R. Chandran, M. Sadasivam, A.E. Serafim Jorge, and M.R. Hamblin. 2014. Physical energy for drug delivery: Poration, concentration and activation. *Advanced Drug Delivery Reviews* 71:98–114.

Lexicomp Online. 2016. Clinical drug information facts & comparisons. http://online.lexi.com/lco.action/home. Wolters Kluwer.

Morgan, S., S. Pullon, and E. McKinlay. 2015. Observation of interprofessional collaborative practice in primary care teams: An integrative literature review. *International Journal of Nursing Studies* 52 (7): 1217–30.

National Collegiate Athletic Association (NCAA). 2015a. NCAA 2015–16 drug-testing exceptions procedures (medical exceptions). www.ncaa.org/health-and-safety/sport-science-institute/2015-16-drug-testing-exceptions-procedures-medical-exceptions.

National Collegiate Athletic Association (NCAA). 2015b. NCAA banned drugs 2015–2016. www.ncaa.org/2015-16-ncaa-band-drugs.

New, S.N., D. Cooley Huff, L.C. Hutchison, T.J. Bilbruck, P.S. Ragsdale, J.E. Jennings, and M. Greenfield. 2015. Integrating collaborative interprofessional simulation into pre-licensure health care programs. *Nursing Education Perspectives* 36 (6): 396–97.

Pedersen, C.A., P.J. Schneider, and D.J. Scheckelhoff. 2012. ASHP national survey of pharmacy practice in hospital settings: Dispensing and administration–2011. *American Journal of Health-System Pharmacy* 69 (9): 768–85.

Rao, R., S. Mahant, L. Chhabra, and S. Nanda. 2014. Transdermal innovations in diabetes management. *Current Diabetes Reviews* 10 (6): 343–59.

Raphael, A.P., O.R.L. Wright, H.A. Benson, and T.W. Prow. 2015. Recent advances in physical delivery enhancement of topical drugs. *Current Pharmaceutical Design* 21 (20): 2830–47.

Rigby, J.H., D.O. Draper, A.W. Johnson, J.W. Myrer, D.L. Eggett, and G.W. Mack. 2015. The time course of dexamethasone delivery using iontophoresis through human skin, measured via microdialysis. *Journal of Orthopedic and Sports Physical Therapy* 45 (3): 190–97.

Roustit, M., S. Blaise, and J.L. Cracowski. 2014. Trials and tribulations of skin iontophoresis in therapeutics. *British Journal of Clinical Pharmacology* 77 (1): 63–71.

United States Anti-Doping Agency. 2015. USADA anti-doping programs. www.usada.org/about/programs.

United States Anti-Doping Agency (USADA). 2016. Independence and history statement. www.usada.org/about/independence-history.

Warner, D.C., G. Schnepf, M.S. Barrett, D. Dian, and N.L. Swigonski. 2002. Prevalence, attitudes, and behaviors related to the use of nonsteroidal anti-inflammatory drugs (NSAIDs) in student athletes. *Journal of Adolescent Health* 30 (3): 150–53.

World Anti-Doping Agency (WADA). 2016. Prohibited list. http://list.wada-ama.org.

Chapter 5

Allen, D.B. 2002. Safety of inhaled corticosteroids in children. *Pediatric Pulmonology* 33 (3): 208–20.

American Hospital Formulary Service. 2016. *American Hospital Formulary Service Drug Information.* Bethesda, MD: American Society of Health-System Pharmacists.

Anderson, S.L., and J.M. Trujillo. 2010. Association of pancreatitis with glucagon-like peptide-1 agonist use. *Annals of Pharmacotherapy* 44 (5): 904–9.

ASHP. 2004. ASHP Therapeutic Position Statement on Strategies for Identifying and Preventing Pneumococcal Resistance. *American Journal of Health System Pharmacy* 61 (22).

Bavry, A.A., F. Thomas, M. Allison, K.C. Johnson, B.V. Howard, M. Hlatky, J.E. Manson, and M.C. Limacher. 2014. Nonsteroidal anti-inflammatory drugs and cardiovascular outcomes in women: Results from the women's health initiative. *Circulation* 7 (4): 603–10.

Bello, A.I, and S. Kwornu. 2014. 5% Ibuprofen iontophoresis compared with transcutaneous electrical nerve stimulation in the management of knee osteoarthritis: A feasibility study. *Open Journal of Therapy and Rehabilitation* 2 (04): 166.

Bhosale, U.A., N. Quraishi, R. Yegnanarayan, and D. Devasthale. 2015. A comparative study to evaluate the cardiovascular risk of selective and nonselective cyclooxygenase inhibitors (COX-Is) in arthritic patients. *Journal of Basic and Clinical Physiology and Pharmacology* 26 (1): 73–79.

Buell, J.., R. Franks, J. Ransone, M.E. Powers, K.M. Laquale, A. Carlson-Phillips, and Association of National Athletic Trainers. 2013. National Athletic Trainers' Association position statement: Evaluation of dietary supplements for performance nutrition. *Journal of Athletic Training* 48 (1):124–36.

Burns, R.D., M. Rosita Schiller, M.A. Merrick, and K.N. Wolf. 2004. Intercollegiate student athlete use of nutritional supplements and the role of athletic trainers and dietitians in nutrition counseling. *Journal of the American Dietetic Association* 104 (2): 246–49.

Cannon, C.P., and P.J. Cannon. 2012. Physiology. COX-2 inhibitors and cardiovascular risk. *Science* 336 (6087): 1386–7.

Clinical Pharmacology Gold Standard. 2016. www.elsevier.com/solutios/drug-database. Elsevier, Inc.

Decker, S.O., M. Wortmann, B.H. Siegler, A. Ulrich, S. Hofer, and T. Brenner. 2015. Metformin-induced lactic acidosis: Severe symptoms with difficult diagnostics. *Metformininduzierte Laktatacidose: Schweres Krankheitsbild mit schwieriger Diagnosestellung.* 64 (4): 292–97.

Dejgaard, T.F., C.S. Frandsen, J.J. Holst, and S. Madsbad. 2016. Liraglutide for treating type 1 diabetes. *Expert Opinions in Biologic Therapy* 16 (4): 579–90.

Díaz-González, F., and F. Sánchez-Madrid. 2015. NSAIDs: Learning new tricks from old drugs. *European Journal of Immunology* 45 (3): 679–86.

Dieu-Donne, O., O. Theodore, Z. Joelle, D. Pierre, O. Smaila, C. Christian, K. Fulgence, and D.Y. Joseph. 2016. An open randomized trial comparing the effects of oral NSAIDs steroid intra-articular infiltration in congestive osteoarthritis of the knee. *Open Rheumatology Journal* 10:8–12.

Estes, K.R. 2015. Skin infections in high school wrestlers: A nurse practitioner's guide to diagnosis, treatment, and return to participation. *Journal of the American Association of Nurse Practitioners* 27 (1): 4–10.

Ferri, F.F. 2016. *Ferri's Clinical Advisor 2016*. Philadelphia: Elsevier.

Hamilton, K., C. Davis, J. Falk, A. Singer, and S. Bugden. 2015. High risk use of OTC NSAIDs and ASA in family medicine: A retrospective chart review. *International Journal of Risk and Safety in Medicine* 27 (4):191–99.

Iannella, H., C. Luna, and G. Waterer. 2013. Inhaled corticosteroids and the increased risk of pneumonia: What's new? A 2015 updated review. *Therapeutic Advances in Respiratory Disease* Aug 7 (4): 225–34.

Kanbayashi, Y., and H. Konishi. 2015. Predictive factors for NSAIDs-related gastrointestinal toxicity: Can COX-2 selective inhibitor prevent it? *Hepatogastroenterology* 62 (140): 787–89.

Lando, H.M., M. Alattar, and A.P. Dua. 2012. Elevated amylase and lipase levels in patients using glucagonlike peptide-1 receptor agonists or dipeptidyl-peptidase-4 inhibitors in the outpatient setting. *Endocrine Practice: Official Journal of the American College of Endocrinology and the American Association of Clinical Endocrinologists* 18 (4):472–77.

Lewis, T., and J. Cook. 2014. Fluoroquinolones and tendinopathy: A guide for athletes and sports clinicians and a systematic review of the literature. *Journal of Athletic Training* 49 (3): 422–27.

Lexicomp Online. 2016. Clinical Drug Information Facts & Comparisons. http://online.lexi.com/lco.action/home. Wolters Kluwer.

Maffulli, N., F. Spiezia, U.G. Longo, V. Denaro, and G.D. Maffulli. 2013. High volume image guided injections for the management of chronic tendinopathy of the main body of the Achilles tendon. *Physical Therapy in Sport* 14 (3): 163–67.

Minze, M.G., M.S. Klein, M.J. Jernigan, S.L. Wise, and K. Fruge. 2013. Once-weekly exenatide: An extended-duration glucagon-like peptide agonist for the treatment of type 2 diabetes mellitus. *Pharmacotherapy* 33 (6): 627–38.

National Collegiate Athletic Association (NCAA). 2015. NCAA Banned Drugs 2015–2016. www.ncaa.org/health-and-safety/sport-science-institute/2015-16-drug-testing-exceptions-procedures-medical-exceptions.

Parsons, J.P. 2014. Exercise-induced bronchoconstriction. *Otolaryngology Clinics of North America* 47 (1): 119–26.

Pasquel, F.J., R. Klein, A. Adigweme, Z. Hinedi, R. Coralli, J.L. Pimentel, and G.E. Umpierrez. 2015. Metformin-associated lactic acidosis. *American Journal of the Medical Sciences* 349 (3): 263–67.

Pelletier, J.P., J. Martel-Pelletier, F. Rannou, and C. Cooper. 2016. Efficacy and safety of oral NSAIDs and analgesics in the management of osteoarthritis: Evidence from real-life setting trials and surveys. *Seminars in Arthritis and Rheumatism* 45 (4 Suppl): S22–27.

Reurink, G., G.J. Goudsuaard, M.H. Moen, A. Weir, J.A. Verhaar, and J.L. Tol. 2014. Myotoxicity of injections for acute muscle injuries: A systematic review. *Sports Medicine* 44 (7): 943–56.

Rigby, J.H., D.O. Draper, A.W. Johnson, J.W. Myrer, D.L. Eggett, and G.W. Mack. 2015. The time course of dexamethasone delivery using iontophoresis through human skin, measured via microdialysis. *Journal of Orthopedic and Sports Physical Therapy* 45 (3): 190–97.

Skoner, D.P. 2016. The tall and the short: Repainting the landscape about the growth effects of inhaled and intranasal corticosteroids. *Allergy & Asthma Proceedings* 37 (3): 180–91.

Soriano-Maldonado, A., L. Klokker, C. Bartholdy, E. Bandak, K. Ellegaard, H. Bliddal, and M. Henriksen. 2016. Intra-articular corticosteroids in addition to exercise for reducing pain sensitivity in knee osteoarthritis: Exploratory outcome from a randomized controlled trial. *PLoS One* 11 (2): e0149168.

Stevens, K.J., J.M. Crain, K.H. Akizuki, and C.F. Beaulieu. 2010. Imaging and ultrasound-guided steroid injection of internal oblique muscle strains in baseball pitchers. *American Journal of Sports Medicine* 38 (3): 581–85.

Svetaz, L.A., A. Postigo, E. Butassi, S.A. Zacchino, and M.A. Sortino. 2016. Antifungal drugs combinations: A patent review 2000–2015. *Expert Opinion on Therapeutic Patents* 26 (4): 439–43.

Trevor, A., B. Katzung, and M. Knuidering-Hall. 2015. *Katzung & Trevor's Pharmacology Examination and Board Review*. 11th ed. New York: McGraw-Hill Education/Medical.

Trinh, K.V., J. Kim, and A. Ritsma. 2015. Effect of pseudoephedrine in sport: A systematic review. *BMJ Open Sport & Exercise Medicine* 1 (1): e000066.

Tscholl, P.M., M. Vaso, A. Weber, and J. Dvorak. 2015. High prevalence of medication use in professional football tournaments including the World Cups between 2002 and 2014: A narrative review with a focus on NSAIDs. *British Journal of Sports Medicine* 49 (9): 580–82.

United States Anti-Doping Agency. 2015. USADA Anti-Doping Programs. www.usada.org/about/programs.

Ussai, S., L. Miceli, F.E. Pisa, R. Bednarova, A. Giordano, G. Della Rocca, and R. Petelin. 2015. Impact of potential inappropriate NSAIDs use in chronic pain. *Journal of Drug Design, Development and Therapy* 9:2073–77.

van Vollenhoven, R.F., M. Petri, D.J. Wallace, D. Roth, C.T. Molta, A.E. Hammer, Y. Tang, and A. Thompson. 2016. Cumulative corticosteroids over 52 weeks in patients with systemic lupus erythematosus: Pooled analyses from the phase III belimumab trials. *Arthritis & Rheumatology* 68 (9): 2184–92.

World Anti-Doping Agency (WADA). 2016. Prohibited list. http://list.wada-ama.org.

Chapter 6

Association of periOperative Registered Nurses. 2014. *Perioperative Standards and Recommended Practices*. Denver, CO: AORN.

Board of Certification. 2016. State regulatory map. Accessed April 14. www.bocatc.org/index.php/state-regulation.

Brolmann, F.W., D.T. Ubbink, E.A. Nelson, K. Munte, C.M. van der Horst, and H. Vermeulen. 2012. Evidence-based decisions for local and systemic wound care. *British Journal of Surgery* 99 (9): 1172–83.

Centers for Disease Control and Prevention. 2016. Infection control in healthcare settings. Accessed April15, 2016. www.cdc.gov/ncidod/dhqp/.

Grimaldi, L., R. Cuomo, C. Brandi, G. Botteri, G. Sisi, and C. D'Aniello. 2015. Octyl-2-cyanoacrylate adhesive for skin closure: Eight years' experience. *In Vivo* 29 (1): 145–48.

Levy, M.J., and Ne. Tang. 2014. Use of tissue adhesive as a field expedient barrier dressing for hand wounds in disaster responders. *Prehospital and Disaster Medicine* 29 (1): 1–3.

Longo, D., A. Fauci, D. Kasper, S. Hauser, J. Jameson, and J. Loscalzo. 2013. *Harrison's Manual of Medicine*. 18th ed. New York: McGraw- Hill.

Perry, A.G., P. Potter, and W.R. Ostendorf. 2014. *Clinical Nursing Skills & Techniques*. 8th ed. St. Louis: Mosby.

Phillips, N. 2013. *Berry and Kohn's Operating Room Technique*. 12th ed. St. Louis: Mosby.

Potter, P., and A.G. Perry. 2011. *Basic Nursing: Essentials for Practice*. 7th ed. St. Louis: Mosby.

Rothrock, J.C. 2016. *Alexander's Care of the Patient in Surgery*. 14th ed. St. Louis: Mosby.

Singer, A.J., L.C. Perry, and R.L. Allen, Jr. 2008. In vivo study of wound bursting strength and compliance of topical skin adhesives. *Academic Emergency Medicine* 15 (12): 1290–94.

Skelhorne, G., and H. Munro. 2002. Hydrogel adhesives for wound-care applications. *Medical Device Technologies* 13 (9): 19–23.

Smith, T.O., D. Sexton, C. Mann, and D. Simon. 2010. Sutures versus staples for skin closure in orthopaedic surgery: Meta-analysis. *British Journal of Sports Medicine* 340:1199.

Chapter 7

Albert, R. 2010. Diagnosis and treatment of acute bronchitis–P1345.pdf. *American Academy of Family Physicians* 82 (11): 1345–50.

Backer, V. 2010. Not all who wheeze have asthma. *Breathe* 7 (1): 16–22.

Ball, J., J. Dains, J. Flynn, B.S. Solomon, and R.W. Stewart. 2014. *Seidel's Guide to Physical Examination*. 8th ed. St. Louis: Mosby.

Barros, M., C. Prinzivalli, and A. Christi. 2016. Asthma, maintenance. In *The 5-Minute Clinical Consult Standard 2016*, edited by Frank Domino, A-17. Philadelphia: Wolters Kluwer.

Boulet, L.P. 2012. Cough and upper airway disorders in elite athletes: A critical review. *British Journal of Sports Medicine* 46 (6): 417–21.

Boulet, L.P., R. Hancox, and K. Fitch. 2010. Exercise and asthma: β_2-agonists and the competitive athlete. *Breathe* 7 (1): 65–71.

Braman, S. 2006. Cough due to acute bronchitis: ACCP evidence-based clinical practice guidelines. *Chest* 129 (1 suppl): 95S–103S.

Bussotti, M., S. Di Marco, and G. Marchese. 2014. Respiratory disorders in endurance athletes—how much do they really have to endure? *Open Access Journal of Sports Medicine* 5:47–63.

Cabry, R., S. Ballyamanda, M. Kraft, and E. Hong. 2013. Understanding paraneoplastic syndromes in athletes. *Current Sports Medicine Report* 12 (1): 33–40.

Carey, D.G., K. Aase, and G. Pliego. 2010. The acute effect of cold air exercise in determination of exercise-induced bronchospasm in apparently healthy athletes. *Journal of Strength and Conditioning Research* 24 (8): 2172–78.

Carver, T. 2009. Exercise-induced asthma: Critical analysis of the protective role of montelukast. *Journal of Asthma and Allergy* 2:93–103.

Coitinho, C., G. Greif, C. Robello, P. Laserra, E. Willery, and P. Supply. 2014. Rapidly progressing tuberculosis outbreak in a very low risk group. [In Eng]. *European Respiratory Journal* 43 (3): 903–6.

Centers for Disease Control and Prevention. 2015. Key facts about seasonal flu vaccine. www.cdc.gov/flu/protect/keyfacts.htm.

Domino, F., R.A. Baldor, J. Golding, and M.B. Stephens. 2016. *The 5-Minute Clinical Consult Standard 2016*. Philadelphia: Lippincott, Williams and Wilkins.

Feden, J.P. 2013. Closed lung trauma. *Clinics in Sports Medicine* 32 (2): 255–65.

Gonzales, R., J. Bartlett, R. Besser, R. Cooper, J. Hickner, J. Hoffman, and M. Sande. 2001. Principles of appropriate antibiotic use for treatment for uncomplicated acute bronchitis: Background. *Annals of Internal Medicine* 134 (6): 479–86.

Havers, F., B. Flannery, J. Clippard, M. Gaglani, R. Zimmerman, L. Jackson, J. Petrie, et al. 2015. Use of influenza antiviral medications among outpatients at high risk for influenza-associated complications during the 2013–2014 influenza season. *Clinical Infectious Disease* 60 (11): 1677–80.

Hayden, M.L., S. Stoloff, G. Colice, N. Ostrom, M. Eid, and J. Parsons. 2011. Exercise-induced bronchospasm: A case study in a nonasthmatic patient. *Journal of the American Academy of Nurse Practitioners* 24:19–23.

Holland, A., C. Hill, A. Jones, and C. McDonald. 2012. Breathing exercises for chronic obstructive pulmonary diseases. *Cochrane Database of Systematic Reviews* 10, no. CD008250.

Hull, J., L. Ansley, P. Robson-Ansley, and J. Parsons. 2012. Managing respiratory problems in athletes. *Clinical Medicine* 12 (4): 351–56.

Intravia, J.M., and T.M. DeBeradino. 2013. Evaluation of blunt abdominal trauma. *Clinics in Sports Medicine* 32 (2): 211–18.

Jarvis, C. 2012. *Physical Examination & Health Assessment*. 6th ed. St. Louis: Elsevier/Saunders.

Johnson-Warrington, V., S. Harrison, K. Mitchell, M. Steiner, M. Morgan, and S. Singh. 2014. Exercise capacity and physical activity in patients with COPD and healthy subjects classified as Medical Research Council dyspnea scale grade 2. *Journal of Cardiopulmonary Rehabilitation and Prevention* 34 (2): 150–54.

Klign, P., A. Van Keimpema, M. Legemaat, R. Gosselink, and H. Van Stel. 2012. Prescribing exercise in advanced COPD: Training smart, not just hard! *European Respiratory Journal* 40 (Suppl 56): 1900.

Korownyk, C., S. Garrison, and M. Kolber. 2015. Antiviral medications for influenza. *Canadian Family Physician* 61 (4): 351.

Krafczyk, M.A., and C.A. Asplund. 2011. Exercise-induced bronchoconstriction: Diagnosis and management. *American Family Physician* 84 (4): 427–34.

Light, R. 2015. Pneumothorax. In *Merck Manual of Diagnosis and Therapy*, edited by R.S. Porter Kenilworth, NJ: Merck.

Little, P., K. Rumsby, J. Kelly, L. Watson, M. Moore, and G. Warner. 2005. Information leaflet and antibiotic prescribing strategies for acute lower respiratory tract infection: A randomized controlled trial. *Journal American Medical Association* 293 (24): 3029–35.

Mensinger, J. 2013. Pneumothorax in a recreational athlete. *International Journal of Athletic Therapy and Training* 27:27–31.

Millward, D., S. Paul, M. Brown, D. Porter, M. Stilson, R. Cohen, E. Olvey, and J. Hagan. 2009. The diagnosis of asthma and exercise-induced bronchospasm in Division I athletes. *Clinical Journal of Sports Medicine* 19 (6): 482–86.

Morris, K. 2010. Management of exercise-induced bronchospasm in adolescents with asthma. *Nurse Practitioner* 35 (12): 18–26.

Nielsen, E., J. Hull, and V. Back. 2013. High prevalence of exercise-induced laryngeal obstruction in athletes. *Medicine and Science in Sports and Exercise* 45 (11): 2030–35.

Ostrom, N., N. Eid, T. Craig, G. Colice, M.L. Hayden, J. Parsons, and S. Stoloff. 2011. Exercise-induced bronchospasm in children with asthma in the United States: Results from the Exercise-Induced Bronchospasm Landmark Survey. *Allergy and Asthma Procedures* 32 (6): 425–30.

Parsons, J. 2010. Current concepts in the diagnosis and management of exercise-induced bronchospasm. *Physician and Sportsmedicine* 38 (4): 48–53.

Parsons, J., D. Cosmar, G. Phillips, C. Kaeding, T. Best, and J. Mastronarde. 2012. Screening for exercise-induced bronchoconstriction in college athletes. *Journal of Asthma* 49 (2): 153–7.

Parsons, J., T. Craig, S. Stoloff, M.L. Hayden, N. Ostrom, N. Eid, and G. Colice. 2011. Impact of exercise-related respiratory symptoms in adults with asthma: Exercise-Induced Bronchospasm Landmark National Survey. *Allergy and Asthma Proceedings* 32 (6): 431–37.

Simpson, A., L. Romer, and P. Kippelen. 2015. Self-reported symptoms after induced and inhibited bronchoconstriction in athletes. *Medicine and Science in Sports and Exercise* 47 (10): 2005–13.

Smoote, M.K., and R.G. Hosey. 2015. Pulmonary infections in the athlete: Current sports medicine reports. *Current Sports Medicine Reports* 8 (2): 71–75.

Sormunen, J., H.M. Bäckmand, S. Sarna, U.M. Kujala, J. Kaprio, T. Dyba, and E. Pukkala. 2014. Lifetime physical activity and cancer incidence—A cohort study of male former elite athletes in Finland. *Journal of Science and Medicine in Sport* 17 (5): 479–84.

Spielmanns, M., C. Fuchs-Bergsma, A. Winkler, G. Fox, S. Kuruger, and K. Baum. 2015. Effects of oxygen supply during training on subjects with COPD who are normoxemic at rest and during exercise: A blinded randomized controlled trial. *Respiratory Care* 60 (4): 540–8.

Stack, M.A., and A. Hakemi. 2011. Diagnosis and treatment of exercise-induced bronchospasm: A review. *Journal of the American Academy of Physician Assistants* 24 (6): 26–30.

Tierney, D., and E.A. Nardell. 2011. Tuberculosis (Tb). In *Merck Manual of Diagnosis and Therapy*, edited by R.S. Porter, 3754. Kenilworth, NJ: Merck.

Uramoto, H., H. Shimokawa, and F. Tanaka. 2012. What factors predict recurrence of a spontaneous pneumothorax? *Journal of Cardiothoracic Surgery* 7:112.

Viets, R. 2015. The evolving influenza test: New options for the management of RIDT. *Medical Laboratory Observer* 47 (9): 30–32.

Chapter 8

American Heart Association. 2013. Facts: every second counts. Accessed October 24, 2013. www.heart.org/idc/groups/heart-public/@wcm/@adv/documents/downloadable/ucm_301646.pdf.

American Heart Association. 2014a. American Heart Association backs current BP treatments. Accessed October 25, 2014. www.heart.org/HEARTORG/Conditions/HighBloodPressure/PreventionTreatmentofHighBloodPressure/American-Heart-Association-backs-current-BP-treatments_UCM_459129_Article.jsp - .Vi1hOOlX_dk.

American Heart Association. 2014b. Peripheral artery disease (PAD). American Heart Association Accessed October 29, 2014. www.heart.org/HEARTORG/Conditions/More/PeripheralArteryDisease/About-Peripheral-Artery-Disease-PAD_UCM_301301_Article.jsp - .VjKGd-lX_dl.

Anderson, S.A., and E.R. Eichner. 2007. Consensus statement: Sickle cell trait and the athlete. In *National Athletic Trainers' Association Consensus Statements*. Available at www.nata.org/sites/default/files/sickle-cell-trait-and-the-athlete.pdf.

Asplund, C.A., and I.M. Asif. 2014. Cardiovascular participation screening practices of college team physicians. *Clinics in Sports Medicine* 24 (4): 275–79.

Ball, J.W., J.E. Dains, J.A. Flynn, B.S. Solomon, and R.W. Stewart. 2015. *Seidel's Guide to Physical Examination*. 8th ed. St. Louis: Elsevier/Mosby.

Betriu, A., J. Tabau, G. Sanz, J. Magrina, and F. Navarro-Lopez. 1980. Relief of angina by periarterial muscle resection of myocardial bridges. *American Heart Journal* 100 (2): 223–26.

Bonow, R.O., M.D. Cheitlin, M.H. Crawford, and P.S. Douglas. 2005. Task force 3: Valvular heart disease. *Journal of the American College of Cardiology* 45 (8): 1334–40.

Booher, M., and B. Smith. 2003. Physiological effects of exercise on the cardiopulmonary system. *Clinics in Sports Medicine* 22 (Jan): 1–22.

Borjesson, M., and A. Pelliccia. 2009. Incidence and aetiology of sudden cardiac death in young athletes: An international perspective. *British Journal of Sports Medicine* 43 (9): 644–48.

Casa, D.J., K.M. Guskiewicz, S.A. Anderson, R. Courson, J.F. Heck, C.C. Jimenez, B.P. McDermott, M.G. Miller, R.L. Stearns, E.E. Swartz, and K.M. Walsh. 2012. National Athletic Trainers' Association position statement: Preventing sudden death in sports. *Journal of Athletic Training* 47 (1): 96–118.

Chappex, N., J. Schlaepfer, F. Fellmann, Z.A. Bhuiyan, M. Wilhelm, and K. Michaud. 2015. Sudden cardiac death among general population and sport related population in forensic experience. *Journal of Forensic and Legal Medicine* 35:62–68.

Charlton, G.A., and M.H. Crawford. 1997. Physiological consequences of training. *Cardiology Clinics* 15 (3): 345–54.

Coleman, J.J., B.L. Zarzaur, C.W. Katona, Z.J. Plummer, L.S. Johnson, A. Fecher, J.M. O'Rear, D.V. Feliciano, and G.S. Rozycki. 2015. Factors associated with pulmonary embolism within 72 hours of admission after trauma: A multicenter study. *Journal of the American College of Surgeons* 220 (4): 731–36.

Delis, K.T., N. Hunt, R.K. Strachan, and A.N. Nicolaides. 2001. Incidence, natural history and risk factors of deep vein thrombosis in elective knee arthroscopy. *Thrombosis and Haemostasis* 86 (3): 817–21.

Drezner, J.A., R. Courson, W.O. Roberts, V.N. Mosesso, M.S. Link, and B.J. Maron. 2007. Inter-association task force recommendations on emergency preparedness and management of sudden cardiac arrest in high school and college athletic programs: A consensus statement. *Journal of Athletic Training* 42 (1): 143–58.

Eichner, E.R. 2010. Iron deficiency anemia. *Current Sports Medicine Reports* 9 (3): 122–23.

Eichner, E.R. 2011. Anemia and blood boosting. Gatorade Sports Science Institute. Accessed October 29, 2011.

www.gssiweb.org/Article/sse-81-anemia-and-blood-boosting.

el Habbal, M.H. 1992. Cardiovascular manifestations of Marfan's syndrome in the young. *American Heart Journal* 123 (3): 752–57.

Gerry, J.L., Jr., L. Morris, and R.E. Pyeritz. 1991. Clinical management of the cardiovascular complications of the Marfan syndrome. *Journal of the Louisiana State Medical Society* 143 (3): 43–51.

Giese, E.A., F.G. O'Connor, F.H. Brennan, P.J. Depenbrock, and R.G. Oriscello. 2007. The athletic preparticipation evaluation: Cardiovascular assessment. *American Family Physician* 75 (7): 1008–14.

Graham, T.P., Jr., D.J. Driscoll, W.M. Gersony, J.W. New-burger, A. Rocchini, and J.A. Towbin. 2005. Task force 2: Congenital heart disease. *Journal of the American College of Cardiology* 45 (8): 1326–33.

Harmon, K.G., D. Klossner, and J.A. Drezner. 2011. Incidence of sudden cardiac death in NCAA athletes. *Circulation* 123 (15): 1594–1600.

Harper, J.L. 2014. Iron deficiency anemia. *Medscape*. Accessed October 29, 2014. http://emedicine.medscape.com/article/202333-overview.

Harris, K.M., M. Tung, T.S. Haas, and B.J. Maron. 2015. Under-recognition of aortic and aortic valve disease and the risk for sudden death in competitive athletes. *Journal of the American College of Cardiology* 65 (8): 860–62.

Hurley, W.L., S.A. Comins, R.M. Green, and J. Canizzaro. 2006. Atraumatic subclavian vein thrombosis in a collegiate baseball player: A case report. *Journal of Athletic Training* 41 (2): 198–200.

Huston, T.P., J.C. Puffer, and W.M. Rodney. 1985. The athletic heart syndrome. *New England Journal of Medicine* 313 (1): 24–32.

Inna, P. 2014. Marfan syndrome. *Medscape*. Accessed October 25, 2014. http://emedicine.medscape.com/article/1258926-overview - a8.

Johnson, J.N., and M.J. Ackerman. 2013. Return to play? Athletes with congenital long QT syndrome. *British Journal of Sports Medicine* 47 (1): 28–33.

Kucera, K.L., D. Klossner, B. Colgate, and R.C. Cantu. 2015. *Annual Survey of Football Injury Research*. Edited by National Center for Catastrophic Sport Injury Research. Chapel Hill, NC: University of North Carolina at Chapel Hill.

MacKnight, J.M. 2003. Exercise considerations in hypertension, obesity, and dyslipidemia. *Clinics in Sports Medicine* 22 (1): 101–21, vii.

The Marfan Foundation. 2015. What is Marfan syndrome? Accessed October 25, 2015. www.marfan.org/about/marfan.

Marijon, E., A. Uy-Evanado, K. Reinier, C. Teodorescu, K. Narayanan, X. Jouven, K. Gunson, J. Jui, and S. Chugh. 2015. Sudden cardiac arrest during sports activity in middle age. *Circulation* 131 (16): 1384–91.

Maron, B.J., M.J. Ackerman, R.A. Nishimura, and R.E. Pyeritz. 2005. Task force 4: HCM and other cardiomyopathies, mitral valve prolapse, myocarditis and Marfan syndrome. *Journal of the American College of Cardiology* 45 (8): 1340–45.

Maron, B.J., R.O. Bonow, R.O. Cannon, M.B. Leon, and S.E. Epstein. 1987. Hypertrophic cardiomyopathy. Implications of clinical manifestations, pathophysiology and therapy. *New England Journal of Medicine* 316 (13): 780–89.

Maron, B.J., J.J. Doerer, T.S. Haas, N.A. Estes, and M.S. Link. 2006. Historical observation on commotio cordis. *Heart Rhythm* 3 (5): 605–6.

Maron, B.J., P.S. Douglas, T.P. Graham, R.A. Nishimura, and P.D. Thompson. 2005. Task force 1: Preparticipation screening and diagnosis of cardiovascular disease in athletes. *Journal of the American College of Cardiology* 45 (8): 1322–26.

Maron, B.J., and N.A. Estes. 2005. Task force 11: Commotio cordis. *Journal of the American College of Cardiology* 45 (8): 1371–73.

Maron, B.J., T.S. Haas, A. Ahluwalia, R.F. Garberich, and N.A. Estes. 2013. Increasing survival rates from commotio cordis. *Heart Rhythm* 10 (2): 219–23.

Maron, B.J., T.S. Haas, C.J. Murphy, A. Ahluwalia, and S. Rutten-Ramos. 2014. Incidence and causes of sudden death in U.S. college athletes. *Journal of the American College of Cardiology* 63 (16): 1636–43.

Maron, B.J., A. Pelliccia, A. Spataro, and M. Granata. 1993. Reduction in the left ventricle wall thickness after deconditioning in highly trained Olympic athletes. *Heart* 69 (2): 125–28.

Maron, B.J., J. Shirani, and L. Poliac. 1996. Sudden death in young competitive athletes. Clinical, demographic, and pathological profiles. *Journal of the American Medical Association* 276 (3): 199–204.

Maron, M.S. 2015a. Family history of sudden death should be a primary indication for implantable cardioverter defibrillator in hypertrophic cardiomyopathy. *Canadian Journal of Cardiology* 31 (11): 1402–6.

Maron, M.S. 2015b. The role of cardiovascular magnetic resonance in sudden death risk stratification in hypertrophic cardiomyopathy. *Cardiac Electrophysiology Clinics* 7 (2): 187–93.

Marsalese, D.L., D.S. Moodie, M. Vacante, B.W. Lytle, C.C. Gill, R. Sterba, D.M. Cosgrove, M. Passalacqua, M. Goormastic, and A. Kovacs. 1989. Marfan's syndrome: Natural history and long-term follow-up of cardiovascular involvement. *Journal of the American College of Cardiology* 14 (2): 422–28; discussion 429–31.

Maumenee, I.H. 1981. The eye in the Marfan syndrome. *Transactions of the American Ophthalmological Society* 79:684–733.

Mitchell, J.H., W. Haskell, P. Snell, and S.P. Van Camp. 2005. Task force 8: Classification of sports. *Journal of the American College of Cardiology* 45 (8): 1364–67.

Moss, A.J., and J. Robinson. 1992. Clinical features of the idiopathic long QT syndrome. *Circulation* 85 (1 Suppl): I140–44.

Musante, R., V. Cupelli, F. Mori, and D.A. Attina. 1987. Ergometric evaluation of physical fitness of athletes affected by mitral valve prolapse: Study of 80 cases. *European Heart Journal* 8 Suppl D: 33–35.

Nagashima, J., H. Musha, H. Takada, and M. Murayama. 2003. New upper limit of physiologic cardiac hypertrophy in Japanese participants in the 100-km ultramarathon. *Journal of the American College of Cardiology* 42:1617–23.

Narayanan, K., A. Uy-Evanado, C. Teodorescu, K. Reinier, G.A. Nichols, K. Gunson, J. Jui, and S.S. Chugh. 2015. Mitral valve prolapse and sudden cardiac arrest in the community. *Heart Rhythm* 13 (2): 498–503.

National Institutes of Health. 2011. Pulmonary embolism. Last modified 2011. Accessed October 29, 2011. www.nhlbi.nih.gov/health/health-topics/topics/pe.

O'Toole, M.T., ed. 2013. *Mosby's Dictionary of Medicine, Nursing & Health Professionals*. 9th ed. St Louis: Elsevier/Mosby.

Parsons, J.T., ed. 2014. *2014–2015 NCAA Sports Medicine Handbook*. Indianapolis: National Collegiate Athletic Association.

Pelliccia, A., B.J. Maron, A. Spataro, M.A. Proschan, and P. Spirito. 1991. The upper limit of physiologic cardiac hypertrophy in highly trained elite athletes. *New England Journal of Medicine* 324 (5): 295–301.

Pelliccia, A., D.P. Zipes, and B.J. Maron. 2008. Bethesda Conference # 36 and the European Society of Cardiology consensus recommendations revisited: A comparison of U.S. and European criteria for eligibility and disqualification of competitive athletes with cardiovascular abnormalities. *Journal of the American College of Cardiology* 52 (24): 1990–96.

Pescatello, L., and J. Kulikowich. 2001. The aftereffects of dynamic exercise on ambulatory blood pressure. *Medicine and Science and Sports Exercise* 33 (11): 1855–61.

Ponamgi, S.P., C.V. DeSimone, and M.J. Ackerman. 2015. Athletes with implantable cardioverter defibrillators. *Clinics in Sports Medicine* 34 (3): 473–87.

Pugh, A., J.P. Bourke, and V. Kunadian. 2012. Sudden cardiac death among competitive adult athletes: A review. *Postgraduate Medical Journal* 88 (1041): 382–90.

Pyeritz, R.E., and V. McKusick. 1976. The Marfan syndrome: Diagnosis and management. *New England Journal of Medicine* 300 (14): 772–76.

Rosendorff, C., D.T. Lackland, M. Allison, W.S. Aronow, H.R. Black, R.S. Blumenthal, C.P. Cannon, et al. 2015. Treatment of hypertension in patients with coronary artery disease: A scientific statement from the American Heart Association, American College of Cardiology, and American Society of Hypertension. *Journal of the American College of Cardiology* 65 (18): 1998–2038

Schreiber, D. 2015. Anticoagulation in deep vein thrombosis. *Medscape*. http://emedicine.medscape.com/article/1926110-overview - a1. Accessed October 29, 2015.

Semsarian, C., J. Sweeting, and M.J. Ackerman. 2015. Sudden cardiac death in athletes. *BMJ* 350:h1218.

Singh, B., S.A. al Shahwan, M.A. Habbab, S.M. al Deeb, and N. Biary. 1993. Idiopathic long QT syndrome: Asking the right question. *Lancet* 341 (8847): 741–42.

Smith, B., and M. Ciocca. 2002. The athletic heart syndrome. In *Principles and Practice of Primary Care Sports Medicine*, edited by W.J. Garrett, D. Kirkendall and D. Squire, 251–59. Philadelphia: Lippincott, Williams & Wilkins.

Solberg, E.E., M. Borjesson, S. Sharma, M. Papadakis, M. Wilhelm, J.A. Drezner, K.G. Harmon, et al. 2015. Sudden cardiac arrest in sports—need for uniform registration: A position paper from the Sport Cardiology Section of the European Association for Cardiovascular Prevention and Rehabilitation. *European Journal of Preventive Cardiology*.

Tamariz, L.J., J. Eng, J.B. Segal, J.A. Krishnan, D.T. Bolger, M.B. Streiff, M.W. Jenckes, and E.B. Bass. 2014. Usefulness of clinical prediction rules for the diagnosis of venous thromboembolism: A systematic review. *American Journal of Medicine* 117 (9): 676-684.

Tang, W.H.W. 2014. Myocarditis. *Medscape*. Accessed October 25, 2014. http://emedicine.medscape.com/article/156330-overview.

Thiene, G., A. Nava, D. Corrado, L. Rossi, and N. Pennelli. 1988. Right ventricular cardiomyopathy and sudden death in young people. *New England Journal of Medicine* 318 (3): 129–33.

Thompson, P.D., G.J. Balady, B.R. Chaitman, L.T. Clark, B.D. Levine, and R.J. Myerburg. 2005. Task force 6: Coronary artery disease. *Journal of the American College of Cardiology* 45 (8): 1348–53.

Toukola, T., E. Hookana, J. Junttila, K. Kaikkonen, J. Tikkanen, J. Perkiomaki, M.L. Kortelainen, and H.V. Huikuri.

2015. Sudden cardiac death during physical exercise: Characteristics of victims and autopsy findings. *Annals of Medicine* 47 (3): 263–68.

Vaidya, A., M.A. Joore, A.J. ten Cante-Hoek, H. ten Cate, and J.L. Severens. 2014. Screen or not to screen for peripheral arterial disease: Guidance from a decision model. *BMC Public Health* 14 (89).

Vettor, G., A. Zorzi, C. Basso, G. Thiene, and D. Corrado. 2015. Syncope as a warning symptom of sudden cardiac death in athletes. *Cardiology Clinics* 33 (3): 423–32.

Vouhe, P. 2015. Anomalous aortic origin of coronary arteries: A frequent and curable cause of sudden death. Bulletin de l'Académie nationale de médecine 198 (3): 465–70; discussion 470–71.

Wells, P.S., D.R. Anderson, J. Bormanis, F. Guy, M. Mitchell, L. Gray, C. Clement, K.S. Robinson, and B. Lewandowski. 1997. Value of assessment of pretest probability of deep-vein thrombosis in clinical management. *Lancet* 350 (9094): 1795–98.

Yasue, H., H. Nakagawa, T. Itoh, E. Harada, and Y. Mizuno. 2008. Coronary artery spasm—clinical features, diagnosis, pathogenesis, and treatment. *Journal of Cardiology* 51 (1): 2–17.

Zipes, D.P., M.J. Ackerman, N.A. Estes, 3rd, A.O. Grant, R.J. Myerburg, and G. Van Hare. 2005. Task force 7: Arrhythmias. *Journal of the American College of Cardiology* 45 (8): 1354–63.

Chapter 9

American Cancer Society. 2014. *Colorectal Cancer Facts & Figures 2014–16*. Atlanta: American Cancer Society.

Anderson, W.D., S.M. Strayer, and S.R. Mull. 2015. Common questions about the management of gastroesophageal reflux disease—American Family Physician. *American Family Physician* 91 (10): 692–97.

Ball, J., J. Dains, J. Flynn, B.S. Solomon, and R.W. Stewart. 2014. *Seidel's Guide to Physical Examination*. 8th ed. St. Louis: Mosby.

Barr, W., and A. Smith. 2015. Acute diarrhea in adults—American Family Physician. *American Family Physician* 89 (3): 180–89.

Bickley, L. 2012. *Bates' Guide to Physical Examination and History-Taking*. 11th ed. Philadelphia: Lippincott Williams & Wilkins.

Brandt, L., W. Chey, A. Foxx-Orenstein, M.Q. Eammon, and L. Schiller. 2009. An evidence-based position statement on the management of irritable bowel syndrome. *American Journal of Gastroenterology* 104 (Suppl 1): S1–S35.

Byrne, G., and C.F. Feighery. 2015. Celiac disease: Diagnosis. *Methods in Molecular Biology* 1326:15–22.

Cars, T., B. Wettermark, R. Lofberg, I. Eriksson, J. Sundstrom, and M. Lordal. 2016. Healthcare utilization and drug treatment in a large cohort of patients with inflammatory bowel disease. *Journal of Crohn's and Colitis* 10 (5): 556–65.

Carter, D., A. Lang, and R. Eliakim. 2013. Endoscopy in inflammatory bowel disease. *Minerva Gastroenterologica e Dietologica* 59 (3): 273–84.

DeFilippis, E.M., and L.M. Callahan. 2013. Atypical presentation of appendicitis in an adolescent cheerleader. *Clinical Journal of Sports Medicine* 23 (6): 494–95.

deOliveria, E.P., R. Burini, and A. Jeukendrup. 2014. Gastrointestinal complaints during exercise: Prevalence, etiology, and nutritional recommendations. *Sports Medicine* 44 (Suppl 1): 79–85.

Domino, F., R.A. Baldor, J. Golding, and M.B. Stephens. 2016. *The 5-Minute Clinical Consult Standard 2016*. Philadelphia: Lippincott Williams & Wilkins.

Ferri, F.F. 2016. *Ferri's Clinical Advisor 2016*. Philadelphia: Elsevier.

Gannon, E.H., and T. Howard. 2010. Splenic injuries in athletes: A review. *Current Sports Medicine Reports* 9 (2): 111–14.

Ha, F., and H. Khalil. 2015. Crohn's disease: A clinical update. *Therapeutic Advances in Gastroenterology* 8 (6): 352–59.

Jensen, L.F., L. Hvidberg, A.F. Pedersen, and P. Vedsted. 2015. Symptom attributions in patients with colorectal cancer. *BMC Family Practice* 16:115.

Juckett, G., and R. Tirivedi. 2011. Evaluation of chronic diarrhea. *American Family Physician* 15 (84): 1119–26.

Kuster, M., B. Renner, P. Oppel, U. Niederweis, and K. Brune. 2013. Consumption of analgesics before a marathon and the incidence of cardiovascular, gastrointestinal and renal problems: A cohort study. *BMJ Open* 3 (4).

Leggit, J.C. 2011. Evaluation and treatment of GERD and upper GI complaints in athletes. *Current Sports Medicine Reports* 10 (2): 109–14.

Lis, D.M., T. Stellingwerff, C.M. Shing, K.D.K. Ahuja, and J.W. Fell. 2015. Exploring the popularity, experiences, and beliefs surrounding gluten-free diets in nonceliac athletes. *International Journal of Sport Nutrition and Exercise Metabolism* 25 (1): 37–45.

Mancini, L., T. Trojian, and A. Mancini. 2011. Celiac disease and the athlete. *Current Sports Medicine Reports* 10 (2): 105–8.

Moghadamyeghaneh, Z., R.F. Alizadeh, M. Phelan, J.C. Carmichael, S. Mills, A. Pigazzi, J.A. Zell, and M.J. Stamos. 2015. Trends in colorectal cancer admissions and stage at presentation: Impact of screening. *Surgical Endoscopy* 30 (8): 3604–10.

Morton, D., and R. Callister. 2015. Exercise-related transient abdominal pain (ETAP). *Sports Medicine* 45 (1): 23–35.

Pelkowski, T.D., and A.J. Viera. 2014. Celiac disease: Diagnosis and management. *American Family Physician* 89 (2): 99–105.

Sapone, A., J.C. Bai, C. Ciacci, J. Dolinsek, P.H. Green, M. Hadjivassiliou, K. Kaukinen, K. Rostami, D.S. Sanders, and M. Schumann. 2012. Spectrum of gluten-related disorders: Consensus on new nomenclature and classification. *BMC Medicine* 10 (1): 13.

ter Steege, R.W., R.H. Geelkerken, A.B. Huisman, and J.J. Kolkman. 2012. Abdominal symptoms during physical exercise and the role of gastrointestinal ischaemia: A study in 12 symptomatic athletes. *British Journal of Sports Medicine* 46 (13): 931–35.

Trivedi, I., and L. Keefer. 2015. The emerging adult with inflammatory bowel disease: Challenges and recommendations for the adult gastroenterologist. *Gastroenterology Research and Practice* 2015 (2015): Article ID 260807.

Viola, T.A. 2010. Evaluation of the athlete with exertional abdominal pain. *Current Sports Medicine Reports* 9 (2): 106–10.

Vivas, S., L. Vaquero, L. Rodriguez-Martin, and A. Caminero. 2015. Age-related differences in celiac disease: Specific characteristics of adult presentation. *World Journal of Gastrointestinal Pharmacology and Therapeutics* 6 (4): 207–12.

Volta, U., G. Caio, F. Giancola, K.J. Rhoden, E. Ruggeri, E. Boschetti, V. Stanghellini, and R. De Giorgio. 2015. Features and progression of potential celiac disease in adults. *Clinical Gastroenterology and Hepatology* 14 (5): 686–93.

Waterman, J.J., and R. Kapur. 2012. Upper gastrointestinal issues in athletes. *Current Sports Medicine Reports* 11 (2): 99–104.

Wilkins, T., C. Pepitone, B. Alex, and R. Schade. 2012. Diagnosis and management of IBS in adults. *American Family Physician* 86 (5): 419–26.

Chapter 10

Adami, H.O. 2010. The prostate cancer pseudo-epidemic. *Acta Oncology* 49 (3): 298–304.

American Cancer Society. 2015. Breast cancer. Last modified January 4, 2016. Accessed January 9, 2016. www.cancer.org/cancer/breastcancer/index.

American Cancer Society. 2016. Cervical cancer. Last modified January 4 2016. Accessed January 7, 2016. www.cancer.org/cancer/cervicalcancer/index.

American Congress of Obstetricians and Gynecologists. 2011a. Ectopic pregnancy. Last modified August 2011. Accessed January 7, 2016. www.acog.org/Patients/FAQs/Ectopic-Pregnancy.

American Congress of Obstetricians and Gynecologists. 2011b. Exercise during pregnancy. Last modified August 2011. Accessed January 7, 2016. www.acog.org/Patients/FAQs/Exercise-During-Pregnancy.

American Congress of Obstetricians and Gynecologists. 2015a. HIV. Accessed January 7, 2016. www.acog.org/About-ACOG/ACOG-Departments/HIV.

American Congress of Obstetricians and Gynecologists. 2015b. Testing for human immunodeficiency virus. Last modified August 2015. Accessed January 7, 2016. www.acog.org/Patients/FAQs/Testing-for-Human-Immunodeficiency-Virus.

Apostolopoulos, N.V., K.I. Alexandraki, A. Gorry, and A. Coker. 2015. Association between chronic pelvic pain symptoms and the presence of endometriosis. *Archives of Gynecology and Obstetrics* 293 (2): 439–45.

Arends, M., A. Wyllie, and C. Bird. 1990. Papillomaviruses and human cancer. *Human Pathology* 21 (7): 686–98.

Baldisserotto, M. 2009. Scrotal emergencies. *Pediatric Radiology Journal* 39 (5): 516–21.

Barkin, J., M.T. Rosenberg, and M. Miner. 2014. A guide to the management of urologic dilemmas for the primary care physician (PCP). *Canadian Journal of Urology* 21 (3): 55–63.

Bennett, J.N. 2015. HIV disease. *Medscape*. Last modified December 15, 2015. Accessed January 8, 2016. http://emedicine.medscape.com/article/211316-overview.

Bernard, J.J. 2009. Renal trauma: Evaluation, management, and return to play. *Current Sports Medicine Reports* 8 (2): 98–103.

Bonci, C.M., L.J. Bonci, L.R. Granger, C.L. Johnson, R.M. Malina, L.W. Milne, R.R. Ryan, and E.M. Vanderbunt. 2008. National Athletic Trainers' Association position statement: Preventing, detecting, and managing disordered eating in athletes. *Journal of Athletic Training* 43 (1): 80–108.

Borrero, E., and L.A. Queral. 1988. A symptomatic abdominal aortic aneurysm misdiagnosed as nephroureterolithiasis. *Annuals of Vascular Surgery* 2 (2): 145–49.

Carter, J.S. 2015. Cervical cancer guidelines. *Medscape*. Last modified May 4, 2015. Accessed January 7. http://emedicine.medscape.com/article/2500003-overview.

Centers for Disease Control and Prevention. 2015a. Breast cancer. Last modified August 20, 2015. Accessed January 7, 2016. www.cdc.gov/cancer/breast/statistics/.

Centers for Disease Control and Prevention. 2015b. Chlamydial infections. Last modified June 4, 2015. Accessed January 8, 2016. www.cdc.gov/std/tg2015/chlamydia.htm.

Centers for Disease Control and Prevention. 2015c. Gonorrhea statistics. Last modified November 17, 2015. Accessed January 6, 2016. www.cdc.gov/std/gonorrhea/stats.htm.

Centers for Disease Control and Prevention. 2015d. HIV/AIDS statistics center. Last modified July 23, 2015. Accessed January 7, 2016. www.cdc.gov/hiv/statistics/.

Centers for Disease Control and Prevention. 2015e. Pelvic inflammatory disease. Last modified June 4, 2015. Accessed January 6, 2016. www.cdc.gov/std/tg2015/pid.htm.

Centers for Disease Control and Prevention. 2015f. Syphilis. Last modified November 12, 2015. Accessed January 8, 2016. www.cdc.gov/std/syphilis/stdfact-syphilis.htm.

Centers for Disease Control and Prevention. 2016. Prostate cancer. Last modified January 4, 2016. Accessed January 4, 2016. www.cdc.gov/cancer/prostate/.

Chandrasekar, P. 2015. Syphilis. *Medscape*. Last modified October 22, 2015. Accessed January 8, 2016. http://emedicine.medscape.com/article/229461-clinical.

Cheungpasitporn, W., S. Rossetti, K. Friend, S.B. Erickson, and J.C. Lieske. 2015. Treatment effect, adherence, and safety of high fluid intake for the prevention of incident and recurrent kidney stones: A systematic review and meta-analysis. *Journal of Nephrology* 29 (2): 211–19.

Daley, E.M., C.A. Vamos, E.R. Buhi, S.K. Kolar, R.J. McDermott, N. Hernandez, and H.J. Fuhrmann. 2010. Influences on human papillomavirus vaccination status among female college students. *Journal of Women's Health (Larchmt)* 19 (10): 1885–91.

Denham, J.W., R. Bender, and W.E. Paradics. 2010. It's time to depolarise the unhelpful PSA-testing debate and put into practice lessons from two major international screening studies. *Medical Journal of Australia* 192 (11): 655.

Duarte, R., D. Fuhrich, and J.D. Ross. 2015. A review of antibiotic therapy for pelvic inflammatory disease. *International Journal of Antimicrobial Agents* 46 (3): 272–77.

Favus, M. 2015. Kidney stone emergencies. In *PubMed*, edited by L.J. DeGoot, P. Beck-Peccoz, G Chrousos, A. Grossman, J.M. Hershman, C. Kochm, R. Rebar, F. Singer, A. Vinik, and M.O. Weickert. National Institute of Health.

Ferri, F.F. 2016. *Ferri's Clinical Advisor*. Philadelphia: Elsevier.

Fink, H.A., T.H. Wilt, K.E. Eidman, P.S. Garimella, R. MacDonald, O.R. Rutks, M. Brasure, R.L. Kane, J. Ouellette, and M. Monga. 2013. Medical management to prevent recurrent nephrolithiasis in adults: A systematic review for the American College of Physicians Clinical Guideline. *Annals of Internal Medicine* 158 (7): 535–43.

Fiore, D.C, and C.L. Cox. 2015. Urology and nephrology update: Recurrent urinary tract infection. *Family Practice Essentials* Jan (416): 30–37.

Gamboa, S., S. Gaskie, M. Atlas, and R. VanZant. 2008. Clinical inquiries. What's the best way to manage athletes with amenorrhea? *Journal of Family Practice* 57 (11): 749–50.

Gearhart, P.A. 2015. Human papillomavirus. *Medscape*. Last modified May 26, 2015. Accessed January 8, 2016. http://emedicine.medscape.com/article/219110-overview.

Gomes, D.O., R.R Vidal, B.F. Foeppel, D.F. Faria, and M Saito. 2015. Cold weather is a predisposing factor for testicular torsion in a tropical country. A retrospective study. *Sao Paulo Medical Journal* 133 (3): 187–90.

Grandi, G., A. Xholli, S. Ferrari, M. Cannoletta, A. Volpe, and A. Cagnacci. 2013. Intermenstrual pelvic pain, quality of life and mood. *Gynecologic and Obstetric Investigation* 75 (2): 97–100.

Greene, M.H., C.P. Kratz, and P.L. Mai. 2010. Familial testicular germ cell tumors in adults: 2010 summary of genetic risk factors and clinical phenotype. *Endocrine-Related Cancers* 17 (2): R109–21.

Heidenreich, A., P.J. Bastina, J. Bellmunt, M. Bolla, S. Joniau, T. van der Kwast, M. Mason, V. Matveev, T. Wiegel, F. Zattoni, and N. Mottet. 2014. EAU guidelines on prostate cancer. Part I: Screening, diagnosis, and local treatment with curative intent—update 2013. *European Urology* 65: 124–37.

Hilibrand, M.J., S. Hammoud, M. Bishop, D. Woods, R.W. Fredrick, and C.C. Dodson. 2015. Common injuries and ailments of the female athlete; pathophysiology, treatment and prevention. *Physician and Sportsmedicine* 43 (4): 403–11.

Iacovides, S., I. Avidon, and F.C. Baker. 2015. What we know about primary dysmenorrhea today: A critical review. *Human Reproduction Update* 21 (6): 762–78.

Karakan, T., M. Bagcioglu, S. Ozcan, O. Telli, H. Turgut, M. Ozkan, and C. Germiyanoglu. 2015. Seasonal preponderance in testicular torsion: Is it a myth? *Archivos Espanoles de Urologia* 68 (10): 750–54.

Kaunitz, A.M. 1999. Oral contraceptive health benefits: Perception versus reality. *Contraception* 59 (1 Suppl): 29S–33S.

Liang, T., P. Metcalfe, W. Sevcik, and M. Noga. 2013. Retrospective review of diagnosis and treatment in children presenting to the pediatric department with acute scrotum. *American Journal of Roentgenology* 200:W444–49.

Lu, Q., G. Zhang, H. Lian, S. Zhang, X. Li, W. Gan, and H. Guc. 2015. Clinical analysis of 49 cases with testicular torsion. *Zhonghua Wai Ke Zhi* 53 (8): 599–602.

Marjoribanks, J., R.O. Ayeleke, C. Farquhar, and M. Proctor. 2015. Nonsteroidal anti-inflammatory drugs for dysmenorrhoea. *Cochrane Database Systematic Reviews* 7:CD001751.

May, L.E., J. Knowlton, J. Hanson, R. Suminski, C. Paynter, and X. Fang. 2015. Effects of exercise during pregnancy on maternal heart rate and heart rate variability. *Physical Medicine Rehabilitation* 8 (7): 611–7.

May, L.E., S.A. Scholtz, R. Suminski, and K.M. Gustafson. 2014. Aerobic exercise during pregnancy influences infant heart rate variability at one month of age. *Early Human Development* 90:33–38.

Mayo Clinic. 2016. Cervical cancer. Accessed January 7, 2016. www.mayoclinic.org/diseases-conditions/cervical-cancer/basics/definition/con-20030522.

Medina-Bombado, D., and A. Jover-Palmer. 2011. Does clinical examination aid in the diagnosis of urinary tract infections in women? A systematic review and meta-analysis. *BMC Family Practice* 12:111–24.

Mohsin, R., and K.M. Siddiqui. 2010. Recurrent urinary tract infections in females. *Journal of Pakistan Medical Association* 60 (1): 55–59.

Mountjoy, M., J. Sundgot-Borgen, L. Burke, S. Carter, N. Constantini, C. Lebrun, N. Meyer, R. Sherman, K. Steffen, R. Budgett, and A. Ljungqvist. 2014. The IOC consensus statement: Beyond the female athlete triad—relative energy deficiency in sport (RED-S). *British Journal of Sports Medicine* 48 (7): 491–97.

National Cancer Institute. 2015. SEER data fact sheets: Testis cancer. National Institutes of Health. Accessed January 3, 2016. http://seer.cancer.gov/statfacts/html/testis.html.

Nuno, V.L., M. Gonzalez, S.M. Loredo, B.M. Nigon, and F. Garcia. 2016. A cross-sectional study of human papillomavirus vaccine utilization among university women: The role of ethnicity, race, and risk factors. *Journal of Lower Genital Tract Disease* 20 (2): 131–4.

O'Toole, M.T., ed. 2013. *Mosby's Dictionary of Medicine, Nursing & Health Professionals*. 9th ed. St Louis: Elsevier/Mosby.

Onoyama, S., L. Qui, H.P. Low, C. Chang, W.C. Strohsnitter, E.R. Norwitz, M. Lopresti, K. Edminston, I. Lee, D. Trichopoulos, P. Lagiou, and C. Hsieh. 2016. Prenatal maternal physical activity and stem cells in umbilical cord blood. *Medicine and Science in Sports and Exercise* 48 (1): 82–89.

Parsons, J.T., ed. 2014. *2014–2015 NCAA Sports Medicine Handbook*. Indianapolis: National Collegiate Athletic Association.

Perales, M., A. Santos-Lozano, F. Sanchis-Gomar, M. Luaces, H. Pareja-Galeano, N. Garatachea, R. Lucia, and A. Barakat, 2015. Maternal cardiac adaptations to a physical exercise program during pregnancy. *Medicine and Science and Sports Exercise* 48 (5): 896–906.

Porter, R.S., and J.L. Kaplan, eds. 2011. *The Merck Manual*. 19th ed. Whitehouse Station, NJ: Merck Sharp & Dohme Corporation.

Qaseem, A., P. Dallas, M.A. Fociea, M. Starkey, and T Denbery. 2014. Dietary and pharmacologic management to prevent recurrent nephrolithiasis in adults: A clinical practice guideline from the American College of Physicians. *Annuals of Internal Medicine* 161 (9): 659–68.

Qureshi, S. 2015. Chlamydial genitourinary infections. *Medscape*. Last modified June 28, 2015. Accessed January 8, 2016. http://emedicine.medscape.com/article/214823-overview.

Rauh, M.J., J.F. Nichols, and M.T. Barrack. 2010. Relationship among injury and disordered eating, menstrual dysfunction, and low bone mineral density in high school athletes: A prospective study. *Journal of Athletic Training* 45 (3): 243–52.

Roque, R., and S.C. Esteves. 2016. A systematic review of clinical practice guidelines and the best practice statements for the diagnosis and management of varicocele in children and adolescents. *Asian Journal of Andrology* 18:1–7.

Rupp, T.J. 2015. Testicular torsion in emergency medicine. *Medscape*. Last modified August 12, 2015. Accessed January 3, 2016. http://emedicine.medscape.com/article/778086-overview.

Saab, M.M., M. Landers, and J. Hegarty. 2016. Testicular cancer awareness and screening practices: A systematic review. *Oncology Nursing Forum* 43 (1): E8–23.

Salvaggio, M. 2015. Herpes simplex. *Medscape*. Last modified September 18, 2015. Accessed February 13, 2016. http://emedicine.medscape.com/article/218580-overview - a6.

Samra-Latif, O.M. 2015. Contraception. *Medscape*. Last modified April 11, 2015. Accessed January 23, 2016. http://emedicine.medscape.com/article/258507-overview.

Shephard, R.J. 2015. Exercise proteinuria and haematuria: Current knowledge and future directions. *Journal of Sports Medicine and Physical Fitness* 55 (4): 267–72.

Tajchner, L., J.O. Larkin, and M.G. Bourke. 2009. Management of the acute scrotum in a district hospital: 10-year experience. *Scientific World Journal* 9:281–86.

Torrone, E., J. Papp, and H. Weinstock. 2014. Prevalence of *Chlamydia trachomatis* genital infection among persons ages 14–39 years—United States, 2002–2012. *Morbidity and Mortality Weekly Report* 63:834–38.

Travis, L.B., C. Bears, J.M. Allan, A.A. Dahl, D.R. Feldman, J. Oldenburg, G. Daugaard, et al. 2014. Testicular cancer survivorship: Research strategies and recommendations. *Journal of the National Cancer Institute* 012 (15): 1114–30.

Varma, P.P., P. Sengupta, and R.K. Nair. 2014. Post exertional hematuria. *Renal Failure* 36 (5): 701–3.

White, W.M. 2015. Varicocele. *Medscape*. Last modified December 3, 2015. Accessed January 3, 2016. http://emedicine.medscape.com/article/438591-overview.

Wong, B. 2015. Gonorrhea. *Medscape*. Last modified June 26, 2015. Accessed January 8, 2016. http://emedicine.medscape.com/article/218059-overview.

Workowski, K.A. 2015. 2015 sexually transmitted diseases treatment guidelines. Centers for Disease Control and Prevention. Last modified June 4, 2015. Accessed January 2, 2016. www.cdc.gov/std/tg2015/urethritis-and-cervicitis.htm.

Yusuf, G.T., and P.S. Sidhu. 2013. A review of ultrasound imaging in scrotal emergencies. *Journal of Ultrasound* 16:171–78.

Zannoli, L., M. Giorgi, E. Spagnolo, G. Montanari, G. Villa, and R. Seracchioli. 2014. Dysmenorrhea absenteeism from school, and symptoms suspicious for endometriosis in adolescents. *Journal of Pediatric & Adolescent Gynecology* 27 (5): 258–65.

Chapter 11

American Heart Association. 2015. Heart disease, stroke and research statistics at a glance. Last modified December 16, 2015. Accessed January 9, 2016. www.heart.org/idc/groups/ahamah-public/@wcm/@sop/@smd/documents/downloadable/ucm_480086.pdf.

Andary, M.T. 2015. Guillain-Barre syndrome. *Medscape*. Last modified July 1, 2015. Accessed January 9, 2016. http://emedicine.medscape.com/article/315632-overview.

Armon, C. 2015. Amyotrophic lateral sclerosis. *Medscape*. Last modified December 30, 2015. Accessed January 10, 2016. http://emedicine.medscape.com/article/1170097-overview.

Barr, W.B. 2001. Methodologic issues in neuropsychological testing. *Journal of Athletic Training* 36 (3): 297–302.

Barr, W.B., and M. McCrea. 2001. Sensitivity and specificity of standardized neurocognitive testing immediately following sports concussion. *Journal of the International Neuropsychological Society* 7:693–702.

Baugh, C.M., E. Kroshus, A.P. Bourlas, and K.I. Perry. 2014. Requiring athletes to acknowledge receipt of concussion-related information and responsibility to report symptoms: A study of the prevalence, variation, and possible improvements. *Journal of Law, Medicine & Ethics* 42 (3): 297–313.

Belanger, H.G., and R.D. Vanderploeg. 2005. The neuropsychological impact of sports-related concussion: A meta-analysis. *Journal of the International Neuropsychological Society* 11:345–57.

Belbasis, L., V. Bellou, and E. Evangelou. 2016. Environmental risk factors and amyotrophic lateral sclerosis: An umbrella review and critical assessment from current evidence from systematic reviews and meta-analyses of observational studies. *Neuroepidemiology* 6 (46): 96–105.

Benson, B.W., G.M. Hamilton, W.H. Meeuwisse, P. McCrory, and J. Dvorak. 2009. Is protective equipment useful in preventing concussion? A systematic review of the literature. *British Journal of Sports Medicine* 43 (Suppl 1): i56–67.

Benson, B.W., A.S. McIntosh, D. Maddocks, S.A. Herring, M. Raftery, and J. Dvorak. 2013. What are the most effective risk-reduction strategies in sport concussion? *British Journal of Sports Medicine* 47 (5): 321–26.

Blake, R.B. 2010. Complex regional pain syndrome (reflex sympathetic dystrophy). American Academy of Orthopedic Surgeons. Last modified June 2010. Accessed January 10, 2016. http://orthoinfo.aaos.org/topic.cfm?topic=a00021.

Bompadre, V., T.M. Jinguji, N.D. Yanez, E.K. Satchell, K. Gilbert, M. Burton, E.U. Conrad, 3rd, and S.A. Herring. 2014. Washington State's Lystedt law in concussion documentation in Seattle public high schools. *Journal of Athletic Training* 49 (4): 486–92.

Boyajian-O'Neill, L., D.O. Cardone, W. Dexter, J. DiFiori, K.B. Fields, D. Jones, R. Pallay, E. Small, F. Reed, W.O. Roberts, R. Wroble, and P. Zinni. 2004. Determining clearance during the preparticipation evaluation. *The Physician and Sportsmedicine* 32 (11): 29–41.

Broglio, S.P., R.C. Cantu, G.A. Gioia, K.M. Guskiewicz, J. Kutcher, M. Palm, T.C. Valovich McLeod, and Association of National Athletic Trainers. 2014. National Athletic Trainers' Association position statement: Management of sport concussion. *Journal of Athletic Training* 49 (2): 245–65.

Broglio, S.P., and T.W. Puetz. 2008. The effect of sport concussion on neurocognitive function, self-report symptoms and postural control: A meta-analysis. *Sports Medicine* 38 (1): 53–67.

Broglio, S.P., S.N. Macciocchi, M.S. Ferrara, 2007. Sensitivity of the Concussion Assessment Battery. *Neurosurgery* 60:1050–58.

Buki, B., M. Eckner, H. Junger, and Y.W. Lundberg. 2013. Vitamin D deficiency and benign paroxysmal position vertigo. *Medical Hypotheses* 80 (2): 105–214.

Casa, D.J., J. Almquist, S.A. Anderson, L. Baker, M.F. Bergeron, B. Biagioli, B. Boden, et al. 2013. The inter-association task force for preventing sudden death in secondary school athletics programs: Best-practices recommendations. *Journal of Athletic Training* 48 (4): 546–53.

Centers for Disease Control and Prevention. 2015a. Epilepsy. Last modified August 10, 2015. Accessed January 9, 2016. www.cdc.gov/epilepsy/basics/fast-facts.htm.

Centers for Disease Control and Prevention. 2015b. Guillain-Barre syndrome and flu vaccine. Last modified October 16, 2015. Accessed January 9, 2016. www.cdc.gov/flu/protect/vaccine/guillainbarre.htm.

Centers for Disease Control and Prevention. 2015c. Prevalence of amyotrophic lateral sclerosis in the United States, 2010–2011. www.cdc.gov/mmwr/pdf/ss/ss6307.pdf.

Chrisman, S.P., M.A. Schiff, S.K. Chung, S.A. Herring, and F.P. Rivara. 2014. Implementation of concussion legislation and extent of concussion education for athletes, parents, and coaches in Washington State. *American Journal of Sports Medicine* 42 (5): 1190–96.

Comer, R. 2015. Bear River girls basketball coach suffers stroke at 27. *Standard Examiner*. www.standard.net/High-School/2015/09/30/Bear-River-girls-basketball-coach-suffers-stroke-at-27.

DeMatteo, C., K. Stazyk, L. Giglia, W. Mahoney, S.K. Singh, R. Hollenberg, J.A. Harper, C. Missiuna, M. Law, D. McCauley, and S. Randall. 2015. A balanced protocol for return to school for children and youth following concussive injury. *Clinical Pediatrics* 54 (8): 783–92.

Dorksen, A. 2015. Ohio HS football player hospitalized after stroke. *Athletic Business*. Last modified October 1, 2015. Accessed January 9, 2016. www.athleticbusiness.com/high-school/ohio-hs-football-player-hospitalized-after-stroke.html.

Eisen, A., and C. Krieger. 2013. Ethical considerations in the management of amyotrophic lateral sclerosis. *Progress in Neurobiology* 110:45–53.

Epilepsy Foundation. 2015. Commercial truck driver. Accessed January 9. www.epilepsy.com/get-help/managing-your-epilepsy/independent-living/employment/safety-sensitive-jobs/commercial-truck.

Ferri, F.F. 2016. *Ferri's Clinical Advisor*. Philadelphia: Elsevier.

Galetta, K.M., L.E. Brandes, K. Maki, M.S. Dziemianowicz, E. Laudano, M. Allen, K. Lawler, B. Sennett, D. Wiebe, S. Devick, L.V. Messner, S.L. Galetta, and L.J. Balcer. 2011. The King-Devick test and sports-related concussion: Study of a rapid visual screening tool in a collegiate cohort. *Journal of the Neurological Sciences* 309 (1–2): 34–39.

Galetta, K.M., J. Morganroth, N. Moehringer, B. Mueller, L. Hasanaj, N. Webb, C. Civitano, D. A. Cardone, A. Silverio, S.L. Galetta, and L.J. Balcer. 2015. Adding vision to concussion testing: A prospective study of sideline testing in youth and collegiate athletes. *Journal of Neuroophthalmology* 35 (3): 235–41.

Gessel, L.M., S.K. Fields, C.L. Collins, R.W. Dick, and R.D. Comstock. 2007. Concussions among United States high school and collegiate athletes. *Journal of Athletic Training* 42 (4): 495–503.

Gibson, T.B., S.A. Herring, J.S. Kutcher, and S.P. Broglio. 2015. Analyzing the effect of state legislation on health care utilization for children with concussion. *Journal of the American Medical Association Pediatrics* 169 (2): 163–68.

Gioia, G.A. 2015. Multimodal evaluation and management of children with concussion: Using our heads and available evidence. *Brain Injury* 29 (2): 195–206.

Gioia, G.A., J.C. Schneider, C.G. Vaughan, and P.K. Isquith. 2009. Which symptom assessments and approaches are uniquely appropriate for paediatric concussion? *British Journal of Sports Medicine* 43 (Suppl 1): i13–22.

Giza, C.C., J.S. Kutcher, S. Ashwal, J. Barth, T.S. Getchius, G.A. Gioia, G.S. Gronseth, et al. 2013. Summary of evidence-based guideline update: Evaluation and management of concussion in sports: Report of the Guideline Development Subcommittee of the American Academy of Neurology. *Neurology* 80 (24): 2250–7.

Gompf, S.G. 2015. Rabies. *Medscape*. Last modified October 8, 2015. Accessed January 10, 2016. http://emedicine.medscape.com/article/220967-overview.

Grindel, S.H., M.R. Lovell, and M.W. Collins. 2001. The assessment of sport-related concussion: The evidence behind neuropsychological testing and management. *Clinical Journal of Sports Medicine* 11:134–43.

Guo, P., and J. Li. 2015. Short and long term effect of quick repositioning maneuver for patients with benign positional vertigo induced in the straight head hanging test. *Zhonghua Wai Ke Zhi* 7 (95):1986-1989.

Guskiewicz, K.M., J. Register-Mihalik, P. McCrory, M. McCrea, K. Johnston, M. Makdissi, J. Dvorak, G. Davis, and W. Meeuwisse. 2013. Evidence-based approach to revising the SCAT2: Introducing the SCAT3. *British Journal of Sports Medicine* 47 (5): 289–93.

Guskiewicz, K.M. 2001. Postural stability assessment following concussion: One piece of the puzzle. *Clinical Journal of Sports Medicine* 11:182–89.

Halstead, M.E., K. McAvoy, C.D. Devore, R. Carl, M. Lee, and K. Logan. 2013. Returning to learning following a concussion. *Pediatrics* 132 (5): 948–57.

Harden, R.N., S. Bruehl, B.S. Galer, S. Slatz, M. Bertram, M. Backonja, R. Gayles, N. Rudin, M.K. Bhugra, and M. Stanton-Hicks. 1999. Complex regional pain syndrome: Are the IASP diagnostic criteria valid and sufficiently comprehensive? *Pain* 83 (2): 211–19.

Harden, R.N., S. Bruehl, M. Stanton-Hicks, and P.R. Wilson. 2007. Proposed new diagnostic criteria for complex regional pain syndrome *Pain Medicine* 8 (4): 326–31.

Harmon, K.G., J. Drezner, M. Gammons, K. Guskiewicz, M. Halstead, S. Herring, J. Kutcher, A. Pana, M. Putukian, and W. Roberts. 2013. American Medical Society for Sports Medicine position statement: Concussion in sport. *Clinical Journal of Sport Med* 23 (1): 1–18.

Harvey, H.H. 2013. Reducing traumatic brain injuries in youth sports: Youth sports traumatic brain injury state laws, January 2009–December 2012. *American Journal of Public Health* 103 (7): 1249–54.

Horer, R.D., K.A. Kamins, J.R. Feussner, S.C. Grambow, J. Hoff-Lindquist, Y. Harati, H. Mitsumoto, et al. 2003. Occurrence of amyotrophic lateral sclerosis among Gulf War veterans. *Neurology* 23 (61): 742–49.

Ilieva, H., M. Polmenidou, and D.W. Cleveland. 2009. Non-cell autonomous toxicity in neurodegenerative disorders: ALS and beyond. *Journal of Cellular Biology* 187 (6): 761–72.

Janes, S.D. 2013. Pediatric stroke often misdiagnosed, treatment delayed. *ABC News.* February 11, 2013. http://abcnews.go.com/Health/pediatric-stroke-misdiagnosed-treatment-delayed/story?id=18444256.

Jauch, E.C. 2015. Acute management of stroke. *Medscape.* Last modified October 14, 2015 Accessed January 9, 2016. http://emedicine.medscape.com/article/1159752-overview.

Karsarskis, E.J., J.H. Lindquist, C.J Coffman, S.C. Grambow, J.R. Feussner, E.Z. Oddone, K.A. Kamins, and R.D. Horner. 2009. Clinical aspects of ALS in Gulf War veterans. *Amyotrophic Lateral Sclerosis* 10 (1): 35–41.

Kinart, C., M. Cuppett, and K. Berg. 2002. National Collegiate Athletic Association: Prevalence of migraines in NCAA Division I male and female basketball athletes. *Headache* 42 (7): 620–29.

Ko, D.Y. 2015. Epilepsy and seizures. *Medscape.* Last modified November 19, 2015. Accessed January 9, 2014. http://emedicine.medscape.com/article/1184846-overview.

Kontos A.P., R.J. Elbin, P. Schatz, T. Covassin, L. Henry, J. Pardini, and M.W. Collins. 2012. A revised factor structure for the post-concussion symptom scale: Baseline and post-concussion factors. *American Journal of Sports Medicine* 40 (10): 2375–84.

Kramer, S.F., L. Johnson, J. Bernhard, and T. Cumming. 2015. Energy expenditure and cost during walking after stroke: A systematic review. *Archives in Physical Medicine and Rehabilitation* 97 (4): 619–32.

Langlois, J.A., W. Rutland-Brown, and M.M. Wald. 2006. The epidemiology and impact of traumatic brain injury: A brief overview. *Journal of Head Trauma Rehabilitation* 21 (5): 375–78.

Leray, E., T. Moreau, A. Fromont, and G. Edan. 2015. Epidemiology of multiple sclerosis. *Revue Neurologique* Dec 21.

Lewis, D.W. 2002. Headaches in children and adolescents. *American Family Physician* 65 (4): 635–36.

Li, J.C. 2015. Benign paroxysmal positional vertigo. *Medscape.* Last modified June 29, 2015. Accessed January 10, 2016. http://emedicine.medscape.com/article/884261-overview.

Luzzio, C. 2015. Multiple sclerosis. *Medscape.* Last modified October 14, 2015. Accessed January 10, 2016. http://emedicine.medscape.com/article/1146199-overview.

Mackenzie, B., P. Vivier, S. Reinert, J. Machan, C. Kelley, and E. Jacobs. 2015. Impact of a state concussion law on pediatric emergency department visits. *Pediatric Emergency Care* 31 (1): 25–30.

Maddocks, D.L., G.D. Dicker, and M.M. Saling. 1995. The assessment of orientation following concussion in athletes. *Clinical Journal of Sports Medicine* 5:32–35.

Makdissi, M., G. Davis, B. Jordan, J. Patricios, L. Purcell, and M. Putukian. 2013. Revisiting the modifiers: How should the evaluation and management of acute concussions differ in specific groups? *British Journal of Sports Medicine* 47 (5): 314–20.

McCrea, M., W. Barr, K.M. Guskiewicz, C. Randolph, S. Marshall, R. Cantu, and J. Onate. 2005. Standard regression-based methods for measuring recovery after sport-related concussion. *Journal of the International Neuropsychological Society* 11:58–69.

McCrea, M. 2001. Standardized mental status testing on the sideline after sport-related concussion. *Journal of Athletic Training* 36 (3): 274–79.

McCrea, M., K.M. Guskiewicz, S.W. Marshall, W.B. Barr, C. Randolph, R.C. Cantu, J.A. Onate, J. Yang, and J.P. Kelly. 2003. Acute effects and recovery time following concussion in collegiate football players: The NCAA Concussion Study. *Journal of the American Medical Association* 290 (19): 2556–63.

McCrea, M., J.P. Kelly, and C. Randolph. 2000. *The Standardized Assessment of Concussion: Manual for Administration, Scoring, and Interpretation.* 2nd ed. Waukesha, WI: CNS Inc.

McCrea, M., J.P. Kelly, C. Randolph, R. Cisler, and L. Berger. 2002. Immediate neurocognitive effects of concussion. *Neurosurgery* 50 (5): 1032–42.

McCrory, P., W. Meeuwisse, M. Aubry, B. Cantu, J. Dvorak, R.J. Echemendia, L. Engebretsen, K. Johnston, J.S. Kutcher, M. Raftery, and A. Sills. 2013. Consensus statement on concussion in sport—The 4th International Conference on Concussion in Sport held in Zurich, November 2012. *Clinical Journal of Sport Medicine* 23 (2): 89–117.

McCrory, P., W. H. Meeuwisse, M. Aubry, R. C. Cantu, J. Dvorak, M. Ruben, J. S. Kutcher, et al. 2013. Consensus statement on concussion in Sport: The 4th International Conference on Concussion in Sport, Zurich, November 2012. *Journal of Athletic Training* 48 (4): 554–75.

Mucha, A., M.W. Collins, R.J. Elbin, J.M. Furman, C. Troutman-Enseki, R.M. DeWolf, G. Marchetti, and A.P. Kontos. 2014. A brief vestibular/ocular motor screening (VOMS) assessment to evaluate concussions: Preliminary findings. *American Journal of Sports Medicine* 42 (10): 2479–86.

National Institute of Neurological Disorders and Stroke. 2015a. NINDS Guillain-Barre syndrome. Last modified November 19, 2015. Accessed January 10, 2016. www.ninds.nih.gov/disorders/gbs/gbs.htm.

National Institute of Neurological Disorders and Stroke. 2015b. NINDS headache information page. Last modified November 3, 2015. Accessed January 9, 2016. www.ninds.nih.gov/disorders/headache/headache.htm.

National Institute of Neurological Disorders and Stroke. 2016. NINDS amyotrophic lateral sclerosis (ALS). Last modified January 8, 2016. Accessed January 10, 2016. www.ninds.nih.gov/disorders/amyotrophiclateralsclerosis/ALS.htm.

National MS Society. 2015. Multiple sclerosis. Last modified December 16, 2015. Accessed January 10, 2016. www.nationalmssociety.org/What-is-MS/MS-FAQ-s.

National Stroke Association. 2016. Act FAST. Accessed January 9, 2016. www.stroke.org/understand-stroke/recognizing-stroke/act-fast.

O'Toole, M.T., ed. 2013. *Mosby's Dictionary of Medicine, Nursing & Health Professionals.* 9th ed. St Louis: Elsevier/Mosby.

Polman, C., S.C. Reingols, B. Banwell, M. Clanet, J.A. Cohen, M. Filippi, K. Fujihara, et al. 2011. Diagnostic criteria for multiple sclerosis: 2010 revisions to the McDonald criteria. *Annuals of Neurology* 69 (2): 292–302.

Pop Warner. 2015. Pop Warner Concussion Policy. www.popwarner.com/safety/concussionpolicy.htm.

Porter, R.S., and J.L. Kaplan, eds. 2011. *The Merck Manual.* 19th ed. Whitehouse Station, NJ: Merck Sharp & Dohme Corporation.

Preparticipation Physical Evaluation Working Group. 2010. *Preparticipation Physical Evaluation.* Edited by D.T. Bernhardt and W.O. Roberts. 4th ed. Elk Grove Village, IL: American Academy of Pediatrics.

Riemann, B.L., and K.M. Guskiewicz. 2000. Effects of mild head injury on postural stability as measured through clinical balance testing. *Journal of Athletic Training* 35 (1): 19–25.

Ruijun, J., L.H. Schwamm, M.A. Perves, and A.B. Singhal. 2013. Ischemic stroke and transient ischemic attack in young adults. *Journal of the American Medical Association Neurology* 70 (1): 51–7.

Sady, M.D., C.G. Vaughan, and G.A. Gioia. 2011. School and the concussed youth: Recommendations for concussion education and management. *Physical Medicine Rehabilitation Clinics of North America* 22 (4): 701–19, ix.

Sarmiento, K., J. Mitchko, C. Klein, and S. Wong. 2010. Evaluation of the Centers for Disease Control and Prevention's concussion initiative for high school coaches: Heads up: Concussion in high school sports. *Journal of School Health* 80 (3): 112–18.

Scopaz, K.A., and J.R. Hatzenbuehler. 2013. Risk modifiers for concussion and prolonged recovery. *Sports Health* 5 (6): 537–41.

Shenouda C., P. Hendrickson, K. Davenport, J. Barber, and K.R. Bell. 2012. The effects of concussion legislation one year later—what have we learned: A descriptive pilot survey of youth soccer player associates. *PMR.*

Smith, E.D., M. Swartzon, and C.A. McGrew. 2014. Headaches in athletes. *Current Sports Medicine Reports* 13 (1): 27–32.

Taylor, D.C. 2015. Vertigo. *MedicineNet.* Last modified May 1, 2015. Accessed January 10, 2016. www.medicinenet.com/vertigo_overview/article.htm.

Thomas, D.G., J.N. Apps, R.G. Hoffmann, M. McCrea, and T. Hammeke. 2015. Benefits of strict rest after acute concussion: A randomized controlled trial. *Pediatrics* 135 (2): 213–23.

Toussirot, E., and M. Bereau. 2016. Vaccination and induction of autoimmune diseases. *Inflammation & Allergy Drug Targets* 4: epub ahead of print.

Valovich McLeod, T.C., D.H. Perrin, K.M. Guskiewicz, R. Diamond, S.J. Shultz, and B.M. Gansneder. 2004. Serial administration of clinical concussion assessments and learning effects in healthy youth sports participants. *Clinical Journal of Sport Medicine* 14 (5): 287–95.

Valovich McLeod, T.C., and G.A. Gioia. 2010. Cognitive rest: The often neglected aspect of concussion management. *Athletic Therapy Today* 15 (2): 1–3.

Valovich McLeod, T.C., and T.D. Hale. 2015. Vestibular and balance issues following sport-related concussion. *Brain Injury* 29 (2): 175–84.

Valovich McLeod, T.C., D.H. Perrin, K.M. Guskiewicz, R. Diamond, S.J. Shultz, and B.M. Gansneder. 2004. Serial administration of clinical concussion assessments and learning effects in healthy youth sports participants. *Clinical Journal of Sport Medicine* 14 (5): 287–95.

Van Kampen, D.A., M.R. Lovell, J.E. Pardini, M.W. Collins, and F.H. Fu. 2006. The value added of neurocognitive testing after sports-related concussion. *American Journal of Sports Medicine* 34 (10): 1630–35.

Wang, M.D., J. Gomes, N.R. Cashman, J. Little, and D. Krewski. 2014. A meta-analysis of observational studies of the association between chronic occupational exposure to lead and amyotrophic lateral sclerosis. *Journal of Occupational Environment Medicine* 56 (12): 1235–42.

WebMD. 2015. Epilepsy health center. *WebMD*. Last modified 2015. Accessed January 9, 2016. www.webmd.com/epilepsy/medications-treat-seizures.

Wheeler, A.H. 2015. Complex regional pain syndrome. *Medscape*. Accessed January 10, 2016. http://emedicine.medscape.com/article/1145318-overview.

Williamson, R.W., D. Gerhardstein, J. Cardenas, D.B. Michael, N. Theodore, and N. Rosseau. 2014. Concussion 101: The current state of concussion education programs. *Neurosurgery* 75 (Suppl 4): S131–35.

Wingerchuk, D.M., and J.L. Carter. 2014. Multiple sclerosis: Current and emerging disease-modifying therapies and treatment strategies. *Mayo Clinic Proceedings* 89 (2): 225–40.

World Health Organization. 2012. Headache disorders. Last modified October 2012. Accessed January 9, 2016. www.who.int/mediacentre/factsheets/fs277/en/.

Young, C.C., B.A. Jacobs, K. Clavette, D.H. Mark, and C.E. Guse. 1997. Serial sevens: Not the most effective test of mental status in high school athletes. *Clinical Journal of Sports Medicine* 7:196–98.

Chapter 12

Aerni, G.A. 2013. Blunt visual trauma. *Clinics in Sports Medicine* 32 (2): 289–301.

Ahmed, F., R.J. House, and B.H. Feldman. 2015. Corneal abrasions and corneal foreign bodies. *Primary Care: Clinics in Office Practice* 42 (3): 363–75.

American Academy of Pediatrics. 2003. Eye examination in infants, children, and young adults by pediatricians: Policy statement. *Pediatrics* 111 (4): 902–7.

Andreoli, C., M. Gardiner, R.G. Bachur, J. Trobe, J.A. Marx, and J.F. Wiley. 2012. Traumatic hyphema: Epidemiology, anatomy, and pathophysiology. Accessed August 27, 2016. www.uptodate.com/contents/traumatic-hyphema-clinical-features-and-diagnosis.

Armstrong, G.W., J.G. Kim, J.G. Linakis, M.J. Mello, and P.B. Greenberg. 2013. Pediatric eye injuries presenting to United States emergency departments: 2001–2007. *Graefe's Archive for Clinical and Experimental Ophthalmology* 251 (3): 629–36.

Ball, J., J. Dains, J. Flynn, B.S. Solomon, and R.W. Stewart. 2014. *Seidel's Guide to Physical Examination*. 8th ed. St. Louis: Mosby.

Bansal, S., D.V. Gunasekeran, B. Ang, J. Lee, R. Khandelwal, P. Sullivan, and R. Agrawal. 2016. Controversies in the pathophysiology and management of hyphema. *Survey of Ophthalmology* 61 (3): 297–308.

Bickley, L. 2012. *Bates' Guide to Physical Examination and History-Taking*. 11th ed. Philadelphia: Lippincott Williams & Wilkins.

Borrione, P., F. Quaranta, V. De Luca, F. Sperandii, E. Ciminelli, E. Cantera, F. Fagnani, and F. Pigozzi. 2015. Ophthalmologic findings in contact sport disciplines. *Journal of Sports Medicine and Physical Fitness* Sep 2 Epub ahead of print.

Cass, S.P. 2012. Ocular injuries in sports. *Current Sports Medicine Reports* 11 (1): 11–15.

Castle, A.M. 2012. *The Use of Safety Eye Protection by Children in Recreational Sports*. Ferris State University.

Chang, H.-Y.P., N. Huynh, and S. Borboli-Gerogiannis. 2012. Eye injuries associated with orbital or periorbital trauma. *Investigative Ophthalmology & Visual Science* 53 (14): 4962.

Coronica, R., and C. Murty. 2015. Ocular emergencies: Screening tool and alert protocol. *Insight* 40 (4): 5–13.

Design, F., N. Barker, R. White, S. Studios, M. Chat, T. Wendell, T. Banks, A. Arbucci, D. Danchuk, and E. Macpherson. 2012. Corneal abrasions: How to prevent a painful tear. *New York Journal of Style and Medicine*. Accessed August 27, 2016. www.nyjsm.com/Medicine/Ophthalmology/Corneal_Abrasions_RanjitR_ShahS.cfm.

Ellis, J. 2013. *Focus on Trauma: Facial Trauma*. AOSSM Sports Medicine and the NFL Boston, MA, May 9, 2013.

Farrington, T., G. Onambele-Pearson, R.L. Taylor, P. Earl, and K. Winwood. 2012. A review of facial protective equipment use in sport and the impact on injury incidence.

British Journal of Oral and Maxillofacial Surgery 50 (3): 233–38.

Ferri, F.F. 2016. *Ferri's Clinical Advisor 2016*. Philadelphia: Elsevier.

Geissler, K.E., and J.R. Borchers. 2015. More than meets the eye: A rapidly progressive skin infection in a football player. *Clinical Journal of Sport Medicine* 25 (3): e54–e56.

Jarvis, C. 2012. *Physical Examination & Health Assessment*. 6th ed. St. Louis: Elsevier/Saunders.

Joondeph, S.A., and B.C. Joondeph. 2013. Retinal detachment due to crossfit training injury. *Case Reports in Ophthalmological Medicine* 2013:189837.

Kriz, P.K., R.D. Zurakowski, J.L. Almquist, J. Reynolds, D. Ruggieri, C.L. Collins, P.A. d'Hemecourt, and R.D. Comstock. 2015. Eye protection and risk of eye injuries in high school field hockey. *Pediatrics* 136 (3): 521–27.

Kuryan, J., A. Cheema, and R.S. Chuck. 2014. Laser-assisted in-situ keratomileusis (LASIK) versus laser-assisted subepithelial keratectomy (LASEK) for the correction of myopia. *Cochrane Database of Systemic Reviews* 4: Art. No.: CD011080.

Liu, M., Y. Chen, D. Wang, Y. Zhou, X. Zhang, J. He, T. Zhang, Y. Sun, and Q. Liu. 2016. Clinical outcomes after SMILE and femtosecond laser-assisted LASIK for myopia and myopic astigmatism: A prospective randomized comparative study. *Cornea* 35 (2): 210–16.

Logothetis, H.D., S.M. Leikin, and T. Patrianakos. 2014. Management of anterior segment trauma. *Disease-a-Month* 60 (6): 247–53.

Mishra, A., and A.K. Verma. 2012. Sports related ocular injuries. *Medical Journal Armed Forces India* 68 (3): 260–66.

Mittal, V., R. Jain, R. Mittal, U. Vashist, and P. Narang. 2015. Successful management of severe unilateral chemical burns in children using simple limbal epithelial transplantation (SLET). *British Journal of Ophthalmology* 100 (8): 1102–8.

Parsons, J.T. 2014. *2014–15 NCAA Sports Medicine Handbook*. Indianapolis: National Collegiate Athletic Association.

Ong, H.S., A. Barsam, O.C. Morris, D. Siriwardena, and S. Verma. 2012. A survey of ocular sports trauma and the role of eye protection. *Contact Lens and Anterior Eye* 35 (6): 285–87.

Peck, K.Y., D.A. Johnston, B.D. Owens, and K.L. Cameron. 2013. The incidence of injury among male and female intercollegiate rugby players. *Sports Health: A Multidisciplinary Approach* 5 (4): 327–33.

Richardson, B. 2013. *Pediatric Primary Care: Practice Guidelines for Nurses*. Boston: Jones & Bartlett.

Riordan-Eva, P., and E. Cunningham. 2011. *Vaughan & Asbury's General Ophthalmology*. 18th ed. New York: McGraw-Hill.

Roat, M.I. 2014. Overview of conjunctival and scleral disorders. *Merck Manual*. Whitehouse Station, NJ: Merck Sharp & Dohme.

Sbicca, J.A., and R.L. Hatch. 2012. Target lesions and other paintball injuries. *The Journal of the American Board of Family Medicine* 25 (1): 124–27.

Sridhar, J., J.S. Chang, S. Liao, K.M. Cavuoto, and A.V. Rachitskaya. 2015. The spectrum of pediatric orbital BB gun injuries: A case series. *Journal of Pediatric Ophthalmology and Strabismus*. 52: E59–E62.

Stacey, A.W., C.N. Czyz, J.A. Foster, and D. Comstock. 2012. Eye injuries in U.S. high school athletes: Results of a six-year epidemiologic study. *Investigative Ophthalmology & Visual Science* 53 (14): 6770.

Vinger, P.F. 2012. *The Mechanisms and Prevention of Sports Eye Injuries*. Protective Eyewear Certification Council.

Wu, F., Y. Liu, and K. Zhang. 2015. Examination of the retina. *New England Journal of Medicine* 373 (25): 2484.

Zimmerman, A.B., K.L. Lust, and M.A. Bullimore. 2011. Visual acuity and contrast sensitivity testing for sports vision. *Eye & Contact Lens* 37 (3): 153–59.

Chapter 13

AAO-HNSF. 2014. AAO-HNSF releases clinical practice guideline on acute otitis externa. *American Family Physician* 90 (10): 731–36.

AAO-HNSF. 2015. AAO-HNSF releases guideline on managing tinnitus. *American Family Physician* 92 (1): 65.

Akhlaghi, F., M. Esmaeelinejad, and P. Safai. 2015. Etiologies and treatments of odontogenic maxillary sinusitis: A systematic review. *Iranian Red Crescent Medical Journal* 17 (12): e25536.

American Cancer Society. 2016. Oral cavity and oropharyngeal cancer. Last modified January 27, 2016. Accessed February 2, 2016. www.cancer.org/cancer/oralcavityandoropharyngealcancer/detailedguide/oral-cavity-and-oropharyngeal-cancer-key-statistics.

Andreeff, R. 2016. Epistaxis. *Journal of the American Academy of Physician Assistants* 29 (1): 46–47.

Araujo, T.M., and M.C. Iorio. 2015. Effects of sound amplification in self-perception of tinnitus and hearing loss in the elderly. *Brazilian Journal of Otorhinolaryngology* 82 (3): 289–96.

Ball, J., J. Dains, J. Flynn, B.S. Solomon, and R.W. Stewart. 2014. *Seidel's Guide to Physical Examination*. 8th ed. St. Louis: Mosby.

Bickley, L. 2012. *Bates' Guide to Physical Examination and History-Taking.* 11th ed. Philadelphia: Lippincott Williams & Wilkins.

Bilge, A., A. Gunes, M. Dagli, F.F. Koybasioglu, and A. Guvey. 2016. The impact of topical and systemic enoxaparin sodium use on traumatic tympanic membrane perforation and myringosclerosis. *European Archives of Otorhinolaryngology* 273 (10): 3035–43.

Burgess, J. 2015. White lesions of the oral cavity. Last modified March 3, 2015. Accessed February 4, 2016. http://emedicine.medscape.com/article/2105120-overview.

Chhetri, S.S. 2014. Acute otitis media: A simple diagnosis, a simple treatment. *Nepal Medical College Journal* 16 (1): 33–36.

Cots, J.M., J.I. Alos, M. Barcena, X. Boleda, J.L. Canada, N. Gomez, A. Mendoza, I. Vilaseca, and C. Llor. 2015. Recommendations for management of acute pharyngitis in adults. *Acta Otorrinolaringológica Española* 66 (3): 159–70.

DeMuri, G.P., J.E. Gern, S.C. Moyer, M.J. Lindstrom, S.V. Lynch, and E.R. Wald. 2016. Clinical features, virus identification, and sinusitis as a complication of upper respiratory tract illness in children ages 4–7 years. *Journal of Pediatrics* 171: 133–9.

Dinc, A.E., M. Damar, M.B. Ugur, Oz, II, S.S. Elicora, S. Biskin, and H. Tutar. 2015. Do the angle and length of the eustachian tube influence the development of chronic otitis media? *Laryngoscope* 125 (9): 2187–92.

Domino, F., R.A. Baldor, J. Golding, and M.B. Stephens. 2016. *The 5-Minute Clinical Consult Standard 2016.* Philadelphia: Lippincott Williams & Wilkins.

Ebell, M.H. 2014. Diagnosis of streptococcal pharyngitis. *American Family Physician* 89 (12): 976–77.

Ferri, F.F. 2016. *Ferri's Clinical Advisor 2016.* Philadelphia: Elsevier.

Fox, R., R. Nash, Z.W. Liu, and A. Singh. 2016. Epistaxis management: Current understanding amongst junior doctors. *The Journal of Laryngology & Otology* 130 (3): 252–5.

Goldman, L., and A. Schafer. 2011. *Goldman's Cecil Medicine.* 24th ed. Philadelphia: Elsevier/Saunders.

Hong, P., M. Bance, and P.F. Gratzer. 2013. Repair of tympanic membrane perforation using novel adjuvant therapies: A contemporary review of experimental and tissue engineering studies. *International Journal of Pediatric Otorhinolaryngology* 77 (1): 3–12.

Jarvis, C. 2012. *Physical Examination & Health Assessment.* 6th ed. St. Louis: Elsevier/Saunders.

Kosaner Kliess, M., R. Zoehrer, B. Schlick, M. Mariacher, and M. Urban. 2015. Subjective outcomes with bone con-duction and middle ear implants for patients with conductive or mixed hearing loss. *Value in Health* 18 (7): A364.

Kraus, F., and R. Hagen. 2015. The traumatic tympanic membrane perforation—aetiology and therapy. *Laryngorhinootologie* 94 (9): 596–600.

Laine, M.K., P.A. Tahtinen, O. Ruuskanen, E. Loyttyniemi, and A. Ruohola. 2015. Can trained nurses exclude acute otitis media with tympanometry or acoustic reflectometry in symptomatic children? *Scandinavian Journal of Primary Health Care* 33 (4): 298–304.

Lee, J.H., J.S. Lee, D.K. Kim, C.H. Park, and H.R. Lee. 2015. Clinical outcomes of silk patch in acute tympanic membrane perforation. *Clinical and Experimental Otorhinolaryngology* 8 (2): 117–22.

Liu, J., Z. Yan, and M. Zhang. 2015. Clinical diagnosis and treatment of allergic pharyngitis. *Lin Chung Er Bi Yan Hou Tou Jing Wai Ke Za Zhi* 29 (15): 1401–5.

Lynch, D. 2014. Oral examination. Last modified December 9, 2014. Accessed February 1, 2016.

Martonffy, A.I. 2015. Oral health: Prevention of dental disease. *Family Practice Essentials* 428:11–15.

Park, H., S.N. Hong, H.S. Kim, J.J. Han, J. Chung, M.W. Seo, S.H. Oh, S.O. Chang, and J.H. Lee. 2015. Determinants of conductive hearing loss in tympanic membrane perforation. *Clinical and Experimental Otorhinolaryngology* 8 (2): 92–96.

Perez, F., and G. Rada. 2016. Is antibiotic prophylaxis in nasal packing for anterior epistaxis needed? *Medwave* 16 (Suppl 1): e6357.

Sanchez, G.V., and L.A. Hicks. 2014. Acute sinusitis and pharyngitis as inappropriate indications for antibiotic use. *Antimicrobial Agents and Chemotherapy* 58 (6): 3572.

Settipane, R., and M. Kaliner. 2013. Chapter 14: Nonallergic rhinitis. *American Journal of Rhinology and Allergy* May-June 27 (Suppl 1): S48–51.

Shy, B.D., and R.J. Strayer. 2014. Nonsteroidal anti-inflammatory drugs are an effective alternative to corticosteroids to treat pain in pharyngitis. *Annals of Emergency Medicine* 64 (6): 686.

Stephen, J.M. 2014. Gingivitis. *Medscape.* Accessed February 1, 2016. http://emedicine.medscape.com/article/763801-overview.

Stoopler, E.T., and T.P. Sollecito. 2014. Recurrent gingival and oral mucosal lesions. *Journal of American Medical Association* 312 (17): 1794–95.

Sur, D., and M. Plesa. 2015. Treatment of allergic rhinitis. *American Family Physician* 92 (11): 985–92.

Taschieri, S., S. Torretta, S. Corbella, M. Del Fabbro, L. Francetti, A. Lolato, and P. Capaccio. 2015. Pathophysiology of sinusitis of odontogenic origin. *Journal of*

Investigative and Clinical Dentistry December 14, Epub ahead of print.

Wald, E., K. Applegate, C. Bordley, D. Darrow, M. Glode, S. Marcy, C. Nelson, R. Rosenfeld, N. Shaikh, M. Smith, P. Williams, and S. Weinberg. 2013. Clinical practice guideline for the diagnosis and management of acute bacterial sinusitis in children aged 1 to 18 years. *Pediatrics* 132 (1): 262–80.

Walling, A.D., and G. Dickson. 2012. Hearing loss in older adults. *American Family Physician* 85 (12): 1150–56.

Wang, J., X. Dou, D. Liu, P. Song, X. Qian, S. Wang, and X. Gao. 2015. Assessment of the effect of deviated nasal septum on the structure of nasal cavity. *European Archives of Otorhinolaryngology* 273 (6): 1477–80.

Wasson, J.D., and M.W. Yung. 2015. Evidence-based management of otitis media: A 5S model approach. *Journal of Laryngology and Otology* 129 (2): 112–19.

Williams, J.V., Y. Kamhieh, and L.J. Cohen. 2015. A simple technique for the single-handed management of anterior epistaxis. *Clinical Otolaryngology* 40 (6): 737.

Wojcik, B.E., W. Szeszel-Fedorowicz, R.J. Humphrey, P. Colthirst, A.C. Guerrero, J.W. Simecek, A. Fedorowicz, S. Eikenberg, G.G. Rogers, and P. DeNicolo. 2015. Risk of dental disease non-battle injuries and severity of dental disease in deployed U.S. Army personnel. *Military Medicine* 180 (5): 570–77.

Zakaria, M., N. Othman, and A.C. Lih. 2016. Is the degree of hearing loss truly dependent on the site of tympanic membrane perforation? *Oman Medical Journal* 31 (1): 83–84.

Chapter 14

American Cancer Society. 2016. Cancer facts and figures, 2016. Last Modified February 1, 2016. Accessed February 20, 2016. www.cancer.org/research/cancerfactsstatistics/cancerfactsfigures2016/.

American College of Rheumatology. 2015. Fibromyalgia. Accessed March 6, 2016. www.rheumatology.org/I-Am-A/Patient-Caregiver/Diseases-Conditions/Fibromyalgia.

American College of Rheumatology. 2016. ACR-endorsed criteria for rheumatic diseases. Last modified 2016. Accessed March 5, 2016. www.rheumatology.org/Practice-Quality/Clinical-Support/Criteria/ACR-Endorsed-Criteria.

American Diabetes Association. 2016. Diagnosing diabetes and learning about prediabetes. Accessed March 5, 2016. www.diabetes.org/diabetes-basics/diagnosis/?loc=db-slab-nav.

Balsamo, S., and L. dos Santos-Neto. 2011. Fatigue in systemic lupus erythematosus: An association with reduced physical fitness. *Autoimmunity Reviews* 10:2011.

Bartels, C.M. 2015. Systemic lupus erythematosus (SLE). *Medscape*. Last modified September 25, 2015. Accessed March 5, 2016. http://emedicine.medscape.com/article/332244-overview.

Boomershine, C.S. 2015. Fibromyalgia. *Medscape*. Last modified October 23, 2015. Accessed March 6, 2016. http://emedicine.medscape.com/article/329838-overview.

Cefalu, W.T. 2016. American Diabetes Association. Standards of medical care in diabetes—2016. *Diabetes Care* 39 (1): S1–S109.

Centers for Disease Control and Prevention. 2015a. Chronic fatigue syndrome (CFS). Last modified April 7, 2015. Accessed March 6, 2016. www.cdc.gov/cfs/.

Centers for Disease Control and Prevention. 2015b. Diabetes. Last modified November 4, 2015. Accessed March 7, 2016. www.cdc.gov/diabetes/home/index.html.

Centers for Disease Control and Prevention. 2015c. Leading Causes of Death. Last Modified January 20, 2015. Accessed February 20, 2016. www.cdc.gov/nchs/fastats/leading-causes-of-death.htm.

Centers for Disease Control and Prevention. 2015d. Lyme disease. Last modified November 18, 2015. Accessed February 21, 2016. www.cdc.gov/lyme/index.html.

Centers for Disease Control and Prevention. 2015e. Systemic lupus erythematosus (SLE). Last modified April 20, 2015. Accessed March 5, 2016. www.cdc.gov/lupus/.

Cheadle, C. 2015. Supporting student-athletes with type 1 diabetes. National Collegiate Athletic Association. Last modified March 17, 2015. www.ncaa.org/health-and-safety/sport-science-institute/supporting-student-athletes-type-1-diabetes.

Colberg, S.R, R.J. Sigal, B. Fernhall, J.G. Regensteiner, B.J. Blissmer, R.R. Rubin, L. Chasan-Taber, A.L. Albright, and B. Braun. 2010. Exercise and type 2 diabetes: The American College of Sports Medicine and the American Diabetes Association joint position statement. *Diabetes Care* 33:147–67.

Cunha, B.A. 2016. Chronic fatigue syndrome. *Medscape*. Last modified February 16, 2016. Accessed March 6, 2016. http://emedicine.medscape.com/article/235980-overview.

Dall'Era, M. 2013. Systemic lupus erythematosus. In *Current Rheumatology Diagnosis and Treatment*, edited by J.B. Imboden, D.B. Hellman, and J.H. Stone. New York: McGraw-Hill.

Draznin, M.B. 2010. Managing the adolescent athlete with type 1 diabetes mellitus. *Pediatric Clinics of North America* 57 (3): 829–37.

DuPrey, K.M. 2015. Lyme disease in athletes. *Current Sports Medicine Reports* 14 (1): 51–55.

Ferri, F.F. 2016. *Ferri's Clinical Advisor*. Philadelphia: Elsevier.

Gardner, T.B. 2015. Acute pancreatitis. *Medscape*. Last modified April 1, 2015. Accessed March 6, 2015. http://emedicine.medscape.com/article/181364-overview.

Hamdy, O. 2015. Hypoglycemia treatment and management. *Medscape*. Last modified September 8, 2015. Accessed March 7, 2016. http://emedicine.medscape.com/article/122122-treatment.

Hansen-Dispenza, H. 2015. Raynaud phenomenon. *Medscape*. Last modified November 17, 2105. http://emedicine.medscape.com/article/331197-overview.

Harris, G.D., and R.D. White. 2012. Diabetes in the competitive athlete. *Current Sports Medicine Reports* 11 (6): 309–15.

Jiao, J., A. Vincent, S.S. Cha, C.A. Luedtke, C.H. Kim, and T.H. Oh. 2015. Physical trauma and infection as precipitating factors in patients with fibromyalgia. *American Journal of Physical Medicine and Rehabilitation* 94 (12): 1075–82.

Khardori, R. 2015a. Type 1 diabetes mellitus. *Medscape*. Last modified October 8, 2015. Accessed March 7, 2016. http://emedicine.medscape.com/article/117739-overview.

Khardori, R. 2015b. Type 2 diabetes mellitus. *Medscape*. Last modified October 8, 2015. Accessed March 7, 2016. http://emedicine.medscape.com/article/117853-overview-a1.

Lantos, P.M. 2015. Chronic Lyme disease. *Infectious Disease Clinics of North America* 29 (2): 325–40.

Lash, B.W. 2015. Hodgkin lymphoma. *Medscape*. Last modified September 18, 2016. Accessed February 20, 2016. http://emedicine.medscape.com/article/201886-overview.

Lee, S.L. 2015. Hyperthyroidism. *Medscape*. Last modified November 3, 2015. Accessed March 7, 2016. http://emedicine.medscape.com/article/121865-overview.

Lisnevskaia, L., G. Murphy, and D. Isenberg. 2014. Systemic lupus erythematosus. *Lancet* 22 (384):1878–88.

Lister, T.A., D. Crowther, S.B. Sutcliffe, E. Glatstein, G.P. Canellos, R.C. Young, S.A. Rosenberg, C.A. Coltman, and M. Tubiana. 1989. Report of a committee convened to discuss the evaluation and staging of patients with Hodgkin's disease: Cotwolds meeting. *Journal of Clinical Oncology* 7 (11): 1630–36.

Meyerhoff, J. 2016. Lyme disease. *Medscape*. Last modified February 10, 2016. Accessed February 21, 2106. http://emedicine.medscape.com/article/330178-overview.

Noel, R.A., Braun D.K., R.E. Patterson, and G.L Bloomgren. 2009. Increased risk of acute pancreatitis and biliary disease observed in patients with type 2 diabetes. *Diabetes Care* 32 (5): 834–38.

Orlander, P.R. 2015. Hypothyroidism. *Medscape*. Last modified February 19, 2015. Accessed March 8, 2016. http://emedicine.medscape.com/article/122393-overview.

Porter, R.S., and J.L. Kaplan, eds. 2011. *The Merck Manual*. 19th ed. Whitehouse Station, NJ: Merck Sharp & Dohme.

Rapaport, L. 2016. Ticks carrying Lyme disease in almost half of U.S. counties. *Medscape*. Last modified January 19, 2016. Accessed February 21, 2016. www.medscape.com/viewarticle/857408.

Sakthiswary, R., and E. Suresh. 2014. Methotrexate in systemic lupus erythematosus: A systematic review of its efficacy. *Lupus* 23 (3): 225–35.

Schaapveld, M., B.M.P. Aleman, A.M. van Eggermond, C.P.M. Janus, A.D.G. Krol, R.W.M van der Maazen, J. Roesink, et al. 2015. Second cancer risk up to 40 years after treatment for Hodgkin's lymphoma. *New England Journal of Medicine* 373:2499–2511.

Schinasi, L., and M.E. Leon. 2014. Non-Hodgkin lymphoma and occupational exposure to agriculture pesticide chemical groups and active ingredients: A systematic review and meta-analysis. *International Journal of Environmental Research and Public Health* 11 (4): 4449–4527.

Segura-Jimenez, V., I.C. Alvarez-Gallardo, F. Estevez-Lopez, A. Soriano-Maldonado, M. Delgado-Fernandez, F.B. Ortega, V.A. Aparicio, A. Carbonell-Baeza, J. Mota, P. Silva, and J.R. Ruiz. 2015. Differences in sedentary time and physical activity between female patients with fibromyalgia and healthy controls: The al-Andalus project. *Arthritis & Rheumatology* 67 (11): 3014–57.

Staud, R. 2006. Are patients with systemic lupus erythematosus at increased risk for fibromyalgia? *Current Rheumatology Reports* 8:430–35.

Sumpton, J.E., and D.E. Moulin. 2014. Fibromyalgia. In *Handbook of Clinical Neurology*, edited by M.S. Berger and M. Weller, pp. 513–27. Philadelphia: Elsevier.

Tench, C., D. Bentley, V. Vleck, I. McCurdie, P. White, and D. D'Cruz. 2002. Aerobic fitness, fatigue and physical activity in systemic lupus erythematosus. *Journal of Rheumatology* 29 (3): 474–81.

Tucker, M.E. 2013. FDA OKs insulin pump with low-glucose suspend feature. *Medscape*. Last modified September 27, 2013. Accessed March 7, 2016. www.medscape.com/viewarticle/811799.

Vinjamaram, S. 2015. Non-Hodgkin lymphoma. *Medscape*. Last modified March 25, 2015. Accessed February 21, 2016. http://emedicine.medscape.com/article/203399-overview.

Wolfe, F., D.J. Clauw, A. Fitzcharles, R.S. Goldenberg, S. Katz, P. Mease, A.S. Russell, J.B. Winfield, and M.B. Yunus. 2010. The American College of Rheumatology preliminary diagnostic criteria for fibromyalgia and measurement of symptom severity. *Arthritis Care and Research* 62 (5): 600–610.

Wolfson, T.S., M.J. Hamula, and L.M. Jazrawi. 2013. Impact of diabetes mellitus on surgical outcomes in sports medicine. *Physician and Sportsmedicine* 41 (4): 64–77.

Wormser, G.P., R.J. Dattwyler, E.D. Shapiro, J.J. Halperin, A.C. Steere, M.S. Klempner, P.J. Krause, et al. 2006. The clinical assessment, treatment and prevention of Lyme disease, human granulocytic anaplasmosis, and babesiosis: Clinical practice guidelines by the Infectious Diseases Society of America. *Clinical Infectious Diseases* 43 (9): 1089–1134.

Wu, L. 2015. Leukemias. *Medscape*. Last modified April 3, 2015. Accessed February 21, 2016. http://emedicine.medscape.com/article/1201870-overview.

Chapter 15

Agel, J., J. Ransone, R.F. Dick, R. Oppliger, and S.W. Marshall. 2007. Descriptive epidemiology of collegiate men's wresting injuries: National Collegiate Athletic Association injury surveillance system, 1988–1989 through 2003–2004. *Journal of Athletic Training* 42 (2): 303–10.

Alexander, J.P., L.E. Chapman, M.A. Pallansch, W.T. Stephenson, T.J. Torok, and L.J. Anderson. 1993. Coxsackievirus B2 infection and aseptic meningitis: A focal outbreak among members of a high school football team. *Journal of Infectious Diseases* 167 (5): 1201–5.

Anderson, A. 2004. Arthropod pests and the diseases they carry: Prevention in the community and athletic settings. *Athletic Therapy Today* 9 (3): 16–21.

Anderson, L.J., and J.F. Seward. 2008. Mumps epidemiology and immunity: The anatomy of an epidemic. *Pediatric Infectious Diseases Journal* 10:S75–79.

Anderson, W.E. 2015. Varicella-zoster virus. *Medscape*. Last modified October 22, 2015. Accessed March 11, 2016. http://emedicine.medscape.com/article/231927-overview.

Anish, E.J. 2004. Viral hepatitis: Sports-related risk. *Current Sports Medicine Reports* 3 (2): 100–106.

Appiah, G.D., L. Blanton, T. M'Mello, K. Kniss, S. Smith, D. Mustaquiim, C. Steffans, et al. 2015. Influenza activity—United States, 2014–15 season and composition of 2015–16 influenza vaccine. *Morbidity and Mortality Weekly Report (MMWR)* 64 (21): 583–90.

Arnot, R. 1998. The evolving efforts to control hepatitis B virus. *Pediatric Infectious Diseases Journal* 17 (7): S26–S29.

Baorto, E.P. 2015. Staphylococcus aureus infection. *Medscape* Last modified August 6, 2015. Accessed March 19, 2016. http://emedicine.medscape.com/article/971358-overview.

Beaschler, R. 2015. Wrestling 2015–16 and 2016–17 Rules and Interpretations. Edited by National Collegiate Athletic Association. Indianapolis, IN: National Collegiate Athletic Association.

Becker, J.A., and J.A. Smith. 2014. Return to play after infectious mononucleosis. *Sports Health* 6 (3): 232–8.

Begier, E.M., M.S. Oberste, M.L. Landry, T. Brennan, D. Mlynarski, P.A. Mshar, K. Frenette, et al. 2008. An outbreak of concurrent echovirus 30 and coxsackievirus A1 infections associated with sea swimming among a group of travelers to Mexico. *Clinical Infectious Diseases* 47 (5): 616–23.

Bonanni, P., J. Breuer, A. Gershon, W. Hryniewicz, V. Papaevangelou, B. Rentier, H. Rumke, et al. 2009. Varicella vaccination in Europe—taking the practical approach. *BioMed Central Medicine* 28 (7): 26.

Buggs, A.M. 2014. Viral hepatitis. *Medscape*. Last modified December 16, 2014. Accessed March 11, 2016. http://emedicine.medscape.com/article/775507-overview.

Buxton, B.P., J.E. Daniell, B.H. Buxton, E.M. Okasaki, and K.W. Ho. 1994. Prevention of hepatitis B virus in athletic training. *Journal of Athletic Training* 29 (2): 107–12.

CAATE. 2015. Standards. Commission on Accreditation of Athletic Training Education. Accessed March 8, 2016. http://caate.net/pp-standards/.

Cauchemez, S., M. Besnard, P. Bompard, T. Dub, P. Guillemette-Artur, D. Eyrolle-Guignot, H. Salje, et al. 2016. Association between Zika virus and microcephaly in French Polynesia, 2013–15: A retrospective study. *Lancet* 387: 2125–132.

Centers for Disease Control and Prevention. 2009. Progress toward the 2012 measles elimination goal—Western Pacific region, 1990–2008. *Morbidity and Mortality Weekly Report (MMWR)* 58 (24): 669–73.

Centers for Disease Control and Prevention. 2014a. Methicillin-resistant *Staphylococcus aureus* (MRSA) infections. Last modified April 30, 2014. Accessed March 19, 2016. www.cdc.gov/mrsa/tracking/index.html.

Centers for Disease Control and Prevention. 2014b. Types of influenza viruses. Last modified April 19, 2014. Accessed April 17, 2016. www.cdc.gov/flu/about/viruses/types.htm.

Centers for Disease Control and Prevention. 2015a. Human papillomavirus (HPV). Last modified January 26, 2015. Accessed March 8, 2016. www.cdc.gov/hpv/parents/vaccine.html.

Centers for Disease Control and Prevention. 2015b. Information on swine influenza/variant influenza viruses. Last modified May 15, 2015 Accessed March 8, 2016. www.cdc.gov/flu/swineflu/index.htm.

Centers for Disease Control and Prevention. 2015c. Measles (rubeola) for healthcare professionals. www.cdc.gov/measles/hcp/index.html.

Centers for Disease Control and Prevention. 2015d. National Notifiable Diseases Surveillance System (NNDSS). Last modified August 19, 2015. Accessed March 9, 2016. wwwn.cdc.gov/nndss/.

Centers for Disease Control and Prevention. 2015e. Selecting viruses for the seasonal influenza vaccine. Last modified October 20, 2015. Accessed April 17, 2016. www.cdc.gov/flu/about/season/vaccine-selection.htm.

Centers for Disease Control and Prevention. 2015f. Surveillance for viral hepatitis—United States, 2013. Last modified June 25, 2015. Accessed April 16, 2016. www.cdc.gov/hepatitis/statistics/2013surveillance/index.htm - tabs-801937-11.

Centers for Disease Control and Prevention. 2015g. Viral hepatitis: hepatitis B. Last modified December 16, 2015. Accessed March 12, 2016. www.cdc.gov/hepatitis/hbv/hbvfaq.htm - overview.

Centers for Disease Control and Prevention. 2016a. Division of Vector-Borne Diseases (DVBD). Last modified February 19, 2016. Accessed March 19, 2016. www.cdc.gov/ncezid/dvbd/.

Centers for Disease Control and Prevention. 2016b. Emergency preparedness and response. Update: Interim guidelines for prevention of sexual transmission of Zika virus—United States 2016. Last modified February 23, 2016. Accessed March 19, 2016. http://emergency.cdc.gov/han/han00388.asp.

Centers for Disease Control and Prevention. 2016c. Immunization schedules. Last modified February 1, 2016. Accessed March 8, 2016. www.cdc.gov/vaccines/schedules/.

Centers for Disease Control and Prevention. 2016d. Influenza (flu). Last modified March 4, 2016. Accessed March 8, 2016. www.cdc.gov/flu/index.htm.

Centers for Disease Control and Prevention. 2016e. Measles cases and outbreaks. Last modified March 8, 2016. Accessed March 11, 2016. www.cdc.gov/measles/cases-outbreaks.html.

Centers for Disease Control and Prevention. 2016f. Meningitis. Last modified March 4, 2016. Accessed March 20, 2016. www.cdc.gov/meningitis/.

Centers for Disease Control and Prevention. 2016g. Meningococcal disease. Last modified March 6, 2016. Accessed March 20, 2016. www.cdc.gov/meningococcal/index.html.

Centers for Disease Control and Prevention. 2016h. Surveillance and control of *Aedes aegypti* and *Aedes albopictus* in the United States. Last modified March 18, 2016. Accessed March 19, 2016. www.cdc.gov/chikungunya/resources/vector-control.html.

Centers for Disease Control and Prevention. 2016i. Vaccine information statements (VIS). Last modified April 1, 2016. www.cdc.gov/vaccines/hcp/vis/index.html.

Centers for Disease Control and Prevention. 2016j. Zika virus. Last modified March 11, 2016. Accessed March 19, 2016. www.cdc.gov/zika/index.html.

Chen, R.T, T.A. Clark, and J.J. Halperin. 2009. The yin and yang of paracetamol and paediatric immunizations. *Medical Journal of Australia* 189 (9): 484–86.

Chen, S. 2015. Measles. *Medscape*. Last modified March 30, 2015. http://emedicine.medscape.com/article/966220-overview.

Croker, C., R. Civen, K. Keough, V. Ngo, A. Marutani, and B. Schwartz. 2015. Aseptic meningitis outbreak associated with ecovirus 30 among high school football players—Los Angeles County, California, 2014. *Morbidity and Mortality Weekly Report (MMWR)* 63 (51): 1228.

Cunha, B.A. 2015. Infectious mononucleosis. *Medscape*. Last modified October 6, 2015. Accessed March 11, 2016. http://emedicine.medscape.com/article/222040-overview.

Cutler, J., E. Schleihauf, T.F. Hatchette, B. Billard, G. Watson-Creed, R. Davidson, Y. Li, N. Bastien, and S. Sarwal. 2009. Investigation of the first cases of human-to-human infection with the new swine-origin influenza A (H1N1) virus in Canada. *Canada Medical Association Journal* 4 (181): 159–63.

Dhawan, V.K. 2015. Hepatitis C. *Medscape*. Last modified August 3, 2015. Accessed March 12, 2016. http://emedicine.medscape.com/article/177792-overview - a5.

Defendi, G.L. 2016. Mumps, *Medscape*. Last modified April 26, 2016. Accessed August 4, 2016. http://reference.medscape.com/article/966678-overview.

Dupont-Rouzeyrol, M., A. Biron, O. O'Connor, E. Huguon, and E. Descloux. 2016. Infectious Zika viral particles in breastmilk. *Lancet* 387: 1051.

Edlich, R.F. 2015. Necrotizing fasciitis. *Medscape*. Last modified July 9, 2015. Accessed March 12, 2016. http://emedicine.medscape.com/article/2051157-overview.

Ewald, A.J., and D.B. McKeag. 2008. Meningitis in the athlete. *Current Sports Medicine Reports* 7 (1): 22–27.

Ezike, E. 2014. Pediatric rubella. *Medscape*. Last modified December 18, 2014. http://emedicine.medscape.com/article/968523-overview.

Ferri, F.F. 2016. *Ferri's Clinical Advisor*. Philadelphia, PA: Elsevier.

Gilroy, R.A. 2016. Hepatitis A. *Medscape*. Last modified January 28, 2016. Accessed March 11, 2016. http://emedicine.medscape.com/article/177484-overview.

Gondim, F. 2015. Meningococcal meningitis. *Medscape.* Last modified September 4, 2015. Accessed March 20, 2016. http://emedicine.medscape.com/article/1165557-overview - a4.

Grohskopf, L.A., L.Z. Sokolow, S.J. Olsen, J.S. Bresee, K.R. Broder, and R.A. Karron. 2015. Prevention and control of influenza with vaccines: Recommendations of the Advisory Committee on Immunization Practices, United States, 2015–16 influenza season. *Morbidity and Mortality Weekly Reports* 64 (30): 818–25.

Harris, K.M., T.S. Haas, E.R. Eichner, and B.J. Maron. 2012. Sickle cell trait associated with sudden death in competitive athletes. *American Journal of Cardiology* 110 (8): 1185–88.

Harris, M.D. 2011. Infectious disease in athletes. *Current Sports Medicine Reports* 10 (2): 84–90.

Hasbun, R. 2016. Meningitis. *Medscape.* Last modified February 16, 2016. http://emedicine.medscape.com/article/232915-overview.

Hayes, E.B. 2009. Zika virus outside of Africa. *Emerging Infectious Diseases* 15 (9): 1347–50.

Hennessey, M., M. Fischer, and J.E. Staples. 2016. Zika virus spreads to new areas—region of the Americas May 2015–January 2016. *Morbidity and Mortality Weekly Report (MMWR)* 65 (3): 55–58.

Herchline, T.E. 2015. Staphylococcal infections. *Medscape.* Last modified August 24, 2015. Accessed March 19, 2016. http://emedicine.medscape.com/article/228816-overview.

Hill, H.R. 2010. Group A streptococcal carrier versus acute infection: The continuing dilemma. *Clinical Infectious Diseases* 50 (4): 491–92.

Howe, W. 2003. Preventing infectious disease in sports. *The Physician and Sportsmedicine* 31 (2): 23–29.

Howes, D.S. 2015. Encephalitis. *Medscape.* Last modified October 12, 2015. Accessed March 19, 2016. http://emedicine.medscape.com/article/791896-overview.

Huang, A.S., M.M. Cortese, and A.T. Curns. 2009. Risk factors for mumps at a university with a large mumps outbreak. *Public Health Reports* 124 (3): 419–26.

Kashiwagi, S., J. Hayashi, H. Ikematsu, S. Nishigori, K. Ishihara, and M. Kaji. 1982. An outbreak of hepatitis B in members of a high school sumo wrestling club. *Journal of the American Medical Association* 9 (248): 3213–14.

Keller, D.M. 2014. Staph aureus scheme cuts surgical infection. *Medscape.* Last modified October 18, 2014. Accessed March 19, 2016. www.medscape.com/viewarticle/833457.

Kelly, H. 2011. The classical definition of a pandemic is not elusive. *Bulletin of the World Health Organization* 89: 540–41.

Khan, Z.Z. 2015. Group A streptococcal infections. *Medscape.* Last modified September 3, 2015. Accessed March 12, 2016. http://emedicine.medscape.com/article/228936-overview - a5.

Lam, W., A. Dawson, and C. Fowler. 2015. Health promotion intervention to prevent early childhood human influenza at the household level: A realist review to identify implications for programmes in Hong Kong. *Journal of Clinical Nursing* 24 (7–8): 891–905.

Lichenstein, R. 2015. Varicella-zoster (shingles) organism-specific therapy. *Medscape.* Last modified October 5, 2015. Accessed March 11, 2016. http://emedicine.medscape.com/article/1966889-overview.

Lindenmayer, J.M., S. Schoenfeld, R. O'Grady, and R. Carney. 1998. Methicillin-resistant *Staphylococcus aureus* in a high school wrestling team and surrounding community. *Archives of Internal Medicine* 158 (8): 895–99.

Lindsey, N.P., J.A. Lehman, J.E. Staples, and M. Fischer. 2015. West Nile virus and other nationally notifiable arboviral diseases—United States, 2014. *Morbidity and Mortality Weekly Report (MMWR)* 64 (34): 929–34.

Mayo Clinic. 2016. Rubella. Last modified 2016. www.mayoclinic.org/diseases-conditions/rubella/basics/definition/con-20020067.

National Athletic Trainers' Association. 2005. Official statement from the National Athletic Trainers' Association on community-acquired MRSA infections (CA-MRSA). Last modified March 1, 2005. www.nata.org/sites/default/files/MRSA.pdf.

National Athletic Trainers' Association. 2007. Official statement from the National Athletic Trainers' Association on communicable and infectious diseases in secondary school sports. Last modified March 2007. www.nata.org/sites/default/files/CommunicableInfectiousDiseasesSecondarySchoolSports.pdf.

National Federation of State High School Associations. 2013. Sports related skin infections position statement and guidelines. Last modified February 9, 2016. Accessed March 20, 2016. www.nfhs.org/sports-resource-content/smac-position-statements-and-guidelines/.

Navalkele, B.D. 2016. Zika virus. *Medscape.* Last modified March 17, 2016. Accessed March 20, 2016. http://emedicine.medscape.com/article/2500035-overview.

O'Connor, T.E., L.J. Skinner, P. Kiely, and J.E. Fenton. 2011. Return to contact sports following infectious mononucleosis: The role of serial ultrasonography. *Ear, Nose and Throat Journal* 8: E21–24.

Office of Disease Prevention and Health Promotion. 2016. Healthy People 2020 evidence-based resources. Office of Disease Prevention and Health Promotion. Last modified

March 8, 2016. Accessed March 8, 2016. www.healthypeople.gov/2020/tools-resources/Evidence-Based-Resources.

Oldfield, B.J, and R.W Stewart. 2016. Common misconceptions, advancements and updates in pediatric vaccination administration. *Southern Medical Journal* 109 (1): 38–41.

Parsons, J.T., ed. 2014. *2014–2015 NCAA Sports Medicine Handbook*. Indianapolis, IN: National Collegiate Athletic Association.

Perloff, S.A. 2014. MRSA skin infection in athletes. *Medscape*. Last modified August 18, 2014. Accessed March 19, 2016. http://emedicine.medscape.com/article/108972-overview.

Porter, R.S., and J.L. Kaplan, eds. 2011. *The Merck Manual*. 19th ed. Whitehouse Station, NJ: Merck Sharp & Dohme Corporation.

Pyrsopoulos, N.T. 2015. Hepatitis B. *Medscape*. Last modified January 11, 2015. http://emedicine.medscape.com/article/177632-overview.

Reuters Health Information. 2016. Zika may linger in semen long after symptoms fade. Last modified February 16, 2016. Accessed March 20, 2016. www.reuters.com/article/health-zika-semen-idUSL2N15R14N.

Rogers, S. 2008. A practical approach to preventing CA-MRSA infections in the athletic training setting. *Athletic Therapy Today* 13 (4): 35–38.

Roy, P.K. 2015. Hepatitis D. *Medscape*. Last modified April 30, 2015. Accessed March 12, 2016. http://emedicine.medscape.com/article/178038-overview.

Salinas, J.D. 2015. West Nile virus. *Medscape*. Last modified July 14, 2015. Accessed March 19, 2016. http://emedicine.medscape.com/article/312210-overview.

Scheler-Faccini, L., E.M. Ribeiro, I.M. Feitosa, D. Horovitz, D.P. Cavalicanti, A. Pessoa, M.J. Doriqui, et al. 2016. Possible association between Zika virus infection and microcephaly—Brazil, 2015. *Morbidity and Mortality Weekly Report (MMWR)* 65 (3): 59–62.

Schweizer, M., H.Y. Chiang, E. Septimus, J. Moody, B. Braun, J. Hafner, M. Ward, et al. 2014. A multicenter intervention to reduce surgical site infection among patients undergoing cardiac operations and total joint arthroplasty (Stop SSI study). IDWeek, Philadelphia, PA, October 8–12, 2014.

Shefer, A., W. Atkinson, C. Friedman, D.T. Kuhar, G. Mootrey, S.R. Bialke, A. Cohn, et al. 2011. Immunization of health care personnel: Recommendations of the Advisory Committee on Immunization Practices (ACIP). *Morbidity and Mortality Weekly Report (MMWR)* 60: 1–45.

Sifton, D, ed. 2002. *PDG guide to biological and chemical warfare response*. Montvale, NJ: Thompson Publishing.

Sinave, C.P. 2015. Streptococcus group D infections. *Medscape*. Last modified October 20, 2015. Accessed March 12, 2016. http://emedicine.medscape.com/article/229209-overview.

Telxeira, M.G., M. Costa, W.K. de Oliveira, M.L. Nunes, and L.C. Rodrigues. 2016. The epidemic of Zika virus–related microcephaly in Brazil: Detection, control, etiology, and future scenarios. *American Journal of Public Health* 106 (4): 601–5.

Tobe, K., K. Matsuura, T. Ogura, Y. Tsuo, Y. Iwasaki, M. Mizuno, K. Yamamoto, T. Higashi, and T. Tsuji. 2000. Horizontal transmission of hepatitis B virus among players of an American football team. *Archives of Internal Medicine* 160: 2541–45.

U.S. National Library of Medicine. 2016. Reportable diseases. Last modified March 2, 2016. www.nlm.nih.gov/medlineplus/ency/article/001929.htm.

Venkataraman, R. 2015. Toxic shock syndrome. *Medscape*. Last modified April 16, 2015. Accessed March 19, 2016. http://emedicine.medscape.com/article/169177-overview.

Wan, C. 2015. Viral meningitis. *Medscape*. Last modified June 23, 2015. http://emedicine.medscape.com/article/1168529-overview.

Waninger, K.N., and H.Y. Harcke. 2005. Determination of safe return to play for athletes recovering from infectious mononucleosis: A review of the literature. *Clinical Journal of Sports Medicine* 15 (6): 410–16.

Woods, C.J. 2015. Streptococcus group B infections. *Medscape*. Last modified October 20, 2016. Accessed March 12, 2016. http://emedicine.medscape.com/article/229091-overview.

World Health Organization. 2015a. Immunization, vaccines and biologicals: Measles. Last modified July 31, 2015. Accessed March 11, 2016. www.who.int/immunization/monitoring_surveillance/burden/vpd/surveillance_type/active/measles/en/.

World Health Organization. 2015b. Rubella. Last modified November 1, 2015. Accessed March 11, 2016. www.who.int/mediacentre/factsheets/fs367/en/.

World Health Organization. 2015. Meningococcal meningitis. Last modified November 2015. Accessed March 20, 2016. www.who.int/mediacentre/factsheets/fs141/en/.

Yohannes, Y. 2015. Acute mumps. *Medscape*. Last modified November 6, 2015. Accessed March 11, 2016. http://emedicine.medscape.com/article/784603-overview.

Chapter 16

Agel, J., J. Ransone, R.F. Dick, R. Oppliger, and S.W. Marshall. 2007. Descriptive epidemiology of collegiate men's wrestling injuries: National Collegiate Athletic Association injury surveillance system, 1988–1989 through 2003–2004. *Journal of Athletic Training* 42 (2): 303–10.

American Academy of Dermatology. 2015a. Sunscreen FAQs. Accessed March 26, 2016. www.aad.org/media/stats/prevention-and-are/sunscreen-faqs.

American Academy of Dermatology. 2015b. Types of skin cancer. Accessed March 26, 2016. www.aad.org/public/spot-skin-cancer/learn-about-skin-cancer/types-of-skin-cancer.

American Academy of Dermatology. 2016a. Melanoma: Biopsy recommendations. Accessed March 26, 2016. www.aad.org/practice-tools/quality-care/clinical-guidelines/melanoma/biopsy.

American Academy of Dermatology. 2016b. Skin cancer. Accessed March 26, 2016. www.aad.org/media/stats/conditions/skin-cancer.

American Cancer Society. 2016a. Cancer facts and figures, 2016. Last modified February 1, 2016. Accessed February 20, 2016. www.cancer.org/research/cancerfactsstatistics/cancerfactsfigures2016/.

American Cancer Society. 2016b. Key statistics about basal and squamous cell skin cancers. Last modified February 2, 2016. Accessed March 26, 2016. www.cancer.org/cancer/skincancer-basalandsquamouscell/detailedguide/skin-cancer-basal-and-squamous-cell-key-statistics.

American Cancer Society. 2016c. Key statistics for melanoma skin cancer. Last modified February 1, 2016. www.cancer.org/cancer/skincancer-melanoma/detailedguide/melanoma-skin-cancer-key-statistics.

Anderson, W.E. 2015. Varicella-zoster virus. *Medscape.* Last modified October 22, 2015. Accessed March 11, 2016. http://emedicine.medscape.com/article/231927-overview.

Arends, M., A. Wyllie, and C. Bird. 1990. Papillomaviruses and human cancer. *Human Pathology* 21 (7): 686–98.

Arnold, T.C. 2016. Brown recluse spider envenomation. *Medscape.* Last modified February 24, 2016. Accessed March 30, 2016. http://emedicine.medscape.com/article/772295-overview.

Ashack, K.A., K.A. Burton, T.R. Johnson, D.W. Currie, R.D. Comstock, and R.P. Dellavalle. 2016. Skin infections among U.S. high school athletes: A national survey. *Journal of the American Academy of Dermatology* 74 (4): 670–684.

Bader, R.S. 2015. Basal cell carcinoma. *Medscape.* Last modified September 15, 2015. http://emedicine.medscape.com/article/276624-overview.

Barry, M. 2015. Scabies. *Medscape.* Last modified November 18, 2015. Accessed March 30, 2016. http://emedicine.medscape.com/article/1109204-overview.

Bhatia, A.C. 2015. Molluscum contagiosum. *Medscape.* Last modified November 17, 2015. Accessed March 29, 2016. http://emedicine.medscape.com/article/910570-overview.

Bradby, C. 2014. Atopic dermatitis in emergency medicine. *Medscape.* Last modified March 5, 2014. Accessed March 26, 2016. http://emedicine.medscape.com/article/762045-overview.

Brodland, D.G. 2010. Mohs micrographic surgery: An overview. Skin Cancer Foundation. Last modified April 28, 2010. Accessed March 26, 2016. www.skincancer.org/skin-cancer-information/mohs-surgery/mohs-overview

Burkhart, C.G. 2016. Tinea versicolor clinical presentation. *Medscape.* Last modified February 9, 2016. Accessed March 29, 2016. http://emedicine.medscape.com/article/1091575-clinical.

Cappaert, T.A., J.A. Stone, J. W. Castellani, B.A. Krause, D. Smith, B.A. Stephens, and National Athletic Trainers' Association. 2008. National Athletic Trainers' Association position statement: Environmental cold injuries. *Journal of Athletic Training* 43 (6): 640–58.

Castellani, J.W., and A.J. Young. 2012. Health and performance challenges during sports training and competition in cold weather. *British Medical Journal* 46:788–91.

Castellani, J.W., A.J. Young, M.B. Ducharme, G.G Giesbrecht, E. Glickman, and R.E. Sallis. 2006. American College of Sports Medicine position stand: Prevention of cold injuries during exercise. *Medicine and Science in Sports and Exercise* 38 (11): 2012–29.

Centers for Disease Control and Prevention. 2010. Parasites–scabies. Last modified 2010. Accessed March 30, 2016. www.cdc.gov/parasites/scabies/index.html.

Centers for Disease Control and Prevention. 2013. Head lice. Last modified September 24, 2013. Accessed March 29, 2016. www.cdc.gov/parasites/lice/head/index.html.

Centers for Disease Control and Prevention. 2015. Skin cancer trends. Last modified May 5, 2015. Accessed March 26, 2016. www.cdc.gov/cancer/skin/statistics/trends.htm.

Cyr, P.R. 2004. Viral skin infections: Preventing outbreaks in sports settings. *The Physician and Sportsmedicine* 32 (7): 33–38.

Daley, E.M., C.A. Vamos, E.R. Buhi, S.K. Kolar, R.J. McDermott, N. Hernandez, and H.J. Fuhrmann. 2010. Influences on human papillomavirus vaccination status among female college students. *Journal of Women's Health (Larchmt)* 19 (10): 1885–91.

Ferri, F.F. 2016. *Ferri's Clinical Advisor.* Philadelphia, PA: Elsevier.

Fromm, L.J. 2015. Epidermal inclusion cyst. *Medscape.* Last modified October 9, 2015. Accessed March 26, 2016. http://emedicine.medscape.com/article/1061582-overview.

Gearhart, P.A. 2015. Human papillomavirus. *Medscape.* Last modified May 26, 2015. Accessed January 8, 2016. http://emedicine.medscape.com/article/219110-overview.

Guenther, L.C. 2016. Pediculosis and pthiriasis. *Medscape.* Last modified February 5, 2016. Accessed March 29, 2016. http://emedicine.medscape.com/article/225013-overview.

Hammadi, A.A. 2016. Psoriatic arthritis. *Medscape.* Last modified January 21, 2016. Accessed March 26, 2016. http://emedicine.medscape.com/article/2196539-overview.

Hennessey, M., M. Fischer, and J.E. Staples. 2016. Zika virus spreads to new areas—Region of the Americas May 2015–January 2016. *Morbidity and Mortality Weekly Report (MMWR)* 65 (3): 55–58.

Janniger, C.K. 2016. Herpes zoster. *Medscape.* Last modified February 1, 2016. Accessed March 29, 2016. http://emedicine.medscape.com/article/1132465-overview.

John, S.M., M. Trakatelli, R. Gehring, K. Finlay, M. Wittlich, M. Augustin, G. Hilpert, D. Barroso, C. L. Ulrich, and G. Pellacani. 2016. Consensus report: Recognizing non-melanoma skin cancer, including actinic keratosis, as an occupational disease—A call to action. *Journal of the European Academy of Dermatology and Venereology* 30 (Suppl 3): 38–45.

Kao, G.F. 2015. Tinea capitis. *Medscape.* Last modified November 19, 2015. Accessed March 29, 2016. http://emedicine.medscape.com/article/1091351-overview.

Landry, G.L., and C.J. Chang. 2004. Herpes and tinea in wrestling: Managing outbreaks, knowing when to disqualify. *The Physician and Sportsmedicine* 32 (10): 34–41.

Landry, G.L., C.J. Chang, and P.D. Mees. 2004. Treating and avoiding herpes and tinea infections in contact sports. *The Physician and Sportsmedicine* 32 (10): 43–44.

Laube, A. 2014. Dermographism urticaria. *Medscape.* Last modified February 11, 2014. Accessed March 26, 2016. http://emedicine.medscape.com/article/1050294-overview.

Lesher, J.L. 2015. Tinea corporis. *Medscape.* Last modified November 17, 2015. Accessed March 29, 2016. http://emedicine.medscape.com/article/1091473-overview.

Levy, J.A. 2004. Common bacterial dermatoses: Protecting competitive athletes. *The Physician and Sportsmedicine* 32 (6): 33–39.

Lewis, L.S. 2015. Impetigo. *Medscape.* Last modified August 16, 2015. Accessed March 27, 2016. http://emedicine.medscape.com/article/965254-overview.

Mechem, C.C. 2015. Emergent management of frostbite. *Medscape.* Last modified October 5, 2015. Accessed March 27, 2016. http://emedicine.medscape.com/article/770296-overview.

Mechem, C.C. 2016. Frostbite. *Medscape.* Last modified February 26, 2016. Accessed March 27, 2016. http://emedicine.medscape.com/article/926249-overview.

Meffert, J. 2016. Psoriasis. *Medscape.* Last modified March 25, 2016. Accessed March 26, 2016. http://emedicine.medscape.com/article/1943419-overview.

Menter, A., N.J. Korman, C.A Elmets, S.R. Feldman, J.M. Gelfand, K.B. Gordon, A. Gottlieb, et al. 2011. Guidelines of care for the management of psoriasis and psoriatic arthritis. Section 6. Guidelines of care for the treatment of psoriasis and psoriatic arthritis: Case-based presentations and evidence-based conclusions. *Journal of the American Academy of Dermatology* 65 (1): 137–74.

Monroe, M.M. 2015. Cutaneous squamous cell carcinoma. *Medscape.* Last modified July 10, 2015. Accessed March 26, 2016. http://emedicine.medscape.com/article/1965430-overview.

National Athletic Trainers' Association. 2005. Official statement from the National Athletic Trainers' Association on community-acquired MRSA infections (CA-MRSA). Last modified March 1, 2005. www.nata.org/sites/default/files/MRSA.pdf.

National Athletic Trainers' Association. 2007. Official statement from the National Athletic Trainers' Association on communicable and infectious diseases in secondary school sports. Last modified March 2007. www.nata.org/sites/default/files/CommunicableInfectiousDiseasesSecondarySchoolSports.pdf.

National Federation of State High School Associations. 2013. Sports related skin infections position statement and guidelines. Last modified February 9, 2016. Accessed March 20, 2016. www.nfhs.org/sports-resource-content/smac-position-statements-and-guidelines/.

National Federation of State High School Associations. 2015a. General guidelines for sport hygiene, skin infections and communicable diseases. Last modified October 2015. Accessed March 27, 2016. www.nfhs.org/sports-resource-content/smac-position-statements-and-guidelines/.

National Federation of State High School Associations. 2015b. NFHS medical release form for wrestler to participate with skin lesion(s). www.nfhs.org/sports-resource-content/smac-position-statements-and-guidelines/.

National Institute for Occupational Safety and Health. 2015. Venomous spiders. Centers for Disease Control and Prevention. Last modified July 30, 2015. Accessed March 30, 2016. www.cdc.gov/niosh/topics/spiders/default.html.

Parsons, J.T., ed. 2014. *2014–2015 NCAA Sports Medicine Handbook.* Indianapolis, IN: National Collegiate Athletic Association.

Perloff, S.A. 2014. MRSA skin infection in athletes. *Medscape.* Last modified August 18, 2014. Accessed March 19, 2016. http://emedicine.medscape.com/article/108972-overview.

Porter, R.S., and J.L. Kaplan, eds. 2011. *The Merck Manual.* 19th ed. Whitehouse Station, NJ: Merck Sharp & Dohme Corporation.

Rao, J. 2015. Acne vulgaris. *Medscape.* Last modified December 11, 2015. Accessed March 27, 2016. http://emedicine.medscape.com/article/1069804-overview.

Richtig, E., G. Langmann, K. Mullner, and J. Smolle. 2004. Ocular melanoma: Epidemiology, clinical presentation and relationship with dysplastic nevi. *Ophthalmologica* 218 (2): 111–14.

Robbins, C.M. 2015. Tinea pedis. *Medscape.* Last modified November 19, 2015. Accessed March 29, 2016. http://emedicine.medscape.com/article/1091684-overview.

Rogers, S. 2008. A practical approach to preventing CA-MRSA infections in the athletic training setting. *Athletic Therapy Today* 13 (4): 35–38.

Salvaggio, M. 2015. Herpes simplex. *Medscape.* Last modified September 18, 2015. Accessed February 13, 2016. http://emedicine.medscape.com/article/218580-overview - a6.

Schwartz, R.A. 2015. Cholinergic urticaria. *Medscape.* Last modified April 28, 2015. Accessed March 26, 2016. http://emedicine.medscape.com/article/1049978-overview.

Simon, S. 2015. FDA proposes new rules for indoor tanning beds. American Cancer Society. Last modified December 18, 2015. Accessed March 26, 2016. www.cancer.org/cancer/news/news/fda-proposes-new-rules-for-indoor-tanning-beds.

Stevens, D.L., A.L. Bisno, H.F. Chambers, E.P. Dellinger, E.J. Goldstein, S.L. Gorbach, J.V. Hirschmann, S.L. Kaplan, J.G. Montoya, and J.C. Wade. 2014. Practice guidelines for diagnosis and management of skin and soft tissue infections: 2014 update by the Infectious Diseases Society of America. *Clinical Infectious Diseases* 59 (2): e10–e52.

Tajirian, A.L. 2014. Solar urticaria. *Medscape.* Last modified August 11, 2014. Accessed March 26, 2016. http://emedicine.medscape.com/article/1050485-overview.

Tan, W.W. 2015. Malignant melanoma staging. *Medscape.* Last modified October 1, 2015. Accessed March 27, 2016. http://emedicine.medscape.com/article/2007147-overview.

Tan, W.W. 2016. Malignant melanoma. *Medscape.* Last modified February 11, 2016. http://emedicine.medscape.com/article/280245-overview.

U.S. Food and Drug Administration. 2015. Beware of bug bites and stings. U.S. Department of Health and Human Services. Last modified July 25, 2015. Accessed March 30, 2016. www.fda.gov/ForConsumers/ConsumerUpdates/ucm048022.htm.

U.S. National Library of Medicine. 2016. Insect bites and stings. *Medline Plus.* Last modified March 16, 2016. Accessed March 30, 2016. www.nlm.nih.gov/medlineplus/insectbitesandstings.html.

WebMD. 2015. Urticaria, cold. Last modified May 28, 2015. Accessed March 26, 2016. www.webmd.com/allergies/urticaria-cold.

Wiederkehr, M. 2015. Tinea cruris. *Medscape.* Last modified November 18, 2015. Accessed March 29, 2016. http://emedicine.medscape.com/article/1091806-overview.

Williams, C., J. Wells, R. Klein, T. Sylvester, and R. Sunenshine. 2015. Notes from the field: Outbreak of skin lesions among high school wrestlers—Arizona, 2014. *Morbidity and Mortality Weekly Report (MMWR)* 64 (20): 559–60.

Winokur, R., and W. Dexter. 2004. Fungal infections and parasitic infestations in sports. *The Physician and Sportsmedicine* 32 (10): 23–33.

Wong, H.K. 2015. Acute urticaria. *Medscape.* Last modified June 19, 2015. Accessed March 26, 2016. http://emedicine.medscape.com/article/137362-overview - a5.

Wysong, A., H. Gladstone, D. Kim, B. Lingala, J. Copeland, and J.Y. Tang. 2012. Sunscreen use in NCAA collegiate athletes: Identifying targets for intervention and barriers to use. *Preventative Medicine* 55:493–96.

Zinder, S.M., R.S. Basler, J. Foley, C. Scarlata, and D.B. Vasily. 2010. National Athletic Trainers' Position Statement: Skin diseases. *Journal of Athletic Training* 45 (4): 411–28.

Chapter 17

American Psychiatric Association. 2013. *Diagnostic and Statistical Manual of Mental Disorders.* 5th ed. Washington, DC: American Psychiatric Association.

Antony, M., and H. Hood. 2012. Evidence-based assessment and treatment of specific phobias in adults. In *Intensive One-Session Treatment of Specific Phobias,* edited by T.E. Davis III, T.H. Ollendick, and L.-G. Öst, 19–42. New York: Springer.

Anxiety and Depression Association of America. 2015. Generalized anxiety disorder (GAD). www.adaa.org/generalized-anxiety-disorder-gad.

Anxiety Disorders Association of America. 2016. Anxiety disorders. Accessed January 15, 2016. www.adaa.org/.

Asnaan, A., J. Richey, R. Dimaite, D. Hinton, and S. Hofmann. 2010. A cross-ethnic comparison of lifetime prevalence rates of anxiety disorders. *Journal of Nervous & Mental Disease* 198 (8): 551–55.

Baron, D., S. Baron, J. Tompkins, and A. Polat. 2013. Assessing and treating depression in athletes. In *Clinical sports psychiatry: An international perspective*, edited by D.A. Baron, C.L. Reardon, and S.H. Baron. Ames, IA: Wiley-Blackwell.

Bratland-Sanda, S., and J. Sundgot-Borgen. 2013. Eating disorders in athletes: Overview of prevalence, risk factors and recommendations for prevention and treatment. *European Journal of Sport Science* 13 (5): 499–508.

Centers for Disease Control and Prevention. 2012. Vital Signs: Binge drinking prevalence, frequency, and intensity among adults—United States 2010. Accessed August 30, 2016. www.cdc.gov/mmwr/preview/mmwrhtml/mm6101a4.htm.

Committee on Quality Improvement: Subcommittee on Attention-Deficit/Hyperactivity Disorder. 2011. Clinical practice guideline for the diagnosis, evaluation, and treatment of attention deficit/hyperactivity disorder in children and adolescents. *Pediatrics* 28 (5):1077-1022.

Giedd, J. 2003. ADHD and substance abuse. *Medscape,* June 4, 2003. www.medscape.com/viewarticle/456199

Gorman, J. 2002. Treatment of generalized anxiety disorder. *Journal of Clinical Psychiatry* 63 (Suppl 8): 17–23.

Hedden, S., J. Kennet, and R. Lipari. 2015. Behavior health trends in the United States: Results from the 2014 National Survey on Drug Use and Health. In *Substance Abuse and Mental Health Services Administration (SAMHSA)*. Washington, D.C.: Department of Health and Human Services.

Larzelere, M., E. James, and M. Arcuri. 2015. Treating depression: What works besides meds? *Journal of Family Practice* 64 (8): 454–59A.

Levine, J., D. Cole, and K. Chengpappa. 2001. Anxiety disorders and major depression, together or apart. *Journal of Depression and Anxiety* 14:94–204.

Manbar, R., J. Allen, and M. Morris. 2002. Alternative treatments for depression: Empirical support and relevance to women. *Journal of Clinical Psychology* 63:628–40.

Martinsen, M., and J. Sundgot-Borgen. 2013. Higher prevalence of eating disorders among adolescent elite athletes than controls. *Medicine and Science in Sports and Exercise* 45 (6): 1188–97.

Merikangas, K.R., J.P. He, and M. Burstein. 2010. Lifetime prevalence of mental disorders in U.S. adolescents: Results from the National Comorbidity Survey Replication—Adolescent Supplement. *Journal of the American Academy of Child and Adolescent Psychiatry* 49 (10): 980–89.

Mitan, L. 2002. Eating disorders in adolescent girls. *Current Women's Health Report* 2:464–67.

Murray, C., and A. Lopez, eds. 1996. *Global burden of disease: A comprehensive assessment of mortality and disability from diseases, injuries, and risk factors in 1990 and projected to 2020*. Cambridge, MA: Harvard University Press.

National Collegiate Athletic Association. 2015. 2015–16 NCAA banned drugs. Last modified 2015. Accessed February 4, 2016. www.ncaa.org/2015-16-ncaa-banned-drugs.

National Institute on Drug Abuse (NIDA). 2016. Trends & statistics. Accessed March 21, 2016. https://www.drugabuse.gov/related-topics/trends-statistics.

National Institutes of Health (NIH). 2015. Prescription drug abuse. Accessed September 1, 2016. www.drugabuse.gov/publications/research-reports/prescription-drugs/what-prescription-drug-abuse.

Neal, T.L., A. Diamond, S. Goldman, D. Klossner, E.D. Morse, D. Pajak, M. Putukian, et al. 2013. Inter-association recommendations for developing a plan to recognize and refer student-athletes with psychological concerns at the collegiate level: An executive summary of a consensus statement. *Journal of Athletic Training* 48 (5): 716–20.

Parsons, J.T., ed. 2014. *2014–2015 NCAA Sports Medicine Handbook*. Indianapolis, IN: National Collegiate Athletic Association.

Prochaska, J.J., S.C. Fromont, C. Wa, R. Matlow, D.E. Ramo, and S.M. Hall. 2013. Tobacco use and its treatment among young people in mental health settings: A qualitative analysis. *Nicotine and Tobacco Research* 15 (8): 1427–35.

Prochaska, J.O., and C.C. DiClemente. 1983. Stages and processes of self-change of smoking: Toward an integrative model of change. *Journal of Consulting Clinical Psychologists* 51 (3): 390–5.

Raevuori, A., A. Keski-Rahkonen, and H.W. Hoek. 2014. A review of eating disorders in males. *Current Opinion in Psychiatry* 27 (6): 426–30.

Roy-Byrne, P., J. Russo, D.C. Dugdale, D. Lessler, D. Cowley, and W. Katon. 2002. Under treatment of panic disorder in primary care: Role of patient and physician characteristics. *Journal of the American Board of Family Practice* 15 (6): 443–50.

Smink, F., D. van Hoeken, and H. Hoek. 2012. Epidemiology of eating disorders: Incidence, prevalence and mortality rates. *Current Psychiatry Reports* 14 (4): 406–14.

Spitzer, R., K. Kroenke, J. Williams, and B. Lowe. 2006. A brief measure for assessing generalized anxiety disorder: The GAD-7. *Archives of Internal Medicine* 166 (10):1092–7.

Wang, J., and S. Patten. 2002. The moderating effects of coping strategies on major depression in the general population. *Canadian Journal of Psychiatry* 47: 167–73.

World Health Organization. 2001. The world health report 2001—Mental health: New understanding, new hope. Last modified 2001. Accessed February 2016. www.who.int/whr/2001/en/.

World Health Organization. 2011. Mental health atlas 2011—United States of America. www.who.int/mental_health/evidence/atlas/profiles/usa_mh_profile.pdf?ua=1&ua=1.

Zung, W.W. 1965. A self-rating depression scale. *Archives of General Psychiatry* 12 (1): 63–70.

Chapter 18

American College of Sports Medicine (ACSM). 2009. *American College of Sports Medicine's exercise management for persons with chronic diseases and disabilities*. 3rd ed. Champaign, IL: Human Kinetics.

Bhambhani, Y. 2002. Physiology of wheelchair racing in athletes with spinal cord injury. *Sports Medicine* 32: 23–51.

Bhambhani, Y., J. Mactavish, S. Warren, W.R. Thompson, A. Webborn, E. Bressan, Y. Vanlandewijck, et al. 2010. Boosting in athletes with high-level spinal cord injury: Knowledge, incidence and attitudes of athletes in Paralympic sport. *Disability and Rehabilitation* 32 (26): 2172–90.

Birrer, R.B. 2004. The Special Olympics athlete: Evaluation and clearance for participation. *Clinical Pediatrics* 43 (9): 777–82.

Boyajian-O'Neill, L., D. Cardone, W. Dexter, J. DiFiori, K.B. Fields, D. Jones, R. Pallay, et al. 2004. The preparticipation examination for the athlete with special needs. *Physician and Sportsmedicine* 32 (9): 13–19, 42.

Casa D., J. DeMartini, M. Bergeron, D. Csillan, R. Eichner, R. Lopez, M. Ferrara, et al. 2015. National Athletic Trainers' Association position statement: Exertional heat illnesses. *Journal of Athletic Training* 59 (9): 986–1000.

Crutchfield, K.E. 2014. Managing patients with neurologic disorders who participate in sports activities. *Sports Neurology* 20 (6): 1657–66.

Dec, K., K. Sparrow, and D. McKeag. 2000. The physically-challenged athlete: Medical issues and assessment. *Sports Medicine* 29 (4): 245–58.

DePauw, Karen, and Susan Gavron. 2005. *Disability sport*. 2nd ed. Champaign, IL: Human Kinetics.

Ferrara, M., and W. Buckley. 1996. Athletes with disabilities injury registry. *Adapted Physical Activity Quarterly* 13: 50–60.

Gee, C., C. West, and A. Krassioukov. 2015. Boosting in elite athletes with spinal cord injury: A critical review of physiology and testing procedures. *Sports Medicine* 45 (8): 1133–42.

Griggs, K., M. Price, and V. Goosey-Tolfrey. 2015. Cooling athletes with a spinal cord injury. *Sports Medicine* 45:9–21.

Hawkeswood, J., R. O'Connor, H. Anton, and H. Finlayson. 2014. The preparticipation evaluation for athletes with disability. *International Journal of Sports Physical Therapy* 9 (1): 103–15.

Hill, T.C., R. Baverstock, K.V. Carlson, E.P. Estey, G.J. Gray, D.C. Hill, C. Ho, R.H. McGinnis, K. Moore, and R. Parmar. 2013. Best practices for the treatment and prevention of urinary tract infection in the spinal cord injured population: The Alberta context. *Canadian Urological Association Journal* 7 (3–4): 122–30.

Jacob, T., and Hutzler, Y. 1998. Sports-medical assessment for athletes with a disability. *Disability Rehabilitation* 20: 116–9.

Karlsson, A. 1999. Autonomic dysreflexia. *Spinal Cord* 37 (6): 383–91.

Klenck, C., and K. Gebke. 2007. Practical management: Common medical problems in disabled athletes. *Clinical Journal of Sport Medicine* 17 (1): 55–60.

Lai, A., W. Standish, and H. Standish. 2000. The young athlete with physical challenges. *Clinics in Sports Medicine* 19 (4): 793–819.

National Center for Educational Statistics. 2014. Accessed January 2016. http://nces.ed.gov/programs/digest/d14/tables/dt14_204.30.asp.

National Federation of State High School Associations (NFHS): NFHS rules changes affecting risk (1982–2014). 2014. Accessed January 2016. www.nfhs.org/media/1014277/nfhs-risk-minimization-rules-changes-1982-2014.pdf.

National Institute of Neurological Disorders and Stroke (NINDS): NINDS post-polio syndrome information page. 2015. Accessed January 2016. www.ninds.nih.gov/disorders/post_polio/.

Oberlander, T.F., and F.J. Symons, eds. 2006. *Pain in children and adults with developmental disabilities*. Baltimore, MD: Brookes.

Parsons, J.T., ed. 2014. Guideline 3a: Protective equipment. In *2014–2015 NCAA Sports Medicine Handbook*. Indianapolis, IN: National Collegiate Athletic Association.

Patel, D., and D. Greydanus. 2010. The pediatric athlete with disabilities. *Pediatric Clinics of North America*. 57: 795–817.

Patel, D., and A. Roth. 2004. Pediatric athletes with physical disabilities. *Athletic Therapy Today* 9 (2): 16–9.

Prentice, W. 2014. *Principles of athletic training: A competency based approach*. 15th ed. Boston: McGraw-Hill.

Price, M.J., and I.G. Campbell. 2003. Effects of spinal cord lesion level upon thermoregulation during exercise in the heat. *Medicine and Science in Sport and Exercise* 35: 1100–7.

Ramirez, M., J. Yang, L. Bourque, J. Javien, S. Kashani, M.A. Limbos, and C. Peek-Asa. 2009. Sports injuries to high school athletes with disabilities. *Pediatrics* 123 (2): 690–6.

Shepherd, R.J. 2003. Boosting of performance in the athlete with high-level spinal injury. *Adapted Physical Activity Quarterly* 20: 103–17.

Sherrill, C. 2004. *Adapted physical activity, recreation and sport: Cross disciplinary and lifespan.* 6th ed. Boston: McGraw-Hill.

Umphred, D., G. Burton, R. Lazaro, and M. Roller. 2013. *Neurological rehabilitation.* 6th ed. St. Louis: Elsevier.

Webborn, N., S. Willick, and J.C. Reeser. 2006. Injuries among disabled athletes during the 2002 Winter Paralympic Games. *Medicine and Science in Sport and Exercise* 38 (5): 811–5.

Winnick, J. 2011. *Adapted physical education and sport.* 5th ed. Champaign IL: Human Kinetics.

World Health Organization. Definition: intellectual disability. 2016. Accessed January 2016. www.euro.who.int/en/health-topics/noncommunicable-diseases/mental-health/news/news/2010/15/childrens-right-to-family-life/definition-intellectual-disability.

INDEX

Note: Page references followed by an italicized *f* or *t* indicate information contained in figures and tables, respectively.

ABOUT THE AUTHORS

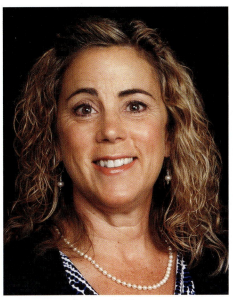

Photo courtesy of Katie Walsh Flanagan.

Katie Walsh Flanagan, EdD, ATC, is a professor and director of the sports medicine and athletic training program in the department of health education and promotion at East Carolina University, where she has worked for more than 20 years. A Board of Certification (BOC) certified athletic trainer, Walsh Flanagan previously worked as a lecturer and assistant athletic trainer at California State University, Fresno, and as the head athletic trainer for the Chicago Power, a men's professional soccer team. She has also assisted as an athletic trainer for various sports in international competitions, including the 1996 Summer Olympic Games and 1987 Pan American Games.

In 2012, Walsh Flanagan was elected to the North Carolina Athletic Trainers' Association Hall of Fame. The organization named her the North Carolina Athletic Trainer of the Year–College/University in 2000 and 2006. She received the Most Distinguished Athletic Trainer award from the National Athletic Trainers' Association in 2010 and their Athletic Trainer Service award in 2006.

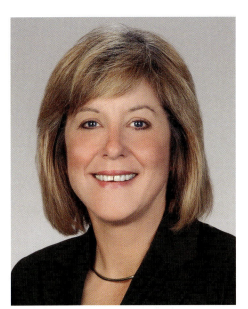

Photo courtesy of Micki Cuppett.

Micki Cuppett, EdD, ATC, is the executive director of the Commission on Accreditation of Athletic Training Education (CAATE) after having served as its president and as a board member. She previously worked for 16 years as a professor of athletic training in the department of orthopedics and sports medicine at the University of South Florida, where she was the athletic training program director. She has also been a professor and director of athletic training education at the University of Nebraska at Omaha.

In addition to her work in academe, Cuppett has been an athletic trainer for three decades, having worked in high school, collegiate, military, and hospital settings. Cuppett is known internationally for her work with human patient simulators and interprofessional education, and she has often been an invited speaker at national and international conferences. She received the Athletic Trainer Service award from the National Athletic Trainers' Association in 2007 and their Most Distinguished Athletic Trainer award in 2012.

CONTRIBUTORS

Tamara C. Valovich McLeod, PhD, ATC, FNATA
Professor
Director of Athletic Training Programs
A.T. Still University
Mesa, Arizona

Monique Mokha, PhD, ATC
Associate Professor
Athletic Training Education and Exercise and
Sport Science Programs
Nova Southeastern University
Davie, Florida

Layne A. Prest, PhD, LIMHP, LMFT
Couple and Family Therapist at PeaceHealth Southwest
Washington
Behavioral Scientist at Family Medicine Residency
Clinical Assistant Professor at University of Washington
Vancouver, Washington

Kevin Sneed, PharmD, CRPh
Senior Associate Vice President at USF Health
Professor and Dean at USF College of Pharmacy
University of South Florida
Tampa, Florida

A special thank you to these contributors for their work on the previous editions:

Joseph Armen, DO
Helen E. Bateman, MD
Larry Collins, PA-C, DFAAPA, ATC
Christine Curran, MD
David Eichenbaum, MD
Richard Figler, MD
Joseph Garry, MD, CAQ, FACSM
Todd L. Kanzenbach, MD, CAQ
Lawrence J. Kusior, MD, FAAOS
Mary H. Lien, MD
Sara McDade, MD
Tiffany O'Connor, MS, ATC/L, OTC
Sally A. Perkins, MS, ATC, CAATE
Arnold M. Ramirez, MD
Dorraine Reynolds, PharmD
Patrick Sexton, Ed D, ATC, CSCS
Charles B. Slonim, MD, FACS
Laurie Small, MD
Bryan W. Smith, MD, PhD
Kevin B. Sneed, PharmD
Daniel J. Van Durme, MD, FAAFP
M. Craig Whaley, MD

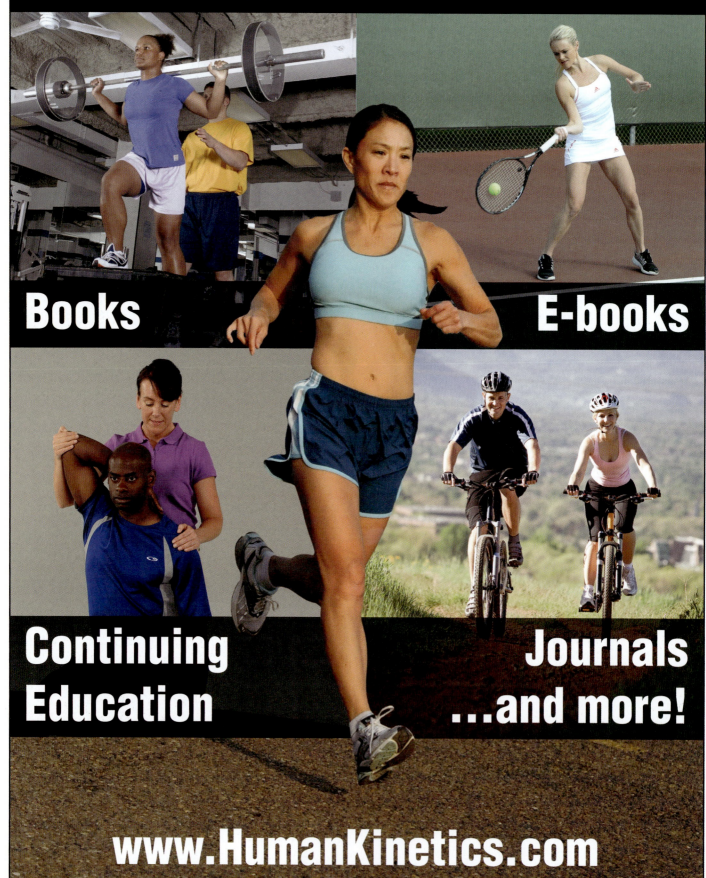

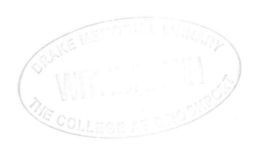